T0173032

IMPROVING GLOBAL HEALTH: FORECASTING THE NEXT 50 YEARS

PATTERNS OF POTENTIAL HUMAN PROGRESS

VOLUME 3

Copyright © 2011 by Frederick S. Pardee Center for International Futures, University of Denver

Published in the United States by Paradigm Publishers, 2845 Wilderness Place, Suite 200, Boulder, Colorado 80301 USA.

Paradigm Publishers is the trade name of Birkenkamp & Company, LLC, Dean Birkenkamp, President and Publisher.

Distributed on the Indian Subcontinent by Oxford University Press India, 1 Jai Singh Road, Post Box 43, New Delhi 110 001 India.

Library of Congress Cataloging-in-Publication Data

Improving global health: forecasting the next 50 years / Barry B. Hughes ... [et al.]. p. ; cm. — (Patterns of potential human progress ; v. 3)

Includes bibliographical references and index.

ISBN 978-1-59451-896-6 (hardcover : alk. paper) — ISBN 978-1-59451-897-3 (pbk. : alk. paper)
1. World health—Forecasting.
2. Twenty-first century—Forecasts.
I. Hughes, Barry, 1945– II.
Series: Patterns of potential human progress ; v. 3.
[DNLM: 1. World Health. 2. Forecasting. WA 530.1 I34 2011]
RA441.I47 2011
362.101'12—dc22
2010025260

Cover design by Bounford.com
Designed and typeset by Bounford.com

Printed and bound in Canada by Friesens Corporation

14 13 12 11 10 5 4 3 2 1

Picture credits

(Photos are from left to right):

Chapter 1
Colette Liddell
© John Greim/fotoLibra
Kelley Burns

Chapter 2
Callen Blackburn
Colette Liddell
Amber Bacca

Chapter 3
© John Greim/fotoLibra
© Joyce Mollet/fotoLibra
© Hazy Sun Images Ltd/fotoLibra

Chapter 4
Thomas De Clerck
Eric Firnhaber
Thomas De Clerck

Chapter 5
Jenny Starkey
Sheryl Ramsey
© John Greim/fotoLibra

Chapter 6
Najim Dost
Eric Firnhaber
Adrielle Knight

Chapter 7
Jason Newcomer
© John Greim/fotoLibra
© John Greim/fotoLibra

Chapter 8
Gretchen Davis
© Mark Gillett/fotoLibra
Teresa Manochhio

Chapter 9
© Hazy Sun Images Ltd/fotoLibra
Thomas De Clerck
© Dave Tait/fotoLibra

Cover Art

The cover art is a representation of an oil painting by Margaret Lawless, artist for the PPHP series. Ms. Lawless is a contemporary abstract artist whose works in various media portray aspects of the human condition, human progress, and the interaction of humans with nature. In this particular painting, she emphasizes the potential inherent within all human beings to experience the full life cycle that health and a healthy environment enable. The S-curve suggested by the red band represents global transitions in health and life expectancy, the further improvement of which is the focus of this volume.

IMPROVING GLOBAL HEALTH:
FORECASTING THE NEXT 50 YEARS

PATTERNS OF POTENTIAL HUMAN PROGRESS

VOLUME 3

Barry B. Hughes

Randall Kuhn

Cecilia M. Peterson

Dale S. Rothman

José R. Solórzano

Barry B. Hughes, Series Editor

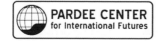

PARDEE CENTER for International Futures

Josef Korbel School of International Studies
University of Denver

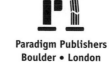

Paradigm Publishers
Boulder • London

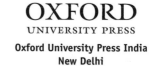

OXFORD
UNIVERSITY PRESS

Oxford University Press India
New Delhi

Preface

Improving Global Health: Forecasting the Next 50 Years is third in the Patterns of Potential Human Progress (PPHP) series, a series that explores prospects for human development and the improvement of the global human condition. Each volume considers one key aspect of how development appears to be unfolding globally and locally, how we would like it to evolve, and how better to move it in desired directions.

The volumes emerge from the Frederick S. Pardee Center for International Futures at the University of Denver's Josef Korbel School of International Studies. The International Futures (IFs) project has worked for more than three decades to develop and use the strongest possible long-term, multiple issue capability for exploring the future of key global issues. The philosophical basis of the IFs project includes these beliefs: (1) prediction is impossible, but forecasting is necessary to help us understand change and to support policy development; (2) analysis should be built around alternative possible futures; and (3) forecasting tools should be as open and transparent as possible.

The first PPHP volume focused on the central issue of global poverty reduction, presenting first a long-range, base case forecast—an elaboration of the path we appear to be on. It then explored an extensive set of variations in that path tied to alternative domestic and international interventions. The second volume provided a long-range, base case forecast for global advances in education participation and attainment, and then developed a normative scenario, looking for aggressive, but reasonable, patterns to enhance global advances in formal education.

This third volume drills down into arguably the most important of all issues for humans: that of health. It recognizes the remarkable epidemiologic and demographic transitions that, while long underway, have gained, lost, and regained momentum in the last 50 years. During that half century to 2010, global life expectancy increased from just over 50 years to approximately 70—yet about 20 countries have a lower life expectancy today than they did two decades ago. This volume explores where the next five decades may take

us. We consider changing mortality and morbidity patterns, including the remarkable ongoing reduction of global deaths from communicable diseases, a pattern that hopefully will be consolidated and extended. We consider also the growing burden of noncommunicable diseases and injuries, especially as populations age nearly everywhere. And we examine possible alternative patterns of 15 specific causes of death and disability and their impacts.

The volume analyzes not only the drivers of change in human health, including advances in income, education, and technology, but also a number of more immediate risk factors (undernutrition, obesity, smoking, road traffic accidents, inadequate water and sanitation, indoor and outdoor air pollution, and climate change) and their health impacts. We focus heavily on the role of human effort in shaping health outcomes, as well as the roles of the natural environment and biological constraints.

Human health interacts closely with broader human development. Therefore, this volume devotes attention not only to the drivers of change in health prospects but also to the ways in which those prospects affect broader demographic and economic futures. Among the advantages of the IFs modeling system is the manner in which it links health forecasting to larger human systems.

Putting these pieces together, this volume uniquely looks forward across half a century at human health for 183 countries and the regions and groupings into which they fall, exploring a broad range of causes of disease and death, probing the deeper and more immediate drivers of change in human health prospects, and linking that analysis to the dynamics of the larger human development system. Our analysis recognizes the great uncertainty around such forecasts and attempts to explore the bases for alternative health futures and their implications. We hope this broad and deep exploration can contribute to the collective effort to assure improved health and well-being for peoples around the world. Those who wish to explore or extend our analysis will find the full IFs system at www.ifs.du.edu.

Acknowledgments

The authors again owe special thanks to Frederick S. Pardee, who conceptualized the Patterns of Potential Human Progress (PPHP) series that this volume continues. We much appreciate Fred's ongoing support for the work of the International Futures (IFs) project and his contribution of energy, enthusiasm, and ideas, including the special responsibility he has taken for the country-specific supporting data tables that accompany the PPHP volumes and appear on-line at the IFs website.

The International Futures simulation modeling system, the core tool of this volume, has been developed over 30 years under the leadership of Barry Hughes at the Josef Korbel School of International Studies, University of Denver. Thanks to the support of the University and the Frederick S. Pardee Center for International Futures, the complete system, including both a downloadable version and an on-line version, is available for all users at www.ifs.du.edu.

IFs, developed originally as an educational tool, owes much to the large number of students, instructors, and analysts who have used or reacted to the system over many years and have provided much appreciated advice for enhancement. The first two volumes of this series provided names of many of those, and without repeating the list we thank them still again (as we do earlier team members, listed also in those two volumes).

IFs team members who made special contributions to this volume include Jonathon Chesebro (data), Brent Corby (data), Eric Firnhaber (photographs), Mariko Frame (photographs), Kia Tamaki Harrold (background working papers), Mohammod Irfan (data and systems support), Josiah Marineau (data and help system), Lisa Matts (supporting research), Jonathan Moyer (web support), Britt Reiersgord (references, photographs, and more), Graham Smith (references), Mark Stelzner (data), Marc Sydnor (photographs and project support on earlier volumes that made this one easier), and Julie Thompson (supporting research). Most especially we express tremendous appreciation to Janet Dickson, who worked closely with the authors throughout the writing and production process. She brainstormed with us, kept us on task, edited the volume, and oversaw the production process.

This volume owes a special debt of gratitude to Colin D. Mathers, Mortality and Burden of Disease Coordinator, Department of Health Statistics and Informatics, World Health Organization, and a founding leader of WHO's Global Burden of Disease project. From our first approach to Dr. Mathers, requesting information about the methods of the GBD project, he was unfailingly helpful. He provided unpublished data from the project and the coefficients used in its formulations, and he patiently answered our questions about the GBD project's methods and approaches. He also reviewed the penultimate manuscript and provided feedback that has saved us from many errors.

We also thank an exceptional group of external reviewers who greatly enhanced this volume through their feedback. They are Jere R. Behrman, William R. Kenan Jr. Professor of Economics and Sociology, University of Pennsylvania; Henk Hilderink, Senior Policy Researcher, Department of Sustainable Development, Netherlands Environmental Assessment Agency (PBL); Gerald Keusch, Professor of Medicine and International Health, Special Assistant for Global Health to the University President, Boston University; Rachel Nugent, Deputy Director of Global Health, Center for Global Development; and Sam Preston, Fredrick J. Warren Professor of Demography, University of Pennsylvania. No one could save us from all of our errors of omission and commission, but they caught many.

Most recent funding for IFs has come from Frederick S. Pardee, the United Nations Environment Programme, the U.S. National Intelligence Council, and the European Commission. Other developments within International Futures have been funded in part by the Strategic Assessments Group of the U.S. Central Intelligence Agency, by the Frederick S. Pardee Center for Longer Range Global Policy and the Future of the Human Condition at RAND Corporation, and by the European Union Center at the University of Michigan. Thanks also to the National Science Foundation, the Cleveland Foundation, the Exxon Education Foundation, the Kettering Family Foundation, the Pacific Cultural Foundation, the United States Institute of Peace, and General Motors for funding that contributed to earlier generations of IFs.

At Paradigm Publishers, Jennifer Knerr, longtime editor and friend of the IFs project, was wonderfully helpful and supportive, and the hands-on editorial guidance provided by Carol Smith and Jeska Horgan-Kobelski was invaluable. At Oxford University Press in New Delhi, we are grateful for the warm support and partnership of Neha Kohli, Associate Development Editor, and Urmilla Dasgupta, Commissioning Editor. We are extremely appreciative of the beautiful design and layout work on all of the series volumes by Trevor Bounford and Denise Goodey of Bounford. com. And with this volume, we were extremely fortunate to welcome Eleanora von Dehsen to our team; we much appreciate her help in standardizing our presentation.

Finally, the authors built on tremendous foundations of work directed toward improving global health. The hope that motivated our work was that we might contribute something to that ongoing stream of effort by exploring the possible trajectory of global health and its broader human development consequences over the next 50 years. Other than the authors, of course, none of the named individuals or institutions bears any responsibility for the current status of the model or for the analysis presented here. Their support is nonetheless greatly appreciated.

Barry B. Hughes
Series Editor

Contents

List of Boxes

List of Figures

List of Tables

Abbreviations and Acronyms

AIDS	acquired immune deficiency syndrome		LEB	life expectancy at birth
ARI	acute respiratory infection		LES	linear expenditure system
ART	Antiretroviral therapy		MDGs	Millennium Development Goals (UN)
BMI	body mass index		MICS	Multiple Indicator Cluster Survey (UNICEF)
BRICs	Brazil, Russia, India, and China			
CDC	Centers for Disease Control		NCDs	noncommunicable diseases
CDs	communicable diseases		NGOs	non-governmental organizations
CEC	Commission for Environmental Cooperation		OAP	outdoor air pollution
CO_2	carbon dioxide		OECD	Organisation for Economic Co-operation and Development
COPD	chronic obstructive pulmonary disease		OLS	ordinary least squares
CRA	Comparative Risk Assessment project (WHO)		PAF	population attributable fraction
CSDH	Commission on Social Determinants of Health (WHO)		$PM_{2.5}$	particulates with a diameter of 2.5 micrometers or less
CVD	cardiovascular disease		PM_{10}	particulates with a diameter of 10 micrometers or less
DALYs	disability-adjusted life years		ppm	parts per million
DHS	Demographic and Health Surveys (USAID)		PPP	purchasing power parity
			RR	relative risk
EC	European Commission		SAM	social accounting matrix
EPP	Estimation and Projection Package		SI	smoking impact
FAO	Food and Agriculture Organization (UN)		SIR	smoking impact ratio
			UNEP	United Nations Environment Programme
GBD	Global Burden of Disease project (WHO)			
GDP	gross domestic product		UNFPA	United Nations Population Fund
GHIs	Global Health Initiatives		UNICEF	United Nations Children's Fund
GISMO	Global Integrated Sustainability Model		UNPD	United Nations Population Division
GMAPS	Global Model of Ambient Particulates		USNIC	United States National Intelligence Council
GNI	gross national income			
GUAM	Global Urban Air quality Model		WDI	World Development Indicators (World Bank)
HDI	Human Development Index		WHO	World Health Organization
HIV	human immunodeficiency virus		WHOSIS	World Health Organization Statistical Information System
IAP	indoor air pollution			
ICD	International Classifications of Disease		WHS	World Health Survey (WHO)
ICSU	International Council for Science		WSH	water, sanitation, and hygiene
IFs	International Futures computer simulation model		YLDs	years lived with disability
			YLLs	years of life lost
IHRs	International Health Regulations			
IIASA	International Institute for Applied Systems Analysis			
IPCC	Intergovernmental Panel on Climate Change			

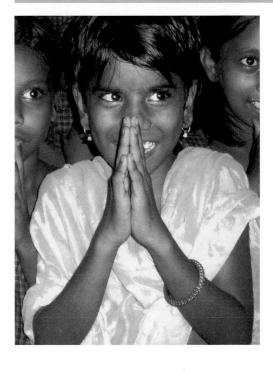

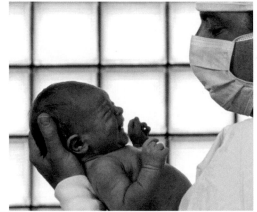

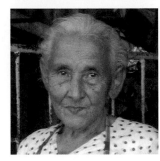

The Story So Far

He who has health has hope
He who has hope has everything.
—Arabic proverb

Health lies at the heart of human development. Our most basic personal and collective decisions reflect our wish to live long, comfortable, and active lives. Yet, for most of human history, the average person's life has been difficult, constrained, and short. When John Graunt first constructed the *Bills of Mortality* for the city of London in 1650, he found that life expectancy was about 27 years (Graunt 1662).[1] In general, up to the time of the industrial revolution in Great Britain, human life displayed a Malthusian pattern of high mortality with transitory deviations, upwards in times of plenty and downwards in times of want or plague.[2]

Since the mid-1700s, however, there has been incredible ongoing advance in human health—Great Britain itself has gained more than one year of life expectancy for every seven calendar years since 1650. Extensions in the length and quality of life first moved across Europe. Especially since World War II, health improvements have spread throughout the world, and the pace has advanced further. Global life expectancy rose from 46 years in 1950 to 69 years in 2007.[3]

This volume explores the story of changes in human health as it might continue to unfold in coming decades. We consider also the variations in that possible story, many associated with human choices. This chapter introduces the foundations of the story and our approach to elaborating it.

Recent Progress and Significant Challenges

Consider what the world has accomplished in recent decades and the challenges that remain, beginning with infant and child mortality. A major reason behind the low life expectancy in Graunt's London was that about 300 per 1,000 children died before the age of five. Between

Since World War II, health improvements have spread across the world at an unprecedented pace.

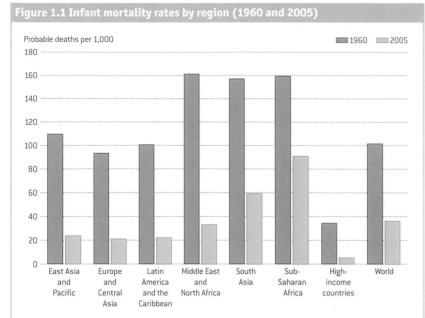

Figure 1.1 Infant mortality rates by region (1960 and 2005)

Probable deaths per 1,000

■ 1960 ■ 2005

Note: Infant mortality refers to children dying before their first birthday; the rates are deaths per 1,000 live births. Throughout this volume, unless otherwise noted, regions are the World Bank geographical groupings of developing countries plus a single high-income category; see Box 4.2 for discussion of country groupings and volume Appendix for lists of region members.

Source: IFs Version 6.32 using data from the World Bank's World Development Indicators (hereafter referred to as WDI).

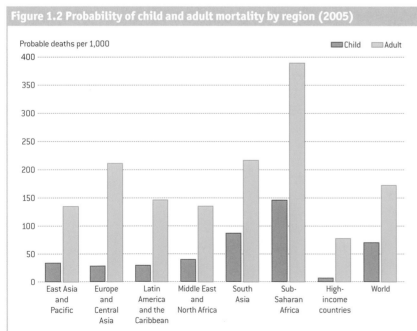

Figure 1.2 Probability of child and adult mortality by region (2005)

Probable deaths per 1,000

■ Child ■ Adult

Note: Child mortality is expressed as the number of children per 1,000 expected to die before their fifth birthday, assuming current age-specific death rates; adult mortality is expressed as the number of 15-year-olds per 1,000 expected to die before age 60, assuming current age-specific death rates.

Source: IFs Version 6.32 using data from multiple sources (see Chapter 3).

1950 and 2006, however, the world's infant mortality rate dropped from 153 to 36 deaths per 1,000 (see Figure 1.1 for regional progress since 1960), and the number of children who die before reaching five years of age has fallen to about 70 per 1,000. This global pace of improvement is unprecedented.

Still, global health problems remain daunting. We estimate that in 2005 about 10.1 million children died before their fifth birthdays, with 99 percent of those deaths occurring in developing countries. That distribution of child deaths illustrates a critical health issue: the great disparity that exists in health prospects across the regions of the world (see Figures 1.1 and 1.2). Had children in poorer countries died at the same rate as those in high-income countries, there would have been about 9 million fewer child deaths (out of the about 10 million globally). The distributions of deaths within countries are also very unequal across income, education, ethnicity, and other social divisions (CSDH 2008: 29).

Communicable diseases claimed about 17 million lives globally in 2005, and they accounted for the vast bulk of child deaths. The communicable disease burden for adults and the elderly is also large. The AIDS epidemic (accounting for about 2 million deaths) heavily affects adults; it lowered life expectancy in all of sub-Saharan Africa by 0.25 years between 1990 and 2000 and contributed to declines of more than 14 years in Botswana and 15 years in Zimbabwe. AIDS is not, however, the only culprit in such setbacks—even with low HIV rates, countries such as Afghanistan and Sierra Leone have experienced recent sustained declines in life expectancy, largely attributable to conflict, political disorganization, and the eventual unwinding of disease control mechanisms (Jamison 2006).

Noncommunicable diseases were responsible for about 32 million deaths globally in 2005; injuries killed another 5 million, and those deaths are rising rapidly with the spread of vehicle ownership. These categories are the primary causes of the death of adults, and they are by far the largest killers in high-income countries. Many developing countries, however, increasingly face a double burden of premature deaths—unnecessarily high rates of both communicable and noncommunicable diseases.

In combination, differences in child and adult mortality probabilities (see Figure 1.2) create a nearly 28-year gap in life expectancy between sub-Saharan Africa and the high-income countries of the world.

A substantial burden of unnecessary mortality and disability also remains in high-income countries. As Figure 1.2 shows, in those countries—where death before the age of retirement is now considered very premature—77 of 1,000 15-year-olds still die before reaching their 60th birthdays. Great effort and investment flow into extending life expectancy everywhere and at all ages, and the story of disease and mortality decline is, hopefully, far from over.

Understanding the Story So Far

Abdel Omran's theory of the epidemiologic transition (Omran 1971) elegantly describes the story of modern improvements in global health. According to this theory, societies experience a transition from high to low levels of population mortality risk concurrent with processes of economic, social, and political development (see Figure 1.3). Economic and educational progress is viewed as resulting in better public health, and vice versa. In other words, the theory asserts that the epidemiologic transition is not merely a result of economic and social change but very much an integrated, dynamic part of it. And in fact, considerable evidence suggests the profound shift from omnipresent mortality risks to delayed and more predictable risks is essential to broader processes of social and economic transformation, including fertility decline, educational investment, better health throughout the course of life, and economic growth (Fogel 1994; Fogel and Costa 1997; Sen 1985; 1987; 1998).

To summarize the health impacts of the epidemiologic transition very briefly, its early stages involve a reduction in infectious and communicable diseases, such as diarrheal and respiratory infections, which largely affect young children and other vulnerable populations. The resulting increased survival of children through the highly vulnerable years of early childhood sets the stage for the large majority of most populations to survive well into adulthood, absent high levels of exposure to violence, accidents, infections of adulthood such as HIV/ AIDS, or the early onset of chronic disease. Thus, the epidemiologic transition implies a shift in the predominant causes of death and morbidity to noncommunicable conditions such as cardiovascular disease, diabetes, and cancer, mostly affecting people at older ages and creating new and different health challenges for society (Omran 1971; Yach et al. 2004).

Near the end of his life, Omran revisited his original 1971 three-stage representation of the epidemiologic transition and added fourth and fifth stages (Omran 1998). He observed a fourth stage (which developed countries began to reach in the 1970s), in which mortality from certain noncommunicable diseases (notably cardiovascular diseases at that time), began to level off and then to decline due to changes in behavior and in medical practice. Omran also envisioned a fifth stage, in which medical advances and declining health differences across social groups could further boost life expectancy, potentially also creating a variety of social challenges associated with prolonged morbidity.[4]

Almost all countries are at least well into the stage of receding communicable disease pandemics, and conditions have rapidly converged in recent decades for all but a small number of countries. For example, in 1950 the gap in life expectancy between the median

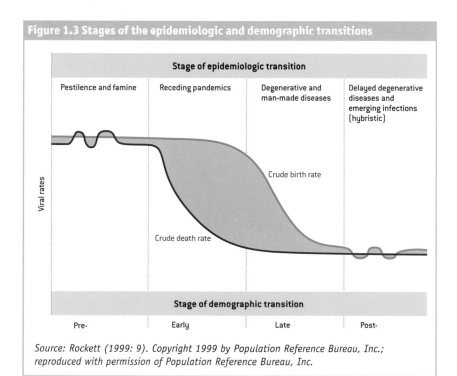

Figure 1.3 Stages of the epidemiologic and demographic transitions

Stage of epidemiologic transition

| Pestilence and famine | Receding pandemics | Degenerative and man-made diseases | Delayed degenerative diseases and emerging infections (hybristic) |

Crude birth rate

Crude death rate

Viral rates

Stage of demographic transition

Pre-   Early   Late   Post-

Source: Rockett (1999: 9). Copyright 1999 by Population Reference Bureau, Inc.; reproduced with permission of Population Reference Bureau, Inc.

country and the country at the 75th percentile stood at about 20 years (45 years to 65 years). By 2000, the margin separating them was a mere five years (69 years to 73 years), and life expectancy in countries at the 25th percentile was 64 years (Jamison 2006). Put another way, people in the world's poorer countries in 2000 were longer-lived than those in wealthier countries of 1950.

Still, very significant gaps remain in health between countries (see again Figures 1.1 and 1.2). At one end, fewer than three of 1,000 infants in Japan die in the first year of life, and a female child born in today's Japan can expect to live 86 years, a level well past what was once thought to be a hard limit to the human life span (Fries 1980), continuing the quite steady growth in life expectancy of women in "best practice societies" (see Figure 1.4).[5] At the other end of the spectrum, in sub-Saharan Africa, more than 90 of every 1,000 infants die in the first year of life, and a female child born in today's sub-Saharan Africa can expect to live only 53 years. And even as we celebrate the tremendous global gains against communicable diseases, we are confronted with the HIV/AIDs epidemic, some endemic diseases, and the possibility of other new or reemerging communicable diseases.

Understanding and Shaping the Story Going Forward

Debates over what determines the health status of individuals and of populations tread on some of the most contested questions of our times, including "nature versus nurture," "individual versus state," and "optimist versus pessimist" (Kunitz 1987; Oeppen and Vaupel 2002). More concretely, some analysts argue that advances in economic growth inevitably lead to longer, healthier lives (McKeown 1976; Pritchett and Summers 1996). The epidemiologic transition might suggest such a relatively automatic process, and economic growth and other deep-driving variables—often called the *distal drivers* of health outcomes—are, in fact, very powerful.

Still, these distal drivers of health leave considerable unexplained variation in health outcomes across countries (Cutler, Deaton, and Lleras-Muney 2006; Preston 1975). Largely preventable diseases continue to kill millions of people each year. Malaria and type 2 diabetes, for instance, do not require expensive or sophisticated cures—the widespread use of bed nets could dramatically decrease malaria, while dietary changes could prevent many cases of type 2 diabetes. Recognizing uncertainties around these and other more immediate causes of health outcomes—typically referred to as *proximate drivers* (which the distal drivers affect but do not fully determine)—alerts us to the substantial difficulties inherent in any attempt to forecast health outcomes. Indeed, the focus of most modern global health action lies with addressing many of these proximate drivers through vaccination, disease eradication, and delivery of basic disease-prevention services, including health education.

Even with the identification of distal and proximate drivers, the picture of changing health remains incomplete. Much of what we want to understand about change in the distal and proximate drivers and the relationships among and between them lies still deeper, at the level of what might be called *super-distal drivers*. Human activity that builds this still-deeper context includes such things as technological advance; human-based change in the natural environment and our exposure to it (including water and sanitation systems, air pollution, and climate change); and change within the social environment (including the development and

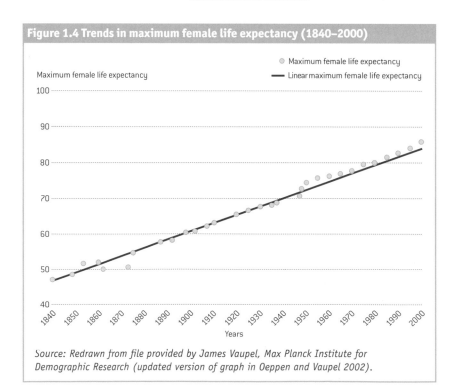

Figure 1.4 Trends in maximum female life expectancy (1840–2000)

Maximum female life expectancy

○ Maximum female life expectancy
— Linear maximum female life expectancy

Years

Source: Redrawn from file provided by James Vaupel, Max Planck Institute for Demographic Research (updated version of graph in Oeppen and Vaupel 2002).

character of health care systems and even the maintenance of efficient markets that may lower drug prices).

Human agency around health often has the aim of providing or acquiring private goods (such as in the doctor-patient relationship). Much conscious and positive collective action, however, is motivated by the fact that a great many advances in health tend to have characteristics of public goods (that is, consumption by one does not preclude consumption by others, and denial to others is difficult). Moreover, there can be many positive social externalities from the good health of others, not least of which is less risk of infection to ourselves. Complicating the organization of human action concerning health is frequent struggle, such as that around intellectual property rights for new drugs or vaccines, over how to draw legal lines between private- and public-good characteristics. Globalization processes, including the spread of smoking and of fast and fatty foods and their obvious negative health consequences, further complicate the private-public debates and push a still broader set of health issues onto the potential global agenda.

A global health agenda has emerged and become more organized and explicit over time, beginning with the statement in the 1948 United Nations Declaration of Universal Human Rights of the right of all peoples to a standard of living adequate for health. A landmark initiative to further human health occurred that same year when the United Nations established the World Health Organization (WHO), whose objective, as stated in its constitution,[6] is the "attainment by all peoples of the highest possible level of health." WHO pursues these goals through coordinating and collaborating with its 193 member governments and other multilateral agencies, by providing technical support, and by developing and maintaining global data systems. While responsive to and financially dependent on its membership, WHO's constitution also mandates a normative role for the organization in developing global health policy (Magnusson 2009; Ruger and Yach 2008/2009). This increasingly includes the use of legal and regulatory mechanisms—such as the legally binding International Health Regulations for communicable disease

surveillance and the 2003 Framework Convention on Tobacco Control—to encourage compliance with international health norms and agreements (Aginam 2002; Magnusson 2009).

While WHO has the key formal leadership role with respect to the global health agenda, global health initiatives reflect a multitude of actors, approaches, and targets (Bettcher, Yach, and Guindon 2000; Brundtland 2004; McMichael 2000). The constituents of what is increasingly referred to as the "global health governance regime"—WHO, private donors and organizations (both formal and informal), and governments and other public entities—have developed a number of global health goals that offer some guideposts for our analysis. The earliest of these goals was the Alma Ata Declaration of 1978, which focused on primary health care and promised "health for all by the year 2000." However, the Alma Ata Declaration offered few measurable objectives.

The global community incorporated a more explicit range of objectives into the Millennium Development Goals (MDGs) for 2015. The explicit MDG health goals include the reduction of infant and child (under-five) mortality rates by two-thirds relative to 1990 and of maternal mortality rates by three-fourths, as well as halting and then reversing growth in the incidence of HIV/AIDS, malaria, and other major diseases (such as tuberculosis). Other MDGs include targets or indicators with respect to proximate health drivers: the MDG for the eradication of extreme poverty and hunger calls for cutting in half between 1990 and 2015 the prevalence of underweight children and the proportion of the total population without access to adequate calorie intake, and the MDG for environmental sustainability calls for a 50 percent reduction in those without access to safe drinking water and improved sanitation over the same period.

The final report of a recent WHO commission, the Commission on Social Determinants of Health (CSDH 2008: 197), has more recently called for goals that both extend the time horizon to 2040 and that focus on the equitable distribution of health outcomes, as exemplified by reducing variations in life expectancy at birth (LEB) within and across countries. With respect to extension of the horizon of existing goals, the Commission urged that all countries reduce the under-five mortality rate by 90 percent between

A complex interplay of underlying ("distal") and more immediate ("proximate") causes or drivers determine health outcomes.

Human activity with respect to technology, the natural environment, and the social environment is a powerful "super-distal" driver of health.

A global health agenda has emerged over the last several decades and is becoming increasingly organized and explicit.

2000 and 2040 and the maternal death rate by 95 percent. With respect to new goals, the Commission urged reducing adult mortality rates in all countries and in all social groups within countries by 50 percent between 2000 and 2040 and reducing by 10 years the gap in LEB between the thirds of countries with the highest and lowest LEB values in 2000 (we estimate the 2000 gap was almost 19 years).

Why This Volume?

Looking forward, not only to the horizons of such goals but also well beyond them, major uncertainties complicate forecasting. A great debate rages about the biological potential of the human genome for continued advance in life expectancy at historical rates, and we certainly cannot rule out major new disease epidemics. A very large portion of our uncertainty, however, revolves around human action—for instance, the advance of our technology, the strength of our health care systems, our will and our access to means to change unhealthy lifestyles, the progress and character of globalization processes, and the extent and impact of environmental change, including air pollution and global warming (Fauci 2001; McMichael, Woodruff, and Hales 2006).

In spite of the complications, we deem the forecasting endeavor necessary. Forecasting helps shape goals that can be attained and then to direct action to them. It helps us anticipate and avoid negative scenarios and decisions that result in misdirected resources. It can also provide insight into the broader economic and social consequences of alternative health futures.

Thus, this volume sets out to tell a story of possible futures for the health of peoples across the world. While recognizing that any modeling approach has many inherent limitations, our dynamic tools allow us to address policy-relevant questions facing countries with differing disease burdens:

- What health outcomes would we expect given current patterns of human development?
- What opportunities exist for intervention and the achievement of alternate, improved health futures?
- How might alternative health futures affect broader economic, social, and political prospects of countries, regions, and the world?

The central tool in the analysis and forecasting of this volume, as in the earlier volumes of the Patterns of Potential Human Progress series treating poverty reduction and advance of education, is the International Futures (IFs) global modeling system. IFs is a computer software tool whose central purpose is to facilitate exploration of possible global futures through the creation and analysis of alternative scenarios. It includes an extensive database for 183 countries for the time period from 1960 to the present. In addition to health, the IFs system incorporates models of population, economics, education, energy, food and agriculture, aspects of the environment, and socio-political change and represents dynamic connections among them. Its interactive interface makes data and scenario analysis relatively straightforward. Chapter 3 will provide considerably more detail concerning the system (and at www.ifs.du.edu we make IFs fully and freely available for use on the web or for download).

Our own health forecasting model within IFs depends heavily on the groundbreaking work of the WHO's Global Burden of Disease (GBD) project.[7] That project, whose first major report appeared in 1996,[8] set out to "provide a comprehensive set of estimates not only of number of deaths by cause but also of total disease burden including [the] burden from disability" (Jamison 1996: xvi). In fact, its forecasts have been the only published global forecasts of regional and cause-specific health outcomes to date (Mathers and Loncar 2006; WHO 2008a). The GBD project has been foundational to our work, and we discuss it at some length in Chapters 2 and 3.

The GBD founders did not, however, design their system to serve as a long-term integrated forecasting tool. Although the GBD project is currently preparing to look further ahead, its most-recent available analyses extend to 2030, now only 20 years distant. Its health forecasts rely on the exogenous input of other forecasts of population and economic growth and do not link health outcomes back to those systems in the feedback loops that we understand to characterize and give dynamic life to the epidemiologic transition. And although WHO has also given rise to the Comparative Risk Assessment project (Ezzati et al. 2004a), a groundbreaking effort mapping key proximate drivers of health and analyzing the impact of reducing health risk factors, the GBD project forecasts rely almost exclusively on three distal drivers of health—income, education, and time (the GBD project treats time primarily as a proxy for technology). As foundational as those distal drivers are, it is attention to proximate drivers that provides most direct leverage of societies on health outcomes. Finally, the GBD forecasts involve limited scenario analysis of the wide range of uncertainty we know to characterize health futures.

In an effort to contribute to the understanding of potential global health futures, we build on and extend the work of the GBD project in a number of ways. The first is time horizon. While accuracy necessarily falls with extended projections, we forecast mortality out to the year 2100 for a number of reasons. One is the recognition that the ongoing epidemiologic transition is a fundamental element of the long-term demographic transition and will help shape the timing and peak of that transition. Another is that longer-term processes (such as global warming) may play an increasingly important part in health futures. More technically, looking at the results of forecasting with models in the longer term helps in understanding their structure and behavior even in the nearer term. Most fundamentally, however, we believe that the global community needs to begin looking and planning well beyond the horizon of the MDGs, at least to the 2040 horizon of the Social Determinants of Health analysis. In this volume we display results primarily for 50 years, to 2060.

Second, although the GBD project's analysis extends to the country level, its published results typically do not. IFs analysis is based at the country level and allows flexible aggregation of country-based results to any country grouping, including those of WHO. The forecasts associated with this volume (including the extensive end tables) add considerably to available health forecasts—in fact, they may be the only health forecasts to which many countries will have access.

Third, we build further on the important work done by GBD authors by embedding mortality and morbidity patterns within larger global systems. In Chapter 4 we explore expected health futures under various conditions of economic growth, education attainment, and technological advance. In Chapter 7 we close the loops and consider the implications of alternative health futures for demographic, economic, and other key human systems. This integrated approach begins to allow a dynamic consideration of the entire human development system around health. Ultimately, a clearer picture of the feedback loops around health, population, and economic factors should allow better understanding of the costs and benefits of intervention, hopefully leading to improved policymaking and better human development outcomes.

Although by no means complete, a fourth way in which we go beyond earlier forecasting is via the important work of beginning to integrate the analysis of proximate drivers into the health forecasting system, resulting in a hybrid health modeling approach that Chapter 3 presents. Health futures for individual countries and the world could be quite significantly different, depending on human action with respect to key behavioral and social factors such as malnutrition, obesity, smoking rates, the extent of improved water and sanitation systems, and indoor or outdoor air pollution. Variation around the world on such proximate drivers is often extremely great, even after controlling for income levels. This suggests much leverage for health-related intervention, which Chapters 5 and 6 explore. Chapter 5 also considers the impact of different futures with respect to vehicle ownership and accident rates, and Chapter 6 further considers the impact of climate change.

The fifth extension of past efforts to forecast global health builds on the individual proximate-driver analyses of alternative potential patterns of health. Clearly, if human leverage is significant on many individual proximate drivers (as well as on the deeper drivers themselves), the aggregate of variation possible in health futures must be very substantial. We map some of that aggregate variation, the space of uncertainty for health futures, returning in doing so also to the uncertainty that surrounds the biological base of health prospects (in our genome and the evolution of pathogens). In Chapter 8 we also consider how our forecasts, rooted in the core GBD model, appear to sit within that space— how optimistic or pessimistic are they?

Analysis with IFs extends the health forecast horizon to 2060 for 183 countries, combining distal, proximate, and super-distal drivers in the analyses.

IFs also explores health futures as they dynamically affect, and are affected by, economic growth scenarios and other components of human development systems.

Conclusion

Considering the fundamental importance of health to humans, it may seem surprising that there has been little forecasting of alternative global health futures. Chapters 2 and 3 will make clearer why that is (for instance, only in recent years have the data become available that enable us to understand even the global health present). And, of course, the wide range of factors that disable or kill us, and the great extent of forces that strengthen or diminish their roles, greatly complicates understanding of possible change. The modeling and analyses that underlie this volume therefore build on a foundation that has been built by others, slowly and laboriously. Our hope is that the dynamic representation of longer-term futures that is the heart of the IFs system will contribute to the understanding of the possible stories of continuing change in global health and to its continued improvement.

1 Wrigley and Schofield (1981) estimated that life expectancy for the United Kingdom in 1700 was about 37 years at birth.

2 Galor and Weil 2000; Oeppen and Vaupel 2002; Preston 1976. The first recorded systematic improvements in human survival were observed among noble populations in Britain in the mid-17th century and population-wide around 1750 (Fogel 1994; Riley 2001; Wrigley and Schofield 1981).

3 Value for 1950 from United Nations Population Fund 1999; 2007 value from World Bank 2009.

4 Martens (2002) has also considered developments beyond the third stage, either in the form of an age of "sustaining health" or an age of medical technology. Simultaneously, Martens has also considered the possibility of a new age of emerging infectious diseases.

5 Life expectancy for men also typically advances in these societies, of course, but frontier analysis normally focuses on women since women's life expectancies are typically longer than men's in today's societies.

6 Available at http://www.who.int/governance/eb/who_constitution_en.pdf.

7 We especially appreciate the generosity of Colin Mathers, Mortality and Burden of Disease Coordinator, Department of Health Statistics and Informatics, World Health Organization, who shared with us the equations and much of the data used in the forecasting work of the GBD project.

8 The 1996 report included estimates for 1990 and projections for 2000, 2010, and 2020.

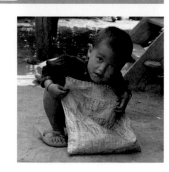

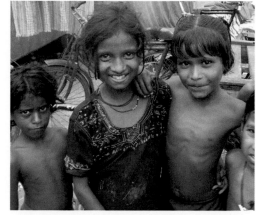

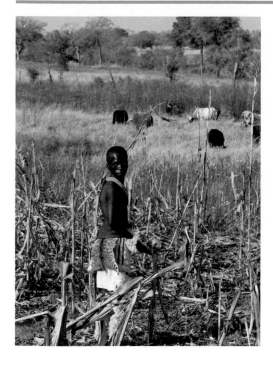

Understanding Health: Concepts, Relationships, and Dynamics

The schema of the epidemiologic transition, which Chapter 1 outlined, describes the general character of change in mortality patterns that richer countries have experienced over the course of two centuries and through which the developing world has been moving very rapidly in recent decades. It also provides some general help in thinking about how human health may change over the next half century. But as a broad framework, it leaves several critical, more specific questions fundamentally unaddressed.

Exactly what is human health? Mortality offers considerable biological clarity and methodological simplicity. All individuals will die, and we can measure the event in a "yes/ no" fashion. In this chapter, and throughout the volume, we pursue the more ambitious goal of classifying the immediate cause of death and of providing at least some understanding of the character of ill-health as well as mortality.

Beyond the most immediate causes or character of death and ill-health, what are the

deeper drivers of population health? In particular, we have an interest in understanding those factors over which we may, as individuals or as societies, exercise some influence. Such exploration in this chapter will necessarily take us well beyond health and demographic systems and into consideration of economic, governance, and environmental systems.

To what does health, in turn, contribute? Amartya Sen's human capabilities framework positions health—and freedom from the burdens, costs, and risks of poor health—as the fundamental element in a constellation of capabilities (including education and political freedom) that are essential to human flourishing (Sen 1985; 1987; 1998). Such a broad perspective on the importance of health leaves us with a wide set of justifications for health promotion: as a right in and of itself, as a marker of a just and well-governed society, as a raw material for productivity and growth, and as the foundation for broader human development.

This chapter provides a conceptual overview of health and begins consideration of health's position within the larger framework of human and environmental systems. The rest of the volume will elaborate and explore the forces that affect health outcomes and also, notably in Chapter 7, the implications of health outcomes for broader human development. We seek to understand a complex web.

Measuring the Disease Burden

When analysts think about current and future levels of health (or as has been more typical, of ill-health), they usually refer to two related categories of outcomes: *mortality* (death) and *morbidity* (illness or disease). The collection of mortality and morbidity statistics by sex, age, and cause dates back to at least the 17th century in some parts of the world. Still, in spite of decades of investment and improvement in data quality, many measurement challenges remain.

Observing mortality

Families and societies have important reasons for the registration of deaths, including ensuring safe disposal of the body, cessation of state benefits provided to the living, and initiation of benefits for survivors. Indeed, almost all states have vital registration systems that nominally collect at least basic mortality information. However, the completeness of the data varies widely between countries.[1]

Though high-quality data remain elusive, the United Nations Population Division (UNPD) uses an array of well-established techniques to estimate all-cause (as opposed to cause-differentiated), age-specific death rates since 1950 in its World Population Prospects database (UNPD 2009b). These data and estimates of mortality from all causes provide a critical anchor or base for estimating and reconciling societal measures of cause-specific mortality and morbidity. In turn, the World Health Organization (WHO) encourages national death registries to categorize deaths according to International Classifications of Diseases (ICD) criteria,[2] which provide highly detailed cause codes for clinicians and public health officials to assign to each death. Recording and reporting inconsistencies and gaps, however, are great.

WHO, in its efforts to systematize understanding of causes of death and their patterns, developed a high-level classification system that organizes the ICD detailed causes of death into three major cause-groups (Murray and Lopez 1996a: 119). These groups, described briefly below, have become the standard high-level classification system of major causes of death and are used extensively throughout this volume.

Group I diseases are primarily *communicable diseases (CDs)* caused by infectious agents outside the body. Group I also includes all other causes of maternal and perinatal mortality as well as nutritional deficiencies. In combination, these are the diseases that tend to prevail in the early stages of the epidemiologic transition. The characteristics that unify them include their preventability (often at low cost), their outsize effect on vulnerable populations (especially the very young and women in childbirth), and the risks of infection to others. While most CDs are short in duration, resulting fairly quickly in either death or recovery, others (such as HIV/AIDS) are becoming increasingly chronic in nature. (As others often do, we use the term *communicable diseases* as shorthand to refer to all of Group I throughout this volume.)

Group II diseases are *noncommunicable diseases (NCDs)* resulting from genetic, cellular, or organic anomalies or degeneration occurring inside the body. While we can thus refer to NCDs as internal causes of death, external forces such as diet, tobacco use, and environmental factors influence many of them.[3] NCDs tend to predominate in later stages of the epidemiologic transition, both because of the progression of underlying risks to health that accompany that transition and because of their tendency to accumulate as an individual reaches older ages. Many also share common characteristics with respect to the relative cost and difficulty of prevention and treatment.

Group III causes of death are *injuries*. Like CDs, injuries are external in cause, yet the external agent interacts with the body's skeletal or organ systems (not the immune system), and the sufferer poses no further risk to the health of others. Group III deaths are most likely among those with high exposure to risk (e.g., in the residence or workplace or through warfare or personal behavior), limited safety precautions, and limited access to treatment.

Limited data are available on cause-specific mortality and morbidity, even at the aggregated "major cause" level of Groups I, II, and III. In a 2005 study, WHO reported that only 23 of its 193 member countries provided "high-quality" cause-of-death data, and 75 member countries had provided no cause-of-death data since 1990 (Mathers et al. 2005). Largely in recognition of this data gap, WHO initiated the

Global Burden of Disease (GBD) study, which in 1990 began providing global estimates of age, sex, and cause-specific mortality and morbidity (Mathers and Loncar 2006; WHO 2008a). For most countries today, the development of cause-specific death rates begins with country cause-of-death registration systems but still relies largely on a series of estimates or imputations (Murray 2007).

Given mortality data or estimates, we can visualize mortality patterns using the J-curve (see Box 2.1 and the left side of Figure 2.1). A J-curve shows age- and sex-specific mortality rates for defined populations for an identified point in time. Plotting multiple J-curves on a single figure allows direct visual comparison across populations, causes of death, or time periods; for instance, the left side of Figure 2.1 compares mortality rates for males and females in Bangladesh from all causes in 2005. Mortality pyramids (see the right side of Figure 2.1) provide a different way to visualize the same data. It is not as easy to plot multiple pyramids

◼ *Gaps in data, and data of varying quality, complicate efforts to measure global mortality— particularly mortality due to specific causes of death.* ◼

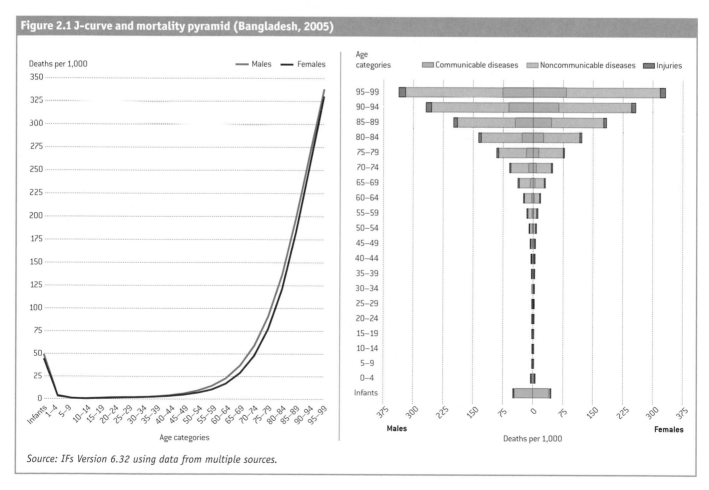

Figure 2.1 J-curve and mortality pyramid (Bangladesh, 2005)

Source: IFs Version 6.32 using data from multiple sources.

Demographers often refer to the mortality curve as the "J-curve," reflecting the characteristic shape of the age-specific mortality pattern in humans and most other mammalian populations. The reproductive requirements of a skill- and resource-intensive species shape the human life cycle. Successful reproduction necessitates relatively predictable and low levels of mortality during the prime ages for childbearing and childrearing (Carey 2003; Kaplan 2006; Olshansky, Carnes, and Brody 2002). Durability in adulthood comes at a cost; humans acquire physical and mental skills over a relatively long period of development and dependency. Some deaths very early in life serve the evolutionary purpose of eliminating the least healthy so that resources can be focused on surviving children.

While the biological complexity necessary for a human's high physical and mental functioning facilitates significant longevity—often well after the childbearing years are concluded—the human body is nonetheless subject to a gradual process of senescence, or the gradual deterioration of cellular and organ function with age. Beginning at about age 25, mortality increases steadily due to the breakdown or obstruction of organs and cells (Carey 2003; Olshansky and Carnes 1994; 1997; Olshansky, Carnes, and Brody 2002). This pattern was first empirically substantiated and mathematically formalized by Benjamin Gompertz, an actuary working in Britain in the mid-19th century. Gompertz (1825) fit an exponential functional form to age patterns of British mortality data from the early 18th century, meaning that he observed that the hazard, or risk, of mortality increased in an accelerating fashion with advancing age from about age 25 through the end of life. This biologically determined age-pattern of mortality can suggest whether societies are reporting too few or too many deaths at certain ages.

on a single figure, but they do facilitate subgroup decomposition, as in the causes of death color-coded in Figure 2.1.

Summarizing mortality

A number of measures exist for summarizing mortality, each of which may paint a somewhat different picture. The most commonly reported measure at the societal level is the *crude death rate* (CDR), defined simply as the total number of deaths divided by the total population (often expressed as deaths per 1,000 people). While CDRs are simple to calculate, they conflate the effects of population distribution with the effects of death rates at any given age. For example, in 2006, the reported crude death rate in Yemen was lower than in Sweden, which reported lower death rates at every age but had a substantially older population (UNPD 2009b).

An alternative approach to summarizing mortality rates is the calculation of life expectancy. Using age-specific mortality rates, a *life table* indicates the survival rate at each age of a hypothetical cohort of people who live their lives according to those rates; in turn, data from the life table can be used to construct a *survival curve* indicating the person-years lived in each of the age categories. Figure 2.2 shows a survival curve based on the estimated 2005–2010 death rates of the Bangladeshi population. We can visualize *life expectancy at birth*, or the average years a newborn could expect to live given current death rates, as the sum of the years of life lived by this population, as indicated at the bottom of Figure 2.2. Life expectancy at birth reflects the pace of mortality throughout the age distribution. For example, only 92 percent of Bangladeshis are expected to reach their 10th birthday, but the 8 percent who died before then nonetheless contribute some years of life; thus, a hypothetical average Bangladeshi can expect to live 9.4 out of 10 possible years through age 10. In older age groups, those dying in earlier periods make no contribution to life expectancy for those groups, and those dying during the period make only a partial contribution. The net result is a life expectancy at birth of 62.9 years for Bangladesh in 2005. As this example suggests, life expectancy is highly sensitive to infant and childhood mortality.

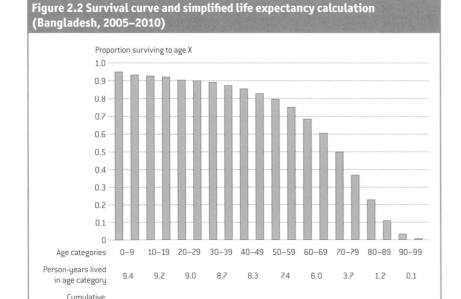

Figure 2.2 Survival curve and simplified life expectancy calculation (Bangladesh, 2005–2010)

Proportion surviving to age X

Age categories	0–9	10–19	20–29	30–39	40–49	50–59	60–69	70–79	80–89	90–99
Person-years lived in age category	9.4	9.2	9.0	8.7	8.3	7.4	6.0	3.7	1.2	0.1
Cumulative person-years lived	9.4	18.5	27.5	36.2	44.5	51.9	57.9	61.6	62.8	62.9

Source: Created by authors using data and estimates from UNPD (2009b).

The same approach can be applied to calculating life expectancy from any particular age. For example, the fact that a 65-year-old Bangladeshi has surpassed the population's life expectancy at birth does not mean that he will die imminently. Rather, given the death rates from that age on, he can expect to live an additional 12.8 years (life expectancy at age 65), or a total average age of 77.8 years.

In an earlier era, when the epidemiologic transition proceeded relatively smoothly from declining child mortality to declining adult mortality, life expectancy could fairly reliably capture a country's position on that path. Today, however, divergent patterns of adult mortality and a reduced correlation between life expectancy and child mortality have diminished the value of life expectancy as a single measure of health. For example, Yemen, the Russian Federation, and Namibia had very similar male life expectancies (60–61) in 2005. Yet the three populations had very different J-curves and survival curves. Yemen had a traditional pattern of high child mortality and high but "typical" adult mortality. On the other hand, the Russian Federation had child mortality levels comparable to a developed country coupled with extraordinarily high adult mortality rates related to noncommunicable diseases and injuries. And in a still different dynamic, Namibia's child mortality was significantly lower than Yemen's, yet high adult mortality due to HIV/AIDS (a Group I disease) brought down its life expectancy.

Other summary measures better capture the age-patterns of mortality. One pair of such measures is child and adult mortality rates. WHO defines the child mortality rate as "the probability of a child born in a specific year or period dying before reaching the age of five";[4] for this reason it is often referred to as the under-five mortality rate. Similarly, WHO defines adult mortality as the probability of surviving from one's 15th to 60th birthdays, a measure that ignores child mortality and old-age survival patterns (de Waal 2002). And studies of longevity sometimes use life expectancy starting from older ages to better isolate the effects of old-age mortality. For instance, the U.S. National Institute of Aging looks at populations 65–84 and 85 and older (sometimes 65–74, 75–84, and 85 and older; see Fries et al. 2000).

Measures such as life expectancy, child mortality, and adult mortality are very useful in conveying information about total mortality. To facilitate the attribution of mortality and changes in mortality to specific causes, however, it is useful to turn to a measure of life expectancy gap such as the *years of life lost* (YLL) measure used in the GBD study. Instead of describing the average years of life lived from birth, the YLL measures the number of years that a person loses upon dying compared to their life expectancy at the age of death. As noted above, one's life expectancy within one's own country can be calculated from any age. But GBD set the standard for how much longer one could have lived not based on one's own population, but based on that of Japan, which has the world's longest-lived population (Murray 1996: 16). Thus, an infant male dying in any country is estimated to have lost 80 years, the life expectancy of a male child born in Japan. The death of a 60-year-old man in any society would be associated with the 22-year life expectancy of a 60-year-old man in the Japanese standard population.

The YLL, which is generally aggregated across the population, offers two useful analytic benefits. First, by ascribing years of life lost at the time of death, we can easily disaggregate the contributions to YLL of specific causes of death just as we do for death rates. Second, the measure of total time lost to mortality is complementary to measures of disease prevalence and duration, to which we turn next.

Observing morbidity

The GBD project's ambitious goals included "generating the first comprehensive and consistent set of estimates of mortality and morbidity by age, sex and region for the world" (Mathers, Lopez, and Murray 2006: 45).

While morbidity (ill-health) and mortality (death) obviously are often related, in practice many individuals are never sick before death (e.g., accident victims) or are sick for very short periods (e.g., with avian influenza), while others experience long periods of morbidity from chronic diseases with widely varying levels of severity. Many of the sick also return to a state of health, though these individuals may differ in a variety of ways from those who were never sick.[5] In all of these cases of sickness,

We need to use measures beyond crude death rates and life expectancy at birth to understand the age-patterns of mortality.

Years of life lost measure an individual's premature death in comparison to a standard (long-lived) population.

the quality of one's existence is (presumably) neither as good as full health nor as bad as death. Put in terms of the earlier YLL example of a man dying at age 60, if he suffered from liver cancer for six years (from age 54), then the six years lost to cancer disability were qualitatively better than his 22 years of premature death, but worse than the preceding 54 years of health.

Clearly it would be desirable to account for the severity of illness in measures of health, yet there are serious conceptual and logistical impediments to doing so. Logistically, the science of collecting population-wide data on the diagnostic and functional dimensions of health remains in its infancy. The Demographic and Health Surveys (DHS) of the United States Agency for International Development and the Multiple Indicator Cluster Survey (MICS) conducted by the United Nations International Children's Fund are indispensable sources of population-wide morbidity data for children and women in most countries. More recently, WHO's World Health Survey (WHS) has begun the process of systematic estimation of reported health burdens and limitations in many countries, a process still largely based on a variety of indirect approaches described below.

Conceptually, severity may be indicated variously by the level of biochemical abnormality that defines a disease, by the extent of functional limitation, by the impact on quality of life, or by the risk of mortality. Each of these factors may vary independently over the course of a particular illness. Indeed, what counts as "healthy" may vary over time and space (Morrow and Bryant 1995). Finally, there is a difficult trade-off between the clarity offered by measuring the occurrence of a specific disease and the comprehensiveness of measuring aggregate morbidity irrespective of the disease. We discuss each of these issues in turn.

Measures of disease occurrence

We divide measures of disease occurrence into *incidence* (new cases of disease among a group at risk) and *prevalence* (presence of disease in a population). In a stock and flow model, incidence is a flow and prevalence is a stock. Prevalence reflects the combined effects of past disease incidence, recovery, and death; that is, it is the sum of those who contracted the disease

less those who recovered and those who died. It thus captures both the societal burden of an illness and the size of the pool of individuals experiencing a higher risk of mortality due to the disease. Although incidence measures are significant for disease surveillance and policy evaluation, collection is often costly and the actual onset of disease is often impossible to observe. The brevity of most acute illnesses poses a special challenge for collecting incidence or prevalence data in most poor countries.

Chronic diseases offer more opportunity to measure morbidity, both in terms of the marginal utility of doing so and their ease of measurement. Many societies, including some middle-income countries, conduct reasonably accurate surveillance of incidence (based on the timing of diagnosis) as well as prevalence. High-quality data are most common for the big three noncommunicable disease risks (cardiovascular diseases, cancers, and diabetes) as well as for HIV/AIDS, the communicable disease of greatest impact in many countries.

Even so, cost and lack of data-collection coverage severely limit development even of prevalence measures. Typically, prevalence data come from hospital reports (preferred) or surveys of individuals, which together systematically undercount prevalence if a significant number of patients have no access to a hospital or no recollection of a diagnosis. Recognizing this, researchers conducting household surveys in poor countries are increasingly assessing disease prevalence through methods such as physical examination and the collection of blood-drawn biomarkers for critical diseases such as HIV/AIDS, cardiovascular diseases, and diabetes. Limitations, however, persist: direct assessments are costly, often cover limited time spans and populations, and typically incorporate data on only a small number of diseases. Nonetheless, they represent a significant step forward, introducing at least the possibility of cross-national disease assessment on a wide scale.

In the end analysis, long-term forecasts are far more likely to employ measures of prevalence than incidence. In the absence of either prevalence or incidence data, analysts often rely on mortality data as either a predictor of, or proxy for, morbidity.

Measures of overall morbidity

Prevalence measures only bring us part of the way to the goal of creating a single morbidity rate that captures the overall burden of morbidity, much as the life expectancy or YLL measures do for mortality. The missing piece, noted earlier, is related to identification and measurement of the severity of each disease.

In order to address this deficiency, researchers with the GBD project developed the concept of a *disability weight* and used it to quantify each disease state along a 0–1 continuum (Lopez et al. 2006b).[6] For example, the disability weight for liver cancer is 0.20 during the diagnostic and therapeutic stage, 0.75 in the metastasis stage, and 0.81 in the terminal stage. In the context of the earlier example, assume that five out of the six years of liver cancer were spent in the diagnostic and therapeutic stage, one year in the metastasis stage, and no significant time in the terminal stage. Thus, we could add 5 * 0.20 = 1 for the first stage and 1 * 0.75 = 0.75 for the final year of life, yielding a total of 1.75. These are referred to as the *years lived with disability* (YLD).

Combining morbidity and mortality into a single measure

The GBD researchers also developed a summary measure designed to combine the impact of both mortality and morbidity into a single statistic: *disability-adjusted life years* (DALYs), which combines years of life lost with years lived with disability.[7] For instance, adding YLD and YLL in our ongoing example case of liver cancer, we find that the combined mortality and morbidity (22 YLL + 1.75 YLD) results in a total DALY estimate of 23.75 years.

While the DALY represents a major step forward in disease burden reporting, it also presents analysts (and especially forecasters) with a number of problems related, first of all, to the disability weights. The base of data for estimating the disability weight for any specific disease remains quite thin. Initially, the disability weights were based on "tradeoff surveys" in which a panel of medical experts was asked to weigh the relative undesirability of particular disorders against one another (Arnesen and Kapiriri 2004); more recently, the estimation of disability weights has incorporated survey results linking key diseases to measures of physical limitation (Mathers, Lopez, and Murray 2006: 50–51). Yet the disability weight concept does not relate to any specific dimension of disease severity, even though the varying effects of diseases on physical functioning, pain, depression, self-efficacy, or productivity could have widely divergent implications for the other dimensions of human progress included in a global health forecast (Anand and Hanson 1997; Arnesen and Nord 1999). Varying relationships between disability weights and the probability of death also complicate the estimation of disability weights; although the disability weight is closely concordant with mortality risk for a wide range of diseases, a number of important conditions (including chronic pain, severe psychiatric conditions, and vision and hearing impairment) carry high disability weights alongside relatively low probabilities of death. In summary, it is often difficult to tell whether the relative importance of certain conditions according to DALYs versus death rates derives from accounting for disability, from counting YLLs instead of deaths, or from two other adjustments applied to most DALY estimates to which we now turn—namely, age-weights and a discount factor.

Most published values of DALYs (and their YLL and YLD components) incorporate age-importance weights and a discount factor (typically 3 percent). The age-weights are primarily intended to reflect the potential impacts or forward linkages from death and disability to such societal functions as labor productivity and parenthood. These adjustments, however, are controversial, given variations in the relevance of different age groups for particular functions and in different societies, not to mention the ethical challenge of placing a value on a life. The choice of the discount rate also raises controversy in terms of what it implies with respect to the value of future life in relation to current life. Some researchers have pointed out that the combination of age-weights and discounting can create perverse cross-societal variations in the value of a life (Arnesen and Kapiriri 2004). While we follow the typical practice of incorporating discounting and age-weighting in our approach, we also make it possible with International Futures (IFs) to look at DALYs and their YLL and YLD components without discounting or age-weighting.

■ Disability-adjusted life years combine the impacts of morbidity and premature death into a single summary measure of disease burden. ■

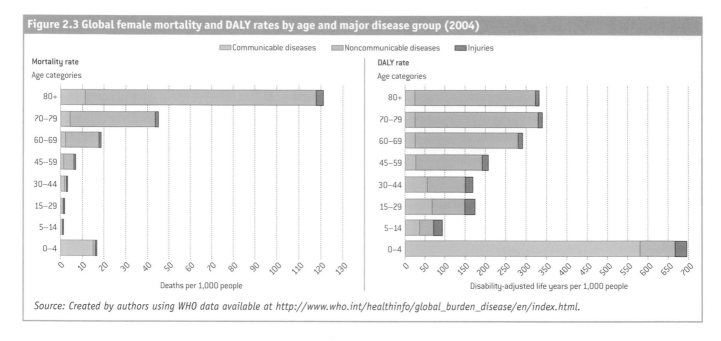

Figure 2.3 Global female mortality and DALY rates by age and major disease group (2004)

☐ Communicable diseases   ☐ Noncommunicable diseases   ■ Injuries

Mortality rate
Age categories

Age	
80+	
70–79	
60–69	
45–59	
30–44	
15–29	
5–14	
0–4	

0 10 20 30 40 50 60 70 80 90 100 110 120 130

Deaths per 1,000 people

DALY rate
Age categories

Age	
80+	
70–79	
60–69	
45–59	
30–44	
15–29	
5–14	
0–4	

0 50 100 150 200 250 300 350 400 450 500 550 600 650 700

Disability-adjusted life years per 1,000 people

Source: Created by authors using WHO data available at http://www.who.int/healthinfo/global_burden_disease/en/index.html.

● *To understand health outcomes, we need to understand distal and proximate causes of health within the context of biology, the natural environment, and human activity.* ●

Finally, there are issues particular to our analysis. One is that it is almost certainly unreasonable to assume that disability weights will not change over time, for instance in response to changing technology specific to the disease or to pain management. A second is that the use of current mortality and morbidity in our broader model already represents some of the forward linkages or impacts by age that are meant to be captured by the age-importance weights and the discount factor.

Though not without problems and limitations, the DALY measure does usefully point our attention to what we miss if we ignore morbidity as a large part of the disease burden. In Figure 2.3, the left panel displays the age and causal structure of mortality for females globally in 2004 by the three broad disease categories reported by the GBD project, while the right panel illustrates the age and causal structure of DALYs in the same year. The two graphs together show that populations experience mortality and morbidity differently. Disease strikes across the age spectrum, with most deaths occurring among the elderly (from noncommunicable causes) or the very young (from communicable causes). The DALY panel not only shows a different age-profile, but also suggests a larger burden of disease from Group I causes than we might expect from the mortality data, especially among infants and children under the age of five.

Understanding Health Outcomes

Assuming that we can conceptualize and measure health outcomes in terms of both morbidity and mortality, the next task becomes understanding what causes differences and changes within them. Figure 2.4 provides a general overview of multiple categories of drivers of health outcomes. *Distal drivers*, or the deep drivers of health outcomes, include those that the GBD project uses in its forecasting, namely, income, education, and time as a proxy for other changes, including technological advance and broader social change. Distal drivers thus refer to societal conditions that do not have direct biological impacts but may enable biological interventions. There are also proximate drivers that more immediately and specifically relate to health outcomes (Lopez et al. 2006b: 2). These drivers often involve action that more directly addresses a human biological outcome, such as vaccination to prevent (or treatment to battle) a specific disease, behavioral changes to reduce obesity, or water-sanitation interventions to reduce exposure to biological agents.[8] While proximate drivers are themselves strongly shaped by distal drivers over time, they suggest points of human leverage that do not require the fundamental restructuring of society (see Soper as edited by Kerr 1970), and many are amenable to intervention in even the poorest of countries.

However, we can only properly understand distal and proximate drivers, and their strengths and limitations, in the broader context of the biological and natural human environments. Health arises from a complex set of biological interactions occurring within our bodies, with other organisms (as in the case of infectious disease), with other humans (as in human-to-human disease transmission and many injuries), and with our broader ecosystem. Human morbidity and mortality would not exist in the absence of our biological vulnerability to external agents such as infectious diseases, physical trauma, and the gradual breakdown of bodily systems due to senescent decline.

A human biological framework also gives rise to the notion of *competing risks*, whereby no intervention can prevent mortality completely—it can only prevent mortality due to a specific cause and delay inevitable death due to some other cause (Cox 1959; Kalbfleisch and Prentice 2002). The deletion of a single cause of death can have a wide range of consequences for all-cause mortality, ranging from almost zero (if everyone dies of something else the next week) to a synergistic effect that saves lives due to multiple causes (if people become healthier in the process).[9] As a result, the distal and proximate drivers of health not only have implications for current health and for health next week (when an epidemic may emerge), but also for longer-term future health.

In addition to the context provided by biology and the human environment and the interplay of distal drivers and proximate risk factors on health outcomes, some health literature makes a further distinction between distal drivers and even broader influencing factors. Smith and Ezzati (2005: 325) used the term *super-distal* to refer to factors that affect "essentially every disease, even if the pathways are not always well understood." The analysis of this volume treats three variables as such super-distal drivers: technology, changes in the natural environment, and the social environment (examples include domestic social action such as health expenditures and global social initiatives such as poverty reduction). The super-distal drivers influence the course of all aspects of human development (e.g., the distal drivers of income and education as well as health outcomes with which income and education are associated). The distinction between distal and super-distal drivers is in

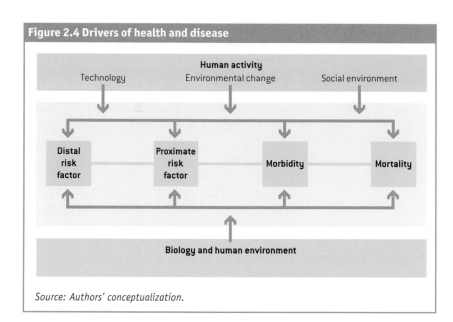

Figure 2.4 Drivers of health and disease

Human activity
Technology   Environmental change   Social environment

Distal risk factor   Proximate risk factor   Morbidity   Mortality

Biology and human environment

Source: Authors' conceptualization.

part a simple broadening and elaboration of the GBD project's distal category, but it is important because measures of income, education, and time alone cannot explain the profound global changes in health outcomes in recent decades.

These conceptual building blocks, including distal and proximate drivers in the context of biology and the super-distal factors linked to human action, provide some foundation for understanding the forces that drive change in human health. The remainder of this chapter, and then the broader volume, explores each in turn.

Distal Drivers of Health

Our current understanding of the distal drivers of health is affected by an ideologically charged debate between a growth-oriented perspective, in which living standards or a proxy such as income are seen as primary drivers of health improvements, and a support-led model in which health systems and interventions are viewed as the primary drivers (Pritchett and Summers 1996; Sen 1998). In the years since the onset of the HIV/AIDS epidemic, we have seen considerable convergence between these two models, driven by evidence of how improved living standards and health systems may interact to produce better outcomes. In fact, living standards, health systems, and health outcomes correlate highly across time, thereby obscuring meaningful understanding of the actual patterns of causation.

In this section, we introduce those distal drivers that the GBD project has thus far used—

WHO's Global Burden of Disease project uses income, education, and time (largely as a proxy for technology) as the distal drivers of health outcomes.

GDP per capita, education, and time—and review the current evidence on other potential drivers. In subsequent sections we move to the proximate drivers that more directly mediate between distal drivers and health outcomes, as well as to the broader biological and human contexts that in turn shape these elements.

Income

For a number of years, the dominant paradigm among leading economists at the International Monetary Fund and at the World Bank suggested that living standards, measured typically by national GDP per capita, were the most important determinant of health. This growth-oriented approach first emerged with the work of Thomas McKeown, an English physician and epidemiologist who analyzed historical data from England and Wales for the period between 1837 and 1990. As a result of his analysis, McKeown attributed 50 percent of the reductions in mortality during this period (much of it preceding the advent of specific medical technologies associated with health improvements) to improved living standards

(McKeown 1976; McKeown and Record 1962). While subsequent research (Sen 1998) revised many of McKeown's findings, his work pointed the way to a simple reality we now know to be consistent across historical periods—namely, that at any single point in time, between 65 and 90 percent of cross-national variation in human life expectancy at birth can be associated with a logged measure of GDP per capita (Filmer and Pritchett 1999; Pritchett and Summers 1996). Figure 2.5 shows this relationship in 2006.

The cross-sectional association is seductive in its simplicity, offering the possibility that one could model all future changes in health simply as a function of change in GDP per capita and that one could emphasize growth as the sole pathway of importance to improving human health outcomes. Yet the cross-sectional relationship is not all that it appears. First and most evidently, even a 65–90 percent correlation leaves considerable room for societies to outperform or underperform the level of health we would anticipate based on income alone. Second, there is uncertainty in the direction of causation and the influence of other factors in the relationship.

Nonetheless, considerable evidence does support a longitudinal, causal relationship between changes in income and subsequent improvements in health outcomes within a single country. The most-studied outcome is infant mortality, and the current "gold standard" estimate comes from Pritchett and Summers (1996). When they lagged infant mortality rates by five years with respect to changes in GDP per capita, Pritchett and Summers found a 24 percent decrease in infant mortality rates with a doubling of GDP per capita; controlling for level of education reduced this impact to 19 percent. Calculations based on these relationships lead them to conclude that "a country at the sample mean GDP would avert one death per 1,000 births if income were higher by 1%" (Pritchett and Summers 1996: 851).[10]

Yet some would argue that, as with the cross-sectional relationship, these within-country studies miss broader and more important trends emerging in the income/health relationship across multiple countries over multiple time periods. In a groundbreaking reconstruction of the relationship between income and health in 1905, 1935, and 1965, Samuel Preston (1975) observed that the

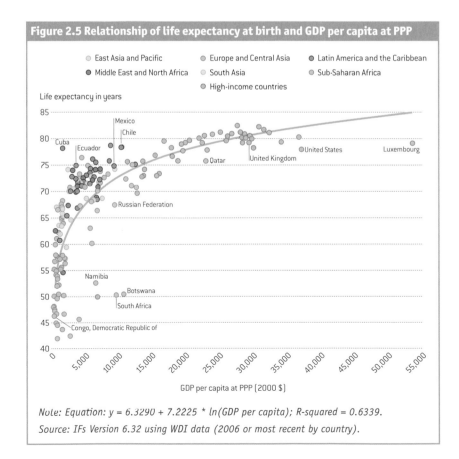

Figure 2.5 Relationship of life expectancy at birth and GDP per capita at PPP

*Note: Equation: y = 6.3290 + 7.2225 * ln(GDP per capita); R-squared = 0.6339.*

Source: IFs Version 6.32 using WDI data (2006 or most recent by country).

elasticity and shape of the cross-country income/health relationship was changing over time. This pattern, shown for four time points in Figure 2.6, clearly suggests that "the relationship between life expectancy and national income per head has shifted upwards during the 20th century" (Preston 1975: 236). Looking vertically, this means that over time the life expectancy associated with a particular GDP per capita has risen dramatically. Looking horizontally, we see that a nation "required an income level approximately 2.6 times higher in the 1930s than in the 1960s" to reach the same life expectancy.

Preston concluded that, over time, variation in income could explain only 10–25 percent of the variation in life expectancy (Preston 1975), and the World Bank's influential 1993 *World Development Report* replicated this finding more recently (World Bank 1993). We thus face a challenging conundrum common to many forecasting efforts. No other single structural determinant of health will approach income's magnitude or consistency across time period, cause, or country—yet it leaves 75–90 percent of the total variation over time unexplained.

Education

The roles of other structural factors such as education, health systems, and culture are potentially important, yet quite difficult to specify, in part because each of them tends itself to be correlated with income. Because living standards are such a powerful predictor of health at any single point in time, a useful entry point to the health systems literature has been to search for common patterns across the list of countries that perform better or worse on health outcomes than would be expected based on income alone. John Caldwell (1986) first used this approach by rank-ordering developing countries in 1983 in terms of income, life expectancy, and infant mortality rate and then qualitatively exploring the countries whose health outcome rankings were higher or lower than their income rankings. His analysis yielded a number of possible common factors relating to culture, gender, health spending, and health systems—factors to which we will return. One dominant theme emerged from the analysis. Better educated societies and societies with a greater tradition of widespread participation in education, particularly of women, had better-

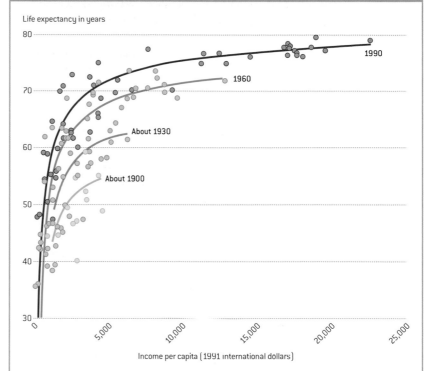

Figure 2.6 Changes in the relationship between life expectancy and income per capita over time

Life expectancy in years

Income per capita (1991 international dollars)

Note: Expressed in 1991 international dollars at PPP for selected countries.

Source: World Bank (1993: 34); reproduced with permission of the International Bank for Reconstruction and Development, World Bank (copyright holder).

than-expected health outcomes. Yet Caldwell's analysis did not pinpoint the existence and direction of causality.

The relationship between education and health outcomes, even after controlling for income, is a strong one. In terms of causal effects, there is considerable evidence from the micro level that, in any society, individuals with higher levels of education attainment will be better able to take care of themselves and—arguably even more important—will be better able to take care of their children. At the macro level, structural regression models have isolated this relationship, with a uniquely identified effect of education on health outcomes (Boehmer and Williamson 1996; Frey and Field 2000; Lena and London 1993). Yet, none of these studies fully identifies the possible causation running from education to health or important confounding factors.

With regard to confounding factors, we note two of particular significance. First, a number of studies have identified that it is not education overall but rather women's education specifically that appears to be associated with better health outcomes (Shen and Williamson 1997; Summers 1994). While this might indicate simply that women's education is of greater causal significance as a determinant of health than men's, it might also indicate that women's education attainment, itself highly correlated with total education attainment, may be a proxy for an unobserved or untested societal factor. One such factor might be a greater degree of gender equity, which might result in narrower health gaps between men and women, or a greater level of women's empowerment, which might enable women to gain better access to prevention and treatment for children (Caldwell 1986; Frey and Field 2000; Nussbaum 2004).

Health and education are also subject to similar forces of demand and supply. Populations that demand greater educational opportunities may also demand greater health opportunities, and so the relationship between education and health may merely capture a societal taste for both outcomes. Similarly, there may be a strong correlation between a society's ability to provide quality educational and health services, whether via government, private, or nonprofit sectors. Thus, the association between education and health outcomes may merely capture the presence of a number of conditions that facilitate both health and educational achievement but do not indicate any kind of causal impact of education on health. We address many of these factors later, while noting that most of them at this time do not provide as consistent a body of evidence to justify inclusion as a distal driver as does education.

Time and its underlying elements

As the above discussion indicates, income and education correlate with a very large portion of the variation in health outcomes across countries. Yet they also leave a great deal unexplained, especially over time. Hence the GBD project has used time as a third variable in its distal-driver formulation. Although time is understood to be most significantly a proxy for technological advance (in close interaction with human biology and biological potential), it also potentially captures other changes related to human action. For instance, sanitation practices (including the

use of soap) involve cultural change even more than they do technology. We will return to this broader context later in the chapter, especially in discussion of super-distal drivers, but first we consider proximate risk factors and the manner in which they mediate between distal drivers and health outcomes.

More Proximate Determinants of Health

The previous section focused on the role of distal drivers—GDP per capita, education, and a time trend (thought to reflect technological change especially)—in determining health outcomes. In and of themselves, however, these factors do not cause health outcomes. Rather, as illustrated generally in Figure 2.4 and specifically in the example for diarrheal disease of Box 2.2, they do so through their effect on proximate risk factors relating to individual behavior and social and environmental conditions. There are very strong relationships between the distal and proximate drivers and health outcomes—so strong that the use of distal drivers alone does offer considerable forecasting power.

Yet simply using broad determinants to forecast health outcomes presents a series of problems. First, any assumption that the relationships across identified distal drivers, proximate risk factors, and ultimate health outcomes will remain stable is almost certainly wrong. Second, by obscuring the more direct or proximate relationships, reliance only on broad determinants offers limited potential for exploring the effects of specific health-related interventions.

It is not difficult to identify intervention points with respect to proximate drivers that suggest at least some degree of potential disconnect between the proximate risks and the distal causes. Clearly the correlations between distal and proximate factors are not perfect. Box 2.2 uses the example of diarrheal diseases to illustrate that although the distal drivers have much impact on the proximate risks, there are also ways in which incremental human effort (as organized, for instance, by national health systems or global initiatives, and targeting nutritional and environmental factors) can modify that relationship.

Over the past 200 years of progress in extending life expectancy, the "best-practice" societies have always been characterized not merely by advanced wealth but also

Box 2.2 Undernutrition and diarrheal disease in developing countries: An example of the interrelationship of distal and proximate drivers of health

Diarrheal infections offer a good example of interrelationships between distal and proximate drivers of health. Diarrheal disease accounts for about one-fifth of child mortality in the world's poorest countries, ranking among the top two or three causes of death in almost all such countries (Black, Morris, and Bryce 2003), yet deaths from diarrheal disease rarely occur in wealthy or middle-income countries. Thus, we can say that the distal driver of income is a major determinant of diarrheal disease, though the pathways linking rising income to reduced diarrheal disease mortality may not be readily apparent. Certainly many diarrheal diseases have treatments that would be easily procured and affordable in rich countries and prohibitively expensive in poor countries. Yet most rich countries drastically reduced diarrheal infections prior to the development of antibiotic drugs (Preston 1975), and few treatments exist for viral causes of diarrhea even today.

Many developing countries, including most "high achievers," have drastically reduced diarrheal disease mortality, both through reductions in incidence and, to a lesser extent, through effective treatment. These successes relate to health systems and to societal education and values, yet we cannot understand the impact of these societal inputs without understanding proximate drivers (Bryce et al. 2003; Jones et al. 2003; Keusch et al. 2006). Effective diarrheal disease interventions can be environmental (reducing the use of unsafe water and improving sanitation), behavioral (improving hygiene and maternal education), and biomedical (diarrheal disease outreach, treatment, and oral rehydration). Most importantly, diarrheal diseases operate in a negative synergy with nutrition; poor nutrition creates greater vulnerability to and severity of infection, and diarrheal infections create nutrient loss and depletion (Mosley and Chen 1984). Most estimates suggest that more than half of all diarrheal disease mortality could be eliminated by ending undernutrition. Similarly, elimination (through vaccination or other means) of non-diarrheal infections such as measles may reduce vulnerability to diarrheal disease.

In summary, diarrheal diseases offer a textbook example of diseases that have a strong relationship to income but are also responsive to multiple proximate-driver-related solutions, such as reduction in undernutrition via provision of food in conjunction with school attendance. Many would argue that as long as global poverty exists, low-cost proximate interventions with respect to diarrheal and other childhood diseases offer a more immediate solution to health improvement than waiting for income to rise, and that such targeted interventions have the potential to produce healthier, better educated, and more productive societies going forward.

by positive environmental and behavioral circumstances and practices. Future mortality gains are likely to become increasingly hard won and possibly even more dependent on a combination of good treatments and good behaviors. Many modern behavioral and nutritional health risks predispose individuals to noncommunicable and some communicable diseases. The consumption of energy-dense foods and increasingly sedentary lifestyles that predispose societies to obesity and other noncommunicable diseases are of particular concern, and environmental stresses may compound these risks. Such concerns are best exemplified by the mortality crisis among men of Russian descent in Russia and former Soviet states, but there are also indications of a rising chronic disease burden and declining life expectancy in many parts of the United States (Ezzati et al. 2008; Rogers et al. 2007).

WHO's ongoing Comparative Risk Assessment (CRA) project provides our starting point for considering the burden of disease associated with proximate risk factors (Ezzati et al. 2004a). The CRA project has used two guiding criteria for including specific risks in its analysis: (1) selecting risks for which sufficient data and scientific understanding exist in order to assess the exposure and health effects associated with the risks; and (2) selecting risks "for which intervention strategies are available or might be envisioned to modify their impact on disease burden" (Ezzati et al. 2004b: xx). Within this framework, the project has tried to provide conceptual and methodological consistency and comparability across the risk factors. Table 2.1 shows the 28 risk factors that the CRA project covered in its most recent report (WHO 2009a) and identifies the subset of those included in IFs forecasts in this volume.

The CRA project and other studies (Laxminarayan, Chow, and Shahid-Salles 2006; Prüss-Üstün and Corvalán 2006) have now provided guidance for identifying links between selected risk factors and specific health outcomes, making possible their inclusion in forecasts of future health. For example, we know that childhood undernutrition is associated with a range of communicable diseases, and obesity with certain chronic diseases (Gaziano et al. 2006; Narayan et al. 2006). However, a number of factors complicate quantitative analysis of proximate risk factors. First, they vary with respect to the size of their impact on health outcomes, their susceptibility to human intervention, and the degree to which they change independently of the distal drivers. Second, existing risk assessment analyses have not fully taken into account competing risks (the possibility that those

WHO's Comparative Risk Assessment project has analyzed the relationship of 28 specific risk factors to health outcomes.

Table 2.1 Proximate health risk factors included in the World Health Organization's Comparative Risk Assessment project

Health category	Risk factor	Attributable mortality (%)	Attributable DALYs (%)
Childhood and maternal undernutrition	Underweight*	3.8	6.0
	Iron deficiency	0.5	1.3
	Vitamin A deficiency	1.1	1.5
	Zinc deficiency	0.1	1.0
	Suboptimal breast feeding	2.1	2.9
Other nutrition-related risk factors and physical activity	High blood pressure	12.8	3.8
	High cholesterol	4.5	2.0
	High blood glucose	5.8	2.7
	Overweight and obesity*	4.8	2.3
	Low fruit and vegetable consumption	2.8	1.0
	Physical inactivity	5.5	2.1
Sexual and reproductive health	Unsafe sex	4.0	4.6
	Unmet contraceptive need	0.3	0.8
Addictive substances	Tobacco use*	8.7	3.7
	Alcohol use	3.8	4.6
	Illicit drug use	0.4	0.9
Environmental risks	Unsafe water, sanitation, hygiene*	3.2	4.2
	Urban outdoor air pollution*	2.0	0.6
	Indoor smoke from solid fuels*	3.3	2.7
	Lead exposure	0.2	0.6
	Global climate change*	0.2	0.4
Occupational risks	Risk factors for injuries	0.6	0.8
	Carcinogens	0.3	0.1
	Airborne particulates	0.8	0.4
	Erogonomic stressors	0.0	0.1
	Noise	0.0	0.3
Other selected risk factors	Unsafe health-care injections	0.7	0.5
	Child sexual abuse	0.1	0.6

Note: Mortality and DALY values are for 2004. Risk factors marked with an asterisk (*) are included as proximate drivers in the IFs health model.

Source: Attributable mortality and DALY rates calculated by authors using data from WHO 2009a (Annex A, Tables A3 and A4, pages 50 and 52.)

saved from one cause of death will simply die from another) in their estimated relationships (Laxminarayan, Chow, and Shahid-Salles 2006). And finally, data for some of the factors are very limited. For these reasons, and because all modeling is time and other-resource limited, we currently incorporate a subset of the CRA proximate risk factors in our forecasts, as indicated by the asterisks in Table 2.1. Chapters 5 and 6 explore the implications of alternative

assumptions about these, independently from their expected evolution in the face of changes in distal drivers.

Super-Distal Drivers and the Broader Uncertainty Context of Health

Figure 2.4 portrayed a general model of changing health outcomes in which two major sets of contextual factors (human biology as part of the broader natural environment and human activity) shape the distal and proximate drivers, their relationships with each other, and their impact on health. We return to those general contextual factors now. As the above discussion indicated, income and education explain a large portion of the variation in health outcomes across countries. Yet they leave a great deal unexplained, especially over time.

Change over time, which almost certainly is in substantial part a proxy for technological change, was the most significant source of non-income variations in Preston's analysis of cross-national mortality differentials (Preston 1975). Clearly such change is associated with improved health outcomes in richer societies, and it also has an enormous impact on the pace at which poorer nations are able to achieve the health outcomes of richer ones. We can point to a number of key technological advances driving health improvements over the past two centuries, including the germ theory of disease. We must also consider the global role of innovations in disease management and technology transfer. In considering Preston's findings, Wilkinson (2007: 1) offered an interpretation that illustrates the challenges of modeling health:

> What we have to explain is why, with the passage of time, the same amount of income buys progressively more health. It is as if the price of health goes down or, as I once put it (Wilkinson 1996), there is a change of gearing between income and health.

While the notion of a change in price or a change in gearing is conceptually helpful, our ability to predict technology as a function of anything other than time is severely limited. In 1945, it would have been difficult to forecast the dramatic global epidemiologic transition that was about to take place. Looking to the future, it remains unclear whether this change in gearing is a permanent feature of human health, whether we have reached the highest gear possible, or whether we will, in fact, see a downshift to lower levels of health relative to living standards. Hence the GBD has used time as a third variable in its distal formulation (and we have adopted that model). Although time is understood to be most significantly a proxy for technological advance (in close interaction with biological context and potential), it also potentially captures change related to human action that more truly represents super-distal drivers, even including cultural evolution.

Overall, many implications of these super-distal drivers are captured via distal or proximate drivers, yet we are left with a great deal of uncertainty with respect to the overall trend of health improvement and the pattern and level of convergence or divergence we might expect between countries whose health outcomes are currently very different. Technology has a particularly complicated place in our schema, partly a distal driver and partly a function of broader human activity, but always also interacting closely with the constraints imposed by biology. We look to that interaction first, before turning to other elements of human activity.

Technology and biological limits

Human action drives advances in technology. Vaccines and antibiotics are prime examples, but the range is huge and the future progression of technological advance is highly uncertain. The most significant source of uncertainty concerning technology relates to the frontiers of human longevity. As discussed in Box 2.3, the arguably plausible range for life expectancy of the longest-lived societies on earth in the year 2100 ranges anywhere from 87 to 105 years (for low estimates see Carnes and Olshansky 2007; and Olshansky, Carnes, and Brody 2002; see Oeppen and Vaupel 2002 for high estimates).

The most plausible forecasts both account for trends in age-specific mortality and attempt to separate extrinsic causes of death that are more amenable to elimination from intrinsic causes of death that are more directly related to human senescence (Bongaarts 2006).[11] Yet age-specific, disease-specific, and even overall mortality

progress may lag during certain periods when they are not a societal investment priority or between technological revolutions, only to once again accelerate. One notable example from recent history involves cardiovascular disease (CVD) mortality rates. Gains in reduction of cardiovascular disease mortality rates stagnated between 1945 and 1968 in the United States as societal investments focused on infectious disease control and the lagged burden of tobacco consumption manifested itself. Between 1968 and 1995, however, cardiovascular disease mortality rates dropped precipitously (Goldman and Cook 1984; Hunink et al. 1997).

That said, a considerable gap between what humans could achieve and what humans actually will achieve will probably continue. The magnitude of mortality reduction necessary to maintain continued linear improvement in life expectancy is staggering. Many of the technology-dependent therapies underlying such improvements would carry considerable financial costs and would confront serious debate surrounding interventions that might violate bioethical or religious standards or could create unanticipated mutation risks. These debates have already begun with respect to stem cell research and treatments and the genetic modification of lower organisms, and they will almost certainly grow louder in the future. Also, there are clearly ethical issues around expenditures directed at the leading edge of longevity advance rather than toward closing large inequalities within and across societies. Thus, economic and ethical constraints might impact the pace of mortality reduction in a putative "best practice" society and in the relative progress of trailing societies, despite technological possibilities.

In addition to issues about technology and health arising from economic and ethical constraints and from uncertainty about the relationship between technology and the limits of human biology, considerable uncertainty prevails in understanding technological prospects in the battle against infectious diseases, particularly in light of lagging progress in a number of countries, the overwhelming HIV/AIDS epidemic, and the emergence or reemergence of a number of drug-resistant infectious diseases.[12]

In Preston's analysis of changes in health over time, the greatest change in the positive

Human activity affecting health has a broader scope than the proximate and distal drivers represent; we need also to consider "super-distal" drivers.

Biological limits restrict what technology can accomplish, but technology may or may not achieve all that is possible.

Human action drives advances in health-related technology and in the transfer of that technology through social systems.

Box 2.3 Prospects for human longevity: A debate

There is heated debate between so-called longevity pessimists and optimists, each garnering a range of epidemiologic, demographic, and biological support. In general, the core pessimistic argument depends first on biological limits to the human life span, and second on the policy difficulties and high costs of preventive mortality, particularly in societies with high levels of behavioral or environmental risk. By this logic, chronic obstructive and metabolic disorders, such as CVDs and diabetes, are more endogenous to the human body than communicable diseases and thus more difficult or expensive to prevent. The pessimist school draws heavily on the "Hayflick limit"—the notion that reproductive and functional life spans of cells are time limited and that human evolution provides no mechanism for selecting for longer life spans (Hayflick 1996). According to this view, as exogenous causes of disease are being gradually eliminated, the remaining causes of death are more likely to result from not easily reversed genetic defects and processes of senescence. Pessimists point to demographic evidence showing the compression of mortality in advanced societies into increasingly narrow age ranges, such that continued mortality improvement would require substantial mortality reductions at ages that only a handful of humans have ever experienced, as well as the near-total elimination of deaths of those 65 to 85 years of age. They argue further that it would require the continued pushing back of causes of death that seemed inevitable until only recently (CVDs, many cancers) and of causes that have even yet to be imagined.

While the pessimist argument is biologically compelling, a considerable array of demographic evidence points to continued improvements in longevity. Over time, pessimistic projections have repeatedly been surpassed, often only shortly after the publication of the purported limit (Oeppen and Vaupel 2002; Wilmoth 1997). Optimists point to tremendous improvements in the survival of the oldest-old (those 85+), which have of late outpaced advance at younger ages, resulting in a dramatic increase in the population over age 100. Optimists supplement the demographic evidence by pointing to specific technological innovations such as cellular regeneration and replacement, nanotechnologies for treatment delivery, tools for reprogramming the human genotype for greater reliability, and genomic analysis for the better application of existing therapies (Carey 2003; Carey and Judge 2001; Oeppen and Vaupel 2002). Thus far, they argue, there is no evidence of a hard limit to life, little evidence of approaching limits to life, and ever more promising technological opportunities.

gearing between income and health resulted not from pushing outward the frontiers of modern technology but rather from the gradual transfer to poor countries of existing technologies, such as antibiotics, vaccination, and chemical spraying of infectious disease vectors (Preston 1975). Thus, improvements were the result not merely of technology itself, but also of efforts to transfer technology, provide technical support, and fund the delivery of technologies, carried out through a robust post–World War II intergovernmental framework embodied in WHO (Henderson 1998; Mosley 1984; Preston 1975; 1980; 1996). While future progress in the fight against communicable disease will certainly depend on the pace of new technologies, our ability as a planet to address the proximate drivers of disease via changes to the broader social environment will also determine much of the progress.

The social environment

The final report of the WHO Commission on the Social Determinants of Health emphasized the indelible imprint that the social environment leaves on human health (CSDH 2008). Some of its effects occur at the national level. For instance, we can observe these relationships in the dramatic decline in male life expectancy in post-Soviet Russia, a crisis whose causes extend not merely into individual and collective risk behaviors (e.g., stress and alcohol consumption) but into the role of broader shocks to political continuity, macroeconomic stability, commodity prices, and national identity. We note also the important role of global factors—the global economy, trade, and health actions—in shaping the national context and in directly shaping human health. For example, systems of global aid, trade, travel, and information affect the availability of pharmaceutical treatments, the transmission of disease vectors across borders, and exposure to hazardous substances such as tobacco and air pollution. While understanding their close interactions, we look, in turn, at the domestic and global elements of the social environment.

Domestic health expenditures and other social influences on health

Inasmuch as a wealthy country completely bereft of health services or health spending would have notably poor health standards, a nation's social and health systems must have an impact on health. Although researchers have found it difficult to pinpoint measurable societal factors (including health services and health spending) that drive health improvements, those countries that achieve better or worse health outcomes than their income and education would lead us to expect have offered a natural starting point in the search for further systemic determinants of health. This literature has tended to focus separately on developed and less-developed countries.

Among developed countries, a great proportion of the deviation from the expected income-health relationship is explained by one country, the United States, which has one of the world's highest incomes per capita but ranks only 38th in infant mortality, 32nd in female life expectancy, and 18th in male life expectancy (UNPD 2009a). Other "Anglo-Saxon" societies such as Canada and the United Kingdom also perform worse than expected, albeit to a much lesser extent. Possible explanations for this Anglo-Saxon deviation include inefficient or poorly managed health systems, high rates of poverty, weak welfare states, high levels of inequality, two-party political systems, and higher rates of behaviors that pose health risks and/or levels of individualism (Berkman et al. 2000; Starfield and Shi 2002; Subramanian, Belli, and Kawachi 2002).

Caldwell's study (1986) of health outcomes in less-developed countries offers a similarly dazzling range of potential sources of structural health variation, some of which are policy-relevant, many of which are not. In addition to education, his findings pointed to the association of the following with positive health outcomes: high levels of health spending or physicians per capita; equity of income or public service availability; a reputation for efficient public service provision; socialist or egalitarian government; a history of civilian, democratic rule; and high levels of gender equity and female autonomy. On the other hand, Caldwell found varying relationships between religious beliefs and practices and health outcomes. Each of his findings has received considerable and often controversial study over the past 25 years.[13]

Perhaps the most interesting and provocative proposition suggests that high levels of societal inequality lead to poor health outcomes, both through the greater prevalence of poverty as well as through higher levels of stress, distrust, violence, and problem behavior (Kawachi, Kennedy, and Lochner 1997; Navarro 2004; Navarro and Shi 2001; Wilkinson and Pickett 2006). However, the inequality hypothesis has been the subject of great debate, offering limited statistical support and few well-understood explanatory pathways (Deaton 2002; 2003; Mellor and Milyo 2001). More generally, Nathanson (1996) offered a framework for understanding the recurring and remarkably stable role over time of broader national norms of social organization and justice in determining health outcomes, identifying three important variables: degree of state centralization, the presence or absence of active grassroots organizations, and societal constructions of risk toward individual versus collective outcomes.

More recently, a number of studies have begun to explore the connection between health outcomes and the more readily forecastable and policy-relevant measure of societal health expenditures, but even this relationship is complicated. We can imagine that, above and beyond the possibility that public health spending would lead to improved health, it would also demonstrate a broader societal commitment to human welfare. Then again, a society with high levels of public health spending might merely be a very sick society (HIV/AIDS has certainly led to increased public health expenditures) or a very inefficient society (as implied by the high levels of health expenditure without noteworthy health outcomes in the United States). Moreover, any analysis that controls for income, the single biggest determinant of health spending, is bound to offer only limited support for the impact of health spending itself.

Despite these complications, some recent studies point to the potential role of health spending and health systems in determining health outcomes, particularly for child health outcomes in poorer countries. Some estimates of the effect of health spending per capita, even after controlling for GDP per capita, have found coefficients in the range of -0.1 to -0.2—meaning that, above and beyond the effect of income, a 1 percent increase in health expenditure will lead to between a 0.1 percent and 0.2 percent decrease in child mortality (Anand and Ravallion 1993; Bidani and Ravallion 1997; Jamison et al. 1996; Nixon and Ulmann 2006; Wagstaff 2002).

Other studies that measured the independent effect of public sector health spending as a percentage of GDP, also after controlling for GDP per capita, tended to find smaller, often insignificant effects (Filmer and Pritchett 1999; Musgrove 1996). Filmer and Pritchett (1999) estimated that a doubling of average health expenditures per capita from 3 percent to 6 percent would reduce the child mortality rate by only 9–13 percent. They also noted that their estimates implied a cost of between $47,000 and $100,000 per child death averted, well above the typical cost associated with prevention of deaths due to specific causes in the societies they studied. After controlling for the effects of factors such as income, education, and ethno-linguistic factors, Filmer and Pritchett noted there was little difference in average health expenditures between the 10 best and

The social environment of health includes domestic health expenditures and policies and— increasingly—global health initiatives, including health governance structures.

the 10 worst achieving countries, as well as considerable variation within those groupings. Filmer, Hammer, and Pritchett (2000; 2002) pointed to a number of factors limiting the effectiveness of public health expenditures, including corruption; ineffectiveness of existing or complementary inputs; redundancy of new services to existing services; and the failure to target incremental spending toward the areas of highest impact—particularly toward health problems affecting the poor (who also tend to have the highest rates of preventable illness and death) and to problems that people would not otherwise address on their own (public goods such as vaccination or sanitation). In conclusion, as it stands, the literature suggests that societal, and possibly governmental, action can influence health, but that systematic effects across society have been relatively small. Many of the most important efforts, however, can be captured through the forecasting of specific proximate drivers of health.

Global health initiatives

Aspects of the global social environment pertaining to health increasingly involve global efforts aimed at both transferring technologies directed at specific proximate risk factors and creating global public goods and a global health governance structure. In particular, in addition to the efforts of the World Health Organization, development agencies, private donors, and the World Bank have increased their global health funding and programmatic efforts. To a great extent, each of these constituencies has placed an emphasis on disease-specific interventions targeting proximate drivers. The World Bank, tasked not with directly promoting health but rather with poverty alleviation and development, became increasingly involved with global health policy beginning in the early 1980s. The Bill and Melinda Gates Foundation, the largest private donor, has focused on all-encompassing disease-specific initiatives aimed at conditions such as polio and on development of new low-cost technologies for communicable disease detection and treatment. These foundations are joined by public-private partnerships or *global health initiatives* (GHIs), involving multiple partners working together to solve a single or small range of issues (e.g., HIV/AIDS, malaria, and tuberculosis). Approximately 100 GHIs currently

exist, and the largest of these—the Global Fund to Fight AIDS, Tuberculosis, and Malaria, the Global Alliance for Vaccines and Immunization, the President's Emergency Plan for AIDS Relief, and the World Bank Multi-Country AIDS Program—contribute substantially to international funding for communicable disease control overall.

Many observers have questioned the long-term sustainability of such efforts to address proximate drivers without targeting health systems and the broader social environment (Garrett 2007), pointing in part to the failures of a previous generation of post–World War II international health actions. Specifically, in countries where those earlier disease-control efforts were successful, communicable disease risks gave way to a new set of life-course health risks (due to noncommunicable diseases and injuries) that required greater expenditures and depended on the development of health systems. In some of the world's more disadvantaged countries, and in isolated or disenfranchised areas of emerging countries, persistent and emerging communicable disease risks posed a challenge that demanded social and political changes on top of technological interventions. Significantly, in 2007 the World Bank refined its health strategy to move away from specific disease control, focusing instead on strengthening national health systems and partnering with private donors to fund initiatives (Ruger 2007). The WHO CSDH report signaled another shift toward programs targeting the social environment. Yet past failures such as the Alma Ata Declaration (which promised "health for all by the year 2000") suggest that the challenges of changing the social environment will be many.

The current generation of efforts to alter the social environment is embodied in a growing push, led by WHO, for global health governance, a term that "refers to the formal and informal institutions, norms and processes which govern or directly influence global health policy and outcomes" (Sridhar 2009: 1366). This broad understanding recognizes that health governance can and does occur at multiple levels (from local to global) and might include a variety of mechanisms (both formal and informal, private and public). In fact, many observers question whether national governments even have the ability to protect and promote adequately the health of their citizens in a rapidly globalizing world (Fidler 2008/2009; Lee et al. 2007). Civil society organizations—including nongovernmental organizations and community organizations that either provide health services directly or lobby for health change— are also playing increasingly important roles in global health agenda setting, monitoring, and enforcement (Doyle and Patel 2008; Sridhar 2009). Combined with the recent march of global economic integration, these emerging global governance efforts[14] constitute a fundamental shift toward a truly global health system. Yet their future impact on health outcomes depends on many things.

The natural environment

One final super-distal driver subject to a number of ongoing global governance efforts is our changing natural environment. Reflecting its ubiquitous nature, Smith and Ezzati (2005: 325) refer to the natural environment as a super-distal risk factor in that it "affects essentially every disease, even if the pathways are not always well understood." Given the role that it plays in the evolutionary mechanisms of mutation and natural selection, a complete consideration of the environment would include not only the environment to which individuals are exposed, but also the environment to which their ancestors were exposed (Smith, Corvalán, and Kjellström 1999). However, for the purpose of this volume— forecasting changes in health outcomes for the next half-century—the focus of our concern is changes in the natural environment that humans induce. These include factors as disparate as the introduction of local water pollutants and climate change. Similarly, an interaction of human and natural systems is shaping the rapid evolution and drug-resistance of many threatening infectious agents, presenting increased risk of emerging and reemerging infectious disease (Fauci 2001; McMichael, Woodruff, and Hales 2006). We attempt to capture some of the uncertainty relating to natural environmental change in Chapter 6.

Conclusion

The preceding sections have offered a survey of the conceptualization and measurement of health and of the drivers of change in health patterns over time and across societies. The chapter has given special attention to the distal and proximate drivers of health outcomes and has also drawn attention to the broader contextual determinants, including human biology and human activity expressed through super-distal elements such as technology, the social environment, and the natural environment.

With respect to distal drivers, national income—as a source of health-seeking resources and a proxy for health-seeking behaviors—offers the most reliable predictor of future changes in health. Yet income cannot explain most national variation in health outcomes over time. Studies also identify the effects of education attainment. The GBD project's representation of distal drivers also includes a time term, often seen to be technology. Yet technological advance is uncertain, dependent on both the biological context for it and the extent of human activity supporting it.

Tremendous uncertainty surrounds the effort to understand alternative global health futures, making attention to only distal and proximate drivers inadequate. Mapping uncertainty is, of course, a critical aspect of forecasting, and this chapter has only begun the process of doing so. Although analysis of past health trends offers some insight into the pace and pattern of technological change, we cannot know whether these trends will continue, and our lack of certainty with respect to physiological constraints on longevity interacts strongly with that uncertainty. Nor can we truly anticipate the extent of continued support for much positive human action beyond the development of technology—for instance, for continued growth in health spending and for large global initiatives to fight communicable diseases.

In addition, there are sources of uncertainty with much more negative overtones. With respect to the biological context, there is, of course, great uncertainty surrounding the continued unfolding of the HIV/AIDS epidemic and the wild-card possibility of other and even more virulent pandemic diseases. With respect to human activity, we are only beginning to map the extent of damage that environmental change, especially global warming, may do generally and to human health specifically. Chapter 8 in particular will return to the issue of uncertainty, but it pervades all of our analysis.

Human-induced changes in the natural environment also act as super-distal drivers of health outcomes.

Tremendous uncertainty surrounds efforts to understand alternative global health futures.

For instance, our discussion of proximate drivers will identify considerable uncertainty around human choices and behavior.

Still another significant source of uncertainty, and one on which this chapter has scarcely touched, relates to the forward linkages from health to other dimensions of human well-being and the feedback loops that those linkages create. The current era of global health action itself stems from a new interest in those relationships. Sen's human capabilities framework (Sen 1998; 1999a; 1999b) outlined such connections and placed health at the foundation of human needs that must be met in order to achieve development and human security. On the negative side, scholars such as de Waal (2002) have pointed out how extremely high mortality due to HIV/AIDS could shift the positive feedback loop between

health and socioeconomic development into reverse, leading to a downward spiral instead of continuing progress. On the positive side, Fogel's theory of technophysio evolution placed human physiology not merely as the basis of increased production but also as the catalyst for subsequent stages of broad economic, technological, and social development (Fogel 1994; Fogel and Costa 1997).

While we wait to elaborate and explore these forward linkages in greatest detail in Chapters 7 and 8, interim chapters will build on the concepts and understanding of change introduced here and will also begin building our maps of that which we understand best about possible global health futures and that which we understand least. We turn first to the tools that we can use for thinking about alternative futures.

---

1   A 2005 WHO study found that mortality registration coverage ranged from 100 percent in the European region to less than 10 percent in the African region. As a result, even all-cause mortality data for some countries are still derived from sample surveys, indirect estimation techniques, and imputations based on "model life tables" for typical populations rather than through registration of deaths (Mahapatra et al. 2007; Setel et al. 2007).

2   The ICD is currently in its 10th revision. For information about the ICD and its history, see http://www.who.int/classifications/icd/en.

3   Some noncommunicable diseases are also driven, at least in part, by communicable diseases, as in the case of human papillomavirus as a principal determinant of cervical cancer.

4   For these and other definitions, see the World Health Organization Statistical Information System (WHOSIS) Indicator Compendium, available at http://www.who.int/whosis/indicators/WHS09_IndicatorCompendium_20090701.pdf.

5   While most would argue that the formerly sick are probably not as healthy as those who were always healthy (referring to a cumulative burden of disease), proponents of the selection hypothesis have argued that those who survive disease, particularly severe life-threatening ones, may have proven their relative fitness and may actually be healthier than individuals who never experienced illness.

6   For specific disease weights and methodology, see Mathers et al. (2003) and Mathers and Loncar (2005).

7   Using the methods developed for determining YLDs and DALYs, WHO also reports healthy life expectancy, defined as the number of years an individual can expect to live in "full health."

8   In practice of course, many drivers instead lead, both intentionally and unintentionally, to increased morbidity and mortality. Among the proximate

drivers, roads, cigarettes, wars, and failed surgical interventions may have negative impacts. Similarly, improved living standards could, though they have not yet been shown to, lead to a net deterioration of health. In all cases, the impacts ultimately operate through biological pathways.

9   A classic example of negative competing risks involves oral rehydration therapies (ORTs), which mitigate the loss of fluids associated with cholera and other watery diarrheal disorders but have no effect on blood dysenteries such as shigellosis. If ORT is the only antidiarrheal intervention in place, many of those not dying from cholera would merely go on to die of shigellosis. By contrast, epidemiologists are constantly in search of the positive competing risks (or synergistic beneficial outcomes) that emerge when a single treatment not only eliminates all deaths due to that particular cause but also improves health in a way that reduces deaths due to other causes. Measles vaccinations, for instance, not only effectively eliminated measles deaths but also led to a reduction in long-term measles-related effects (e.g., blindness, micronutrient deficiency, and cognitive impairment), thereby further reducing mortality and morbidity rates.

10   Pritchett and Summers also cited a number of other country-level studies reporting statistically significant elasticities linking rising income to declining infant mortality and other health measures. For infant mortality these include: -0.19 from Flegg (1982); -0.161 (after controlling for education, safe water, and physicians per capita) from Hill and King (1992); -0.21 from Subbarao and Raney (1995); and -0.27 when Pampel and Pillai (1986) looked only at developed nations. Comparable estimates have been found for child mortality (Pritchett and Summers 1996; Wagstaff 2002) and maternal mortality (Bokhari, Gai, and Gottret 2007).

11   Bongaarts (2006) pursued one of the more cogent efforts to remove extrinsic causes of mortality

and deaths related to smoking from a standard demographic forecast and concluded that the best case high-end life expectancy in 2050 would be about 97.

12   We should note that the reversal of the pre-1990s trend of mortality reduction is observable only in sub-Saharan Africa for communicable diseases and in Eastern Europe for noncommunicable diseases. Other regions remain on trend, though a number of specific countries affected by long-running conflicts have seen sustained reversals (e.g., Iraq and Afghanistan).

13   Governance variables have offered a particularly contentious, and inconclusive, arena for macro health research. A slew of studies have addressed relationships between governance and health outcomes. A number of studies have found small but significant effects of democracy on improved health (Besley and Kudamatsu 2006; Franco, Álvarez-Dardet, and Ruiz 2004; Navia and Zweifel 2003; Przeworski et al. 2000; Shandra et al. 2004; Szreter 1997), but an equal number have found no effects (Ross 2006) or even negative ones (Gauri and Khaleghian 2002; Khaleghian 2004). Most of the confusion surrounds how exactly one defines a democracy. A line of research with more consistent findings relates to the impact of governance efficacy on health (de la Croix and Delavallade 2009; Gupta, Verhoeven, and Tiongson 2002; Kaufmann, Kraay, and Mastruzzi 2004; Rajkumar and Swaroop 2008; Shen and Williamson 1997; 2001). In particular, measures of government accountability, stability, violence, effectiveness, corruption, and legal institutions have been found to have a strong impact on infant mortality (de la Croix and Delavallade 2009; Gupta, Verhoeven, and Tiongson 2002; Shen and Williamson 1997; 2001).

14   One example is the International Health Regulations (IHR) enacted in 2007. The IHR is a legally binding instrument that requires the 194 WHO member countries to report certain disease outbreaks and public health events to WHO.

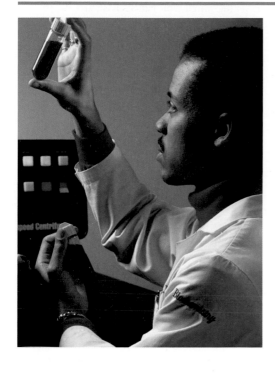

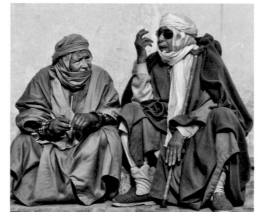

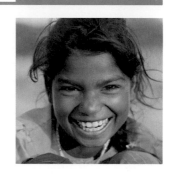

Forecasting Global Health

As a bridge between the largely conceptual discussion of Chapter 2 and the forecasting analyses to come, this chapter turns to the more technical topic of how we can best forecast global health futures. We can differentiate tools for looking at the future of global health on several dimensions of coverage and aggregation: whether they are country-specific or multi-country; whether they focus on morbidity, mortality, or both; whether they treat health in the aggregate or consider specific causes of morbidity and mortality; whether they forecast for 10 years or 25 years or even more.

We can also talk about them with respect to their concern with, and treatment of, related human development issue areas: whether they consider demographics, economics, and socio-political characteristics explicitly and dynamically in interaction with health; whether they consider primarily the impact of such other issues on health or also look to the implications of health for other aspects of human development. Further, we can

distinguish tools and models in terms of their basic methodological characteristics—whether they focus on very select driving variables or more broadly and structurally portray multiple interacting determinants of human health; whether they tend primarily to be accounting systems that exogenously (externally) provide assumptions about change or whether they more dynamically and endogenously represent households, governments, and other potential agents in interaction.

As always in thinking about the future, the most important dimension on which to understand tools and their use is their purpose. We can identify at least three interrelated purposes of health forecasting systems, very much related to the purposes of this volume:

1. to understand better where patterns of human development appear to be taking us with respect to global health, giving attention to the distribution of disease burden and the patterns of change in it

2. to consider opportunities for intervention and achievement of alternative health futures, enhancing the foundation for decisions and actions that improve health
3. to prepare society for the demographic and other broad (for instance, economic and socio-political) impacts of changing health patterns

This chapter reviews many of the existing forecasting tools and identifies strengths and weaknesses relative to such purposes. It also explains the approach of this volume using the International Futures (IFs) modeling system. We begin with some information about that system because it provides the broader context of our health model and analysis with it.

Integrating Health with Broader Human Development: The Larger IFs System

IFs is a large-scale, long-term, integrated global modeling system. It represents demographic, economic, energy, agricultural, socio-political, and environmental subsystems for 183 interacting countries.[1] In support of this series on Patterns of Potential Human Progress, we have added models of education and health. The central purpose of IFs is to facilitate exploration of global futures through alternative scenarios.

The goals that motivated the design of IFs fall generally into three categories: human development, social fairness and security, and environmental sustainability. Across these domains, the project draws inspiration from seminal writers such as Sen (1999a) with his emphasis on freedom and individual development, Rawls (1971) with his emphasis on fairness within society, and Brundtland (World Commission on Environment and Development 1987) with her seminal definition of sustainability. In combination, these emphases provide a philosophical framework for the exploration of human beings as individuals, of human beings with one another, and of human beings with the environment.

Fundamentally, IFs is a thinking tool, allowing variable time horizons through 2100 for exploring human leverage in pursuit of key goals in the face of great uncertainty. IFs assists with:

- understanding the state of the world and the future that appears to be unfolding
  - identifying tensions and inconsistencies that suggest political, economic, or other risk in the near and middle term (a "watch list" functionality);
  - exploring longer-term trends and considering where they might be taking us;
  - working through the complex dynamics of global systems.
- thinking about the future we want to see
  - clarifying goals and priorities;
  - developing alternative scenarios ("if-then statements") about the future;
  - investigating the leverage we may have in shaping the future.

Human systems fundamentally involve agents (economists often represent them as individuals in households or firms; political scientists add governments) interacting with one another in various structures (economists focus on markets; political scientists look to action-reaction systems and international regimes; sociologists add societies and demographic structures; anthropologists focus on cultures; physical scientists extend the reach to ecosystems). In general, scientists seek to understand the co-creation and evolution of agent behavior and structural characteristics.

IFs attempts to capture some of that richness. It is a structure-based (with extensive representation of underlying accounting systems such as demographic structures and the exchanges of goods, services, and finance), agent-class driven (so as to provide a basis for representing change), dynamic modeling system. That is, IFs represents typical behavior patterns of major agent-classes (households, governments, firms) interacting in a variety of global structures (demographic, economic, social, and environmental). The system draws on standard approaches to modeling specific issue areas whenever possible, extending those as necessary and integrating them across issue areas. For instance, the demographic model uses the typical "cohort-component" representation, tracking country-specific populations over time by age and sex (extended by education). Within that structural or accounting framework, the model represents the fertility decisions of households

● *The central purpose of IFs is to facilitate exploration of global futures through alternative scenarios.* ●

● *IFs is a structure-based and agent-class driven integrated modeling system, producing forecasts for 183 countries through the year 2100.* ●

(influenced by income and education) as well as mortality and migration patterns. Similarly with respect to health, we have attempted to build on existing approaches to its forecasting—particularly those of the World Health Organization's Global Burden of Disease (GBD) project—extending those as possible and integrating them with the larger IFs system.

As well as being rooted in the theory of various disciplines and subspecializations, IFs is heavily data based. Data come from the various member organizations of the United Nations family and many other sources. The database underlying IFs, and integrated with the system for use by others, includes data for 183 countries over as much of the period since 1960 as possible. The model system itself runs in annual time-steps from its initial year (currently 2005).[2] The menu-driven interface of the IFs software system allows the display of historical data since 1960 in combination with results from a base case and from alternative scenarios over time-horizons from 2005 through 2100, facilitating user-interventions flexibly across time, issue area, and geography. It provides tables, standard graphical formats, and a basic Geographic Information System or mapping capability. It also provides specialized display formats, such as age-sex and age-sex-education cohort structures and social accounting matrices.

Figure 3.1 shows the major conceptual blocks of the IFs system. The elements of the technology block are, in fact, scattered throughout the model. The named linkages between blocks and the linkages themselves are a small illustrative subset, not an exhaustive listing.

The two models within the IFs system that interact most closely with the health model are the population and economic models. Some of the key characteristics of the population model are that it:

- represents 22 age-sex cohorts to age 100+ in a standard cohort-component structure (but computationally spreads the 5-year cohorts initially to 1-year cohorts and calculates change in 1-year time-steps);
- calculates change in cohort-specific fertility of households in response to income, income distribution, infant mortality (from the health model), education levels, and contraception use;

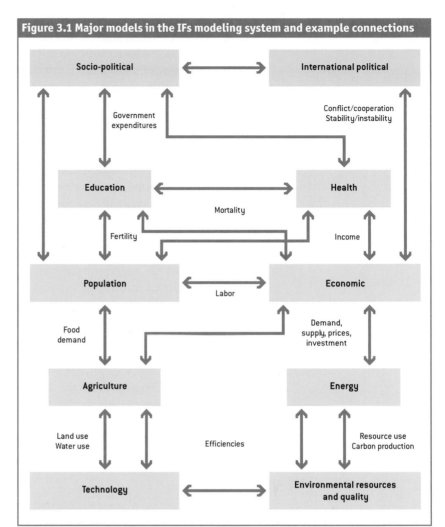

Figure 3.1 Major models in the IFs modeling system and example connections

- uses mortality calculations from the health model;
- separately represents the evolution of HIV infection rates and deaths from AIDS;
- computes average life expectancy at birth, literacy rate, and overall measures of human development;
- represents migration, which ties to flows of remittances.

Some of the most important characteristics of the economic model are that it:

- represents the economy in six sectors: agriculture, materials, energy, industry, services, and information/communications technology;
- computes and uses input-output matrices that change dynamically with development level;

- is a general equilibrium-seeking model that does not assume exact equilibrium will exist in any given year; rather it uses inventories as buffer stocks and to provide price signals so that the model chases equilibrium over time;
- contains a Cobb-Douglas production function that (following insights of Solow and Romer) endogenously represents contributions to growth in multifactor productivity from human capital (education and health), social capital and governance, physical and natural capital (infrastructure and energy prices), and knowledge development and diffusion (research and development [R&D] and economic integration with the outside world);
- uses a linear expenditure system (LES) to represent changing consumption patterns;
- utilizes a "pooled" rather than a bilateral trade approach for international trade;
- has been imbedded in a social accounting matrix (SAM) envelope that ties economic production and consumption to representation of intra-actor financial flows.

The socio-political model also interacts with the health model as well as with the economic, demographic, and education models. Some of its relevant features are that it:

- represents fiscal policy through taxing and spending decisions;
- shows six categories of government spending: military, health, education, R&D, foreign aid, and a residual category;
- represents changes in social conditions of individuals (such as fertility rates, literacy levels, and poverty), attitudes of individuals (such as the level of materialism/post-materialism of a society from the World Values Survey), and the social organization of people (such as the status of women);
- represents the evolution of democracy;
- represents the prospects for state instability or failure.

The environmental model of IFs, important in many ways for our health analysis, is not as developed as that of many integrated assessment models, but among its capabilities it:

- forecasts exposure to indoor air pollution from the use of solid fuels for heating and cooking;

- computes outdoor particulate concentrations for urban areas;
- forecasts atmospheric accumulations of carbon dioxide from fossil fuel use and deforestation and replicates findings from more extensive general circulation models to compute associated changes in temperature and precipitation, which in turn affect crop yields.

Although initially developed as an educational tool, IFs increasingly supports research and policy analysis. It was a core component of a project exploring the New Economy sponsored by the European Commission (EC) in the TERRA project and a subsequent EC project on information and communication technology and sustainability. Forecasts from IFs supported Project 2020 (*Mapping the Global Future*) of the National Intelligence Council (USNIC 2004) and *Global Trends 2025* (USNIC 2008). IFs also provided driver forecasts and some integrating analysis for the *Global Environment Outlook-4* of the United Nations Environment Programme (UNEP 2007).

The system facilitates scenario development and policy analysis via a "scenario-tree" that simplifies changes in framing assumptions and agent-class interventions. Users can save scenarios for development and refinement over time. Standard framing scenarios (such as those from the United Nations Environment Programme's *Global Environmental Outlook-4*), are available with the model for users to explore and potentially develop further.

IFs is freely available to all users on-line at www.ifs.du.edu and in a somewhat richer downloadable version at the same address. The model's help system contains primary documentation, and the website provides extended reports and publications.

Before turning to the modeling of global health futures within IFs, we first review the foundations provided by other models, including aggregate mortality models and structural health models. We then discuss at some length the hybrid approach we have developed.

All-Cause Mortality Models
In a very real sense, health forecasting began as part of population forecasting, as the size and age structure of a population depend

on the relationship between fertility and mortality. As part of population or demographic forecasting, the emphasis has generally been on mortality as an event (e.g., mortality from all causes) rather than on specific causes of death, but there have been exceptions, such as special attention to HIV/AIDS.

The standard approach to forecasting future population size is the *cohort-component method*, which traces the movement of each *population cohort* through the life span of its members, subtracting out deaths at each age and adding new births to the bottom of the cohort structure. The key drivers of population change, beyond the simple mechanical process of aging (and setting aside the dynamics of migration), are age-specific mortality and fertility rates. Age-specific mortality rates determine life expectancy at any given year, including the typical specification of life expectancy at birth. Models that use cohort-component methods can also begin their analysis with specifications of change in life expectancy and then work backward to modify the age-specific mortality patterns according to mortality schedules standardized for typical populations (Coale and Demeny 1983). In either case, these methods tend to be primarily extrapolative (Bongaarts 2005), although expert judgment may also shape them substantially.

The United Nations Population Division (UNPD) produces the most widely used country-level population forecasts. With the exception of extended attention to HIV/AIDS, its forecasts do not deal with causes of death but instead focus on life expectancy as an aggregate measure. UNPD has summarized its approach as follows:

> Mortality is projected on the basis of models of change of life expectancy produced by the United Nations Population Division. These models produce smaller gains the higher the life expectancy already reached. The selection of a model for each country is based on recent trends in life expectancy by sex. For countries highly affected by the HIV/AIDS epidemic, the model incorporating a slow pace of mortality decline has generally been used so as to reflect a slowdown in the reduction of mortality risks not related to HIV/AIDS. (UNPD 2009a: 24)

The United States Census Bureau also produces basically extrapolative global population forecasts by country. Its methodology for forecasting changes in life expectancy at birth involves the fitting of a logistic or S-shaped curve to the most recent estimate for life expectancy; analysts fit mortality by age to the forecast through interpolation between past rates and rates representing especially low mortality.[3]

The International Institute of Applied Systems Analysis (IIASA) uses a somewhat different but still fundamentally aggregate method for forecasting mortality within a cohort-component model. IIASA describes its method as "expert argument-based probabilistic forecasting," that is, the use of Delphi-like processes[4] across multiple sources and expert surveys to map ranges of likely fertility and mortality (Lutz, Sanderson, and Scherbov 2004: 20). The efforts of the IIASA World Population Program are of special interest because of their purpose, namely, the linking of demographics to broader aspects of human development, such as education and health, and to policy-relevant aspects of demographics, such as the speed of population aging (Lutz, Sanderson, and Scherbov 2008; Lutz and Scherbov 2008), and population impacts on environmental sustainability.[5]

While these aggregate mortality models focus on population forecasting rather than on health forecasting, they alert us to some of the important characteristics that policy analysts and scientists increasingly want to see. For instance, the emphasis of the UNPD on HIV/AIDS as a critical uncertainty in population forecasting draws attention to the desirability of differentiating mortality by cause, especially when death rates from one or more specific causes may be rising and therefore behaving contrary to larger background patterns. And IIASA's emphasis on linking the analysis of population change to other human systems draws attention to both backward and forward linkages in the analysis of population and health.

Health forecasting began with mostly extrapolative forecasts of mortality and life expectancy as necessary components of population forecasting.

The Emergence and Development of Structural Models

Samuel Preston, in his foreword to a major study published in 2006 (Lopez et al. 2006a: xv), noted that "before 1990, the global disease landscape was perceived 'through a glass darkly.'" Analysts had data on cause of death with relative accuracy for only a small number of countries, and "nowhere were estimates of disease incidence, prevalence, survival, and disabling sequelae consistently combined into population-level profiles of morbidity and mortality."

Circumstances began to change in the early part of the 1990s through the combined efforts of the World Health Organization (WHO) and the World Bank. At that time, WHO, through its Global Burden of Disease project, was building an emerging global database of health statistics, and the first major study of global health, *Disease Control Priorities in Developing Countries* (Jamison et al.), was published in 1993. The Disease Control Priorities project was sponsored by the World Bank, and served as the backdrop for the World Development Report of that year, *Investing in Health* (World Bank 1993). The World Bank reports were geared toward identifying priorities for interventions to achieve rapid health improvements in developing countries with constrained public resources, and they used the emerging WHO database in their analyses of the disease burden of developing countries and targeted interventions. Meanwhile, WHO was developing protocols for estimating and projecting disease-specific mortality and morbidity, and produced *The Global Burden of Disease* (Murray and Lopez 1996b) in 1996. This truly landmark study included 1990 data and provided global projections of mortality and morbidity for over 100 specific diseases through 2020 using new techniques, as discussed in the next section.

A stream of ongoing studies and reports from both WHO's GBD project and the World Bank's Disease Control Priorities project have appeared since those first reports,[6] and a major new GBD study updated with 2005 data is due for release late in 2010. As a result of these projects, a foundation for a structural approach to understanding current global health conditions and thinking about their dynamics in coming years has been established, consolidated, and extended.

Global burden of disease

The GBD project broke new ground not only by focusing specifically on global health, but also through its methodology and approach. First, rather than relying heavily on extrapolative techniques, it identified and used independent variables (income, education, and time) to understand and anticipate health outcomes and changes in them. Second, it disaggregated total mortality into multiple causes of death, important because the driver-outcome relationships vary with cause of death as well as with age and sex. Together these changes made possible a shift to a structural approach to understanding and forecasting health.

In the first GBD report (Murray and Lopez 1996b), the GBD researchers took a major step by building on data for 1990 to forecast the burden of disease in 2000, 2010, and 2020. As we discussed in Chapter 2, they also developed a measure of years lived with disability (YLD) and added it to years of life lost (YLL) to early mortality to create an aggregate measure of disability-adjusted life years (DALYs). Because Murray and Lopez used structural models of disease driven primarily by income and education, they were also able to develop three alternative scenarios of the future mortality and morbidity for over 100 diseases based on differing income and education assumptions for the eight global regions of their analysis.

Mathers and Loncar (2006) built on that path-breaking work in several ways. In addition to drawing on newer and far more extensive disease data and estimates from 2002, they updated driver-variable forecasts; separated diabetes from other noncommunicable diseases (reflecting expectations of increasing overweight and obesity); created regression models specifically for low- and lower-middle-income countries; and developed separate projection models for HIV/AIDS, tuberculosis, lung cancer, and chronic respiratory diseases. They also undertook analysis at the country level rather than at the regional level (although aggregating back to the regional level for presentation of results), and they extended the forecast horizon to 2030. A subsequent update with 2004 data and estimates was published in 2008 (WHO 2008a).

The major-cause typology of disease in the GBD approach builds from three broad cause-groups (Groups I, II, and III; see again Chapter 2) and major clusters within them. Beginning with the 2002 update (Mathers and Loncar 2006), all communicable diseases and maternal, perinatal, and nutritional conditions, with the exception of HIV/AIDS, constitute one cluster. Within Group II (noncommunicable diseases and conditions) the clusters are malignant neoplasms (excluding lung cancer), type 2 diabetes, cardiovascular diseases, digestive disorders, chronic respiratory conditions, and other noncommunicable diseases. And within Group III (injuries) the clusters are road traffic accidents, other unintentional injuries, and intentional injuries. In all, in the GBD projections accompanying the 2002 update, Mathers and Loncar (2006) developed models to forecast mortality and morbidity for 10 major-cause clusters and 132 specific causes within them, including HIV/AIDS. The same clusters and specific diseases were included in the 2004 GBD update (WHO 2008a).

As we discussed in Chapter 2, the conceptual foundation for GBD forecasting has been the use of broad distal drivers rather than directly causal independent variables; those drivers explain very high proportions of the variation in health outcomes. The specific distal drivers used for forecasting were GDP per capita (at purchasing power parity); years of education attainment of adults (extrapolated from the database of Barro and Lee 1996); and a time coefficient that in large part captures technological improvement. The GBD modelers also developed a measure of smoking impact. The GBD project's use of smoking impact in a selected subset of disease formulations reflected the delayed impact of smoking on the incidence of smoking-related diseases, as well as population-specific smoking patterns that the GBD researchers found were not well forecast by distal-driver formulations alone.

The GBD approach has enabled very significant progress with respect to the first major purpose for health forecasting, namely, the desire to understand better possible future changes in health. However, because the driving variables (with the exception of smoking) are not directly causal and therefore do not constitute points of immediately accessible leverage or intervention, the approach does not as directly as we might desire support the second purpose—providing a basis for understanding leverage and informing decision and action. To move in that direction, we now turn to discussion of more proximate drivers of change in the disease burden.

Comparative risk assessment and forecasting

Supplementing the work of the GBD forecasters and moving closer to the level of human choice and action, WHO's Comparative Risk Assessment (CRA) project has identified major disease risk factors and analyzed the burden of disease observed in a population with a given distribution of those risk factors, relative to that in a population with an alternative and theoretically minimal distribution of the risk factors, in order to quantify the impact of risk factors on diseases (Ezzati et al. 2004a; WHO 2009a). The project has identified 28 risk factors (see Table 2.1) grouped in seven categories: childhood and maternal undernutrition; other nutrition-related risk factors and physical activity; sexual and reproductive health; addictive substantives; environmental risks; occupational risks; and other selected risks.

Although the CRA project has not done so, theoretically, one could use the analysis that connects these risk factors to disease burden to forecast change in that disease burden. It would, of course require the development and use of models that represented risk factors. And the effort would struggle with the complex interactive effects of the risk factors (their effects are not simply additive) and with missing risks (it would never be possible to represent all of them). We return to these issues later in this chapter in the discussion of the IFs forecasting approach.

To date, the GBD project has not incorporated comparative risk assessments into its forecasting formulations except in the cases of (1) smoking impact on noncommunicable respiratory diseases, and (2) body mass index (BMI) on diabetes. Instead, efforts to explore choices and interventions tied to proximate risks have focused to a greater degree on detailed analysis of specific diseases and associated intervention options (including some attention to the role of larger health systems) without moving to the

The GBD approach has used broad distal drivers to analyze and forecast health outcomes for 132 specific diseases and conditions.

WHO's Comparative Risk Assessment project has identified 28 major disease risk factors and analyzed their relationship to disease burdens.

level of forecasts.[7] In short, there remains a gap between the GBD project's health forecasting approach and the attention of those interested in analyzing proximate action options. The gap exists with respect to the level of aggregation of disease types in the forecasting and, to an even greater extent, with respect to the drivers used in the forecasting formulations. Specialized models of specific diseases are now being developed and are partially closing that gap.

Specialized disease-cause models and systems dynamics approaches

Even in the aggregate forecasting of the UNPD and the distal-driver-based work of the GBD, the projects relied in some instances on more specialized treatment of specific diseases and health risks, such as the separate modeling of HIV/AIDS in the otherwise aggregate mortality analysis of the UNPD and of smoking impact in the structural analysis of the GBD project.

The Spectrum system of the Joint United Nations Programme on HIV/AIDS (UNAIDS) is an important example of a specialized model.[8] It differentiates the prevalence of HIV (the stock of those afflicted) from the incidence of new infections, mirroring the common distinction between stocks and flows in the structural analysis of systems. It further represents the transition or flow rates from the prevalence of HIV to the manifestation of AIDS, as well as the rate of deaths of those with AIDS (in part as a function of the availability of antiretroviral therapy).

Although not explicitly using the terminology and computer software associated with systems dynamics, the UNPD, GBD, and UNAIDS modeling and forecasting of HIV/AIDS implicitly draws on that approach. Other efforts to examine specific diseases have drawn more explicitly on systems dynamics. For instance, Homer et al. (2004) described a diabetes model developed under the auspices of the United States Centers for Disease Control (CDC). Beginning with a generic model of chronic disease (with separate stocks representing the general population, the vulnerable population, those afflicted without complications, and those afflicted with complications), they proceeded in sessions with CDC staff to develop a specific model for diabetes. The model developers obtained data and parameters from a variety of sources and

developed a base case that simulated well the historical growth of diagnosed adult diabetes in the United States after 1980. They also presented the model with the appropriate caveats that apply to systems dynamics models, including the difficulty of specifying the full initial condition and parameter sets and the resulting caution required in interpreting specific numerical output as opposed to more general system behavior.

Regardless of the caveats and the difficulties that would face any attempt to generalize this diabetes model to countries around the world, it illustrates the potential for a deeper and, in a significant sense, more truly structural approach to health forecasting than that of the distal-driver models.[9] Such an approach can conceivably serve the purpose (number 2 in our earlier list) of those interested in choices and action, rather than simply forecasting patterns of change (our purpose 1). Such systems dynamics–like approaches also have the clear advantage of explicitly representing morbidity (the stocks of disease prevalence) as a stage of disease progression rather than an aggregate correlate of mortality.

One can begin to imagine a hybrid system of modules to forecast and study health, some of which might be relatively simple distal-driver formulations, some of which may tap knowledge about specific risk factors, and some of which may be more deeply and richly structural with respect to the progression of a disease. Such a system could help bridge the gap between the desire to fully understand patterns of morbidity and mortality and the desire to move the forecasting enterprise toward the goals of aiding choice and action. The development of such a system is a theme that this chapter will continue to develop.

GISMO: Integrating structural and dynamic representations

The Global Integrated Sustainability Model (GISMO) of the Netherlands Environmental Assessment Agency (Hilderink and Lucas 2008) is an emerging model with a number of the characteristics that allow bridging the forecasting of changes in human health with more detailed exploration of the determinants of such changes. The GISMO modeling system forecasts distal forces (such as GDP per capita)

● Hybrid health models could combine formulations based on distal drivers and risk analysis with more richly structural approaches. ●

● The GISMO model of the Netherlands Environmental Assessment Agency has begun to build a hybrid model that links environmental risks and health outcomes. ●

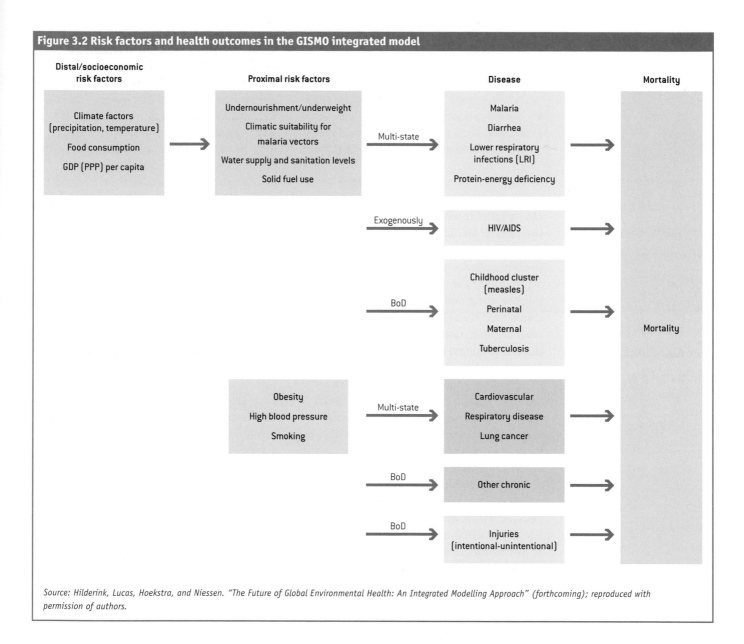

Figure 3.2 Risk factors and health outcomes in the GISMO integrated model

| Distal/socioeconomic risk factors | Proximal risk factors | | Disease | | Mortality |

Distal/socioeconomic risk factors:
Climate factors (precipitation, temperature)
Food consumption
GDP (PPP) per capita

Proximal risk factors:
Undernourishment/underweight
Climatic suitability for malaria vectors
Water supply and sanitation levels
Solid fuel use

Multi-state → Malaria, Diarrhea, Lower respiratory infections (LRI), Protein-energy deficiency

Exogenously → HIV/AIDS

BoD → Childhood cluster (measles), Perinatal, Maternal, Tuberculosis

Proximal risk factors:
Obesity
High blood pressure
Smoking

Multi-state → Cardiovascular, Respiratory disease, Lung cancer

BoD → Other chronic

BoD → Injuries (intentional-unintentional)

Mortality

Source: Hilderink, Lucas, Hoekstra, and Niessen. "The Future of Global Environmental Health: An Integrated Modelling Approach" (forthcoming); reproduced with permission of authors.

and uses those to drive change in a number of risk factors that then link to specific causes of death. Figure 3.2 illustrates the process.

Because of the environmental focus of GISMO's home institution, many of its pathways tend to emphasize driving variables, risk factors, and specific diseases related to the environment. Those risk factors and mortality outcomes are modeled using a multi-state approach, distinguishing proximal and distal determinants. Other health outcomes are modeled in GISMO using the GBD project's methodology (shown as BoD in Figure 3.2).

Although Figure 3.2 does not show it, the linkages in GISMO flow not just from driving

modules to health outcomes but also from health outcomes back to other modules, notably the demographic one. This embedding of a health module in a broader system begins to help the system also serve the third purpose of health modeling identified earlier, namely, the exploration of how the future of health may affect broader demographic, economic, and even socio-political systems.

Returning to the general purposes of existing forecasting approaches

The beginning of this chapter identified three general and interrelated purposes of health modeling and forecasting:

- understanding better where patterns of human development appear to be taking us with respect to global health
- considering opportunities for intervention and achievement of alternative health futures
- preparing society for the broader (for instance, demographic, economic, and socio-political) impacts of changing health patterns

Different forecasting approaches serve different purposes, and hybrid models have the greatest potential to address multiple purposes.

No model is likely to serve all of these purposes well, and we have seen that the forecasting efforts have generally been quite limited in their intent. The GBD project's distal-driver models have opened the door for addressing the first purpose—mapping changing disease burdens. They also provide some foundation for thinking about decisions and actions to shape alternative futures because they quantify, by cause of death, the magnitude of current and (forecasted) future mortality and morbidity.

More specialized models potentially offer more targeted help with the allocation of resources and other interventions both across and within death-cause categories, because they can distinguish different stages of disease with potentially variable associated costs and benefits of intervention. Truly meeting the desires of those who wish to use a model to make cost-benefit decisions about alternative health interventions almost certainly requires a level of detail in representation that is at least at that of the CDC diabetes model referred to earlier. Moving to that level of detail generally means, however, that such modeling sacrifices any attempt to map the complete disease burden, as well as any effort to look at aggregate social implications.

The aggregate mortality models are perhaps currently best suited to helping with the third purpose, namely, the exploration of alternative mortality futures (with age-sex specificity) so as to help society paint, with quite a broad brush, the possible wide implications of different health futures. For example, those who think about financial requirements of pension systems regularly use such models. Analysis of forward linkages could potentially also further enrich the basis for action by providing information about the more indirect costs and benefits of alternative health futures. In reality, the level of aggregation in their treatment both of disease types and of social implications tends to limit analysis to large-scale demographic impacts.

Building a hybrid, integrated system

Although no model can do everything, the association of different approaches with different contributions suggests that a somewhat more hybrid and integrated model form could help with all three forecasting purposes and could provide a richer overall picture of alternative health futures. Figure 3.3 shows the general structure that such a system might take. Formulations based on distal drivers could remain at its core. Again, such a core structure is especially useful in accomplishing the first purpose, because the distal-driver formulations of the GBD offer an existing treatment of health outcomes that is comprehensive with respect to diseases and their related mortality and morbidity.

There is no inherent reason, however, that income, education, and time should be equally capable of helping us forecast disease in each of the major categories (let alone each of the specific diseases) that the GBD models examine. For example, distal-driver formulations tend to produce forecasts of constantly decreasing death rates. Yet we know that smoking, obesity, road traffic accidents, and their related toll on health tend to increase in developing societies among those who first obtain higher levels of income and education, and that only with further societal spread of income and education do smoking and road traffic deaths (and perhaps also obesity) typically decline.[10]

Richer structural models might help us capture such more complex patterns. Many death cause-specific distal formulations would

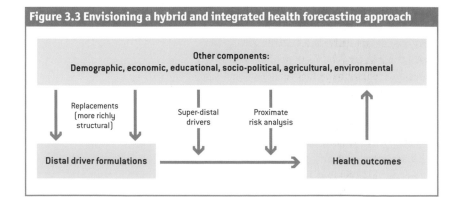

Figure 3.3 Envisioning a hybrid and integrated health forecasting approach

Other components:
Demographic, economic, educational, socio-political, agricultural, environmental

Replacements (more richly structural)

Super-distal drivers

Proximate risk analysis

Distal driver formulations

Health outcomes

benefit from modifications and, in some cases, replacement. Deeper and richer structural formulations, like those for specific diseases such as HIV/AIDS or diabetes, are examples. So too, our exploration toward mid-century and beyond of forecasts of deaths from road traffic accidents generated by the distal-driver formulation of the GBD project suggested that a variety of floor and ceiling effects need consideration in the longer term, and that a more richly structural formulation could limit perverse forecasting behavior. (We should, of course, not expect GBD distal formulations that were built for forecasting 25–30 years to be fully capable of use over time-horizons of 50 years or more.)

A hybrid model of the form we wish to see also should contribute to the second purpose of health forecasting, as more specialized structural representations may help us identify opportunities for interventions to improve health futures. These interventions might occur either in the form of super-distal drivers (for example, policy-driven human action with respect to health systems) or the amelioration of proximate risk factors through changes in the behavior of individuals, or in the combination of super-distal drivers and proximate risk factors. As an example, the socio-political and environmental modules in IFs act, in part, as super-distal foundations for variables such as undernutrition and indoor air pollution, which in turn facilitate analyses of proximate risk factors and human action around them.

Finally, with respect to the third purpose (the connections of health with other human systems), representation of these connections would allow health outcomes to feed back to broader human development systems, closing the loop. Many linkages of all of these broader system elements with health should be bi-directional.

Modeling Health in IFs

The IFs health model system is a modularly hybrid and integrated system of the kind that Figure 3.3 sketches. Like any model, it has many limitations; it is an evolving and improving system. In the remainder of this chapter we describe its current form, and in Chapter 4 we will explore the behavior of the system in and

of itself and in comparison with the health forecasts of others.

The IFs health model forecasts 15 individual and clustered causes of death and disability. We list them below, grouped by the GBD major cause categories:

Group I—diarrheal diseases; HIV/AIDS; malaria; respiratory infections; other communicable diseases

Group II—cardiovascular diseases; diabetes; digestive disorders; malignant neoplasms; mental health; respiratory conditions and diseases; other noncommunicable diseases

Group III—intentional injuries; road traffic accidents; other unintentional injuries

The GBD (mostly distal driver) model foundation in IFs

The IFs model begins with the driver outcome formulations developed by the GBD project for its analyses.[11] Mathers and Loncar (2006) built a general distal-driver formulation and applied it to selected major disease clusters (elaborating their forecasting to many other diseases with regressions linked to the major clusters). We applied their major-cause formulation to largely the same major clusters and elaborated a small subset of additional detailed cause-of-death categories (namely, malaria, respiratory infections, and mental health) in accordance with our needs for this volume (discussed below).[12] The core Mathers and Loncar formulation that we implemented is:

$$\ln(M_{a,k,i,r}) = C_{a,k,i} + \beta_1 * \ln(Y_r) + \beta_2 * \ln(HC_r) + \beta_3 * (\ln(Y_r))^2 + \beta_4 * T + \beta_5 * \ln(SI_{a,k,r})$$

where
M is mortality level in deaths per 100,000 for a given age group a, sex k, cause i, and country or region r; C is a constant; Y is GDP per capita at PPP; HC is total years of completed education for adults 25 and older; T is time (year = 1900); and SI is smoking impact.

Some important differences in our approach relative to that of the GBD required

● *Richer structural models might help us capture the complex patterns between health drivers, health outcomes, and forward linkages from health.* ●

● *We are building and using a hybrid model that combines distal formulations, treatment of risk, extended structures, and integration with broader human development.* ●

● *The IFs health model has at its core the distal-driver outcome formulations developed by the GBD project.* ●

development of algorithms for computation of initial conditions and small multiplicative adjustments to formulations. Specifically, we begin forecasts in the base year of 2005, we maintain five-year age categories up through 100+, and we represent infants as a separate category. In contrast, the initial data we obtained from the GBD project provided country, sex, and cause-specific mortality, but from the year 2004 and in more aggregated categories at the youngest and oldest ages.[13] Moreover, we have our own sources of data for GDP per capita and education attainment level, which we forecast using our own models.

To reconcile our approach with data used by the GBD project and with GBD formulations we:

- computed a set of initial scaling parameters (by country, sex, and cause of death) that assure consistency of total deaths forecast using the GBD formulations and our 2005 values of driving variables with the cause-specific mortality data in the GBD's detailed death file;[14]
- calculated a second set of scaling or normalization parameters (by country, sex, and age category) that force the sum of all deaths to be the same as the UNPD mortality data for each five-year age and sex category for the year 2005. This process also spreads the more highly aggregated 2004 mortality data of the GBD project[15] into five-year age categories.[16] This process assures that we have initial conditions consistent with UNPD mortality data in our base year.[17]

These adjustments mean that, except for total mortality by age and sex from the UNPD, our numbers in the 2005 base year will not match other data precisely, but that the overall pattern of deaths by cause should be quite close to the GBD data.[18] In the forecasts themselves, we keep the multiplicative scaling and normalization parameters constant over time because there is no clear reason for changing them.

Lumped within the major cause categories forecast with the formulation above are certain diseases we wish to deal with explicitly. These include three diseases in the category "communicable diseases other than HIV/AIDS"—diarrheal diseases, malaria, and respiratory infections—and two diseases under "other

noncommunicable diseases"—chronic respiratory conditions (discussed later in conjunction with proximate-driver and relative-risk analysis) and mental health (for which we represent constant death rates). For the first three, the GBD project (Mathers and Loncar 2005 and 2006) provides a distal-driver formulation for detailed causes of mortality that we also use.

The regression equations for the detailed causes take the form:

$$\ln(M_{a,k,i,d,r}) = C_{a,k,i,d,r} + \beta_{a,k,i,d,r} * \ln(M_{a,k,i,r})$$

where

M is mortality rate in deaths per 100,000 for age group a, sex k, general cause i, and country or region r; calculated using the Mathers and Loncar formulation for the major cause category; d is the specific disease.

For the base year, the death rates for the specific diseases are calculated using the above equation.[19] For future years, given the form of the equation, a 1 percent change in the mortality rate for the general cause-group is associated with a ß percent change in the mortality rate for the detailed cause.[20] As an example, the ß for diarrheal diseases for males in the 0–4 age group is 1.493 (Mathers and Loncar 2005: 115). Thus, a 1 percent decline in the mortality rate for communicable diseases other than HIV/AIDS for males in the 0–4 age group in a specific country implies a 1.493 percent decline in the mortality rate for diarrheal diseases for the same group.

In an early phase of model development, we replicated the basic GBD distal-driver models (with the above selected breakouts of detailed causes) and then analyzed forecasts made with our drivers from the integrated IFs system, both in order to compare our results with those of the GBD and also to explore the behavior of the formulations beyond the time-horizon for which they were initially estimated and used. Although our primary focus is 2060 (a 50-year horizon), we pushed the horizon to 2100 in order to understand better the behavior of the equations. The extensions, modifications, and replacements of distal-driver-only functions that we made and describe below resulted from our desire to improve long-term forecasting capability.

● *We modified or replaced some GBD distal-driver functions to improve forecasting capability over our longer forecast horizon.* ●

Specialized structural model formulations and approaches in IFs

The distal-driver formulation serves well for many disease and death categories. The approach serves less well in other cases, particularly those in which mortality rates tend not to monotonically increase or decrease, often because a complex and perhaps sequential set of factors drive morbidity and mortality patterns. In such cases, still richer structural models can be helpful. One example is smoking, where the GBD approach uses an alternative smoking impact series, but a forecast of smoking rates itself as a driver of impact could be very useful. Another example, which drove the GBD project itself to look for an alternative approach, is HIV/AIDS. We needed either to do as the GBD did and rely on the forecasts of others (such as UNAIDS) or to develop our own approach, which might ultimately allow us to build more scenario "handles" into our own analysis; we chose the latter course. A third example is road traffic accident deaths, where our work with the formulation of the GBD suggested inadequate ceiling effects (upper limits beyond which a forecast should not reasonably go) and long-term forecasts of deaths that appeared unrealistic. A fourth example is health spending as it relates to communicable disease deaths of children. Although subject to significant debate, as Chapter 2 discussed, there is much reason to represent the possibility that health expenditures augment the distal drivers in affecting at least some health outcomes.

Smoking, smoking impact, and chronic diseases

In 1992 Peto et al. proposed a method for calculating the proportion of deaths caused by smoking that was not dependent on statistics on prevalence of tobacco consumption. This method involved developing an indicator for accumulated smoking risk, termed the *smoking impact ratio* (SIR). Ezzati and Lopez (2004: 888) defined the SIR as "population lung cancer mortality in excess of never-smokers, relative to excess lung cancer mortality for a known reference group of smokers." In other words, the ratio is derived by comparing actual population lung cancer mortality with the expected lung cancer mortality in a reference population of nonsmokers. Because the SIR is derived from age-sex lung cancer mortality

it can also provide an indication of the "maturity" of the smoking epidemic (the extent to which the population had been exposed to tobacco in the past) (Ezzati and Lopez 2004: 888). Once the SIR has been determined, one can then use it to estimate the proportions of deaths from other diseases attributable to smoking (Peto et al. 1992).

For the GBD project, Mathers and Loncar developed country-level smoking impact (SI) projections to 2030 (Mathers and Loncar 2006; and Mathers and Loncar, Protocol S1 Technical Appendix, n.d.) and used them as part of their distal-driver formulation. The SI projections rely on expert judgment, and it was not possible for the IFs project to improve on them; thus, we used those projections without change. Forecasting beyond 2030 required, however, that the IFs project extend those series, taking into account a long lag between smoking rates and smoking impact. We therefore wanted smoking rates themselves to drive our approach. The development of a structural forecast system for those rates involved several main steps. First, we created a historical series of estimated smoking rates. This was necessary because historical smoking rate data are exceptionally sparse, and we needed to understand the patterns and trajectory of smoking behavior over time. We built the historical imputed smoking series on the most recent smoking rate data point of each country and the smoking impact forecasts of the GBD. Assuming a direct 25-year lag between smoking rate and smoking impact,[21] we used year-to-year percentage changes in the smoking impact series to change smoking rates before and after our smoking data point.[22] In spite of the simplicity of this approach, and the fact that smoking impact reflects more than smoking rates,[23] we found that the constructed series tended to match relatively well when more than one historical point for smoking rate existed.

Second, we constructed cross-sectional relationships that suggest expected rates of smoking based on GDP per capita at PPP for males and females separately:

$$ExpSmoking\_Rate_{Males} = 0.00224 * GDPPCP^2 - 0.3386 * GDPPCP + 38.3996$$

> ● *Our representations of smoking impact, HIV/AIDS, road traffic accidents, and health spending differ from or augment those of the GBD.* ●

$$ExpSmoking\_Rate_{Females} = -0.00573 * GDPPCP^2 + 0.6893 * GDPPCP + 5.6634$$

Third, we initialized a moving average rate of change in smoking rate with the compound rate of change between 1995 and 2005. We advanced that moving average over time by slowly changing the moving average toward the expected values of the cross-sectional formulations (weighting the expected value 1/10 of the moving average value each year). We introduced a number of other algorithmic rules to produce what appeared to be reasonable forecasts of smoking rates given the general notion of a bell-shaped curve (or rise and then fall) of smoking with income and time. These included bounding the expected value formulations at $30,000 for females and $50,000 for males so as to avoid complete collapse of smoking rates at high income levels.

Finally, for forecasting we used the same process in reverse that we had earlier used to estimate the smoking series. With the year-to-year percentage change in smoking rate forecasts from 2005 forward, we changed the year-to-year values of the smoking impact series 25 years later.

HIV/AIDS

The ultimate objective of the calculations around HIV infections and AIDS is to forecast annual deaths from AIDS by age category and sex. We began, however, by forecasting country-specific values for the HIV prevalence rate ($HIVRATE$).[24] For the period from 1990–2007 we have reasonably good data and estimates from UNAIDS (2008) on prevalence rates and have used values from 2004 and 2006 to calculate an initial rate of increase ($hivincr$) in the prevalence rate across the population (which for most countries is now negative).[25]

There will be an ultimate peak to the epidemic in all countries, so we need to deal with multiple phases of changing prevalence: continued rise where rates are still growing steadily, slowing rise as rates peak, decline (accelerating) as rates pass the peak, and slowing rates of decline as prevalence approaches zero in the longer term. In general, we need to represent something of a bell-shaped pattern, but one with a long tail because prevalence will persist for the increasingly long lifetimes of those infected and if pockets of transmission linger in selected population subgroups.[26] As a first level of user-control over the pattern, we add scenario specification via an exogenous multiplier on the prevalence rate ($hivm$).

The movement up to the peak involves annual compounding of the initial growth rate in prevalence ($hivincr$), dampened as a country approaches the peak year. Thus, we can further control the growth pattern via specification of peak years ($hivpeakyr$) and prevalence rate in those peak years ($hivpeakr$), with an algorithmic logic that gradually dampens growth rate to the peak year:[27]

$$HIVRATE_r^t = HIVRATE_r^{t-1} * (1 + hivincr_r^t) * \mathbf{hivm_r}$$

where

$hivincr_r^t = F(\mathbf{hivincr_r^{t=1}}, \mathbf{hivpeakyr_r}, \mathbf{hivpeakr_r})$; t is time (shown in this chapter only when equations reference earlier time points); and r is country (geographic region in IFs terminology). Here and elsewhere, names in bold are exogenously specified parameters.

As countries pass the peak, we posit that advances are being made against the epidemic, both in terms of social policy and technologies of control, at a speed that reduces the total prevalence rate by a certain percentage annually ($hivtadvr$). To do this, we apply to the prevalence rate an accumulation of the advances (or lack of them) in a technology/social control factor ($HIVTECCNTL$). In addition, if decline is already underway in the data for recent years, we add a term based on the initial rate of that decline ($hivincr$), in order to match the historical pattern; that initial rate of decline decays over time and shifts the dominance of the decline rate to the exogenously specified rate ($hivtadvr$). This algorithmic formulation generates the slowly accelerating decline and then slowing decline of a reverse S-shaped pattern with a long tail:

$$HIVRATE_r^t = HIVRATE_r^{t-1} * (1 - HIVTECCNTL_r^t)$$

where

$$HIVTECCNTL_r^t = HIVTDCCNTL_r^{t-1} * (1 + \mathbf{hivtadvr} * t/100) + F(\mathbf{hivincr_r^{t=1}})$$

Finally, calculation of country- and region-specific numbers for HIV prevalence is simply a matter of applying the rates to the size of the population (POP) number.

$$HIVCASES_r^t = POP_r^t * HIVRATE_r^t$$

The rate of death of those with HIV would benefit from a complex model in itself, because it varies with the medical technology available, such as antiretroviral therapy (ART) and the age structure of prevalence. We have simplified such complexities because of data constraints, while maintaining basic representation of the various elements. Because both the manifestation of AIDS and deaths from it lag considerably behind the incidence of HIV, we link the death rate of AIDS (*HIVAIDSR*) to a 10-year moving average of the HIV prevalence (*HIVRateMAvg*). We also posit an exogenously specified technological advance factor (*aidsdrtadvr*) that gradually reduces the death rate of infected individuals (or inversely increases their life span), as ART is doing. And we allow the user to apply an exogenous multiplier (*aidsratem*) for further scenario analysis:

$$AIDSDRATE_r^t = HIVRateMAvg_r^t * HIVAIDSR_r^{t=1}$$
$$* (1 - \textbf{aidsdrtadvr}_r^t / 100) * \textbf{aidsratem}_r^t$$

where
$$HIVRateMAvg_r^t = F(HIVRATE_r^t, \text{last 10 years})$$

We spread this death rate across sex and age categories. We apply a user-changeable table function to determine the male portion as a function of GDP per capita at PPP, estimating that the male portion rises to 0.9 with higher GDP per capita.[28] To specify the age structure of deaths, we examined data from large numbers of studies on infections by cohort in Brazil and Botswana (in a U.S. Census Bureau database) and extracted a rough cohort pattern from those data.

Road traffic accident deaths

Deciding that the distal-driver formulation alone was producing unrealistic estimates of deaths from road traffic accidents in the long-term, we replaced the distal formulation with a more deeply structural one tied to the growth of the vehicle fleet (occurring pretty much around the world with income growth but saturating at higher income levels) and the declining rate of accidents and deaths per vehicle (which occurs also at higher income levels). Thus, the overall forecast pattern is one of rather rapid growth in road traffic death rates when the vehicle fleet is growing most rapidly, followed by slowing growth of road traffic death rates and ultimately by their decline.

We based our forecast of vehicles per capita (*VEHICLFLPC*) on the formula of Dargay, Gately, and Sommer (2007):

$$VEHICLFLPC = (852 - RF) * e^{(-5.987 * e^{(-0.2 * GDPPCP(R))})}$$

where

GDPPCP is GDP per capita at PPP (thousand dollars) and RF is an adjustment factor (changing over time) to compensate for different land densities, taking the United States as the base. We computed the adjustment factor using the formula from Dargay, Gately, and Sommer:

$$RF = 38.8 * \left(\frac{POP(R)}{LANDAREA(R)} - \frac{POP(USA)}{LANDAREA(USA)} \right)$$

where

RF is the adjustment factor, POP is the population (millions) of country R, and LANDAREA is the total land area (10,000 square kilometers) of country R. We computed the adjustment factor only when country R had higher density than the United States.[29]

Deaths per vehicle tend to fall with income. R. J. Smeed originally proposed a quite widely accepted relationship, now labeled Smeed's Law,[30] which in his notation and without units relates deaths to vehicle ownership:

$$D = 0.0003(np^2)^{\frac{1}{3}}$$

where

D is annual road deaths, n is number of vehicles (which we compute from vehicles per capita above), and p is population. We spread deaths across age categories using information from the GBD project's detailed death tables.

> ● Distal drivers influence health outcomes through their effects on health risk factors (proximate drivers) rather than directl.●

Public spending on health

The GBD project's distal-driver formulation does not take public spending on health into account. However, we add a term to the basic GBD distal-driver formulation to incorporate the relatively consistent inverse relationship of public spending on health with child mortality rates in poor countries (Anand and Ravallion 1993; Bidani and Ravallion 1997; Nixon and Ulmann 2006; Wagstaff 2002). For countries having a GDP per capita (at PPP) of $15,000 or less, our model applies a simple elasticity for the effects of government health expenditure as a percentage of GDP on all-cause mortality for the 0–4 age group from the distal-driver formulation (the base calculation that health expenditures adjust):

$$\ln(_5q_0{}^{adj}) = \ln(_5q_0{}^{base}) - 0.06 * HealthExp\%$$

where

$_5q_0$ is the mortality rate for age 0–4.

In IFs this formalized version becomes

$$MortAdj^t_{j = 0-4, r, k = 1} = Mort^t_{j = 0-4, r, k = 1} * (1 + HlExpFct^t_r)$$

where

$$HlExpFct^t_r = \textbf{elhlmortspn} * (100 * GDS^t_{r, g = health} / GDP^t_r) - GDSHI^{t = 1}_r)$$

where

$$GDSHI^{t = 1}_r = GDS^{t = 1}_{r, g = health} / GDP^{t = 1}_r * 100$$
$$\textbf{elhlmortspn} = -0.06$$

GDS is government expenditure; GDSHI is initial government expenditure; HlExpFct is health expenditure factor; elhlmortspn is the elasticity of mortality with health spending; j is age category; r is country/region; k is cause (1 is communicable); t is time-step

In this calculation we use health expenditure as a percentage of GDP, rather than health expenditure per capita, to avoid any confounding with the distal driver for GDP per capita. We established this coefficient for all-cause mortality in the 0–4 age category on the basis of multivariate regressions using the GBD distal-driver specifications as a base model and compared the coefficient with the results of existing studies (Anand and

Ravallion 1993; Filmer and Pritchett 1999; Wagstaff 2002).[31]

Model extensions to include proximate drivers in IFs

As we have noted previously, the distal drivers do not, in and of themselves, cause health outcomes. Rather, they influence mortality and morbidity through their effects on a host of proximate risk factors. If these factors move in parallel with the distal drivers—that is, if changes in the distal drivers fully capture the risk factors and the efficacy of the health systems—then it would be reasonable to forecast solely on the basis of the distal drivers. To the extent that this is not the case, however, dealing with risk factors more explicitly may improve forecasts. Moreover, the proximate drivers provide some analytical leverage with respect to ways in which we might improve future health outcomes, the second forecasting purpose identified earlier. In summary, forecasting based on proximate drivers and risk factors brings us closer to the level of targeted human interventions.

In this section, we describe a method for modifying forecasts based solely on the distal drivers (and our specialized structural extensions to them) by addressing a number of the risk factors identified in WHO's CRA project discussed earlier (Ezzati et al. 2004a). We have not addressed all risk factors, or all health outcomes related to the selected risk factors, because of limitations of data, knowledge, and time. Still, the procedure we describe does allow us to deal with some of the more important risk factors and provides a foundation on which we and others can build further.

The basic proximate-driver approach in IFs

We build our approach on an understanding of two basic concepts used in the CRA project, specifically *relative risk* (RR) and *population attributable fraction* (PAF).

A relative risk is a "measure of the risk of a certain event happening in one group compared to the risk of the same event happening in another group."[32] We follow the approach taken by the CRA study, comparing our forecast population at risk to an "ideal" population with a "theoretical minimum" level of risk. For example, WHO estimates that children under five who are moderately or severely underweight are almost

> ● Based on concepts from the CRA project, we extended the IFs health model to include selected health risks as proximate drivers of health outcomes. ●

nine times more likely to die from communicable causes than is a population of "normal-weight" children (Blössner and de Onis 2005).

As its name suggests, a PAF reflects the degree to which a specific risk factor is associated with the occurrence of a specific health outcome. Formally, it is the proportional reduction in disease or death rates for the total population (including those with and without the risk factor) that we would expect if we reduced a particular risk factor to a theoretically minimum level (Murray et al. 2004). The further the current situation is from the ideal, the closer the value of the PAF will be to 1.

A PAF is calculated as:

$$(\sum RR(x)P(x) - \sum RR(x)P'(x) \,/\, \sum RR(x)P(x)) = 1 - \sum RR(x)P'(x) \,/\, \sum RR(x)P(x)$$

where

$RR(x)$ is relative risk at exposure level x; $P(x)$ is the population distribution in terms of exposure level, that is, the shares of the population exposed to each level of exposure; $P'(x)$ is the theoretical minimum population distribution in terms of exposure level. For certain risks this is defined as no exposure; where this is not realistic, WHO defines an international reference population

Following this definition, multiplying the mortality from a particular disease by the PAF yields an estimate of the number of people who would not have died had the risk factor been at its theoretical minimum level. If we assume that the values of $RR(x)$ and $P'(x)$ for particular risk factors and diseases do not differ across countries or change over time,[33] then changes in the PAF are solely a function of changes in $P(x)$, the exposure of the population to the particular risk factor. Thus, it is necessary to be able to forecast the future levels of the risk factors. Later sections of this chapter describe how this is done for specific risk factors.

Since our forecast of health outcomes from distal drivers implicitly suggests certain proximate-driver levels, we are really interested in the effect of a difference in (1) estimates of the future levels of a risk factor based only on distal drivers, and (2) estimates based on a more complete set of drivers. Again,

assuming this is possible, we can calculate two versions of the PAF, namely, PAF_{Full} and PAF_{Distal}. Defining $Mortality_{Distal}$ as the mortality calculated using only the distal drivers and $Mortality_{Final}$ as the mortality after accounting explicitly for the risk factor, we can state that:

- $Mortality_{Distal} * PAF_{Distal}$ represents the number of people who would not have died had the risk factor been at its theoretical minimum level using the distal formulations for mortality and the proximate risk factor; and
- $Mortality_{Final} * PAF_{Full}$ represents the number of people who would not have died had the risk factor been at its theoretical minimum level using a more complete formulation for mortality and the proximate risk factor.

If we assume that no other factors influence the difference in total mortality between the distal formulation and that using the full model, then:

$$Mortality_{Final} - Mortality_{Distal} = Mortality_{Final} * PAF_{Full} - Mortality_{Distal} * PAF_{Distal}$$

Yields:
$$Mortality_{Final} = Mortality_{Distal} * ((1 - PAF_{Distal}) \,/\, (1 - PAF_{Full})) = Mortality_{Distal} * \sum RR(x)P_{Full}(x) \,/\, \sum RR(x)P_{Distal}(x)$$

The adjustment factor is the ratio of the weighted average relative risks based on the distributions using the distal-only versus the full formulations for estimating the value of the risk factor. A higher weighted average RR based on the full formulation implies that the distal drivers overestimate the improvement (or underestimate the deterioration) in the risk factor. Thus, the mortality forecast needs to be adjusted upward. Alternatively, if the weighted average RR is lower based on the full formulation than on the distal formulation, the mortality forecast will be adjusted downward. Note that this property of the calculation actually obviates the need to know the theoretical minimum population.

Mapping proximate drivers to diseases and age categories
We used this approach to modifying distal-driver forecasts by forecasts of proximate risks for

eight proximate risk factors (refer back to Table 2.1 for the broader list of factors included in the WHO CRA project and to Chapters 5 and 6 for the eight IFs analyses). Table 3.1 shows the particular diseases and age groupings that each of the risk factors in IFs affects.

An example of the proximate-driver approach in IFs: Undernutrition

We elaborate here the process for specification of the adjustment factor linking a proximate driver (in this case, undernutrition as measured by underweight) and disease (in this case, all communicable diseases other than HIV/AIDS) for children under five. For elaboration of our approach to the other proximate drivers included in this volume, please see the specific sections in Chapters 5 and 6 and the technical documentation of the health model at www.ifs.du.edu.

Fishman et al. (2004) discuss the many risks of death and disease that undernutrition, in the form of being underweight, poses to children under the age of five and to women of reproductive age. They point, in particular, to the potential consequences for children

Our treatment of childhood undernutrition illustrates the IFs approach to modeling individual proximate drivers.

under the age of five from communicable diseases other than HIV/AIDS, one of the general cause-groups included in the GBD project. They break this category down into diarrhea, pneumonia (respiratory infections), malaria, measles, and a combined group of these and all other communicable diseases except HIV/AIDS, providing specific relative risks for each of the four specific disease groups, as well as for the combined group. As noted earlier, we also separate out diarrhea, respiratory infections, and malaria but define our fourth group to include measles as well as other communicable diseases except HIV/AIDS. Thus, we are able to estimate mortality rates, Mortality$_{Distal}$, for each of three separate and one combined cause-groups, as described earlier in this chapter.[34]

Fishman et al. (2004) specified the risk factor for undernutrition in terms of weight-for-age using an "average" population, with a given mean and standard deviation. For any particular country, children under five years of age are assigned to one of four categories: severely underweight (more than three standard deviations [SDs] below the mean weight for the "average" population), moderately underweight (3SDs to 2SDs below the mean weight for the "average" population), mildly underweight (2SDs to 1SD below the mean weight for the "average" population), and normal weight (no more than 1SD below the mean weight for the "average" population). This constitutes the population distribution in terms of exposure level, specified as P(x) in earlier discussion of the proximate-driver approach in IFs. Fishman et al. (2004) also described the theoretical minimum distribution, P'(x). Using their all-cause category as an example (Fishman et al. 2004: 64), children who are severely underweight are 8.72 times as likely to die from communicable diseases as those with a normal weight; those who are moderately underweight are 4.24 times as likely to die; and those who are mildly underweight are 2.06 times as likely to die.

In order to calculate the adjustment factor for the effect of undernutrition on children's mortality from communicable diseases, we need to know the population distributions (P) of undernutrition based on both the distal drivers, P$_{Distal}$(x), and the full model,

Table 3.1 Risk factors and their disease impacts in IFs

Risk factor	Diseases impacted in IFs	Age group impacted in IFs
Childhood underweight	Diarrheal diseases Respiratory infections Malaria Other communicable diseases	<5?
Body mass index	Cardiovascular diseases Diabetes	30+
Smoking	Malignant neoplasms Cardiovascular diseases Respiratory diseases	30+
Unsafe water, sanitation, and hygiene	Diarrheal diseases	All ages
Urban air pollution	Respiratory infections Respiratory diseases Cardiovascular diseases	30+
Indoor air pollution from household use of solid fuels	Respiratory infections Respiratory diseases	<5 (infections) 30+ (diseases)
Global climate change	Diarrheal diseases Respiratory infections Malaria Other communicable diseases	<5
Vehicle ownership and fatality rates	Road traffic accidents	All ages

Note: In IFs, global climate change affects the listed diseases for children under five years of age through its impact on childhood underweight.

Source: IFs project.

$P_{Full}(x)$. Using historical data, we developed formulations for calculating both of these. The latter draws on IFs representation of the food system. Most directly, it is a function of available calories per capita within a country, which reflects dynamics around income levels and food prices that, in turn, respond to land resources and use, crop yields, fish catch and aquaculture, energy prices, and more.[35]

The population distributions and relative risks provide all the information necessary to calculate the adjustment factor and the adjusted mortality, Mortality$_{Full}$, using the equation specified earlier in the section titled "The basic proximate-driver approach in IFs." Since we deal only with a single risk factor in this case, the formulation requires nothing further.

Dealing with multiple risk factors

Sometimes more than one risk factor will be linked to a particular disease. In theory, this requires estimating joint relative risks and exposure distributions. Under certain circumstances, however, a simple method can be used to calculate a combined PAF that involves multiple risk factors (Ezzati et al. 2004a):

$$PAF^{combined} = 1 - \prod(1-PAF^i)$$

where
   PAF^i is the PAF for risk factor i

The logic here is as follows: 1-PAF^i represents the proportion of the disease that is not attributable to risk factor i. Multiplying these 1-PAF^i terms yields the share of the disease that is not attributable to any of the risk factors, and subtracting this product from 1 leaves the share of the disease that is attributable to the set of risk factors considered.

Say that we have two risk factors:[36]

$$PAF^{combined} = 1 - (1-PAF^1)(1-PAF^2)$$

Following from the discussion above, the combined adjustment factor can be calculated as:

$$((1-PAF^{combined}_{Distal}) / (1-PAF^{combined}_{Full})) =$$
$$[(1-PAF^1_{Distal})(1-PAF^2_{Distal})] / [(1-PAF^1_{Full})$$
$$(1-PAF^2_{Full})]$$

$$= [(1-PAF^1_{Distal}) / (1-PAF^1_{Full})] * [(1-PAF^2_{Distal}) /$$
$$(1-PAF^2_{Full})]$$

$$= [\sum RR^1(x)P^1_{Full}(x) / \sum RR^1(x)P^1_{Distal}(x)] *$$
$$[\sum RR^2(x)P^2_{Full}(x) / \sum RR^2(x)P^2_{Distal}(x)]$$

In other words, the combined adjustment factor is a simple multiplication of the individual adjustment factors.

Other proximate-driver modifications of distal formulations

In limited cases, GBD researchers decided that model behavior necessitated proximate-driver modifications to the distal-driver approach. For example, while distal relationships suggest falling rates of noncommunicable disease over time, the popular assumption that BMI levels will continue to increase over the next decade(s) indicates that diabetes mortality might actually rise in the near to mid-future.[37] Similarly, in the GBD 2002 update, Mathers and Loncar (2006) introduced an adjustment factor related to smoking to re-estimate chronic respiratory–related mortality (a subset of other noncommunicable disease), citing concerns that distal-driver projections alone did not adequately reflect assumptions of decreasing smoking rates in high-income countries (Mathers and Loncar, Protocol S1 Technical Appendix, n.d.: 6). We generally followed the GBD approach to these two disease categories, with slight modifications for endogenizing our BMI forecasts into diabetes as described below.

Diabetes. For a population at a "theoretical minimum" level of BMI (mean 21 and one standard deviation), we assume that diabetes-related mortality will decrease over time at 75 percent of the rate of other noncommunicable disease–related mortality, following the logic employed by the GBD researchers (see again Mathers and Loncar, Protocol S1 Technical Appendix, n.d: 5). For a population with levels of BMI above the theoretical minimum, however, we compute a country-, age-, and sex-specific shift factor (labeled "diabetes relative risk" in the IFs model) that modifies this expected decrease in other noncommunicable disease–related mortality rates in order to

■ We used the approach of the CRA project to deal with multiple (interacting) risk factors. ■

determine the expected diabetes-related mortality rate.

For each unit of BMI increase, the relative risk of diabetes-related mortality (compared to a theoretical minimum population) ranges from approximately 1.4 for females and 1.2 for males, depending on age group.[38] Since we do not forecast age-specific BMIs in IFs (due largely to a lack of historical data), we initialize our diabetes shift factor to match those provided by the GBD project. However, in forecasts after 2005 we use our assumptions around future BMI to drive projections.

Respiratory diseases. The two subsets of chronic respiratory conditions—chronic obstructive pulmonary disease (COPD) and other chronic respiratory conditions—are computed separately from other noncommunicable diseases, and both follow the same formulation:

$$Mort = LN(SIR*RR + 1-SIR) *(Exp(ONCD\_Mort)^{0.75})$$

SIR is a "smoking impact ratio," calculated as smoking impact divided by an adjustment factor that is specific to age, gender, and to some regional differentiation.[39] Relative risks (RR in the above equation) are also specific to gender, age, and type (COPD or other respiratory disease) and were provided by the GBD authors. ONCD_Mort is other noncommunicable disease mortality.

Disability and DALYs

To represent morbidity, we followed the path of Mathers and Loncar (2005 and 2006) and linked change in years of living with disability over-time to change in years of life lost over-time. In general, the GBD approach posits that disability declines at a rate that is some fraction of decline in mortality rates (from 0 or no decline in disability to 100 percent, or fully comparable decline). As Mathers and Loncar explained:

> YLD projections were generally derived from the YLL projections by applying the ratio of YLD to YLL for 2002. For ischaemic heart disease and stroke, future incidence rates were assumed to decline at 50% of their mortality rate declines reflecting

declining case fatality rates as well as incidence rates. For causes where there is little or no mortality, age-sex-specific YLD rates per capita were generally assumed to remain constant into the future. For certain mental disorders, musculoskeletal conditions, and hearing loss, disability weights were assumed to decline somewhat with improvements in income per capita reflecting increasing treatment coverage. YLD rates for nonfatal communicable diseases and nutritional deficiencies were assumed to decline at between 50% and 100% of the mortality rate declines for Group I causes. (2006: 2016)

Table 3.2 shows the relative rates of decline that the IFs project adapted from the GBD discussion. In all cases, the rate of decline in morbidity rate is posited to be equal to or less than the decline in mortality rate, frequently only half as much. One of the strong implications of the approach and of the coefficients that are less than 100 percent is that the forecasts will generate an ongoing shift of total disease burden from mortality to disability.

In contrast to this expeditiously simple approach to forecasting disability in IFs, existing evidence provides a complicated picture of the relationship between declining mortality and morbidity. For chronic diseases such as cardiovascular diseases, reductions in cause-specific mortality result from treatment as well as from prevention, meaning that decreased mortality should be associated with relatively less decline in the incidence of the disease (Mathers and Loncar, Protocol S1 Technical Appendix, n.d.). As a greater proportion of incident cases survive and continue to be affected by the disease, prevalence rates should rise, an expectation confirmed by empirical data (CDC and The Merck Company Foundation 2007; Robine and Michel 2004). In other words, the decline in incidence or prevalence of a disease associated with a mortality decline should be determined by the relative prominence of prevention (reducing both incidence and prevalence) versus treatment (which should not affect incidence and should increase prevalence).

● *IFs forecasts disability rates from disease-specific relationships between morbidity and mortality.* ●

Moreover, the basic logic of the current approach in IFs does not address changes in disease severity as mortality declines. While the survival of those who would otherwise have been most likely to die might increase the average severity of disease among surviving cases, it is also quite possible that the very treatments that reduce mortality would also reduce disease severity across the entire distribution of illness. In fact, most recent evidence points to reductions in morbidity (as measured by self-rated health status and performance on the activities of daily living) that outstrip the pace of mortality reduction, meaning that even as populations grow older, they spend a greater proportion of those extra years in good health (Crimmins 2004; Payne et al. 2007; Robine and Michel 2004). In other words, even as prevalence increases due to greater survivorship, reductions in the average severity of disease may be so great as to reduce the overall burden of morbidity (Crimmins 2004; Mathers et al. 2004). See further discussion on this issue in Chapter 7.

Conclusion

Considering the importance of health to us individually and as societies, modeling and forecasting health outcomes is a remarkably new activity. Movement beyond attention to life expectancy and age-specific mortality in the aggregate to the exploration of future multiple-cause mortality extends back only about two decades. The Global Burden of Disease project broke much important new ground in its analyses of causes of mortality and disability and in its two major sets of projections, each extending about 30 years.

We have been fortunate in being able to build significantly on the GBD project's distal-driver approach in our IFs work. There is, however, reason to believe that the future of forecasting will turn increasingly to a more hybrid, integrated analysis of systems, more regularly supplementing distal-driver analysis with attention to the kind of proximate-driver and elaborated structural representations that better allow modelers to connect forecasting with policy analysis. Moreover,

almost inevitably there will be increasing efforts to integrate health modeling with the modeling of demographic and economic systems (minimally), and probably with some representation of environmental, socio-political, and other specialized systems, such as agriculture and energy.

We cannot pretend to feel highly confident in our efforts to construct and use such a hybrid, integrated health model in a broader modeling system. Nonetheless, the foundations do exist upon which to at least tentatively explore the possible futures of global health in larger context. The next chapter lays out a base case forecast of global health as a foundation, before it and subsequent chapters turn to exploration of possible alternative health futures.

Table 3.2 Percent changes in disability relative to declines in mortality by cause in IFs

	Percent changes in disability with changes in mortality
Communicable diseases	
Diarrheal diseases	75
HIV/AIDS	75
Malaria	100
Respiratory infections	100
Other communicable diseases	75
Noncommunicable diseases	
Cardiovascular diseases	50
Diabetes	100
Digestive disorders	100
Malignant neoplasms	100
Respiratory diseases	100
Other noncommunicable diseases	100
Injuries	
Intentional injuries	75
Road traffic accidents	75
Other unintentional injuries	75

Note: Mortality refers to years of life lost and disability to years of living with disability; IFs also represents mental health but does not model a mortality/morbidity relationship for it.

Source: Except for HIV/AIDs, IFs project estimates for communicable and noncommunicable diseases are based primarily on Table 6 (page 19) of Mathers and Loncar Protocol S1 Technical Appendix [n.d.]; the estimates for HIV/AIDs and injuries are IFs project assumptions.

1 For introduction to the character and use of the model, see Hughes and Hillebrand 2006.

2 More technically, the model structure is recursive (it computes equations sequentially in each time-step without simultaneous solution). It combines features of systems dynamics (notably the accounting structures with careful attention to both flows and stocks) and econometrics (using estimated equations for the dynamic behavior of the agent-classes).

3 The broader population forecasting methodology is available at www.census.gov/ population/www/ documentation/twps0038.pdf. The method uses fixed-point logistic models.

4 The full Delphi method involves multiple and systematic iterations across a group of experts to map (and generally narrow) disagreement and establish a central tendency (Gordon and Helmer-Hirschberg 1964).

5 Although IIASA historically forecast population by global region, it has moved to country and even intra-country analysis.

6 See, for example, Jamison et al. 1993; Jamison et al. 2006; Lopez et al. 2006a; Mathers and Loncar 2006; Murray and Lopez 1996b; WHO 2008a; 2009a; and World Bank 1993.

7 See the individual chapters in the recent Disease Control Priorities project report for examples of this approach (Jamison et al. 2006).

8 See http://data.unaids.org/pub/Presentation/2009/ 20090414_spectrum_2009_en.pdf and also Stover et al. 2008.

9 Similarly, Homer and Hirsch (2006) developed a systems dynamics model to explore the role of public health systems in prevention and care of chronic disease.

10 It is partly for this reason that the creators of the GBD models added exogenous specification of smoking impact to the otherwise mostly monotonically (one-direction only) changing specifications.

11 We are indebted to Dr. Colin Mathers, who generously shared with us his original database and regression models and provided responses to our many queries about them. We regret and accept full responsibility for any errors we may have made in our use of them.

12 Using the GBD historical data, we re-estimated the formulation for cardiovascular diseases in order to correct for a discrepancy in the direction of the coefficient for female smoking at older ages.

13 IFs represents populations in five-year intervals up through 100+, whereas the oldest age category in the GBD data combined all ages from 85+. In addition, we are able to represent infants separately (as well as within the 0–5 age category), and the GBD project only included them in the 0–5 group.

14 The GBD's detailed death file of mortality rates for 2004 was provided by Dr. Colin Mathers.

15 We began by spreading the same death rates for all five-year age categories within larger categories, but then used smoothing procedures for the initial spread so as to represent better the changing patterns of mortality by cause of death across five-year categories. We normalized the death rates across disease types so as to make the total death rates of countries consistent with UNPD data for each five-year category.

16 As we noted earlier, Mathers and Loncar (2006) did not separately estimate infants (those under one year of age); we used their coefficients for the under-five age category for infants also.

17 We used the UNPD's 2008 revision for initialization.

18 Complicating initialization further, the UNPD presents its data in five-year ranges, including 2000–2005 and 2005–2010. The age- and sex-specific survivor-table values in those ranges therefore do not correspond to specific years like our base of 2005. After correspondence with Kirill Andreev of the UNPD, which we acknowledge appreciatively, we decided to average the mortality values in the two five-year ranges ending and beginning with 2005.

19 Since Mathers and Loncar did not provide coefficients specifically for diarrheal diseases and malaria, we use those provided for the more general category of infectious and parasitic diseases. They provide separate coefficients for gender and seven age categories but not region. We calculate the adjustment factors in the same way as for other diseases, as described later in this chapter.

20 In theory, if $\beta > 1$ ($\beta < 1$) and the mortality rate for the general cause-group increased (decreased) sufficiently, the mortality rate for the detailed cause could exceed the mortality rate for the general cause-group. Furthermore, if $\beta > 1$ and the mortality rate for the general cause-group decreased, the mortality rate for the detailed cause theoretically could fall below zero. As these would represent illogical results, we checked to make sure that these situations did not occur in the actual projections or, if they did, we—as Mathers explained to us the GBD researchers did—adjusted the sum of the specific causes to match the projected general cause-group rate.

21 Mathers and Loncar in their Protocol S1 Technical Appendix (n.d.: 8) said that their approach assumed 25-year time lags between tobacco consumption and smoking impact.

22 The IFs smoking impact forecast is age-cohort specific, while our smoking rate is not; thus, we needed a weighted average growth rate. The weighting used the population-cohort sizes in 2005.

23 There is not a one-to-one relationship, of course, between smoking rate and smoking impact based simply on a lag. Many other factors, including what is smoked and how (including frequency), will affect smoking impact. Treatment might also be an impact, although the GBD time/technology variable in the distal formulation could pick up some of that. We further understand that our historical smoking series is stylized.

24 The IFs approach does not use an incidence-based model, which would be an alternative. Such a model would also allow specification of mother-to-child transmission and of treatment coverage and success.

25 The IFs pre-processor calculates initial rates of HIV prevalence and annual changes in it using the middle estimates of the UNAIDS 2008 data. When middle estimates do not exist, as in the case of the Democratic Republic of Congo, it uses an average of high and low estimates. The system uses data for total population prevalence but also includes HIV prevalence for those 15–49.

26 A more satisfactory approach would use stocks and flows and would have a more strongly systems dynamics character. It would track infected individuals, presumably by age cohorts, but at least in the aggregate. It would compute new infections (incidence) annually, adding those to existing prevalence numbers, transitioning those already infected into some combination of those manifesting AIDS, those dying, and those advancing in age with HIV. But the data do not seem widely available to parameterize such transition rates, especially at age-category levels.

27 Table 17 of the Annex to "World Population Prospects: The 2002 Revision" (UNPD 2003: 77–78) provided such estimates for 38 African countries and selected others outside of Africa; the IFs project has revised and calibrated many of the estimates over time as more data have become available. By 2004–2006, however, quite a number of countries had begun to experience reductions, and this logic has become less important except in scenario analysis for countries where prevalence is still rising.

28 Early epidemic data from sub-Saharan Africa and the United States supported this assumption.

29 Dargay, Gately, and Sommer (2007) also describe an adjustment factor related to the percentage of a total population residing in urban areas; we did not implement that factor.

30 Http://en.wikipedia.org/wiki/Smeed%27s_law. See Adams (1987) and Smeed (1949). Others have disputed the law.

31 For each age-sex-cause-specific regression, HealthExp% was added and tested for significance. After considering Ordinary Least Squares (OLS), random-effects, and fixed-effects models, only the HealthExp% effect on all-cause mortality for the age 0–4 age group was considered sufficiently robust. Because HealthExp% effects are specified as linear, they could be quite large for countries with extraordinarily high levels of HealthExp%, particularly when combined with low GDP per capita. Few such cases exist within the existing distribution, however. For today's countries with GDP per capita below $15,000, HealthExp% has a mean of 6.3%, a standard deviation of 1.6%, and a range from 2.4% to 10.5%. HealthExp% also tends to be somewhat higher for wealthier countries in this group. Using the results implied by these regressions and sensitivity testing of the IFs base model, we find that the effect of a one standard deviation change in HealthExp% on $_5q_0$ (about 2.6% lower) is about one-fifth as large as the effect of a one standard deviation change in GDP per capita (about a 14% reduction).

32 "Dictionary of Cancer Terms," National Cancer Institute, http://www.cancer.gov/dictionary/ (accessed January 2010).

33 This is very reasonable for $P'(x)$ by its definition. With respect to $RR(x)$, we assume these to be the same for all countries unless otherwise specified in the CRA reports. Any change over time is likely to be picked up in other parts of our model dealing with changes in technology and the efficiency of health care systems.

34 The mortality rate for the residual category consisting of measles and other communicable diseases is calculated as the difference between the mortality rate for the general category "communicable diseases other than HIV/AIDS" as a whole and the sum of the separate mortality rates for diarrhea, respiratory infections, and malaria.

35 We present further details on these formulations in Chapter 5 in the section on undernutrition and in the technical documentation of the IFs health model at www.ifs.du.edu.

36 In the sequence of our calculations we decompose this equation in practice by finding the individual PAFs, computing their individual independent effects with (1-PAFDistal)/(1-PAFFull), and multiplying mortality independently and cumulatively.

37 In the CRA study on overweight and obesity, James et al. (2004: 498) reported that 58 percent of the global burden of type 2 diabetes was attributable to increases in BMI. Note that the study's assumption of rising BMI rates over time is not always replicated in IFs forecasts.

38 Relative risk estimates taken from Kelly et al. (2009).

39 Dr. Mathers provided us with the GBD project's adjustment factors, which remain constant over time in the forecast (although, since smoking impact changes over time, SIR does change with year). China and a subset of countries in Southeast Asia (Bangladesh, Bhutan, Democratic People's Republic of Korea, India, Maldives, Myanmar, and Nepal) were treated separately from one another and from the single "world" category in which all other countries were combined.

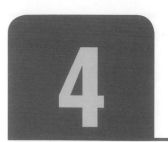

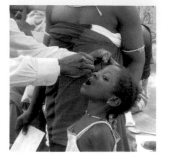

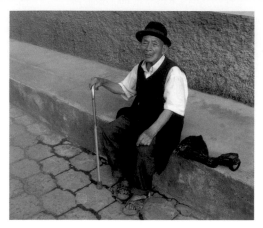

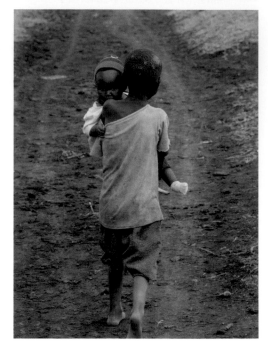

The Current Path as It Seems to Be Unfolding

■ *How might global patterns of health change as this century unfolds?* ■

Assuming that historical relationships among income, education, and health outcomes remain relatively stable, how might global patterns of health change as this century unfolds? Should countries currently beset mostly by communicable diseases expect more of the same or instead (or additionally) start to prepare themselves for an onslaught of chronic diseases? In higher-income countries how rapid might be the seemingly inexorable rise in the portion of citizens who are retired and how long might they live in good and ill health? How could health outcome forecasts vary with different projections of income or education? Such questions matter greatly for policymakers and stakeholders seeking to develop systems that best support population health and well-being.

The attempt to explore changing patterns of health drives both this chapter and the rest of this volume. This chapter begins by presenting the International Futures (IFs) base case or reference case forecasts of global health

(where current conditions of the system and its dynamics appear to be taking us).[1] We also compare our base case with other forecasts, to the extent that such are available.

We know, of course, that forecasts even 10 years into the future will be wrong. Thus, we must not only present our base case but also direct attention in this analysis to some of the greatest uncertainties with respect to that forecast—uncertainties with respect to the key drivers of health and their relationships with health systems, uncertainties with respect to leverage of human interventions, and uncertainties that could result from even greater surprises in the system. This chapter begins the analysis of uncertainty, and subsequent chapters will continue it.

The Base Case

While distal or broad factors such as income or education do not directly cause mortality and morbidity, historical relationships between these factors and outcomes provide a starting point for thinking about probable health futures. Thus, as discussed in Chapter 3, we begin our exploration of the path of global health with analyses rooted in the distal-driver formulations created for the 2002 and 2004 versions of the Global Burden of Disease (GBD) analysis (Mathers and Loncar 2006; WHO 2008a), supplemented by inclusion of selected health risk factors. Most of our results extend the IFs base case (see Box 4.1) to 2060, and in some cases to the end of the century. (In Chapters 5 and 6, we will turn our attention to the potential impact of alternative forecasts of the proximate risk factors.)

Life expectancy

We begin by looking at the most widely used aggregate health measure, that of life expectancy. Figure 4.1 shows historical increases in life expectancy separately for females and males since 1960 and the IFs forecast through 2100 for each World Bank developing region and a single high-income country grouping (see Box 4.2 for discussion of country groupings). The long horizon of Figure 4.1 provides context for subsequent analyses focusing on the period until 2060.

The historical patterns themselves are of considerable interest. They clearly show the power of disruptive events and periods, three in particular. First, in East Asia and Pacific there was a substantial jump in life expectancy in the earliest years of the historical period. In 1960, the life expectancy of China had fallen to 36 years because of the horrendous turmoil associated with the ironically named "Great Leap Forward." By 1967, it had rebounded to nearly 60 years. Given China's sizable population, the impact on regional and even global averages was substantial. Second, the HIV/AIDS epidemic is clear in the pattern of sub-Saharan Africa. The probable peaking of AIDS deaths (to which we will return) explains the reversal in the early years of the post-2005 forecast of the dip in life expectancy we see in the late years of the historical series. For instance, in Botswana life expectancy fell from 64 years in 1985–1990 to 48 years in 2000–2005; the United Nations Population Division forecasts a return to 55 years in the 2005–2010 period (UNPD 2009b: 13). Third, in Europe and Central Asia (which in the absence of the high-income countries

consists mostly of former communist countries), life expectancy was fundamentally flat across the historical period, with male life expectancy actually dropping in the post-Soviet era. Again, some reversal of the decline is underway. Collectively, these historical patterns constitute a warning with respect to the forecasts—the future is unlikely to unfold as smoothly as those lines suggest.

More generally, these historical patterns also show us how regional stories can change quite significantly over a period of a few decades. In 1960, life expectancies of countries in developing Europe and Central Asia and in the high-income grouping were very nearly the same, as were those in sub-Saharan Africa and South Asia. By 2005, however, the regions in each of these pairings had diverged. On the other hand, over the same period the Middle East and North African region had quite dramatically narrowed its gap with the high-income countries.

Looking forward, several issues of interest are apparent in the historical and forecast series of life expectancy by region, shown from 1960 through 2100 in Figure 4.1. One is the gap between the rich and poor of the world, which the figure clearly shows to be narrowing, but nonetheless quite slowly until well into the century. A second concerns the unfolding of HIV/AIDS, especially given the recent character of the possible peaking of the epidemic; more

Box 4.1 The base case of IFs

The base case is not a simple extrapolation of variables in multiple issue areas, including health, but rather the dynamic, nonlinear output of the fully integrated IFs system. The integrated system of the base case includes the health model that Chapter 3 described, with both its distal and proximate formulations activated. Thus, health forecasts respond to demographic, economic, education, and other models of IFs and, in turn, affect their behavior. Among the most obvious consequences of this integration are that changes in health result in changes in population and GDP, which can either accelerate or retard further changes in health outcomes (via positive and negative feedbacks). Chapter 7 will explore these linkages and dynamics in some detail.

The forecasts that other IFs system models produce of key drivers, such as GDP per capita and educational attainment of adults, are thus foundational underpinnings of its health forecasts. Hughes et al. (2009: 56–71) explored those forecasts, comparing them to other forecasts such as those of the UNPD and World Bank. As a general rule, the IFs base case produces behavior that tends to be quite similar to medium variant or base forecasts of such analyses (see also Hughes 2004 and 2006). We note that our forecasts of African economic growth tend to be slightly more optimistic than most other analyses. We note too that we build in the "great recession" with International Monetary Fund-based assumptions, beginning in 2007 and ending for most of the world by 2011, and we forecast peak global oil production between 2030 and 2040, with some consequences for economic growth of oil producers and consumers.

generally, the rate of decline in communicable diseases will especially affect the forecasts for the developing regions. A third issue is the rate of potential expansion in life expectancy of those countries and populations at the leading edge of the fight against chronic diseases. In Figure 4.1, especially for males, there is a slowing in the forecasted growth pattern of the rates of extension in life expectancy in the high-income countries between the historical pattern and the forecasts.

Following the lead of the Commission on Social Determinants of Health (CSDH 2008) in looking at the gap in life expectancy at birth (LEB) between the sixty countries with the longest and shortest LEBs, Figure 4.2 shows that gap historically and in our base case forecast (life expectancies in 2005 define the two country sets). The CSDH goal is a reduction of that gap by 10 years between 2000 and 2040. Figure 4.2 suggests the complications of attaining that goal and the very great improbability that we will do so. One historical complication is that, after several decades of decline, the gap began increasing in the 1990s as a direct result of the HIV/AIDS epidemic.

The epidemic may have peaked (to be discussed below), but the recentness of that turn gives us less confidence than we would like in the forecast that the historical rate of decline in the gap after 1960 will resume, perhaps even with some catch-up. Another factor that makes goal achievement difficult is more positive—life expectancies of high-income countries continue to advance. Even with renewed decline in the gap, movement of the difference in life expectancy from 18.8 years in 2000 to 8.8 appears unlikely to happen until after 2060 (in fact, not until near the end of the century). The goal, unfortunately, appears overly ambitious.

The forecasts of advance in regional life expectancy in Figure 4.1 and of reduction in the global gap in Figure 4.2 depend on what will happen with respect to advances against communicable and chronic diseases. With respect to communicable diseases, there are many wild cards, including the possible mutation of known diseases and/or emergence of new ones that are not responsive to existing modes of prevention and treatment. The best-recognized wild card is the continued unfolding

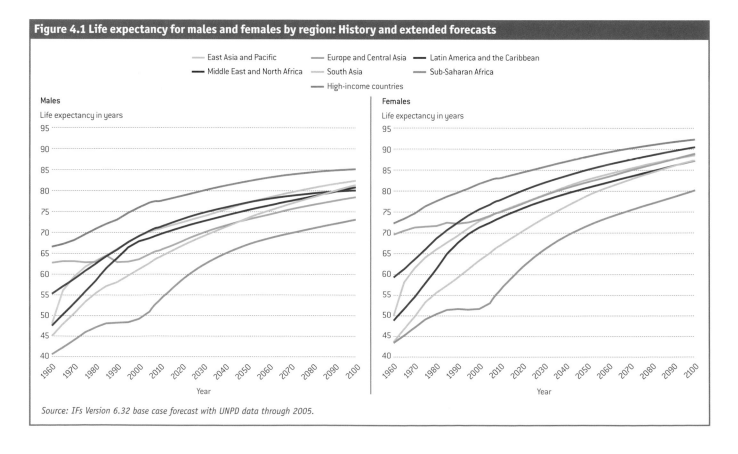

Figure 4.1 Life expectancy for males and females by region: History and extended forecasts

East Asia and Pacific — Europe and Central Asia — Latin America and the Caribbean
Middle East and North Africa — South Asia — Sub-Saharan Africa
High-income countries

Males
Life expectancy in years

Females
Life expectancy in years

Year

Year

Source: IFs Version 6.32 base case forecast with UNPD data through 2005.

● *Overall, our forecasts for continued decline in deaths from communicable diseases are very encouraging (about 70 percent by 2060).* ●

of the HIV/AIDS epidemic. Globally, annual deaths due to AIDS rose very rapidly from about 225,000 in 1990 to 2 million just 14 years later. Although UNAIDS estimates of deaths drop from that peak in 2004 to 1.85 million in 2007, forecasts are very challenging.

As we turn to Figure 4.3, recall that we use the term "communicable diseases" to refer to all Group I diseases or conditions even though the category also includes maternal and perinatal conditions and nutritional deficiencies (about 75 percent of Group I diseases are communicable, and the large majority of the remainder are perinatal conditions). In Figure 4.3 we show separate IFs base case forecasts of deaths for four major communicable diseases (AIDS, diarrhea, malaria, and respiratory infections) and a combined category—"other communicable diseases"—modeled in the aggregate, which includes deaths from maternal and perinatal conditions and nutritional deficiencies as well as other communicable diseases (e.g., tuberculosis, measles, and parasitic infections). Our forecast of deaths in the combined category is slightly less than the sum of deaths from the four separately modeled categories.

Overall, our forecasts for decline in global deaths from all communicable diseases are very positive, with a reduction of just over 40 percent by 2030 and almost 70 percent by 2060. This is generally consistent with historical patterns of progress against most of the diseases. The greatest uncertainty most likely

attends the magnitude of decline we forecast for AIDS deaths; our forecast for decline in deaths from malaria may also be somewhat optimistic given the disease's historical persistence and propensity for resurgence. Importantly, with forecasted continuing increases in population, communicable disease mortality rates (not shown) are forecast to drop even more rapidly than numbers of deaths.

Whereas our forecasts for deaths from communicable disease might appear optimistic, our forecasts for mortality more generally

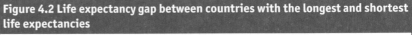

Figure 4.2 Life expectancy gap between countries with the longest and shortest life expectancies

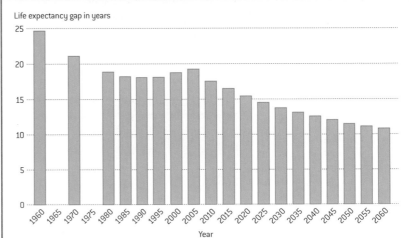

Life expectancy gap in years

Note: The comparison is between populations in the 60 longest-lived countries and those in the 60 shortest-lived countries; country groupings are based on 2005 data.

Source: IFs Version 6.32 base case forecast using all available UNPD data through 2005.

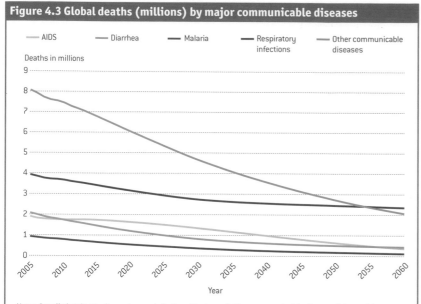

Figure 4.3 Global deaths (millions) by major communicable diseases

— AIDS   — Diarrhea   — Malaria   — Respiratory infections   — Other communicable diseases

Deaths in millions

Year

Note: Recall that in IFs discussion and displays the term "other communicable diseases" is used to describe all Group I diseases that we do not forecast separately. Thus, the term as we use it includes maternal and perinatal conditions and nutritional deficiencies as well as the communicable diseases that we do not forecast separately. Tuberculosis and perinatal conditions are the major diseases in our undifferentiated category.

Source: IFs Version 6.32 base case forecast.

exceed that of the nearest following population by more than a full year, even catch-up by other countries will be challenging, much less the forging of a faster pace of increase.[2]

One key reason that life expectancy gains may slow is that the room for further dramatic reduction of infant and child mortality due to communicable diseases and maternal and perinatal diseases (key reasons for past major advances in life expectancy even in high-income countries) has greatly decreased. Future mortality reductions need to come from adult and older adult populations, where they have historically been more difficult to achieve and where they proportionately add many fewer years of life expectancy. And they require attention to a different kind of disease burden—that caused primarily by noncommunicable diseases.

Changing disease burden

The nature of the global burden of disease is changing. As the previous section indicated, a rapid reduction is underway, and forecast to continue, in death rates and deaths from communicable diseases. Figure 4.4 reinforces this point by comparing communicable disease death rates in sub-Saharan Africa with those in high-income countries at three different points in time. According to the base case forecast, by 2060 communicable disease death rates in sub-Saharan Africa will have declined dramatically and almost reached the extremely low death rates forecast for those of the high-income countries.

Figure 4.5 shows a similar comparison for noncommunicable disease death rates, again contrasting those of sub-Saharan Africa with

● At the same time, we forecast a slowing of life expectancy gains for system leaders. ●

may appear more pessimistic. Our base case forecasts suggest that, after a long period of quite steady gains, countries and regions on the leading edge of life expectancy may experience decreasing incremental gains in future decades (see Table 4.1).

Such slowing of gains by system leaders may not be unreasonable, especially given 2005 data that indicate the pace of increase for the life expectancy of Japanese women had already slowed significantly relative to the rate of the prior decade. Moreover, given that the life expectancy of Japanese women has come to

● The global burden of disease is shifting to noncommunicable diseases and conditions. ●

Table 4.1 Life expectancy of females in globally leading country: History and forecast

	Expected years of life	Increase in years per decade	Globally leading country
1960	76.1		Iceland
1970	77.6	1.5	Norway
1980	79.8	2.2	Iceland
1990	82.5	2.7	Japan
2000	85.7	3.2	Japan
2010	86.8	1.1	Japan
2030	89.3	1.3	Japan
2060	92.5	1.1	Japan

Source: IFs Version 6.32 base case forecast with UNPD data through 2000.

those of high-income countries. The gaps between the two groups today are much less dramatic than those for communicable diseases. While we forecast progress in both country groupings over the period, we also forecast a more modest rate of decline than for communicable diseases. We also expect that the smaller inter-regional gaps will close much more slowly than those for communicable diseases.

Rooted in these changing patterns of death rates, the aggregate global burden of disease (see the Forecast Tables at the end of this volume for country and regional values) is changing in several ways, including (1) the relative balance of disease types, and (2) the

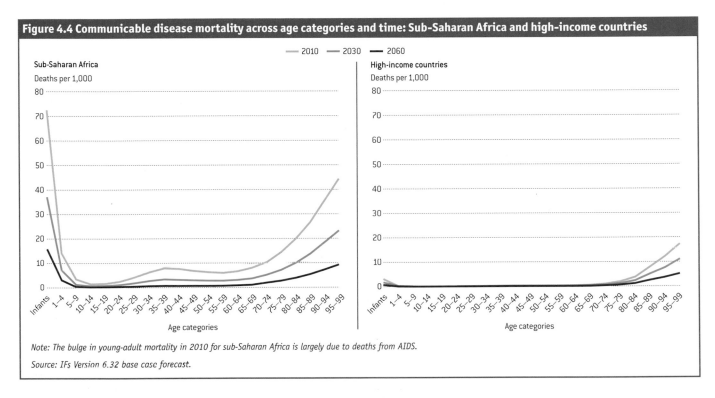

Figure 4.4 Communicable disease mortality across age categories and time: Sub-Saharan Africa and high-income countries

Note: The bulge in young-adult mortality in 2010 for sub-Saharan Africa is largely due to deaths from AIDS.

Source: IFs Version 6.32 base case forecast.

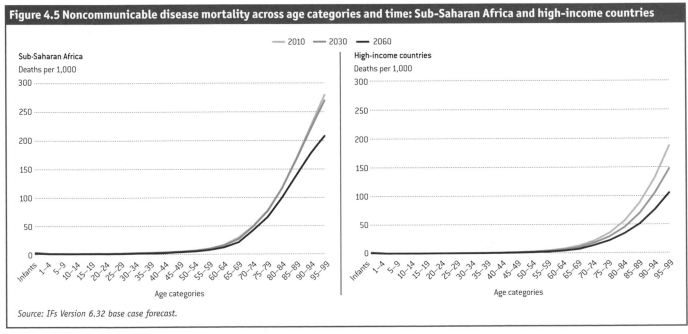

Figure 4.5 Noncommunicable disease mortality across age categories and time: Sub-Saharan Africa and high-income countries

Source: IFs Version 6.32 base case forecast.

balance between mortality and morbidity. Figure 4.6 shows the changing relative burden of global disease across the major disease groups.

In the top panel of Figure 4.6, global deaths in millions show the rapid ongoing shift away from deaths due to communicable diseases to deaths from noncommunicable diseases (already the major cause category in 2005). Even in sub-Saharan Africa, the balance will shift to the latter around 2030 in the base case, and in 2060 sub-Saharan Africa's deaths from noncommunicable diseases will outnumber those from communicable diseases by more than 5 to 1. These shifts reflect changing death rates (as illustrated in Figures 4.4 and 4.5) in combination with a changed (older) population structure.

The picture is rather different, however, when we turn to years of life lost (discounted and age-weighted), calculated in IFs as the number of years between the age at death and the gender-specific life expectancy in the country with the longest life span at that time. Communicable diseases cause most deaths in the early years of life (see again Figure 4.4) and therefore result in more years of life lost per individual. The middle panel of Figure 4.6 shows that they currently account for most years of life lost, and that it will not be until the 2020s, and then only if communicable diseases continue the forecasted dramatic decline, that noncommunicable diseases will cause the majority of years of life lost worldwide (and not until the early 2050s in sub-Saharan Africa). The balance is, however, shifting very rapidly.

The third panel in Figure 4.6 provides still another perspective on change in

global disease burden. When we consider years of living with disability (again with discounting and age-weighting), chronic diseases heavily dominate the global pattern. In fact, by the late 2030s, injuries are projected to create a heavier total disability burden than do communicable diseases, one reason to be increasingly concerned with road traffic accidents. (The reality is that the methodology for forecasting change in disability rates is sufficiently simple and uncertain that we should read these as indications of possible tendencies rather than as forecasts per se.)

Overall, Figures 4.4, 4.5, and 4.6 show the remarkable transition we expect will occur around the world during the first half of this century in the burden of disease (Box 4.3 and Table 4.2 look at the likely progress of Brazil, Russia, India, and China). Whereas the story historically has been the fight against communicable diseases, the world is now in the midst of a dramatic shift to chronic conditions as the primary source of death and disability—a shift that is occurring also in sub-Saharan Africa, despite its very large remaining communicable disease burden.

Attention to global goals

In recent years, the health indicators that have received the most attention have been those of the Millennium Development Goals (MDGs), which explicitly call for reduction of infant and child (under-five) mortality rates by two-thirds between 1990 and 2015 and maternal mortality rates by three-fourths. The goals also call for halting and reversing growth in incidence of malaria, HIV/AIDS, and tuberculosis by 2015.

With respect to the disease-specific goals, our forecasts do suggest major reductions in those disease rates (see again Figure 4.3). However, with respect to the age-specific goals,

Box 4.3. Will the large and rapidly developing BRICs (Brazil, Russia, India, and China) catch up with the high-income countries?

Yes and no. Setting aside child mortality, which by 2060 will likely drop to the quite low level of about three children per 1,000 dying before reaching age five, we can focus on the probability of a 15-year-old dying before reaching the age of 60. Table 4.2 suggests that the BRICs will substantially narrow the absolute gap between themselves and the high-income countries, but that even so their probability of such death will remain about twice as high in 2060, and that even then the BRICs will not have reached the level of the high-income countries in 2010. In short, although their aggregate economic size will likely have passed that of the high-income countries, they will lag behind system leaders in important aspects of human development. Moreover, there is great variation among the BRICs now (the probable number of 15-year-olds dying before age 60 is now about 280 per 1,000 in Russia versus 124 per 1,000 in China), and the variation is likely to remain high in 2060.

Table 4.2 Probable number of 15-year-olds per 1,000 dying before age 60: BRICs and high-income countries

	2010	2030	2060
BRICs	165	133	97
High-income countries	76	62	48

Source: IFs Version 6.32 base case forecast.

the left panel of Figure 4.7 suggests that not a single region of the world is likely to meet the infant mortality goal—and therefore, by implication, the child mortality goal with which it is closely correlated. Latin America and the Caribbean and East Asia and Pacific are likely to come reasonably close, with reductions near 60 percent. Europe and Central Asia, South Asia, Middle East and North Africa, and the high-income countries are all likely to post close to 50 percent reductions over that period. Sub-Saharan Africa, although it will likely make substantially greater absolute progress than any other region, will have, in the base case experience, a reduction closer to one-third (about the rate of reduction between 1960 and 1990). Rates of reduction in the next 25-year period, between 2015 and 2040, are likely to be quite a bit faster for sub-Saharan Africa but slower in other regions than in recent years (as the values get very low in other regions, rates of progress will logically begin to decline).

More recently, WHO's Commission on Social Determinants of Health (CSDH 2008) called for 90 percent reductions in under-five mortality between 2000 and 2040. In the case of sub-Saharan Africa that would require a decrease from about 150 per 1,000 to 7.5 per 1,000, and our base case forecast for 2040 is several times higher than that. In fact, that target rate is about the level of high-income countries today, and our forecasts show it unlikely to be attained in sub-Saharan Africa until near the end of the century.

Although there is no set global goal around it, another widely watched number is the global number of deaths of children under five years of age. Only recently has that number fallen below the widely watched figure of 10 million per year (Black, Morris, and Bryce 2003). In the base case we see that figure dropping to 5.8 million in 2040 and 3.2 million in 2060, a remarkable potential accomplishment. As context for these numbers, IFs forecasts a global total of 623 million children in 2005, 621 million in 2040, and 577 million in 2060.

Earlier (Figure 4.2) we saw that the CSDH's goal for closing the gap in life expectancy at birth between longest- and shortest-lived country sets was unlikely to be met. The CSDH also called for halving adult morality rates in all countries, and in all social groups within them, between 2000 and 2040 (CSDH 2008: 107).

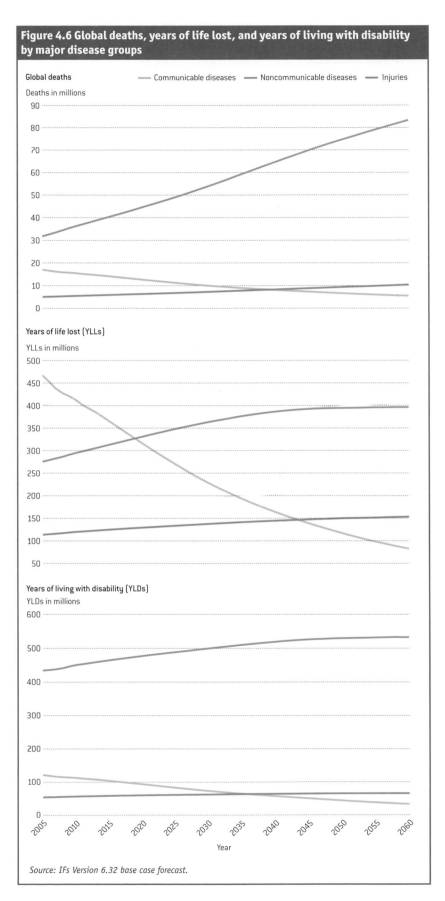

Figure 4.6 Global deaths, years of life lost, and years of living with disability by major disease groups

Global deaths

— Communicable diseases   — Noncommunicable diseases   — Injuries

Deaths in millions

Years of life lost (YLLs)

YLLs in millions

Years of living with disability (YLDs)

YLDs in millions

Year

Source: IFs Version 6.32 base case forecast.

Even though it does not include 2000, the right panel of Figure 4.7 suggests that sub-Saharan Africa may well meet that goal at a regional level, with a reduction from 380 per 1,000 in 2005 to 186 per 1,000 in 2040, partly because there is such considerable room for reduction. Such reduction would require significant progress against AIDS as well as a variety of other adult death causes, because the base case shows essentially no decline in the region's age-specific cardiovascular death rates (forecast patterns of the effects of both smoking and obesity work against progress there). The adult mortality goal is, however, unlikely to be met in any other region (Europe and Central Asia and South Asia will likely have one-third or more reductions), in part because the adult mortality rates in most other regions are very considerably below the current high levels of sub-Saharan Africa.

Although there is much room for progress in reducing adult mortality, the process has proceeded quite far in many parts of the world, especially in high-income countries. Adult mortality rates through age 59 have been pushed to quite low levels, with mortality then jumping considerably for those 60 and older, making the right-hand corner of the J-curve more of a right-angle (a process called *rectangularization*). As that process continues, we would expect rates of gain for adults below the age of 60 to slow.

In spite of likely failure to meet most established global health goals, it is important to end this discussion of the base case with some very positive statements about the story of improvements in global health (in particular, reductions in communicable diseases). Progress with respect to reducing disease has been remarkably fast in recent decades and appears to be on track to continue at a strong pace. Although HIV/AIDS and the resurgence of malaria have devastated many countries and communities and obviously slowed the narrowing of the life expectancy gap across countries in the last two decades, progress in narrowing the gap also appears likely to resume, thanks to a great many strong local and global efforts. The fact that many global goals appear unlikely to be met reflects in part an understandable sense of urgency with respect to health progress and a desire to assure that targets are high. It also reflects the quite recent emergence of global health forecasting as a foundation for realistic targeting. Goal setting, if it includes consideration of aggressive but reasonable forecasts, can and almost certainly will improve.

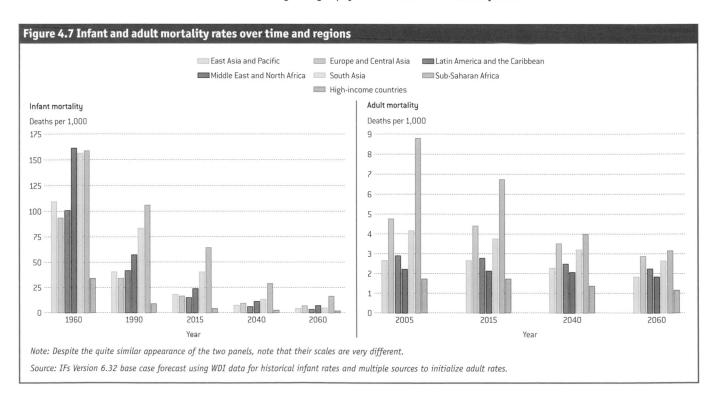

Figure 4.7 Infant and adult mortality rates over time and regions

Legend:
East Asia and Pacific — Europe and Central Asia — Latin America and the Caribbean — Middle East and North Africa — South Asia — Sub-Saharan Africa — High-income countries

Infant mortality
Deaths per 1,000

Adult mortality
Deaths per 1,000

Note: Despite the quite similar appearance of the two panels, note that their scales are very different.

Source: IFs Version 6.32 base case forecast using WDI data for historical infant rates and multiple sources to initialize adult rates.

Comparison with Other Forecasts

Chapter 3 reviewed alternative approaches for providing forecasts relevant to understanding the future of global health, including aggregate (mainly extrapolative) analyses, integrated structural approaches, and specialized disease-specific forecasts. To provide some context for the base case forecasts of IFs, which rely heavily on the distal-driver approach of the GBD project, we compare IFs forecasts with others in each of the three major approaches, considering both the magnitude of differences and the reasons for them.

Life expectancy forecasts: United Nations Population Division

In recent years IFs forecasts of life expectancy have been somewhat higher than those used in the UNPD's population forecasts because the IFs forecasts of AIDS deaths have been lower (we will return to this comparison later). However, the UNPD substantially lowered its forecasts of AIDS deaths in its 2008 revision (UNPD 2009a), and now the magnitude of difference between the two forecasts of life expectancy has declined. As Table 4.3 shows, IFs forecasts a global life expectancy in 2050 of almost two years more than the UNPD projects (the fact that the UN forecast is a period rather than a point forecast complicates exact comparison).[3] Most

of this difference results from more optimistic forecasts in IFs for developing regions, but some also arises from somewhat more optimistic forecasts in more developed regions. With respect to Africa, where the difference is the greatest (three full years), both the economic and the education forecasts of IFs for Africa are somewhat more optimistic than those of many analysts, and these two variables heavily shape the distal-driver health formulations used in the IFs base case.

Earlier we pointed out that patterns of growth in the global average of life expectancy reflect a combination of growth in life expectancy at the leading edge and of the extent of convergence of populations with low life expectancies toward the longer life expectancies at the leading edge. Table 4.4 compares the UNPD forecast for life expectancy of the 10 countries that it anticipates will have the highest values in 2050 with the numbers produced by IFs for the same 10 countries. IFs identifies six of the same 10 countries as likely candidates for the top 10 list (adding France, Norway, Singapore, and the United Kingdom). In general, the expectations from IFs are slightly above those of the UNPD.

Probing more deeply into the basis for forecast differences in life expectancy, we see that recent UNPD forecasts for reductions in

IFs forecasts of life expectancy are somewhat more optimistic than those of the UNPD, particularly for Africa.

Table 4.3 UNPD and IFs life expectancy forecasts in years by region

	UNPD		IFs	
	2005–2010	2045–2050	2005	2050
Africa	54.1	67.4	55.3	70.4
Asia	68.9	76.8	69.3	78.2
Europe	75.1	81.5	75.8	82.7
Latin America and Caribbean	73.4	79.8	73.7	81.2
Northern America	79.3	83.5	79.3	85.2
Oceania	76.4	82.1	76.8	82.2
More developed regions	77.1	82.8	77.2	83.8
Less developed regions	65.6	74.3	67.0	76.3
Least developed countries	55.9	68.5	56.7	70.0
World	67.6	75.5	69.0	77.3

Note: Rather than the World Bank regions commonly displayed in this volume, for comparative purposes this table is organized by the standard UN regions and groupings used in UNPD forecasts.

Source: UNPD (2009: 11) and IFs Version 6.32 base case forecast.

Table 4.4 UNPD and IFs forecasts of countries with longest life expectancies

	UNPD	IFs
	2045–2050	2050
Australia	86.0	86.9
Canada	85.3	85.6
Hong Kong	86.7	84.7
Iceland	86.1	87.4
Israel	85.4	86.0
Japan	87.1	87.7
Macao	85.7	NA
Spain	85.4	85.4
Sweden	85.2	87.0
Switzerland	86.1	86.8

Note: Males and females combined.

Source: UNPD (2009a: 72) and IFs Version 6.32 base case forecast.

under-five mortality are more conservative than those of IFs. Specifically, in 2009 the UNPD's forecast for 2050 of deaths of children under five was about 65 per 1,000 births for sub-Saharan Africa (reading from Figure 6 in UNPD 2009a: 16) and just over 30 for the world as a whole. The corresponding values from IFs are 41 for sub-Saharan Africa and 20 for the world as a whole. The difference for sub-Saharan Africa would account for a substantial portion of IFs higher life expectancy forecasts.

In summary, the forecasts from the IFs base case are slightly more optimistic than those of the UN. In particular, our forecasts for sub-Saharan Africa (and therefore for the reduction of its communicable disease burden) are more positive. We will return to this issue later in this chapter and also in Chapter 8.

Death and disability forecasts: GBD project

The GBD project's 2004 update (WHO 2008a) provides regional forecasts of deaths by age, sex, and cause out to 2030. As we might expect, given the similarities in our base case approach with the GBD approach and our use of their death data to initialize our model, base case forecasts from IFs largely mirror those that the GBD project produced (Table 4.5 summarizes them by region and major disease category). On the whole, the IFs model forecasts somewhat higher total mortality in terms of numbers of deaths. This could reflect some differences in underlying population forecasts, which differ between GBD and IFs.

Table 4.6 turns to disability-adjusted life years (DALYs), and compares the GBD project's forecasts with those of IFs in 2008 and 2030. Because DALYs combine years of life lived with disability (YLD) with years of life lost (YLL), and because of the difficulty in forecasting YLDs (see again Chapter 3), considerable differences in GBD

Table 4.5 GBD and IFs forecasts of regional deaths (millions) in 2030 by major disease group

	Communicable diseases		Noncommunicable diseases		Injuries	
	GBD	IFs	GBD	IFs	GBD	IFs
East Asia and Pacific	1.2	1.3	15.9	16.6	1.5	1.9
Europe and Central Asia	0.3	0.1	4.6	4.5	0.3	0.4
Latin America and the Caribbean	0.4	0.4	4.0	4.0	0.6	0.5
Middle East and North Africa	0.4	0.2	2.4	2.1	0.4	0.3
South Asia	2.4	2.6	10.9	11.2	1.9	1.9
Sub-Saharan Africa	4.3	4.7	5.1	4.9	1.6	1.3
High-income countries	0.5	0.6	8.8	10.3	0.6	0.6
World	9.4	9.9	51.6	53.7	6.8	7.0

Notes: Region members are not identical in the GBD and IFs forecasts because of movement of some countries out of developing regions into the high-income category in the most recent World Bank classifications.

Source: WHO projections of mortality and burden of disease, 2002–2030, available at http://www.who.int/healthinfo/global_burden_ disease/projections/en/index.html (see Mortality-Baseline Scenario, World Bank regions Excel download) and IFs Version 6.32 base case forecast.

Table 4.6 GBD and IFs forecasts of DALYs (millions) in 2030 by major disease group

DALYs in 2008	Communicable diseases		Noncommunicable diseases		Injuries	
	GBD	IFs	GBD	IFs	GBD	IFs
East Asia and Pacific	59.6	59.9	210.2	208.8	44.0	41.1
Europe and Central Asia	12.6	10.7	69.0	64.6	14.0	12.8
Latin America and the Caribbean	17.6	18.3	63.0	63.5	15.6	14.7
Middle East and North Africa	18.4	13.5	37.0	29.5	13.0	6.6
South Asia	158.1	169.6	182.7	173.2	51.9	48.4
Sub-Saharan Africa	252.5	259.5	87.4	85.2	35.6	36.0
High-income countries	6.2	7.4	102.0	111.6	9.1	9.5
World	525.1	539.0	751.1	739.9	183.9	169.2

DALYs in 2030	Communicable diseases		Noncommunicable diseases		Injuries	
	GBD	IFs	GBD	IFs	GBD	IFs
East Asia and Pacific	26.3	27.4	242.3	243.6	33.7	42.2
Europe and Central Asia	6.9	4.9	56.8	57.8	7.3	10.1
Latin America and the Caribbean	8.4	8.9	77.7	77.8	18.4	17.4
Middle East and North Africa	11	6.1	51.2	38.8	15.0	8.7
South Asia	68.2	75.9	236.8	216.6	51.7	55.9
Sub-Saharan Africa	146.8	171.3	131.2	119.7	55.2	52.4
High-income countries	4.1	5.1	103.6	121.7	9.7	10.0
World	271.6	299.6	899.6	880.9	191.1	196.7

Notes: Region members are not identical in the GBD and IFs forecasts because of movement of some countries out of developing regions into the high-income category in the most recent World Bank classifications.

Source: WHO projections of mortality and burden of disease, 2002–2030, available at http://www.who.int/healthinfo/global_burden_disease/projections/en/index.html (see Mortality-Baseline Scenario, World Bank regions Excel download) and IFs Version 6.32 base case forecast.

and IFs forecasts might be expected. However, they are again generally comparable, with the exception of the forecasts for DALYs from communicable diseases in sub-Saharan Africa and in Middle East and North Africa in 2030.

Child mortality and death cause forecasts: GISMO

The Global Integrated Sustainability Model (GISMO) of the Netherlands Environmental Assessment Agency forecasts mortality rates for males and females separately for 27 world regions and 13 age groups (see Chapter 3 for more detail). The system covers environmental health risks especially well, and those make a disproportionate contribution to the disease burden for children under five.

Using assumptions from the World Bank and the Food and Agricultural Organization of the United Nations on economic growth

and food consumption, the GISMO team produced forecasts through 2030 for the health measures in the Millennium Development Goals (Hilderink, Lucas, and Kok 2009). We focus here on their forecasts of child mortality (see Figure 4.8) and see that while the GISMO team forecast substantial progress in reducing child mortality rates, it also forecast that none of the developing regions will fully meet its MDG target for 2015 (although East Asia and Pacific and Latin America and the Caribbean would be very close) and that South Asia and sub-Saharan Africa will still be far from their targets.

The GISMO team also concluded that many of the risk factors related to the environment, such as food, water, energy, and climate, will still make a relatively high contribution to health loss in 2030. Of these factors, water supply and sanitation are forecast to show the greatest

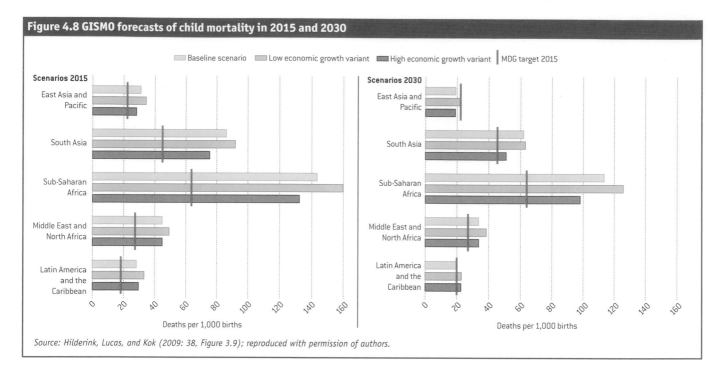

Figure 4.8 GISMO forecasts of child mortality in 2015 and 2030

Baseline scenario   Low economic growth variant   High economic growth variant | MDG target 2015

Scenarios 2015

Deaths per 1,000 births

Scenarios 2030

Deaths per 1,000 births

Source: Hilderink, Lucas, and Kok (2009: 38, Figure 3.9); reproduced with permission of authors.

● Similar patterns
in infant and child
mortality are
suggested by IFs
and GISMO, including
child deaths
specifically related
to diarrhea. ●

progress, partly due to continuing urbanization and the generally higher rates of access to improved water and sanitation in urban areas. On the other hand, inadequate food intake is forecast to still exact a high toll among children. Projected population growth partly offsets the progress in rate reductions, such that in 2030, analysis with GISMO anticipates that 1.2 million children will still die of pneumonia caused by indoor air pollution and that 0.8 million children will still die of diarrhea related to unsafe drinking water and sanitation. And as Figure 4.8 indicates, sub-Saharan Africa is expected to still have by far the highest child death rates.

While Figures 4.7 and 4.8 are not directly comparable (Figure 4.7 shows IFs forecasts of infant mortality rates and Figure 4.8 shows GISMO's forecasts of child mortality rates), nonetheless a comparison of the figures and the discussion around them suggests very similar conclusions from the two models with respect to likely progress by 2015 on reducing infant and child mortality.

The GISMO model also identifies deaths by a variety of specific causes (as does IFs), and Figure 4.9 compares its forecasts for child deaths from diarrhea with those of IFs. The declines forecast by the two models are very similar, both trending to a total of about 0.8 million annual deaths in 2030.

HIV and AIDS forecasts: UNAIDS

The future course of the AIDS epidemic is one of the greatest unknowns in thinking about the future of global health and, because of its importance, even in the forecasting of global population more generally. UNAIDS has produced the forecasts of AIDS deaths to which other forecasters have been widely attentive in recent years, including the UNPD in its population reports and revisions.

As the HIV/AIDS epidemic has evolved, so also have the data, modeling, and forecasting emerging from UNAIDS and used in the UNPD reports.[4] For example, in comparison to the forecast in the 2004 Revision (UNPD 2005), the UNPD's 2006 Revision (UNPD 2007) foresaw 32 million fewer deaths between 2005 and 2020 in 62 countries. Even with that adjustment, assumptions regarding possible alternative scenarios spanned an extreme range, consistent with great uncertainty. The alternative scenarios were forecasts around a No-AIDS assumption; a High-AIDS assumption (no decline in high-risk group membership rates or infection rates ["force of infection"] among those individuals); and an AIDS-vaccine assumption (with a perfectly effective vaccine posited to be fully available by 2010 and therefore cutting new HIV infections to zero).

Further refinements in the UNAIDS tools are reflected in the UNPD's 2008 Revision (UNPD

2009a), which builds on 2007 UNAIDS estimates and forecasts. The 2007 estimates focused on 58 countries, compared to 62 in the 2006 Revision.[5] Fifty-three were countries with HIV prevalence rates of 1 percent or more, and five were countries with lower prevalence rates but populations large enough to result in more than 500,000 people with HIV. The 2007 UNAIDS estimates changed some parameters in the projection methodology. Specifically, the major changes in parameters were an assumption that every 20 years there will be a 50 percent decline in the movement of new individuals into high-risk groups and that every 30 years there will be a 50 percent decline in the chances of transmission due to changes in behavior among those at risk and increases in access to treatment for those infected. Elaborative analyses gave special attention to mother-to-child transmission and to the coverage levels of antiretroviral therapy. For instance, the UNPD's 2008 forecasts reflected the assumption that 26 of the 58 focus countries would achieve levels of antiretroviral treatment of 70 percent or more by 2015 and that those receiving treatment would survive 27.8 years, versus 11.7 years for those not receiving it (UNPD 2009a: viii and 24).

The result both of rapidly changing patterns of the HIV/AIDS epidemic and of changing understandings of it (including refinement in estimation and projection methodologies) was a substantial downward adjustment in the estimates in the 2008 Revision (UNPD 2009b) of those infected with HIV (from 39.5 million to 33.2 million) and strikingly reduced projections of cumulative AIDS deaths from 2005 and 2020 (from 42 million to 26 million).

Overall, it appears that the newest generation of forecasts of AIDS deaths emerging from the UN is moving toward relatively stable numbers until about 2015 with decline thereafter, and that is roughly the pattern in the forecasts of IFs also. The cumulative global death forecast for IFs is 27.8 million between 2005 and 2020, not surprisingly somewhat higher than the total reported in the 2008 Revision, which is focused on the most afflicted 58 countries. The IFs project has taken the medium estimates of historical and current HIV prevalence and AIDS deaths and built its own forecasting model taking those into account (see Chapter 3). For several years, however, the forecasts of IFs were

lower than those published in the UNPD reports, so with the recent UN revisions the two sources of forecasts have increasingly converged.

Turning to specific highly affected countries, it is possible to use the UNAIDS Estimation and Projection Package (EPP) and Spectrum model to forecast HIV/AIDS through 2015, and we have done that. Table 4.7 compares the results of those forecasts with values in IFs; although they are generally quite similar, there are instances of large differences (the largest differences are in the HIV rate of Kenya and AIDS deaths in Mozambique). Again, we note the uncertainty that attends HIV/AIDS forecasting.

The year 2015 is not, however, a very long forecasting horizon, so in addition Table 4.7

■ Much uncertainty attends HIV/AIDS forecasting, and there are both similarities and differences between IFs and UNAIDS forecasts. ■

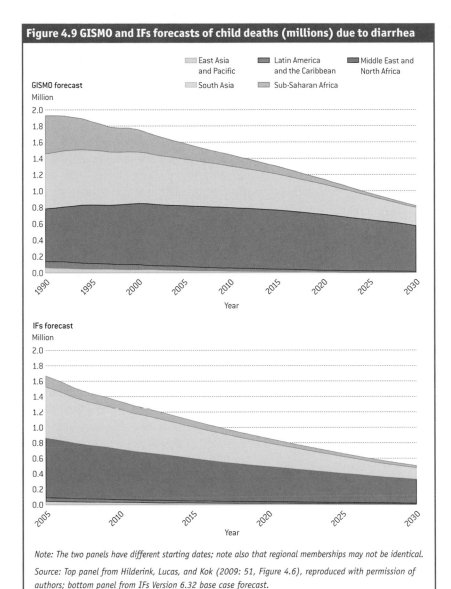

Figure 4.9 GISMO and IFs forecasts of child deaths (millions) due to diarrhea

Note: The two panels have different starting dates; note also that regional memberships may not be identical.

Source: Top panel from Hilderink, Lucas, and Kok (2009: 51, Figure 4.6), reproduced with permission of authors; bottom panel from IFs Version 6.32 base case forecast.

includes forecasts from IFs for 2040. Those values show the very long tail that the HIV epidemic could have, even if the assumptions of its current peaking are correct. The overall profile of it in the long term now appears to be that of extremely sharp rise in the 1980s and 1990s, some leveling in the 2000s, and then the long tail of decline. Once again, however, a caution about very great uncertainty is in order. For instance, if the death pattern for South Africa of Table 4.7 were to unfold, it would mean that a little less than 13 million South Africans would die of AIDS between 2005 and 2060. In a population that is likely to range from 50 to 55 million at any one time over this period, that is a quite incredible prospective burden of morbidity and mortality.

Road traffic accident deaths: World Bank and GBD

Chapter 3 discussed the significant differences that moving from aggregate to structural models, with their explicit representation of drivers, can make in forecasting capabilities and results. There are, however, very different kinds of structural models, representing drivers and causality in very different ways.

The GBD project followed the same approach to forecast road traffic deaths as it did deaths in all but a very small number of cases—that is, through regression-based distal-driver structural formulations rooted in income, education, and a time term.

As we have stated before, the GBD researchers did not intend for their formulations to be used beyond 2030. In contrast, a World Bank study by Kopits and Cropper (2005) used a more deeply structural approach—in which they forecast vehicles per person and fatalities per vehicle—that can reasonably be extended across a longer time span. Although income change remains the key driver in their approach, they capture the saturation of vehicle ownership and combine that with decreasing fatality rates per vehicle above an income threshold. As we indicated in Chapter 3, our desire to extend the GBD approach beyond 2030 led us to adopt the more structural approach of Kopits and Cropper for IFs, with our own formulations of vehicle ownership and fatality rates per vehicle.

Table 4.8 shows the results. The top half compares the rate of growth in road traffic deaths from 2000 to 2020 from Kopits and Cropper with the rate of growth from 2005 (the initial year) to 2025 from IFs. The initial data are obviously not comparable, even taking into account different starting years; for Kopits and Cropper (2005: 177) they come from yearbooks of the International Road Federation, and for IFs they are rooted in the GBD 2004 detailed update of deaths. The global growth patterns are quite similar, but many regional ones differ considerably. Relative to Kopits

Table 4.7 Spectrum and IFs forecasts of HIV prevalence and AIDS deaths for countries with highest numbers of deaths					
	HIV prevalence rate (percent)			AIDS deaths (thousands)		
	Spectrum	IFs		Spectrum	IFs	
	2015	2015	2040	2015	2015	2040
Ethiopia	1.3	1.2	0.6	59	62	44
Kenya	1.6	2.8	1.5	81	77	47
Mozambique	7.4	6.2	3.4	120	59	39
Nigeria	1.9	1.8	1.0	194	136	90
South Africa	12.3	11.2	6.1	370	391	167
Tanzania	3.7	3.4	1.9	95	95	65
Uganda	2.4	2.8	1.5	55	66	48
Zambia	9.1	8.0	4.4	68	57	40
Zimbabwe	6.1	7.4	3.9	47	42	19

Note: Prevalence rates are expressed as a percent of the total population.

Source: UNAIDS Spectrum system at http://www.unaids.org/en/KnowledgeCentre/HIVData/Epidemiology/EPI_software2009.asp and IFs Version 6.32 base case forecast.

Table 4.8 Estimates and forecasts of road traffic fatalities (thousands) by region using three forecasting systems

	Kopits and Cropper			IFs		
	2000	2020	% change	2005	2025	% change
East Asia and Pacific	188	337	79.3	358	694	93.9
Europe and Central Asia	32	38	18.8	74	81	9.5
Latin America and the Caribbean	122	180	47.5	96	141	46.9
Middle East and North Africa	56	94	67.9	68	127	86.8
South Asia	135	330	144.4	231	473	104.8
Sub-Saharan Africa	80	144	80.0	222	358	61.3
High-income countries	110	80	(27.3)	98	102	4.1
World	723	1,204	66.5	1,149	1,979	72.2
	GBD formulation in IFs			IFs		
	2005	2100	% change	2005	2100	% change
East Asia and Pacific	358	274	(23.5)	358	527	47.2
Europe and Central Asia	74	41	(44.6)	74	45	(39.2)
Latin America and the Caribbean	96	88	(8.3)	96	135	40.6
Middle East and North Africa	68	180	164.7	68	251	269.1
South Asia	231	622	169.3	231	1,043	351.5
Sub-Saharan Africa	222	4,279	1827.5	222	1,286	479.3
High-income countries	98	50	(49.0)	98	68	(30.6)
World	1,149	5,535	381.7	1,149	3,355	192.0

Note: The GBD formulations were not intended for forecasting beyond 2030 and are shown for illustrative purposes only, using IFs distal-driver forecasts.

Source: Kopits and Cropper (2005: 176); GBD formulation forecasts by IFs system; IFs Version 6.32 base case forecast.

and Cropper, IFs provides generally lower growth rates for the lowest-income regions and somewhat higher values for middle- and high-income regions.

Framing Scenario Analysis

Although base case forecasts (see again Box 4.1 for a brief discussion of the key characteristics of the IFs base case) are a useful device for beginning to think about the future of global health, the uncertainty surrounding such forecasts requires that we fairly quickly extend thinking to alternative possible futures. To a very large degree, human action will shape those alternatives through behavioral choices and through the development and transfer of medical technology. Before the coming chapters in which we begin to explore alternative health futures tied to variations in assumptions concerning

more proximate drivers (and the specific causes of death that they influence), it is useful here to use the distal-driver formulations to think about the range of alternatives that the distal drivers themselves might generate.

Alternative futures for GDP per capita and education

Alternative assumptions about the future of the three key distal drivers in the GBD and IFs formulations generate quite different health forecasts. The exploration of alternative assumptions also shows that the three drivers have inherent characteristics that strongly shape their own likely variation and therefore the degree to which they might give rise to alternative health forecasts.

Most significant, perhaps, is the difference in character of GDP per capita and years of

Relative to a World Bank study, IFs tends to forecast lower traffic accident growth rates for low-income regions and higher ones for middle- and high-income regions.

education in an adult population. As a general rule, there is considerably more uncertainty around the magnitude of future GDP per capita than there is around adults' educational levels. GDP per capita is an annual flow variable (that is, it is generated anew each year), driven by multiple underlying stocks, such as capital supply, years of adult education, and multifactor productivity. Scenarios for the future annual growth rate of the global GDP can reasonably be a percentage point higher or lower than the base case over prolonged periods of time (and several percentage points different over shorter time horizons, such as the years of the global recession that began in 2008). Such variation can set in motion feedbacks to a substantial number of underlying stocks and can create significant long-term divergence of future paths.[6] Between 2005 and 2060 the base case takes global GDP per capita at purchasing power parity from $7,700 to $25,000. Alternative scenarios with one percentage point lower and one percentage point higher GDP growth rates set up a range in 2060 from $13,600 to $37,900, a 2.8 factor of difference.

Figure 4.10 shows the possible implications of the three alternative economic growth scenarios for global life expectancy (which we understand, of course, to represent not the impact of

income itself, but the wide range of health improvements income makes possible). The scenarios set up a spread of almost three years in life expectancy by 2060. Not surprisingly, the high-growth scenario, relative to the low-growth scenario, has a greater impact on low-income regions than on middle- and high-income regions. The greatest impact is on South Asia, with a life expectancy gap of 3.4 years between the low- and high-growth scenarios; in sub-Saharan Africa the difference is nearly three years. In sub-Saharan Africa, differing impacts across economic growth scenarios on the rate of reduction in communicable diseases lead to the greatest and rather dramatic differences in years of life lost. Between 2005 and 2060, the high-growth scenario reduces cumulative years of life lost in sub-Saharan Africa by a rather astounding 2,267 million years relative to the low-growth scenario, a reduction of 16 percent. A significant portion of that reduction is, however, not a direct result of reduction in mortality rates, but rather an indirect effect that results from reduced fertility and population size associated with higher economic growth (Chapter 7 returns to an analysis of the larger, complex systems in which health sits).

In rather sharp contrast to analysis of economic futures, the variation in likely educational futures is much less. Countries around the world invest heavily in education and are increasing their flow of students through primary, secondary, and tertiary programs at relatively steady rates (in recent years very rapidly by historical standards). It takes, however, more than 40 years, even in countries with relatively low life expectancies, for those who complete secondary education to pass through their life span, carrying with them their formal education attainment levels (represented in both the GBD and IFs models by the common indicator of years of attainment by adults 25 years of age and older; see Barro and Lee 1996; 2000; and 2001). Thus, the difference between the base case for the advance of education attainment levels in sub-Saharan Africa and an "aggressive but reasonable" normative scenario, which accelerates enrollment rates significantly, is not that great—in fact, levels of attainment differ by less than one year and therefore by about 10 percent in 2060 (see Dickson, Hughes, and Irfan 2010 for extended exploration of

> ● *Exploring health impacts of alternative assumptions about the future of our distal drivers helps us frame uncertainty.* ●

Figure 4.10 Global life expectancy forecasts across three economic growth-rate scenarios

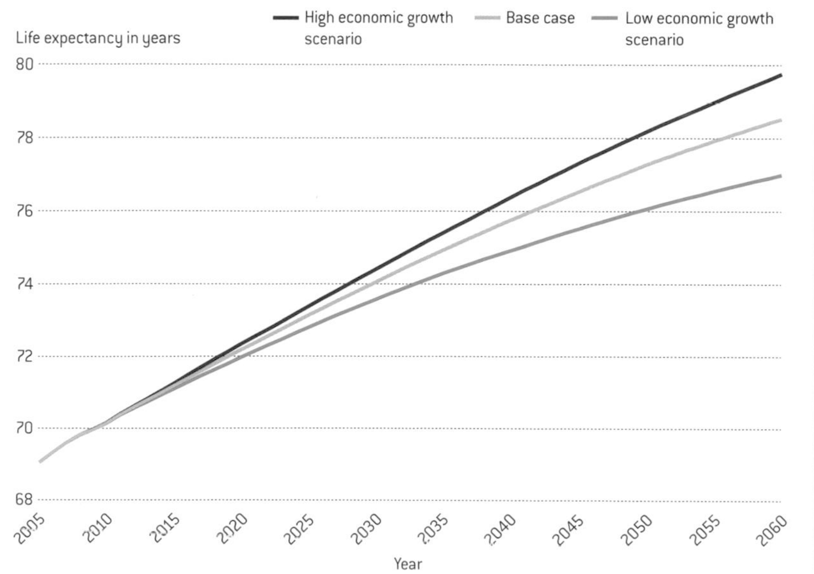

Source: IFs Version 6.32 base case forecast and high and low economic growth rate scenarios.

educational futures and the normative scenario; were we also to explore a low-growth scenario for education, the full range of results would be roughly twice those reported here). The resultant impact on life expectancy in 2060 is proportionately modest. At the global level it is only 0.5 years, and even in sub-Saharan Africa, where the normative education scenario creates the greatest difference in adults' years of education, the incremental life expectancy in 2060 is only 1.1 years—hardly insignificant, but quite modest in comparison to the differences across economic scenarios. (Education has, of course, other important health-related impacts in the IFs model, including its implications for fertility and overall population growth; see again Dickson, Hughes, and Irfan 2010.)

It is probable that the uncertainty around the parameterization of the contribution of education attainment in the GBD model and the IFs base case approach (or the parameterization of the other distal drivers for that matter), is a greater source of uncertainty in the overall contribution of education to health than the difference between the base case and the normative scenario. The complex structure of the distal-driver equations, however, makes true sensitivity analysis very complicated (see Box 4.4).

Alternative futures for time/technology

In addition to GDP per capita and education, the third principal distal driver in the GBD project's formulations is time. The coefficients on the time term reduce mortality by steady annual amounts (albeit different amounts across geography, cause of death, and age or gender) independent of the impacts of income and education.

The time-term is often understood to be a proxy in substantial part for technology, but it is in reality a catchall term for all else beyond income and education that is changing dynamically in the system, including change in any of the super-distal drivers described in Chapter 2. Thus, for example, the term could pick up ideational and associated behavioral changes, such as changed dietary, exercise, or smoking patterns in response to new knowledge about their health impacts. It could also pick up negative dynamics, such as increasing social violence related to changed mores and/or greater inequality.

The relationship between rising income and declining mortality is as challenging to forecast as it is to theorize. Alternative forecasting commonly looks to changes in parameters of the forecasting formulations. We might wish, for instance, to explore the "change in gearing" in the income-mortality relationship (Wilkinson 2007) that helps give rise to the tendency for the gap between rich and poor countries to narrow over time. If the income-mortality relationship were based on a single coefficient we could simply change it. That is not the case, however.

The GBD project's regressions for each age-sex-cause cluster include separate terms for the log of GDP per capita (LGDPC) and a square term (LGDPCSQ), a combination that defies any simple interpretation of individual relationships. Whatever the theory might say about the overall relationships, many regressions fail to produce a simple relationship between income increase and mortality decrease. Most communicable diseases are negatively related to LGDPC and unrelated to LGDPCSQ. In contrast, death rates for most noncommunicable disease groups actually rise with LGDPC before declining with LGDPCSQ, creating a set of parabolic relationships that often peak at relatively high levels of income. Accidents and violence rise monotonically with LGDPC (giving rise to the high road traffic fatality numbers for Africa discussed earlier).

Income effects are further confounded by the fact that the other distal drivers, most notably education, also tend to rise with income. Further, the income coefficients for the same disease in one age-sex group might look quite different from those for another age-sex group. Finally, the separate GBD formulations for rich and poor countries would yield stagnating life expectancy gains for today's poor countries if we did not throw a switch to move countries into the high-income group (discussed in Chapter 3).

Therefore, our analysis throughout this volume is tied to variation in the distal drivers (or around alternative values of proximate drivers, to be discussed in Chapters 5 and 6), rather than to change in the parameters that relate income or education to health outcomes.

To explore the sensitivity of health outcomes to this representation of the impact of technological and other time-related changes, we arbitrarily considered the implications of increasing or decreasing the annual change by 50 percent. The impact on global life expectancy of that significant percentage change is very considerable, even somewhat larger than that associated with economic growth. In 2060, global life expectancies in the high and low time-term scenarios differ by 3.5 years—the high time-term scenario increases life expectancy by about 1.5 years relative to the base case and the low time-term scenario reduces it by 2 years relative to the base case. The difference between the high and low time-term cases varies across country groupings, reaching 4.5 years in South Asia, compared to 2.5 years in Latin America and the Caribbean.[7]

The gains in life expectancy from accelerating the impact of the time term are seen in reduced mortality from communicable and noncommunicable diseases. In contrast, accelerating the impact of time has negative consequences for mortality from injuries. Globally, the cumulative years of life lost due to injuries between 2005 and 2060 are more than 13 percent higher in the high time-term scenario than in the low one. Because deaths in that cause-group are lower than those from noncommunicable diseases and close to those from communicable diseases, the higher years of life lost to injuries do not offset the combined reductions in communicable and noncommunicable disease deaths, but they do hold down the overall improvement in life expectancy, particularly because many deaths from injuries occur in the middle years of life. The increase in mortality from injuries in the high time-term scenario is almost entirely from intentional injuries (such as murders), not from unintentional injuries or road traffic accidents. Clearly, growing levels of gun and other violence in recent decades in many areas of the world (including sub-Saharan Africa and North America) influenced the sign of the coefficients on the time term for the injury category. It is, of course, uncertain whether such increases will continue.

Overall, this analysis of uncertainty around the distal drivers of health outcomes suggests there is the potential for interventions around each of them to improve health futures. It also suggests, however, that the greatest uncertainty, and therefore potential leverage, exists around the economic growth and time/technology drivers and perhaps, somewhat surprisingly, that there may be considerably less potential leverage around education. It is important to emphasize, however, that we must treat carefully and somewhat skeptically estimates of model coefficients in areas where variables are highly correlated, such as GDP per capita and education.

Conclusion

The health forecasts of the IFs base case—relying heavily on the methodology of the GBD forecasters but extended in a number of ways that Chapter 3 discussed (including the addition of eight proximate risk factors)—

portray a world through 2060 in which health outcomes continue on a path of rapid and generally positive change, albeit with significant differences from historical patterns. Life expectancy continues to rise, but at a slowing pace (a slowing that Chapter 2 discussed as being somewhat controversial). While death rates continue to fall in the aggregate, opportunities for progress with respect to reducing deaths at younger ages from communicable diseases play out largely before 2060—in fact, that is a key reason that gains in life expectancy become harder to attain.

The primary causes of death nearly everywhere are now noncommunicable diseases, and the shift to that pattern will become more pronounced. As a result of this shift to dominance of deaths from noncommunicable causes, global patterns of death will increasingly converge.

Relatively few forecasts of health outcomes exist. The aggregate life expectancy forecasts of the UNPD and the cause-specific projections of the GBD modelers are the most notable. Not surprisingly, given the rooting of the IFs distal-driver health formulations in those of the GBD project, the forecasts of IFs tend to be similar to them. Still, the IFs forecasts provide both an extended time horizon and the value of some specialized structural formulations. In addition, the IFs forecasts offer the value of dynamic interactions across IFs demographic, health, economic, and education models. These interactions have allowed us to begin exploring the range of uncertainty in some of our base case forecasts (recognizing of course that uncertainties related to specification and estimation throughout the model may dwarf those related to drivers such as educational attainment).

Most health policy does not focus on increasing GDP or educational attainment, however. Instead, it is more closely tied to what the health community and the framework used in this volume term proximate drivers. We turn next to that analysis.

> ● With our formulations, alternative income and time/technology scenarios impact health outcomes more than the education scenarios. ●

1 For a more extended discussion of forecasting with IFs and the meaning and use of base case analysis, see Hughes et al. 2009 (especially Chapter 5).

2 In technical terms this pattern of declining gains at the leading edge of life expectancy partly reflects the logarithmic functional form of the GBD forecasting equations in which incremental gains in income and education have decreasing marginal impacts on mortality.

3 Forecasts from the UNPD, the GBD project, and other projects use different country groupings and cover varying time periods and specific points of time, and we match the groupings and time frames of the individual projects in our comparisons with them.

4 The UNAIDS Reference Group on Estimates, Modeling and Projections has refined over time its tools for forecasting HIV prevalence and AIDS deaths. The EPP projects prevalence, which the Spectrum suite of models can use to calculate forecasted AIDS cases, deaths, and other variables. See http://www.unaids.org/en/KnowledgeCentre/ HIVdata/Epidemiology/epi_software2007.asp.

5 Gambia, Madagascar, Moldova, Myanmar, and Niger moved out of the 1 percent or more prevalence group, and Mauritius moved into it.

6 One percentage point higher or lower GDP growth is fairly widely used in scenario sets for the analysis of long-term economic, energy, or other impacts. We close the loops from health back to the population and economy (see Chapter 7) in order to analyze the full effects of the difference.

7 This seems counterintuitive and should be reviewed in future model work.

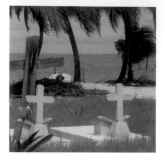

5

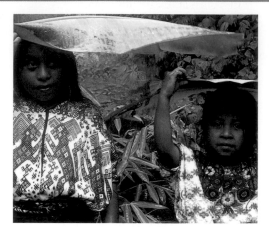

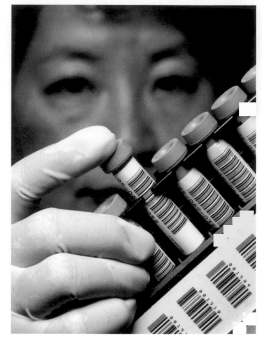

Analysis of Selected Proximate Risk Factors

■ Changes in disease-predisposing behaviors can have powerful impacts on overall health. ■

When communities or governments seek to improve health outcomes across both broad populations and specific population subgroups, they most often focus on specific health risk factors over which they can exercise leverage. Efforts to reduce obesity and lower smoking rates are examples of attempts to reduce the prevalence of noncommunicable diseases, such as cardiovascular diseases and cancer. Similarly, distributing information about safe sex practices and providing access to contraceptives are examples of efforts in the fight against sexually transmitted infectious diseases. Positive changes in such disease-predisposing behaviors (in this case, poor nutrition, smoking, and unsafe sex), while often difficult to achieve in practice, can have powerful impacts on overall health.

While behaviorally linked proximate risks are certainly related to the distal drivers explored in Chapter 4, the relationship is mutable; collectively and individually people can quite possibly alter at least some aspects of their

risk factor profile at any level of development.[1] This observation raises critical questions for those seeking to understand and improve population health outcomes. For example, what relationships exist between proximate and distal factors currently, and how might those change over time? And how might our forecasts of mortality change with favorable (or unfavorable) changes in exposure to specific risks?

This chapter and the next therefore introduce alternative levels of proximate risk factors into the forecast of health outcomes. Specifically, we look further at the relationship between proximate risks and both distal drivers and mortality outcomes, exploring how our base case health forecasts might change if the extent of various risk factors changes.

We chose four such risk factors to explore in this chapter: childhood undernutrition, adult overweight and obesity, tobacco use, and road traffic safety. In Chapter 6, we turn to selected risk factors in the physical environment—namely, water and sanitation, indoor air pollution, urban outdoor air pollution, and climate change. Then at the end of Chapter 6 we step back and look at health impacts across the proximate-driver scenarios explored in both chapters.

Health Risk Transition

We can situate a health risk transition within the broader epidemiologic transition (see Figure 5.1 in relationship to Figure 1.3). Traditional risk factors—such as undernutrition, indoor air pollution, and unsafe water, sanitation, and hygiene—begin at very high levels in the first phase of the epidemiologic transition and decline across phases. Modern risks—such as smoking and obesity—rise across the phases and reach high levels only in the third phase. Other risks tend to rise and then fall as the epidemiologic transition proceeds and might best be called "transition risks." For example, both urban outdoor air pollution and road traffic accidents tend to rise sharply in the first and/ or second phase of the epidemiologic transition and then fall gradually in subsequent phases.

Time itself is obviously not the true driver of the risk transition, and many factors interact to give rise to changing patterns of risks. Income tends to increase over time and influences risk-related behaviors and societal contexts. Social change provides (and is marked by) new options and choices (including in sexual behaviors). Health systems and their technologies evolve. Energy systems, economic structures, and other aspects of infrastructure transform quite dramatically, giving rise to changing physical environments (and a related environmental risk transition to which we will return in Chapter 6) as well as helping shape new lifestyles. It is within this framework of changing health risks over time and across a range of circumstances that we begin our exploration of proximate health risks.

Risk Analysis with IFs

As Chapter 3 explained, the International Futures (IFs) health model has a hybrid character that combines the distal- and proximate-driver formulations, the former as a foundation for forecasting and the latter as a way of exploring variations in risk relative to expectations consistent with the distal variables. Chapter 4 explored the implications for health futures of alternative assumptions concerning the distal drivers. This chapter and the next

do the same with respect to proximate drivers across the phases of the risk transition.

We focus on a subset of proximate health risks. As discussed in Chapter 3, WHO's Comparative Risk Assessment (CRA) project within the broader Global Burden of Disease (GBD) project has provided a map for estimating the mortality and burden of disease associated with individual and joint risk factors. The CRA project's 2004 update (WHO 2009a) included 24 risk factors across seven risk categories,[2] selected from a much larger potential set of risks because of their clear connection to health outcomes, potential for global impact, data availability, and potential for modification through interventions (see again Table 2.1 for a list of the risk categories and risk factors in the CRA 2004 update).

From the CRA project's list, we selected seven for initial inclusion in the IFs health model: childhood undernutrition (as measured by childhood underweight); overweight and obesity (as measured by high body mass index [BMI]); smoking (a subset of smoking and oral tobacco use); unsafe water, sanitation, and hygiene; urban air pollution; indoor air pollution from household use of solid fuels; and global climate change. All but global climate change were within the top 14 risk factors in terms of global deaths in 2004 according to the CRA 2004 update (WHO 2009a: 10).[3] To these seven we added road traffic safety, identified as a modern risk in the CRA report's depiction of the health

Different health risk factors tend to be associated with different stages of the epidemiologic transition, leading to the concept of a "health risk transition."

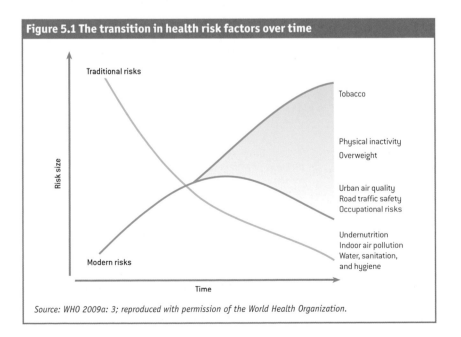

Figure 5.1 The transition in health risk factors over time

Source: WHO 2009a: 3; reproduced with permission of the World Health Organization.

risk transition (see again Figure 5.1) but not included in the CRA's list of 24 quantified risks.[4]

At this time, we have not modeled alcohol use or sexual and reproductive health risk behaviors, despite their very significant mortality and morbidity impacts. Nor have we directly treated

physical (in)activity. In addition to the influence of magnitude of deaths on our choice of factors to explore in this volume, historical and cross-sectional data for most of the risks that we do not treat are more limited than for those we analyze. Future extension of the hybrid modeling approach of this volume will hopefully push further into this more difficult terrain.

Our approach to exploration of proximate drivers, as in our earlier analysis of distal drivers, involves exploring high and low scenarios around the base case forecasts of the various drivers. In order to frame reasonable magnitudes for the high and low scenarios, we considered contemporary variation in risks across countries; Box 5.1 and Figure 5.2 serve as an example by elaborating our approach with respect to undernutrition at different levels of national income. Presumably such variation encompasses and reflects both good and bad health practices. We posit that increasing risks by one standard error above those forecast in the base case constitutes a reasonable basis for a high-risk scenario, while decreasing them by one standard error similarly can represent a low-risk scenario. And as a general rule, we assumed that such shifts in risk relative to initial conditions (and a dynamically changing base case) could not occur instantaneously, however lenient or intense policy might be with respect to such shifts. We therefore phase in the shifts over a 25-year period ending in 2030.

Four of our risk factors (childhood undernutrition, overweight and obesity, smoking, and road traffic safety) are the subject of this chapter, and Chapter 6 groups and presents the analysis and forecasts of the four environmental risk factors. We begin the analysis of proximate risks in this pair of chapters by exploring childhood undernutrition. As in our discussion of other risks, we seek to understand its historical evolution, its key drivers, and the possible health implications around the world of alternative high- and low-risk scenarios.

Childhood Undernutrition

While far from perfect, the nutritional status of most populations today is much improved from historical experience. The foundational approach to nutritional sufficiency in developing countries lies in increasing available calories per capita, with the caveats that increases can eventually lead to overnutrition and that people may eat

---

Box 5.1 Risk factor variability and exploring potential impacts of interventions in IFs

Risk factor estimates often vary quite dramatically across countries at the same general level of development. Figure 5.2 shows, for example, the percentage of children who are underweight relative to GDP per capita. Contrast India and Honduras. In 2005, both had GDP per capita of just over $3,000 at purchasing power parity. Yet the most recent WHO estimates of childhood undernutrition differ strikingly for the two countries—43.5 percent in India (2006) compared to 8.6 percent in Honduras in the same year. The reasons for unexpectedly high or low undernutrition rates in relation to per capita income in particular regions or countries often remain unclear; historically South Asia has been a particular outlier.

One way to quickly summarize the extent of cross-country variation for a risk factor is the standard error relative to the regression line (the equivalent of the standard deviation relative to a mean) in a relationship such as that of Figure 5.2. The standard error of 8.50 compared to a mean underweight percentage of 16.1 suggests that values for undernutrition frequently vary by about 50 percent above or below the values we would expect based on GDP per capita. In contrast, relative to income-based expectations, the variation around female smoking, where the relationship with income is extremely weak, is nearly 80 percent.

High and low proximate-driver scenarios in Chapters 5 and 6 draw on analyses of cross-national variation in the individual risk factors, such as that shown here for childhood underweight. Specifically, the high and low scenarios for undernutrition are 50 percent (or roughly one standard deviation) above and below the base case, and the range of variation for other interventions is similarly linked to the magnitude of the standard errors of those risk factors.

Figure 5.2 Underweight children (percent) as a function of GDP per capita at PPP

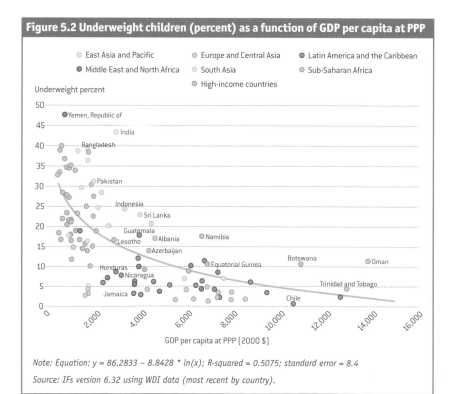

Note: Equation: y = 86.2833 − 8.8428 * ln(x); R-squared = 0.5075; standard error = 8.4

Source: IFs version 6.32 using WDI data (most recent by country).

a sufficient amount of food but fail to absorb the nutrients due to diarrheal disease or other disorders (Fogel 2004b). As recently as the late 1960s and early 1970s, people in many regions of the world had, on average, fewer than 2200 calories available per day and experienced severe nutritional shortfalls. In sub-Saharan Africa and South Asia, available calories remained fairly low through the 1990s, and calorie availability actually fell for the transition countries of Europe during the 1990s (FAO 2006). Still, people in developing countries had an average of over 500 more calories available in 2006 than they did in the mid-1970s, moving on average from 2110 to 2650 (FAO 2006: 3).

The problem of global malnutrition is, however, very far from solved, as we can see from cross-national data on body size. Generally defined, malnutrition describes a condition in which dietary energy or nutrient supply to the body is insufficient, excessive, or imbalanced (resulting from food insecurity, food excess, and/or vitamin and mineral deficiency). Here we use the term undernutrition to describe a physiological state of inadequate nutrition. For children under five years of age, the rate of undernutrition in a population is measured through weight, and underweight is defined as two or more standard deviations below the international reference weight.[5] Recent WHO figures report the percentage of children classified as underweight to be more than 30 percent for 18 countries and more than 20 percent for 40 countries (WHO Statistical Information System, accessed August 2009).[6] Sharply rising prices from 2005 through 2008 (FAO 2008: 6) exacerbated food insecurity in many parts of the world, as did the subsequent economic crisis.

Childhood undernutrition is a major contributor to the overall global burden of disease—in fact, the GBD project has determined childhood underweight to be the single leading global cause of disability-adjusted life years (Ezzati et al. 2006). Although undernutrition is rarely listed as a direct cause of death, analysis suggests that it is an underlying determinant in between 22 and 35 percent of all deaths for children younger than five years of age worldwide (Black et al. 2003).[7, 8]

A study by Pelletier, Frongillo, and Habicht (1993) greatly advanced understanding of the role of childhood malnutrition in disease. The authors reanalyzed data from six population-based studies of childhood malnutrition and demonstrated a number of significant points. First, their analysis confirmed that the risk of mortality is inversely related to weight-for-age (Pelletier 1994). In other words, the analysis showed conclusively that the more malnourished children are, the higher their risk of early death. Importantly, Pelletier, Frongillo, and Habicht demonstrated that mortality risk among children is not limited to those affected by the most severe malnutrition; instead, there is a spectrum of risk associated with all grades of malnourishment, and even mild and moderate forms are associated with an elevated risk of mortality. In fact, because of the high proportion of children falling into the mild-to-moderate range of malnourishment, the number of associated deaths in that population was much higher than the number of child deaths resulting from severe malnutrition (Pelletier, Frongillo, and Habicht 1993: 1132). The results of their study also confirmed that undernutrition has a multiplicative rather than an additive effect on mortality, a finding that has far-reaching implications for child survival strategies at policy and programmatic levels:

> If these associations are causal, an increase or decrease in the prevalence of malnutrition will have a bigger impact on mortality in populations with already high mortality levels than in those populations with low mortality levels. Efforts to lower child mortality would therefore be most effective if attention is given to improving health and nutritional status simultaneously and if such efforts are targeted towards populations with the highest mortality levels. (Pelletier 1994: 2058S)

Drivers and forecasts of undernutrition in children

The determinants of childhood undernutrition are highly complex, multidimensional, and difficult to encapsulate in a single theory. Undernutrition is most directly a result of dietary inadequacy, the effect of an infectious disease on energy absorption, or an interaction between the two. The interaction with infectious

In this chapter we explore high and low scenarios around four risk factors: childhood undernutrition, overweight and obesity, smoking, and road traffic accidents.

Childhood underweight has been identified as the single leading global cause of disability-adjusted life years.

diseases, including diarrheal diseases, links undernutrition strongly to the availability of safe water and sanitation systems, and those are key driving variables in the IFs formulation (we discuss this link in Chapter 6).

Clearly, however, calorie availability is fundamentally important. The number of available calories depends strongly on the interaction of two factors: income (including its distribution) and food price. Long-term trends in calorie availability reflect fairly rapidly rising incomes in most parts of the world and slowly falling real food prices. Both of those trends have seen periods of significant interruption. Famines in 1974 (especially in Bangladesh and Ethiopia) arose in periods of sharply higher-than-normal world food prices in interaction with more localized natural disasters. The "lost decade" of the 1980s in Latin America, with debt crises giving rise to economic stagnation, led to a long flattening of calorie availability levels, just as the fall of incomes in the former communist countries (and the elimination of safety nets) more recently led to a decline in calories available there.[9] Similarly, the sharp rises in world food prices from 2005 through 2009, with a doubling from early 2006 to early 2008 (FAO 2008: 6; FAO Food Price Index data, accessed August 2009)[10] resulted in reports of rapid and significant rises in undernutrition. On average, however, incomes swing much less widely than do food prices. Therefore, the long-term rise in incomes has been a foundational force for dietary

improvement, while food prices have been especially important in the shorter term.

The interaction of supply and demand substantially determines the course of food prices. On the supply side, increased production around the world—as a function primarily of technological advance since the 1950s and primarily of cultivation expansion before that—has been critical. On the demand side, rising incomes translate quite directly into food demand. In fact, the earliest definitions of extreme poverty (living on less than $1 per day) relate quite directly to undernutrition (the Ahluwalia, Carter, and Chenery 1979 poverty level was associated with roughly 2,250 calories per day), and the global numbers of those who are extremely poor and those who are severely malnourished are very comparable. As incomes advance, of course, food demand continues to grow and to change in character, and it has in part been the rapid rise of the global middle class and its demand for improved diets, especially in China and India, that has driven the pressure on food prices since 2000. Another critical factor has been the increased demand on agricultural production for biofuels as an alternative energy source. This pressure depends significantly on the price of energy, as well as on subsidies and policy mandates, and the future course of it is uncertain.

IFs represents the demand and supply interaction in its forecast of calorie availability and nutrition levels. Even taking into account

■ *In the IFs base case, childhood undernutrition falls by 2060 to 5 percent or less in all but South Asia and sub-Saharan Africa, where it remains at 7–8 percent.* ■

Table 5.1 FAO and IFs forecasts of available calories per capita by region

	2015		2030		2050	
	FAO	IFs	FAO	IFs	FAO	IFs
Developing countries	2860	2782	2960	2944	3070	3098
East Asia	3110	3028	3190	3232	3230	3410
Latin America and Caribbean	2990	2961	3120	3084	3200	3217
Near East and North Africa	3080	3062	3130	3153	3190	3245
South Asia	2660	2577	2790	2806	2980	3057
Sub-Saharan Africa	2420	2311	2600	2477	2830	2674
Industrial countries	3480	3505	3520	3545	3540	3603
Transition countries	3030	3116	3150	3227	3270	3265
World	2950	2897	3040	3030	3130	3161

Notes: While the table displays regional categories used by the FAO, the IFs forecasts are for descriptively comparable World Bank regions; there may be small differences in the regionalization of the FAO and IFs forecasts. Calorie estimates from the FAO are based on national Food Balance Sheets rather than food consumption surveys. Thus, they refer to average available calories rather than consumed calories, and are reasonably assumed to be greater than consumed calories.

Source: FAO 2006: 8 and IFs Version 6.32 base case forecast.

the global disruption of income growth resulting from the economic crisis that began in 2008, the analysis with IFs suggests that the longer-term trend in available calories per capita (and thus reduction in undernutrition) continues to appear positive. Forecasts of available calories per capita in IFs are largely very similar to those that the UN Food and Agricultural Organization (FAO) projected in 2006 (see Table 5.1).

Given expectations of increasing calories per capita, IFs forecasts that childhood undernutrition will continue to fall around the world in the base case scenario (Figure 5.3 shows the pattern across country economy categories). At a regional level, the most acute reduction appears in South Asia, where the historical prevalence of undernutrition stands in marked contrast to its expected future of quite rapid economic development (especially in India). By mid-century, projected childhood undernutrition falls to 5 percent or less in all but two regions (South Asia and sub-Saharan Africa), where it remains at 7–8 percent.

Childhood undernutrition and mortality: Alternative scenarios

How might an expansion of policies and programs focused on reducing childhood undernutrition decrease child mortality relative to our base case forecast? Alternatively, how might rising hunger, perhaps in conjunction with unexpected conflict or political turmoil, increase child deaths? To explore these questions, we created high and low scenarios within IFs in which the rate of childhood undernutrition either increases or decreases by 50 percent of its base case expected value by 2030 (see again Box 5.1 for discussion of the foundation for potential variation in undernutrition rates).[11]

On a global basis, the forecast difference between the two scenarios in under-five deaths totals as much as 1.82 million in peak year 2026 (see Figure 5.4). We project the greatest impact in sub-Saharan Africa, where the child mortality rate across our forecast horizon varies by five deaths per 1,000 (e.g., 11.2 versus 16.2 in 2030), and almost 500,000 fewer child deaths occur in the low-undernutrition scenario (as compared to the high scenario) every year from 2020 to 2060. Significant differences also occur in South Asia, where we forecast nearly 600,000 fewer child deaths in peak years (late-

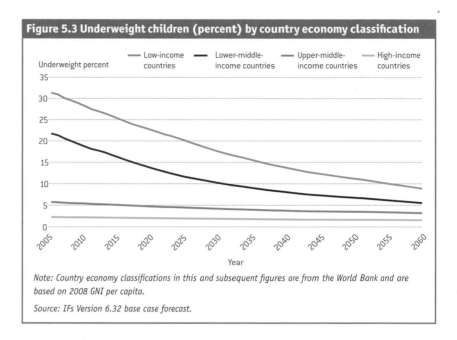

Figure 5.3 Underweight children (percent) by country economy classification

Note: Country economy classifications in this and subsequent figures are from the World Bank and are based on 2008 GNI per capita.

Source: IFs Version 6.32 base case forecast.

2020s). In short, alternative undernutrition rates result in tremendous differences in forecasts of child mortality.

While differences between scenarios peak in the late 2020s, we forecast that child mortality will generally fall across all regions over time. Because child mortality steadily decreases in the base case, the impact of alternative undernutrition scenarios gradually

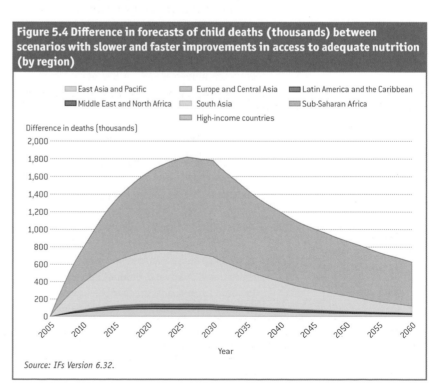

Figure 5.4 Difference in forecasts of child deaths (thousands) between scenarios with slower and faster improvements in access to adequate nutrition (by region)

Source: IFs Version 6.32.

● In our low
undernutrition
scenario, we
forecast as many
as 1.8 million
fewer deaths of
children under five
in 2026 (the year
of peak difference)
than in our high
scenario. ●

● The global
number of adults
considered
overweight
surpassed
those who were
underweight for
the first time in
2000. ●

erodes. The impact of alternative futures for undernutrition would be even somewhat greater but for the fact that the low undernutrition scenario is responsible for a substantial increase in global population by 2060 (about 21 million) compared to the high undernutrition scenario, increasing the population at risk and placing some pressure on food systems (a topic that we explore in our forward linkages in Chapter 7).

Overweight and Obesity

Historically, those concerned about nutrition, and especially about nutrition in the developing world, focused on undernutrition. More recently, there has been increasing awareness of a spectrum of malnutrition extending across insufficiency, excess, and poor or incomplete nutritional quality. Unfortunately, simply being able to eat more and gain weight does not necessarily translate into good health.

Increased body mass can mask serious deficiencies in vitamins, minerals, and other important nutrients. More directly, however, numerous studies relate the growing burden of many noncommunicable diseases to a worldwide escalation of overweight and obesity. As body weight rises, so does the risk of cardiovascular diseases, type 2 diabetes, osteoarthritis, and some cancers.

Overweight and obesity are generally measured in terms of body mass index (see endnote for a description of how BMI is calculated).[12] WHO defines 21–22 as the optimum universal BMI. A BMI equal to or greater than 25 describes overweight, while a BMI equal to or greater than 30 classifies an individual as obese (James et al. 2004).

In 2000, for the first time the global number of adults considered overweight surpassed those who were underweight (Caballero 2007: 1). The prevalence of obesity began rising in high-income countries in the 1930s; the explosion in overweight and obesity appeared more recently and is occurring much more rapidly in low- and middle-income countries (Popkin and Gordon-Larsen 2004). In some Latin American countries, the annual increase in overweight and obesity prevalence rates throughout the 1990s was more than 1 percent—a growth rate four times that of the United States during the same period (Popkin 2002). While data on prevalence and trends in

much of the world remain scarce, studies suggest similarly large increases throughout the 1990s in overweight and obesity for parts of the Middle East, Asia, and even sub-Saharan Africa (Popkin 2002). Many of these countries may bear a double nutritional burden, with excess calorie intake among some population segments even as others remain undernourished.

Drivers and forecasts of obesity

Fundamentally, weight gain results when an individual consumes more energy than the body is using. Yet behind this fairly simple insight lies a more complex web of causality, as suggested by the recognition that interventions aimed at changing eating and/or physical activity patterns often fail to produce sustained results (Hill 2006). Rather, a combination of genetic, nutritional, environmental, and economic factors must converge to produce the rapid increases in population overweight and obesity observed over the past few decades.

Evidence suggests (Peters et al. 2002) that humans evolved to contend with an environment in which food was often unavailable and survival required extensive physical activity (and hence high calorie intake). The environment has changed much more quickly than human physiology; as described in the section on undernutrition, available calories have risen quickly throughout most of the world. Moreover, the composition of available calories has changed over time. Paradoxically, today the (over)production of the cheapest foods, such as vegetable oils and sugar, contribute to a world marked both by oversupply and undernutrition, as individuals consume energy-dense rather than nutrient-dense foods (Elinder 2005; Swinburn et al. 2004). In both high- and some middle-income countries, obesity impacts especially the poorest socioeconomic classes, in part because nutrient-dense foods (such as whole fruits and vegetables) tend to cost more than energy-dense fast foods (Tanumihardjo et al. 2007).[13]

Popkin and Doak (1998) describe a *nutrition transition*, analogous to the demographic and epidemiologic transitions, in which populations abandon traditional ethnic foods and eating practices in favor of a "Western" diet filled with animal products, refined grains, sugar, and fat. Multiple factors drive the nutrition transition, including rising incomes; food prices (themselves influenced by government agricultural policies and agricultural technology); urbanization; and food marketing (Elinder 2005; Popkin and Doak 1998; Swinburn et al. 2004).[14] The factors influencing the nutrition transition also tend to change a population's physical activity patterns, reducing needed calorie intake. Economic development often leads to more sedentary employment, to automobiles replacing bicycles as a primary mode of transportation, and to increased opportunity for sedentary leisure time.

Published forecasts of body mass index often extrapolate from historical trends, due in large part to a paucity of analytical foundations on which to base forecasts (James et al. 2004). However, given the very large increases in both mean BMI and obesity in the recent past, extrapolative methods tend to produce extremely alarming estimates. For example, a recent study estimates that in the United States, where the prevalence of individuals with BMIs over 25 jumped from 47 percent in 1960 to 66 percent in 2003 (Wang, Colditz, and Kuntz 2007), 78 percent of men and 71 percent of women will be overweight in 2020, and over 40 percent of both sexes will be classified as obese (Ruhm 2007). Similarly, WHO forecasts obesity rates of more than 40 percent for many countries by 2015 (https://apps.who.int/infobase/index.aspx).

For a long-range forecast in which body weight modifies health outcomes, such trend forecasting makes little sense as a baseline trajectory. As populations recognize the health effects of poor diet and limited physical activity, they will likely respond in ways that halt or at least slow further weight gain, even if long-term interventions demonstrate mixed results with respect to weight loss. In fact, we currently see some evidence of both government- and consumer-initiated changes, including health promotion campaigns and regulations on food, in both high- and middle-income countries (Popkin 2002).

Of course, exactly how such efforts may ultimately impact body-weight trends remains highly speculative. We are aware of no long-term forecasts of BMI (at least on a global scale) that attempt to model the impact of potential interventions. Instead, projections often vary trend assumptions exogenously. For example, the GBD project's mortality forecast for diabetes (which incorporates BMI) uses time-trend

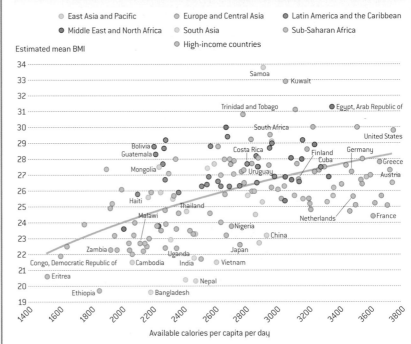

Figure 5.5 Body mass index as a function of calorie availability for females age 30 and older

Legend:
- East Asia and Pacific
- Europe and Central Asia
- Latin America and the Caribbean
- Middle East and North Africa
- South Asia
- Sub-Saharan Africa
- High-income countries

Estimated mean BMI

Available calories per capita per day

Notes: Equation: $-29.44927 + 7.0156 * \ln(x)$; R-squared = 0.2839; SE = 2.15; SE/mean = 0.083. Second-order polynomial has better fit and shows saturation more clearly, but not for males; correlation with calories considerably higher for males (R-squared = 0.51).

Source: IFs Version 6.32 using FAO and WHO data for available calories and BMI respectively (most recent by country).

projections from the WHO's Surf2 report (WHO Global Infobase Team 2005) but modifies them somewhat—after 2010, the GBD project models BMI flattening to 2015 and then remaining constant to 2030.[15]

Rather than extrapolation or exogenous specification of future patterns, IFs uses a driver-based approach, relating adult mean BMI to projections of available calories per capita, the demand for which responds to a function estimated cross-sectionally with income. From forecasts of mean BMI we calculate the population percentage of obesity, using sex-specific linear equations published by CRA authors.[16] Cross-sectional analysis indicates an apparent saturation of calorie availability near 3500 calories per capita per day at higher levels of income. Albeit less clearly, Figure 5.5 also suggests a beginning of saturation of BMI rise with increased calorie availability (especially in Europe).

As a result of saturating calorie availability, and to a lesser degree saturating BMI in high-calorie countries, our base case forecasts of

Our base case forecasts that average BMI and obesity will rise fairly slowly but steadily across all regions through 2060.

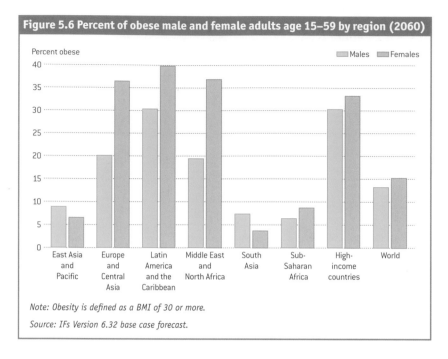

Figure 5.6 Percent of obese male and female adults age 15–59 by region (2060)

Percent obese

Legend: ■ Males ■ Females

Regions (x-axis): East Asia and Pacific; Europe and Central Asia; Latin America and the Caribbean; Middle East and North Africa; South Asia; Sub-Saharan Africa; High-income countries; World

Note: Obesity is defined as a BMI of 30 or more.

Source: IFs Version 6.32 base case forecast.

the lower-middle- and upper-middle-income countries, where there is a combination of significant existing and rising levels of obesity.

There are clear sex differences in population BMI, with contemporary female obesity rates far exceeding those of males across all regions (WHO Global Infobase Team 2005). This trend generally continues throughout our forecasts, though our somewhat slower forecast increase in female (compared to male) average BMI results in slightly higher male obesity rates for the East Asia and Pacific and South Asia regions by 2060. However, for the majority of regions projected to experience a high burden of obesity, female rates will remain between 10 and 20 percent higher than male obesity rates. These observations and forecasts suggest that women could suffer disproportionately from the major ill-health outcomes related to overweight and obesity.

Adult BMI and related mortality: Alternative scenarios

Associations exist between elevated BMI and a host of disease outcomes, including ischaemic heart disease, type 2 diabetes, hypertensive disease, breast cancer, colon and rectal cancers, endometrial cancer, osteoarthritis, and cerebrovascular disease (James et al. 2004). However, quantifying the relationship between BMI and cause-specific mortality becomes complicated by the long lag, typical with chronic diseases, between risk factor, disease

average BMI and obesity rise fairly slowly but steadily across all regions through 2060 (see Figure 5.6). Regionally, IFs projects the fastest rise in Latin America, where an estimated 26 percent obesity rate in 2005 may increase to over 35 percent by 2060. At the other extreme, the obesity rate in sub-Saharan Africa is forecast to rise only from 5.2 percent in 2005 to 7.6 percent in 2060. In fact, in coming decades the biggest news with respect to health implications of the global obesity epidemic will likely be in

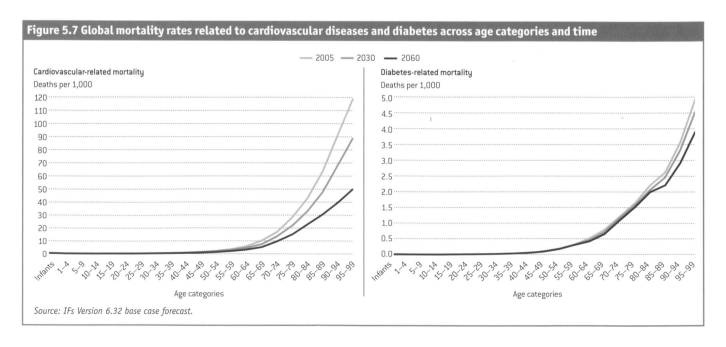

Figure 5.7 Global mortality rates related to cardiovascular diseases and diabetes across age categories and time

Legend: — 2005 — 2030 — 2060

Cardiovascular-related mortality
Deaths per 1,000

Diabetes-related mortality
Deaths per 1,000

Age categories

Source: IFs Version 6.32 base case forecast.

incidence, and eventual death. Still, in the case of two main cause-groups, cardiovascular diseases and type 2 diabetes, significant research exists to allow us to use BMI to modify mortality using published relative-risk estimates (Danaei et al. 2009; McGee and DPC 2005). For cardiovascular-related mortality we use the relative-risk estimates of Danaei et al. (2009: 13), increasing relative risk by 1.02 to 1.14 (depending on age) for every unit of BMI over 21. Our approach to diabetes-related mortality was described earlier in Chapter 3.

In the base case, IFs forecasts that age- and sex-specific cardiovascular mortality rates will generally fall, through mid-century, across regions.[17] Diabetes-related mortality rates also generally decrease over time, though the trend is somewhat less clear for specific age/sex groups in the high-income countries and in the Europe and Central Asia region. At a global level, the decline in our base case mortality rates over time is decidedly more dramatic for cardiovascular-related mortality as compared to diabetes (see Figure 5.7). This reflects the negative impact of rising population BMI on diabetes, which moderates improvements in other distal drivers even in the base case.

As with undernutrition, the prevalence of overweight and obesity varies significantly across countries independent of per capita income and calorie availability. A number of factors might explain the positive cases, including favorable genetics and behavioral interventions that encourage people to make healthy choices around diet and exercise. In addition, technological advances, such as successful pharmaceutical intervention (already being pursued by private industry driven by lucrative market potential), could conceivably alter the obesity landscape dramatically. Obesity could surprise us negatively as well. The spread of processed foods and rapid urbanization of populations are among the factors that could cause it to rise at even faster than historical rates.

Therefore, we consider again high and low scenarios, in which average BMI rises or falls by 10 percent relative to the base case between 2005 and 2030 and remains at that relative level (Box 5.1 discusses the foundation for such rates of intervention). Even the low BMI scenario results in a population average well above international recommendations; for

example, in three regions (Europe and Central Asia, Latin America and the Caribbean, and high-income countries) average BMI in the IFs "low" scenario hovers around 27, just between overweight and obese.

Yet even this modest change in BMI, which in our model impacts only adults over 30 years of age, results in dramatic differences in total mortality. Figure 5.8 shows the differences between the high and low scenarios for cardiovascular- and diabetes-related mortality combined. Globally, the low BMI scenario results in a forecast of nearly 2.8 million fewer annual deaths (compared to the high BMI scenario) throughout the 2030s. Mortality differences are spread across all regions, though we might note especially the impact on low- and middle-income regions. In sub-Saharan Africa, for example, limiting the spread of overweight and obesity becomes increasingly important over our forecast horizon.

In fact, while we often associate overweight and obesity with high-income countries, our scenario forecasts suggest that moderating or reversing BMI trends may particularly benefit low- and middle-income countries. As shown in Figure 5.9, life expectancy differences

In the 2030s, adults over 30 have nearly 2.8 million fewer annual cardiovascular and diabetes-related deaths between the favorable and unfavorable BMI scenarios.

Figure 5.8 Difference in forecasts of deaths (thousands) of adults 30 years of age and older related to cardiovascular diseases and diabetes under high versus low BMI scenarios (by region)

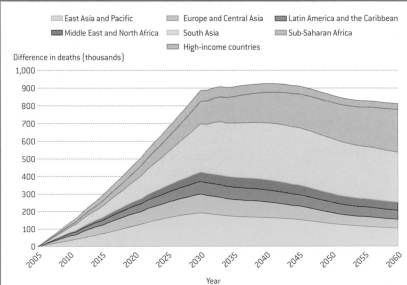

Note: Cardiovascular-related mortality far outstrips diabetes-related mortality in both total and difference comparisons. However, the general shape of their patterns is similar.

Source: IFs Version 6.32.

Figure 5.9 Difference in forecasts of life expectancy between high and low BMI scenarios by country economy classification

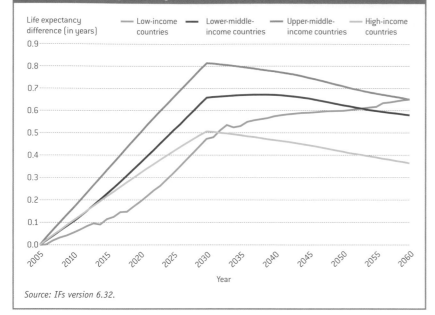

Life expectancy difference (in years)

— Low-income countries — Lower-middle-income countries — Upper-middle-income countries — High-income countries

Source: IFs version 6.32.

between the two scenarios are initially largest in upper-middle-income countries, but by mid-century even people in low-income countries gain somewhat more than one-half year of life expectancy due to reduced BMI.

Tobacco Use

As a recent WHO report on the global tobacco epidemic noted, since its popularization and rapid rise in consumption at the start of the 20th century, tobacco has become one of the world's most significant risk factors for premature death and disability and the single leading preventable cause of death worldwide (WHO 2008c). Cigarette smoking, more than any other form of tobacco use, causes the majority of adverse health effects of tobacco, including cardiovascular disease, chronic obstructive lung disease, and lung cancer (Doll 2004; WHO 2002). Despite increasing global awareness of these adverse effects, the number of deaths attributable to tobacco continues to rise. If current smoking patterns persist, annual tobacco-related deaths are projected to exceed 8 million by the year 2030, still exceeding any other single cause (Jha and Chaloupka 2000; Mathers and Loncar 2006; WHO 2008c).

By the end of World War II, manufactured cigarettes had surpassed all other means of tobacco consumption (Doll 1998: 88; Goodman

■ The World Health Organization has described tobacco use as the single leading preventable cause of death worldwide. ■

1993: 92). In Great Britain, 80 percent of men were regular cigarette smokers (Doll 1998: 88), and in the United States it is estimated that over 50 percent of men were smokers; this number increased to 70 percent in some urban areas by 1950 (Harris 1980). It was also during the war years that tobacco consumption among women in the United States and Great Britain began its trend upward, as cigarettes came to symbolize female independence and emancipation. By the mid-20th century, an estimated 40 percent of adult British women and 28 percent of women in the United States smoked cigarettes (Thun and Henley 2004: 19).

Following an earlier expansion of tobacco use, the decades after World War I saw a marked acceleration in incidence of lung cancer, as well as heart attacks.[18] Lung cancer, formerly an extremely rare disease representing only 1 percent of all cancers in the late 19th century, had by 1940 become a major cause of death (Doll et al. 2004: 1). By the 1950s, it had become the most common form of cancer in the United States and Britain, and by 1990 it had replaced stomach cancer as the most common form of cancer in the world (Cantor and Timmermann 2005: 320).

Evidence of the deleterious effects of tobacco continued to accumulate throughout the 1950s, contributing to a growing scientific consensus that smoking was causally related to lung cancer as well as responsible for a number of other diseases (Doll 1998: 102 103; Thun and Henley 2004: 23–25). This consensus was further strengthened in the 1960s with the release of numerous other case control and cohort studies from various health ministries and research institutes, all of which explicitly concluded that cigarette smoking is causally related to lung cancer. Ultimately, as Doll (1998: 102–103) and Thun and Henley (2004: 24) noted, it was the widely publicized reports of the World Health Organization in 1960, the Royal College of Physicians of London in 1962, and the Advisory Committee to the United States Surgeon General in 1964 that effectively ended any serious counter-arguments, outside of the tobacco industry itself, regarding the causal implications of cigarette smoking.

Drivers and forecasts of tobacco use

Several factors led to the 20th-century popularization of the cigarette. Not inconsequential was the tobacco industry's ability to capitalize on the prevailing sentiments of the time in associating the cigarette with powerful images of patriotism, courage, and heroism during World War I and modernity, sophistication, and autonomy in the 1920s (Rudy 2005: 148). Innovations in technology, including the mechanization of cigarette rolling by machine (invented in 1881), allowed for mass production of a more versatile and affordable mode of tobacco use. Furthermore, milder forms of tobacco had been developed that allowed tobacco smoke to be more easily inhaled (Proctor 2001: 31). These new industrial developments, combined with new marketing strategies (packaging, advertising, and branding) and the power of the images that had come to be associated with the cigarette, created mass demand in markets that had historically preferred tobacco in the form of snuff or chew (Goodman 1993).

In step with rising incomes, much of the worldwide increase in tobacco use now comes from the developing world—especially China. Studies suggest that the income elasticity of demand for tobacco products ranges from between 0.2 and 0.8, with the higher elasticities found in developing countries (FAO 2003). The retail price of tobacco also matters greatly, especially in low-income countries. Given that taxation can heavily influence price, public policy emerges as a further driver of tobacco use.

Still, while the prevalence of smoking in high-income countries could perhaps once be blamed on ignorance of ill-health effects, clearly most users worldwide are now at least somewhat aware of the dangers. What, then, accounts for growing consumer demand among individuals in middle- and low-income countries? A clue may lie in the observation that teenagers make up the bulk of new tobacco users. In fact, many studies suggest that most individuals who avoid smoking in early adulthood never become smokers (Jha and Chaloupka 2000). Young people may underestimate the addictiveness of tobacco, later finding it very difficult to give up. Thus, increased consumer demand in the developing world may result from a mix of habit formation, lax public policy that does not adequately discourage initial use, and growing populations overall. Overcoming that mix of factors leads to falling demand in high-income countries.

In the mid-1990s, Lopez, Collishaw, and Piha (1994) described four stages that characterize adult smoking prevalence and associated mortality, by sex, over time in industrialized countries; smoking rises slowly in stage one and rapidly in stage two, peaks in stage three, and falls through stage four. Ploeg, Aben, and Kiemeney (2009) adopted this stylized model to represent historical smoking patterns and to project future tobacco use for various countries and regions. They placed sub-Saharan Africa in stage one, much of Asia (including China and Japan) in stage two, Eastern and Southern Europe in stage three, and Western Europe and the United States in stage four, with a nearly 100-year period separating the beginning of stage one from the downturn of male smoking deaths in stage four (at which point female smoking deaths are still rising).

Most observers agree with this stylized representation of tobacco use over time. Indeed, a widely cited analysis (Shibuya, Inoue, and Lopez 2005: 481) of four high-income economies (Australia, Canada, the United Kingdom, and the United States) described the historical progression in these countries past stage three (peak use) to the continually diminishing use of stage four, anticipating that the smoking rates in these four countries will decline to around 5 percent by 2035. In spite of these stylized understandings, both the historical and future paths of smoking prevalence around the world, especially for developing economies, remain very unclear. Historical data are very sparse. The IFs project constructed a historical series around the sparse data with "backcasting" based on the smoking impact forecasts of WHO (discussed in Chapter 3). Our constructed historical series and base case forecast appear in Figure 5.10.

The general forecasting approach of IFs is greatly complicated for smoking (in contrast to undernutrition and obesity) by the fact that the relationship of smoking to GDP per capita is very weak. Even the rise and fall of smoking that the four-stage model attempts to capture is not consistently related to income but has been shaped historically by the power of the tobacco industry, transmission of usage patterns internationally, and changing understandings of (and attitudes with respect to) health implications. For males, the R-squared across all countries is effectively zero. Within high-income countries it is 0.15 around a slowing downward slope that

As income increases, smoking tends to increase up to a point and then to begin to decline; males have historically smoked at higher rates than females.

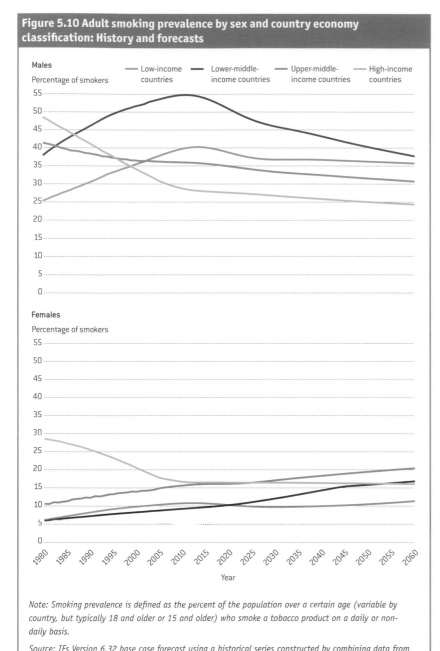

Figure 5.10 Adult smoking prevalence by sex and country economy classification: History and forecasts

Males
Percentage of smokers

Legend: Low-income countries — Lower-middle-income countries — Upper-middle-income countries — High-income countries

Females
Percentage of smokers

Year

Note: Smoking prevalence is defined as the percent of the population over a certain age (variable by country, but typically 18 and older or 15 and older) who smoke a tobacco product on a daily or non-daily basis.

Source: IFs Version 6.32 base case forecast using a historical series constructed by combining data from WDI and WHO with Mathers and Loncar's smoking impact series (Mathers and Loncar 2006: see Chapter 3 of this volume for IFs methodology).

everywhere except in high-income countries. It is possible, for example, that rates in East Asia and Pacific could rise especially sharply (in China, current rates for men are over 50 percent and those for women are under 10 percent). In contrast to the health disadvantage that women have with respect to obesity, they have historically had an advantage with respect to smoking. That is now eroding, especially in middle-income countries. Yet, stronger and better publicized evidence exists today to detail the ill-health effects of smoking. Policy initiatives, such as the global tobacco treaty, may slow initial and/or continued use in many areas. In short, any forecast of tobacco use is open to significant modification and human intervention. See the technical documentation of the IFs health model (Hughes et al. 2010) and Chapter 3 of this volume for our approach.

Tobacco use and related mortality: Alternative scenarios

For several reasons, it is not appropriate to use data on the current prevalence of smoking to obtain smoking-attributable mortality estimates. Due to rapidly changing patterns in tobacco consumption, cross-country comparable data on smoking prevalence are often unavailable or inaccurate, and therefore cannot provide a reliable indicator of attributable risk. Furthermore, the health effects of smoking are related to an exposure history that is influenced in many different ways, including the number of cigarettes smoked per day, at what age smoking began, the degree of inhalation, and the characteristic of the cigarette itself (that is, tar and nicotine content, filter type, and amount of tobacco in one cigarette). And importantly, as we noted in Chapter 3, the lag between smoking and its health impacts appears to be about 25 years.

Future smoking rates remain open to human intervention. Policy initiatives can aim to change individual behavior, raise prices, limit production and export, and create environmental conditions less hospitable to smoking, such as the restrictions on public smoking passed in many countries in recent years. Therefore, we explore a "reduced smoking scenario" in which smoking prevalence falls steadily for males to 50 percent of its

would suggest rates in 2035 closer to 20–25 percent than the 5 percent forecast of Shibuya, Inoue, and Lopez (2005: 481). In spite of relatively low income levels, male smoking rates in many other regions of the world, including East Asia and Pacific, where they are currently especially high, may be near their peaks.

For females, the slope of the again weak relationship of smoking to income is actually upward. Female rates are rising almost

base case rate by 2030 and to 25 percent of the gender-specific base rate for females. The 75 percent reduction for females introduces a greater range of variability for them because, relative to a function with income, female cross-country variability is even greater than it is for males (see again Box 5.1 for discussion of the relationship between cross-country variability and scenario intervention values). In contrast to the more symmetrical high and low interventions that we introduced for malnutrition and obesity, we raise smoking for both sexes by only 25 percent in the high case, in part because our base case forecast already is a bit high relative to Shibuya, Inoue, and Lopez (2005) and because global momentum to reduce smoking has been growing steadily.

Figure 5.11 shows the impact separately for females and males that the high and low smoking scenarios have on mortality related to malignant neoplasms, cardiovascular diseases, and chronic respiratory diseases and conditions. The figure shows regional differences in deaths between the high and low smoking scenarios for the year 2060 only; due to the lagged effect of our smoking interventions, smoking-related deaths in 2030 differ very little between the two scenarios since they are heavily determined by smoking patterns in years already behind us. Interestingly, while our low smoking scenario is more aggressive for females than for males, men still benefit most (in terms of total deaths averted) from reducing smoking. This largely reflects higher current and projected smoking rates for men over women.

Globally, for men and women across the three cause-groups and all age categories, we forecast 1.9 million fewer deaths in 2060 from the low smoking scenario as compared to the high one. Most of the impact (79 percent) results from averted and delayed mortality from malignant neoplasms. The mortality rate reduction is smallest for chronic respiratory diseases and conditions. In combination with the increase in overall population size in the low smoking scenario, the relatively small rate reduction in chronic respiratory conditions results in a marginally greater number of deaths from respiratory diseases, especially among those over 70 years of age, in the low smoking scenario.

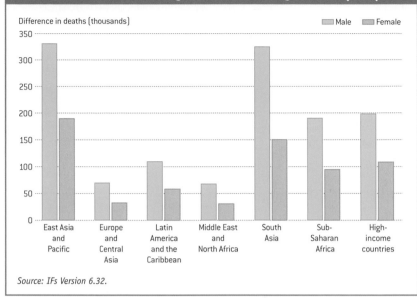

Figure 5.11 Difference in forecasts of deaths (thousands) by region related to malignant neoplasms, cardiovascular diseases, and chronic respiratory conditions and diseases under high versus low smoking scenarios (2060)

Source: IFs Version 6.32.

Vehicle Ownership and Safety

WHO forecasts that by 2030 road traffic accidents will become the fifth-largest cause of mortality, contributing to approximately 2.4 million deaths a year (WHO 2009b). Although road traffic safety is often not included in analyses of major health risks (see the CRA listing in Table 2.2), this large death toll makes patterns of vehicle ownership and safety key risk factors. The discussion around Figure 5.1 identified them as a transitional (rather than traditional or modern) risk factor because they loom largest fairly early in development transitions, and the World Bank projects that fatalities will increase in every region except high-income economies (Kopits and Cropper 2005). Another rather unique characteristic is that the impact of road traffic accidents is concentrated on adults age 15–59 rather than on children or older adults. They therefore merit some of our attention for many reasons.

Drivers and forecasts of vehicle ownership

Mortality related to road traffic accidents depends primarily on two factors: vehicle ownership rates (vehicles per capita) and vehicle fatality rates (deaths per vehicle). Vehicle ownership tends to increase with rising GDP per capita; in contrast, fatalities per vehicle tend to decline as income rises past a relatively low level.

Globally in 2060, we forecast 1.9 million fewer deaths from malignant neoplasms and cardiovascular and respiratory diseases in the low smoking scenario compared to the high one.

These relationships, in combination, suggest that overall mortality will first increase along with income, before declining as income continues to rise. Consistent with this pattern, since the 1970s vehicle ownership in high-income countries has risen more slowly than the vehicle fatality rate has fallen, and overall mortality rates have decreased. In developing countries, however, traffic-related mortality has increased dramatically (Kopits and Cropper 2005).

Focusing on vehicle ownership, Dargay, Gately, and Sommer (2007: 24, Table 4) report that middle-income countries such as China are experiencing growth in vehicle ownership of as much as two times income growth (an elasticity of 2) or even somewhat more. In contrast, they anticipate that the elasticity for high-income countries will be 0.42 between 2002 and 2030. Overall, demand follows an S-shaped (or Gompertz) curve with ownership rising slowly at low income levels, quickly at middle income levels (between $3,000 and $10,000), and then leveling off at the highest income levels (Dargay, Gately, and Sommer 2007). In addition to income, variables that increase or decrease overall vehicle ownership costs (such as fuel prices) may also encourage or discourage ownership. Policy choices and demographic factors play a role as well. Increased urbanization and population density may encourage the development of alternative transportation. However, if governments choose to build more roads instead, vehicles will come.

The number of fatalities per vehicle relates to characteristics of vehicles, drivers, and the larger environment. Studies credit advances in vehicle safety (such as the introduction of the three-point seat belt), driven largely through government regulation, with most proximally reducing accident death rates (O'Neill 2009). Others note that having a large proportion of either very young or very old drivers can increase the probability of a fatal accident (Williams and Shabanova 2003). Environmental and policy factors, such as road maintenance and the imposition of speed limits, may also influence mortality outcomes (Kopits and Cropper 2005; Richter et al. 2005).

Estimates of future fatality rates per vehicle depend heavily on both technological advances and policy decisions. In their forecast for the World Bank, Kopits and Cropper (2005) assume that historical cross-sectional relationships between vehicle fatality rates and income will continue to 2020. Specifically, they expect that deaths per vehicle will rise at very low levels of GDP per capita, decline rapidly at middle income levels, and then decline more modestly at high income levels.[19] IFs uses a variation of this relationship based on Smeed's Law (Adams 1987; Smeed 1949) that represents the downward slope only, generally appropriate because almost all the world is already past the point at which the decline begins. Chapter 3 elaborated the approach, and Chapter 4 compared IFs forecasts of fatalities with those of Kopits and Cropper and the GBD project (see Table 4.8).

Vehicle ownership, fatality rates, and related mortality: Alternative scenarios

Figure 5.12 shows the IFs base case forecast of adult mortality probabilities from road traffic accidents resulting from our interacting forecasts of vehicle numbers and fatalities per vehicle. The mortality probability is substantially lower than that from cardiovascular diseases, but for adults it is still significant. A 15-year-old has 5 to 10 chances per 1,000 of dying from an accident before reaching the age of 60, depending on

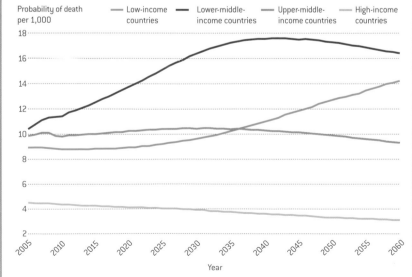

Figure 5.12 Adult mortality probability from road traffic accidents by country economy classification

Note: Adults defined as age 15-59; probability is of a 15-year old dying before age 60 from causes related to road traffic accidents.

Source: IFs Version 6.32 base case forecast.

where he or she lives. Those rates are now rising quite sharply in lower-middle-income countries such as China and India, and after 2030 they are likely to do the same in low-income countries. Regionally, IFs forecasts that the biggest increases in probability of mortality will be in East Asia and Pacific, Middle East and North Africa, and South Asia, with some increase also in sub-Saharan Africa. Levels in high-income countries are likely to trend slowly down, followed by those in Europe and Central Asia, then Latin America and the Caribbean.

Government policy choices can significantly change base case forecasts. The promotion of alternative transportation or high fuel taxes would almost certainly lower vehicle ownership. Alternatively, vehicle ownership might increase under policies designed to encourage individuals to buy cars (such as programs in many countries during the global recession following 2007). Similarly, regulations around road and vehicle safety could result (as they have in many high-income countries) in far fewer accidents per vehicle and/or deaths per accident.

Therefore, we explore the potential impact of alternative scenarios concerning vehicle ownership and vehicle fatality rates. Relative to income levels, there is a great deal of cross-country variation in both of those variables. In the "favorable road traffic safety scenario," vehicle ownership steadily decreases to 50 percent of base case values by 2030 and the fatality rate per vehicle does the same. In the instance of this proximate driver, we compare the favorable scenario with the base case (rather than an unfavorable scenario) because higher values look unlikely in the face of rising energy prices with a concomitant push toward public transport, as well as increasing vehicle safety worldwide.

Figure 5.13 shows the impact of the favorable vehicle accident scenario relative to the base case. In contrast to interventions such as reduction of undernutrition, obesity, or smoking rates, which translate only partially into reductions of death from any single disease or disease cluster (there are always other risk factors), reductions in either vehicle numbers or fatalities per vehicle translate directly into mortality reduction. Thus, while the probability of dying from a traffic accident is generally much less than

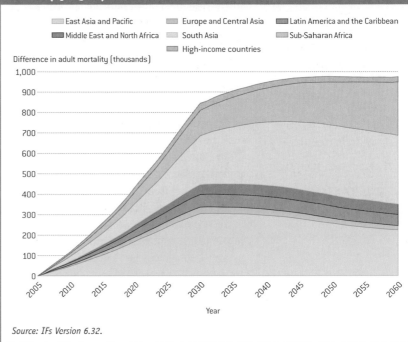

Figure 5.13 Difference in forecasts of adult deaths (thousands) related to road traffic accidents under road traffic safety favorable scenario versus base case forecast (by region)

Source: IFs Version 6.32.

the probability of dying from other causes, the total number of deaths that might be averted in a "favorable road traffic safety scenario" is quite substantial. The difference between the base case and the favorable scenario becomes especially important over time in low- and middle-income countries, where we project significant increases in vehicle ownership.

Conclusion

As detailed throughout this chapter, significant opportunities exist to change health outcomes. We do not pretend to offer solutions for implementing successful interventions, nor can we fully understand how a reduction in one cause of death might ultimately shift the burden of disease to other death causes. However, alternative scenario analysis emerges as a useful tool for thinking about the costs and benefits of policies aimed at specific risk factors affecting population health.

The proximate risk factors highlighted (undernutrition, obesity, smoking, and road traffic safety) represent some of largest sources of avoidable mortality at the beginning of the 21st century. In the base case scenario, on a global basis we forecast a continuing decline

● Road traffic deaths result from two interacting factors that relate to income in opposite ways: vehicle ownership increases with income but fatalities per vehicle decline. ●

in the rate of child undernutrition from 17.6 percent in 2005 to 5.6 in 2060. Although undernutrition is resistant to rapid reduction in the near term, even sub-Saharan Africa is making progress. Yet, our scenario analysis of undernutrition suggests that considerably more rapid progress could avert about 1.8 million child deaths annually at its peak impact in 2026 compared to a more pessimistic scenario. Undernutrition will almost certainly remain one of the leading killers globally for at least the next two to three decades.

In contrast to declining rates of undernutrition, adult obesity rates will likely climb globally from 11 to 14 percent, making it a steadily growing health threat. On a regional basis, our base case suggests that middle- and high-income regions could all have rates near or above 30 percent by 2060 (their rates tend to be near 25 percent already). Our base case forecast of obesity is actually lower than other projections based more on trend extrapolation. Scenario analysis clearly suggests making a priority of interventions aimed at limiting overweight and obesity as well as continuing to fight undernutrition. In the year 2060, the IFs model forecasts 2.5 million fewer deaths globally from cardiovascular-related causes alone in the lower obesity scenario compared to the higher one.

We anticipate in the base case that global adult smoking rates will decline from 28 percent to about 25 percent in 2060, in spite of increases in some developing regions, especially sub-Saharan Africa. Reducing such anticipated smoking levels, especially among males in parts of the developing world, might result in much lower chronic disease mortality; the reduced smoking scenario forecasts approximately 1.6 million fewer global deaths (compared to the high smoking forecast) due to noncommunicable diseases in 2060. For females in developing countries, who at the beginning of this century smoke far less than their male counterparts, prevention seems a reasonable goal. Experience

in high-income countries, where smoking prevalence has fallen significantly from historically high levels, can provide some guidance to countries that wish to attenuate or to avoid progressing through all stages of a smoking epidemic.

Road traffic safety offers another area in which low- and middle-income countries will hopefully benefit from the experience of their high-income neighbors. On a global basis, the base case suggests that accidents per vehicle may decline by about 70 percent between 2005 and 2060. Vehicle ownership will almost certainly increase with income, however, and our base forecast is for a global increase in vehicles per capita that pretty closely offsets the decline in deaths per vehicle. Low- and lower-middle-income countries are at special risk as a result of a rapid rise in vehicle ownership and relatively high death rates per vehicle. Because road traffic accidents are a leading cause of death among 15- to 29-year-olds (WHO 2009b: 3), the adoption of stronger vehicle and road safety standards than are implicit in the base case could provide a unique opportunity to reduce mortality in this population and morbidity across a lifetime. In 2060, IFs forecasts more than 275,000 fewer deaths globally in this age group alone when comparing an increased road traffic safety scenario to the base case model.

This chapter has provided an introduction to possible leverage points available to policymakers looking for opportunities to reduce health risks and associated mortality and morbidity (which is closely related to mortality even though the chapter did not discuss it explicitly), across the age, sex, and regional spectrum. Chapter 6 will continue this exploration, looking at environmental links to health and further potential points of intervention. It will conclude with comparative analysis of health implications of all risk factors treated in both Chapters 5 and 6.

1 For the most part, we focus on behavioral risks rather than on pathophysiological risks (the mechanical, physical, or biochemical precursors or markers of disease or injury, such as elevated blood pressure and cholesterol levels).

2 Earlier CRA studies included 22 risk factors; suboptimal breast feeding and high blood glucose were added to bring the total to 24; occupational risks were combined in one category for a total of 24 risk factors rather than the 28 that would have resulted from looking at each of the five occupational risks separately (WHO 2009a: 5).

3 In making our choices, we also considered areas in which WHO and others are currently attempting major initiatives such as the Framework Convention on Tobacco Control and the Global Strategy on Diet, Physical Activity, and Health (Magnusson 2009).

4 Chapter 3 explained that our distal-driver formulations already include the impact of tobacco (through the smoking impact variable) on certain diseases. The diabetes forecast also adjusts for BMI, an indicator of overweight and obesity. However, the distal-driver formulations only implicitly capture other risk factors to the extent that they are correlated with changes in the distal drivers.

5 WHO adopted new international weight reference standards in 2006. For more detailed information on both the standard and the latest data, see the WHO Global Database on Child Growth and Malnutrition website (http://www.who.int/nutgrowthdb/en/).

6 Data available at http://www.who.int/whosis/en/index.html.

7 This estimate also includes the impacts of maternal undernutrition by taking into account the impacts on children of intrauterine growth restriction and suboptimal breast-feeding.

8 As Chapter 3 described, in IFs the country levels of childhood undernutrition modify under-five mortality related to all communicable diseases other than HIV/AIDS.

9 In some cases, of course, changes of diet under pressure of income reduction can improve health.

10 Data publically available at http://www.fao.org/worldfoodsituation/FoodPricesIndex/en/.

11 For a region such as sub-Saharan Africa, where the base case forecast projects relatively high levels of childhood undernutrition continuing into mid-century, the scenarios change undernutrition forecasts significantly: from 7.7 percent (low scenario) to 23.2 percent (high scenario) in 2030, and from 4.1 percent (low scenario) to 13.0 percent (high scenario) in 2060.

12 Body mass index, defined as weight in kilograms divided by the square of height in meters (kg/m^2), is the generally accepted index measure for classifying overweight and obesity in adults.

13 Weight gain may result from both total calorie overconsumption and macronutrient composition. For example, studies suggest that the proportion of intake derived from dietary fat may influence weight gain even as calories remain constant (Mosca et al. 2004).

14 The ways in which globalization interacts with obesity through global food trade policies and practices and developing countries' dependence on foreign aid is the subject of recent research and concern (see Cassels 2006 for the example of the Federated States of Micronesia).

15 Mathers and Loncar, Protocol S1 Technical Appendix (n.d.).

16 Males (% obese) = 205.1 − 20.4x(mean BMI) + 0.5x(mean BMI)2; Females (% obese) = 168.5 − 17.4x(mean BMI) + 0.4x(mean BMI)2. See James et al. 2004: 519.

17 Both males and females aged 70 and older in sub-Saharan Africa are the exception. For these groups, cardiovascular-related mortality rates peak in the early 2030s.

18 Doll (1998: 94) noted the surprising absence in the historical medical literature of reference to a relationship between bronchial disorders and smoking, despite the high prevalence in smokers of a persistent "smoker's cough."

19 Kopits and Cropper (2005: 174) estimate that fatalities per vehicle begin to decline above $1,000 per capita and especially after reaching $1,200 (1985 dollars), and that total traffic fatalities tend to decline in the range of about $6,100–$8,600. IFs currently forecasts decline in fatalities per vehicle at even lower levels.

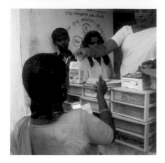

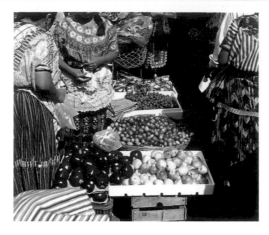

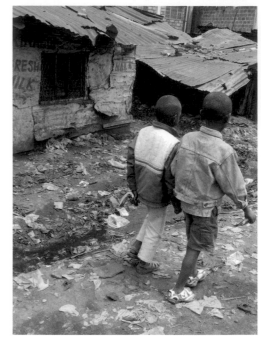

Analysis of Selected Environmental Risk Factors

● *Both traditional and modern environmental risks affect human health.* ●

People have recognized the relationship between the state of the environment and human health for many years. Dr. John Snow, considered the father of modern epidemiology, is best remembered for linking the 1854 London cholera outbreak to the local drinking water supply (McMichael 2001). The smog episodes in Donora, Pennsylvania, in late October 1948 and in London in December 1952 (Davis 2002), as well as Rachel Carson's work on the effects of agricultural chemicals (Carson 1962) were key events in initiating the modern environmental movement. In recent years, concern about the implications of the environment for health has expanded to include such emerging threats as climate change, stratospheric ozone depletion, antibiotic resistance, and the potential effect of hormonally active agents in the environment (Daily and Ehrlich 1996; Diamanti-Kandarakis et al. 2009; National Research Council 1999; WHO 2008b).[1]

Smith and Ezzati (2005), in their concept of an environmental risk transition, captured the

progression from more local and traditional to more global and modern environmental threats to human health as societies develop. In this chapter, we explore the changing relationships between selected aspects of environment and human health and how these may play out in the context of environmental change. In doing so, we must cope with significant uncertainty, not only in identifying the specific roles that the environment plays as a determinant of human health, but also in incorporating environmental change into our projections of health outcomes. As Corvalán and Campbell-Lendrum noted, while

we often know enough about environmental influences to make either quantitative or qualitative projections of eventual health outcomes ... even for relatively well studied exposures, it is possible to make only approximate and incomplete projections, because we will always lack quantitative information on some of the multiple inter-linkages between environmental drivers and health. (2005: 23–24)

This problem is compounded by the fact that in many cases we also lack quantitative information on the environmental drivers themselves and on the numerous other factors that mediate the effect of the environment on human health. Still, there is much we can and need to say about the role of the environment in human health.

Environmental Risk Factors and the Environmental Risk Transition

In Chapter 2, we placed human health into a more general framework of human-environment relationships (see again Figure 2.4). Reflecting the environment's ubiquitous nature, Smith and Ezzati (2005: 325) referred to the environment as a super-distal risk factor in that it "affects essentially every disease, even if the pathways are not always well understood." In a similar vein, Huynen (2008) identifies the many roles that the environment can play as a driver of human health outcomes at the contextual,[2] distal, and proximate levels. The effects include direct impacts from exposure to physical (e.g., temperature and radiation), biotic (e.g., disease pathogens), and chemical (e.g., pollution) factors, as well as indirect impacts related to effects of the environment and environmental change on other drivers of human health. An example of the latter would be the potential impact of climate change on food production and, consequently, its effects on childhood underweight and associated diseases.

As we noted in Chapter 2, given the role that environment plays in the evolutionary mechanisms of mutation and natural selection, a complete consideration of the environment would ideally include not only the environment to which individuals are exposed but also the environment to which their ancestors were exposed (Smith, Corvalán, and Kjellström 1999). Such a broad exploration of the role of the environment would take us well beyond the scope of the present analysis. It would also bring us up against the boundaries of society's present understanding of the linkages between the environment and human health, especially in terms of our ability to quantify these linkages. This is frustrating, particularly as it limits our

capacity to address many of the most significant and growing concerns about the environmental drivers of human health in the future. These include the effects of the growing chemical body burden associated with modern economies (Thornton, McCally, and Houlihan 2002); the growth of antibiotic resistance (Martínez 2009); and the (re-)emergence of old and new infectious diseases (Jones et al. 2008).

Most of the analysis presented in this chapter draws from and builds on the work of the World Health Organization's (WHO) Comparative Risk Assessment (CRA) project. Recall from Chapter 2 that the CRA limited its focus to "risk factors for which there was good potential for satisfactory quantification of population exposure distributions and health effects using the existing scientific evidence and available data, and for which intervention strategies are available or might be envisioned to modify their impact on disease burden" (Ezzati et al. 2004b: xx). As such, the CRA project has included the following specific environmental risk factors: unsafe water, sanitation, and hygiene; urban air pollution; indoor smoke from solid fuels; lead exposure; and climate change (Ezzati et al. 2004a). Even these analyses have been somewhat limited in scope; for example, the quantitative estimates for urban air pollution have extended only to the effects from particulate matter in urban areas with populations over 100,000 and national capitals on three health outcomes: acute respiratory infections in children under five, and lung cancer and selected cardiovascular diseases for adults over 30 (Cohen et al. 2004).

As part of its work on the environmental burden of disease, WHO has expanded this assessment to include solar ultraviolet radiation and mercury among other risk factors, as well as paying attention to the relationships between the environment and malnutrition and between the environment and poverty.[3] The assessments also often include occupational risk factors as part of their consideration of environmental risk factors, which we have chosen not to do. Furthermore, they consider a much wider range of health outcomes (Prüss-Üstün and Corvalán 2006). All of this is important to keep in mind when interpreting WHO's quantitative estimates of the environmental burden of disease, to which we turn in the next section.

In Chapter 5, we introduced the concept of a transition in health risks over time (see Figure 5.1) in which the work of Smith (1990) was seminal. While Smith paid special attention to environmental issues from the start, he soon developed the specific concept of an *environmental risk transition* (Smith 1997). As a complement to the concepts of demographic and epidemiologic transitions, this concept can help us structure our thinking about the evolution of environmental health risks over time. The basic premise is that as societies develop, environmental risks have a tendency to move from the household (e.g., poor water, sanitation, and hygiene and indoor air pollution), to the community (e.g., outdoor air pollution), and then to the globe (e.g., climate change and stratospheric ozone depletion), in what Smith (2001) has referred to as a "sequential housekeeping effort" (see Figure 6.1). In the case of the move toward global environmental risks, it is important to note that these are defined not only by where the impacts occur but also by where the risks originate. For example, the emission of greenhouse gases from the burning of fossil fuels, the primary driver of global climate change, shows a clear increase with income even as the potential effects are expected to fall primarily on persons in poorer countries.

A number of important aspects of the environmental risk transition may not be evident from this simple description, and are not captured in Figure 6.1. First, both the absolute level of health risk from environmental factors and the share of the total burden of disease attributable to the environment are expected to fall as societies proceed along the risk transition. Second, as societies proceed through the risk transition, in addition to moving from more local to more global scales, there is a tendency for an increasing time delay between what causes the risk and the emergence of the risk, as well as between the emergence of the risk and its subsequent health effects. Chapters 3 and 5 discussed this issue of *latency period* with respect to smoking, but it is also significant with respect to environmental pollutants such as airborne lead and the effects of ozone depletion and climate change. Third, the health impacts realized along the risk transition have a tendency to increasingly reflect multiple stresses, making it harder to draw a clear association between the cause and the effect. In addition, there is an increasing potential for low-probability, high-consequence events, as is currently being discussed in relation to climate change. Finally, recalling the double burden of disease discussed in previous chapters, during the environmental risk transition there will be periods of overlap, where groups continue to be affected by traditional risks even as exposure to modern risks is increasing. A clear example of this occurs in the slums of rapidly growing urban areas, where there is frequently a low level of access to improved sources of drinking water and sanitation combined with urban air pollution.

The first and second of these characteristics highlight the significant uncertainty surrounding environmental risk factors and their importance for determining human health, while the latter three tell us we should expect to find differences across countries and groups. Underlying all of this is a further, more fundamental question. What, if any, is the trade-off in terms of human health, between pursuing economic development and addressing environmental concerns?

The Environment and Human Health: The Empirical Evidence

WHO's work on the environmental burden of disease provides some of the only, and certainly the most comprehensive and

Figure 6.1 The environmental risk transition

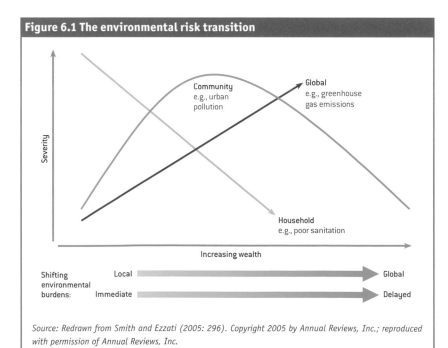

Source: Redrawn from Smith and Ezzati (2005: 296). Copyright 2005 by Annual Reviews, Inc.; reproduced with permission of Annual Reviews, Inc.

consistent, quantitative information on the importance of the environment to human health.[4] In *Preventing Disease Through Healthy Environments: Towards an Estimate of the Environmental Burden of Disease*, Prüss-Üstün and Corvalán (2006) presented, for the year 2002, the first comprehensive estimates of the impact of the environment on 85 disease and injury categories. They derived these results using a combination of methods developed in the CRA project, other estimates from the literature, and a survey of 100 experts. More recently, in *Global Health Risks: Mortality and Burden of Disease Attributable to Selected Major Risks* (WHO 2009a) and on an associated website,[5] they provide estimates for the year 2004; the 2004 estimates are based on the methods developed in the CRA project only.

Table 6.1 summarizes the estimated attributable deaths and disability-adjusted life years (DALYs), as well as the share of specific diseases attributable to each listed risk factor (PAF), at the global level for the year 2004. The authors argued that these should be considered as conservative estimates of the total burden of disease from the environment for the following reasons. First, they included only the major environmental risk factors. Second, the disease burden attributable to environmental factors is not always quantifiable, even where health impacts are readily apparent and fairly well understood. Third, as they themselves noted, their definition of the environment is not comprehensive, because it only includes those aspects of the natural environment that are

● *The burden of disease from environmental risk factors most affects children and the elderly in poorer regions.* ●

Table 6.1 Global deaths and DALYs attributable to environmental risk factors in 2004

Risk factor and major associated diseases		Deaths		DALYs	
		Total (thousands)	PAF	Total (thousands)	PAF
Unsafe water, sanitation, and hygiene	Total	1,908		64,240	
	Diarrheal diseases	1,908	88.2%	64,240	88.3%
Indoor smoke from solid fuels	Total	1,965		41,009	
	Chronic obstructive pulmonary disease	1,058	35.0%	9,817	32.5%
	Lower respiratory infections	872	20.9%	30,854	32.6%
Urban outdoor air pollution	Total	1,152		8,747	
	Ischaemic heart disease	341	4.7%	2,451	3.9%
	Cerebrovascular disease	298	5.2%	1,938	4.2%
	Chronic obstructive pulmonary disease	168	5.5%	990	3.3%
	Lower respiratory infections	118	2.8%	1,522	1.6%
	Trachea, bronchus, lung cancers	108	8.2%	931	7.9%
Lead exposure	Total	143		8,977	
	Ischaemic heart disease	64	0.9%	824	1.3%
	Cerebrovascular disease	53	0.9%	629	1.3%
	Hypertensive heart disease	19	1.9%	212	2.6%
	Mental retardation, lead-caused	0	0.0%	7,189	75.2%
Global climate change	Total	141		5,404	
	Diarrheal diseases	65	3.0%	2,175	3.0%
	Malaria	27	3.0%	1,041	3.1%
	Lower respiratory infections	17	0.4%	592	0.6%
Total		**5,309**		**128,378**	

Notes: Totals for risk factors in each grouping include diseases in addition to those listed, so may exceed the sum of the risk factors for the listed diseases; PAF is the "population attributable fraction," or the share of the burden of each disease attributable to the risk factor with which it is listed.

Source: Data from WHO risk factor estimates for 2004, available at http://www.who.int/healthinfo/global_burden_disease/risk_factors/en/index.html

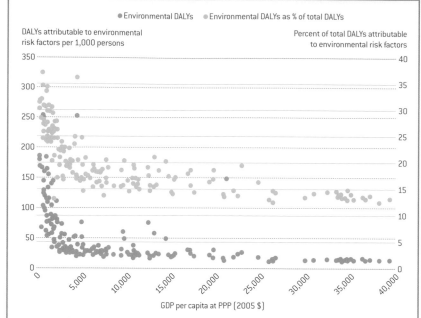

Figure 6.2 Number and percent of global DALYs attributable to environmental risk factors by country income level (2004)

● Environmental DALYs   ● Environmental DALYs as % of total DALYs

DALYs attributable to environmental risk factors per 1,000 persons

Percent of total DALYs attributable to environmental risk factors

GDP per capita at PPP (2005 $)

Note: See endnote 6 for details on specific risk factors and health outcomes included.

Source: Compiled from WHO country profiles of environmental burden of disease (available at http://www.who.int/quantifying_ehimpacts/national/countryprofile/intro/en/index.html) and WHO disease and injury country estimates (available at http://www.who.int/entity/healthinfo/global_burden_disease/gbddeathdalycountryestimates2004.xls).

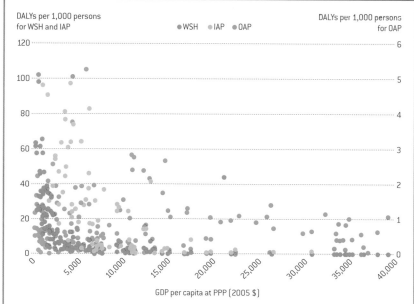

Figure 6.3 Global DALYs attributable to water, sanitation, and hygiene (WSH), indoor air pollution (IAP), and outdoor air pollution (OAP) by GDP per capita (2004)

DALYs per 1,000 persons for WSH and IAP

● WSH   ● IAP   ● OAP

DALYs per 1,000 persons for OAP

GDP per capita at PPP (2005 $)

Note: See endnote 6 for details on specific health outcomes included.

Source: Compiled from country profiles of environmental burden of disease (available at http://www.who.int/quantifying_ehimpacts/national/countryprofile/intro/en/index.html).

modifiable with solutions that are already available (Prüss-Üstün and Corvalán 2006: 27).

Unsafe water, sanitation, and hygiene (WSH) and indoor air pollution constitute the most significant environmental risk factors, each accounting for nearly 2 million annual deaths and more than 40 million DALYs. Prüss-Üstün and Corvalán estimated further that urban outdoor air pollution accounts for more than a million deaths, but approximately the same number of DALYs as lead exposure. Although lead exposure and global climate change currently represent much smaller risks in terms of mortality, there is much greater concern about the potential of the latter to become increasingly important in future years, both directly and through its influence on other risk factors.

In interpreting the results in Table 6.1, it is important to note that the values for total deaths and DALYs conflate the extent to which the environment contributes to a specific disease and the total burden represented by that disease. For some diseases, such as intestinal nematode infections, trachoma, schistosomiasis, dengue, and Japanese encephalitis, more than 95 percent of the disease burden can be attributed to environmental risk factors, but the total incidence of these diseases is so small that they contribute only a small amount to the total burden of disease attributable to environmental risk factors. Alternatively, even though only 14 percent of the total incidence of cardiovascular diseases is attributable to environmental factors, they rank first among all diseases in terms of total global deaths attributable to the environment because cardiovascular diseases are much more common (Prüss-Üstün and Corvalán 2006).

There are significant differences in the distribution of the burden of disease from environmental risk factors across regions and age groups. The risks most affect children and the elderly in poorer regions. This differs to some degree based on the specific risk factor and disease, as we will see later in this chapter.

Returning to our earlier discussion of the environmental risk transition, Figures 6.2 and 6.3, using cross-sectional data for the year 2004, lend support to two of its main hypotheses. Figure 6.2 shows that not only do total DALYs decline with increasing income but so does the share of total DALYs attributable to environmental risk factors.[6] A similar graph using deaths instead of DALYs would show the same pattern. Figure 6.3 illustrates a pattern similar to that shown in Figure 6.1—namely, a clear downward trend with income for unsafe water, sanitation, and hygiene and indoor air pollution, which are characterized as household environmental risks. For outdoor air pollution, a community environmental risk, there is some suggestion of an increase as incomes move from a very low to a medium level, followed by a decline at higher income levels. The significant amount of deviation from these general patterns, however, points to the importance of factors other than average income as determinants of environmental risk (see again Box 5.1).

Environment and Human Health: Risk Factors Now and in the Future

Identifying, much less quantifying, the current and future effects of the environment on human health can be a daunting task. Our general approach to quantification is to start with WHO's work on the current environmental burden of disease and to extend this dynamically so as to forecast how selected environmental risk factors might affect the future burden of disease.

Following the categorization laid out by Smith (1990), we start with household risk factors (unsafe water, sanitation, and hygiene and indoor air pollution), then move to a community risk factor (outdoor air pollution), and then explore a global risk factor (climate change). We have not included lead exposure, due to both its relatively small and decreasing role compared to the other risk factors and the difficulty in adapting the methods used by WHO to estimate the burden of disease associated with this risk factor. This is not to minimize its importance. More generally, we recognize that we are addressing an incomplete set of environmental risk factors and diseases (we focus mostly on traditional risks affecting developing countries). Certainly, there is a much larger set of risk factors and pathways through which the environment has and will play a role in determining human health.

Water, sanitation, and hygiene

Water is fundamental to human health. We use it to clean ourselves, our food, our clothes, and our general surroundings; we ingest it directly; we are largely made of it. At the same time, it provides a breeding ground and source of transmission for a number of disease vectors. Thus, it is not surprising that access to clean water, or more commonly the lack of it, has been a focus of attention in the discussion of health and the environment. The Millennium Development Goals reflect this—target 3 of MDG 7 is to halve, between 1990 and 2015, the proportion of the population without sustainable access to safe drinking water and basic sanitation (UN 2009).

Prüss-Üstün et al. (2004: 1322), in defining unsafe water, sanitation, and hygiene (WSH) as a human health risk, included "the ingestion of unsafe water, lack of water linked to inadequate hygiene, poor personal and domestic hygiene and agricultural practices, contact with unsafe water, and inadequate development and management of water resources or water systems." Thus, there are many transmission pathways by which unsafe water, sanitation, and hygiene present a risk to health. The diseases most associated with unsafe water, sanitation, and hygiene fall into two general categories: (1) those primarily affected by water supply, sanitation, and hygiene—diarrheal diseases, intestinal nematode infections, diseases related to malnutrition, schistosomiasis, trachoma, and lymphatic filariasis; and (2) those primarily affected by poor water resources management—malaria, onchocerciasis, dengue, and Japanese encephalitis. Unsafe water, sanitation, and hygiene has a further, indirect, health impact through its impact on the level of childhood underweight and associated diseases. As noted in the previous chapter, even when children have access to adequate amounts of food, if they suffer from diseases such as diarrhea they do not retain the full calories they consume.

WHO estimated that globally nearly 2 million deaths and over 64 million DALYs related to diarrheal diseases were attributable to unsafe water, sanitation, and hygiene in 2004 (see again Table 6.1). These represented approximately 88 percent of the total burden of disease from diarrheal diseases, and 3.2 percent of all deaths and 4.2 percent of all DALYs. Including all diseases, Fewtrell et al. (2007) estimated that 6.3 percent of all deaths and 9.1 percent of all DALYs were attributable to unsafe water, sanitation, and hygiene in 2002.

We explore the health effects of alternative scenarios for unsafe water, sanitation, and hygiene; indoor air pollution; urban outdoor air pollution; and climate change.

In 2004, nearly 2 million deaths related to diarrheal diseases were attributable to unsafe water, sanitation, and hygiene; most of them were children under five.

Prüss-Üstün et al. (2004) and Fewtrell et al. (2007) described the methods used to estimate these figures. It is only for diarrheal diseases that they spelled out a detailed methodology for estimating the share of the diseases attributable to unsafe water, sanitation, and hygiene. They assumed that all incidences of intestinal nematode infections, schistosomiasis, trachoma, and some vector-borne diseases (e.g., Japanese encephalitis and dengue in certain regions) result from unsafe WSH. They did not include other vector-borne diseases—malaria, lymphatic filariasis, onchocerciasis, and dengue in certain regions—but for future estimates they recommended expert judgment based on local circumstances. This is also the case for malnutrition.

We adapt their methodology for diarrheal diseases in order to get a sense of how changes in the access to improved drinking water and sanitation may influence future health outcomes. Since our methodology and analysis are limited to diarrheal diseases, the results presented here are necessarily underestimates of the health impacts of inadequate WSH.

Drivers and forecasts of access to improved drinking water and sanitation

The development of infrastructure providing access to improved drinking water and

sanitation has been a fundamental component of development in modern times, particularly in urban areas. Yet only since 2000, with the Global Water Supply and Sanitation Assessment (WHO and UNICEF 2000) and the WHO/UNICEF Joint Monitoring Programme (WHO and UNICEF 2008), have there been comprehensive data on levels of access in most countries.

Rather than forecasting actual levels of access to improved drinking water and sanitation, most studies identify a target level, as has been done for the MDGs (see, for example, OECD 2006). In one of the only examples providing future projections, WHO (Prüss-Üstün et al. 2004) assumed that the number of people who acquired coverage between 2000 and 2030 would follow the trend of 1990 to 2000, except for countries in Central and Eastern Europe, which actually saw declines during that decade. For these countries, they assumed no change in coverage. In total, they projected the share of the global population without access to improved water would decrease from 23 percent in 2000 to 7 percent in 2030, and those without access to improved sanitation would fall from 51 percent in 2000 to 17 percent in 2030.

Lacking an existing formulation, we estimated separate cross-sectional relationships between access to improved drinking water and sanitation

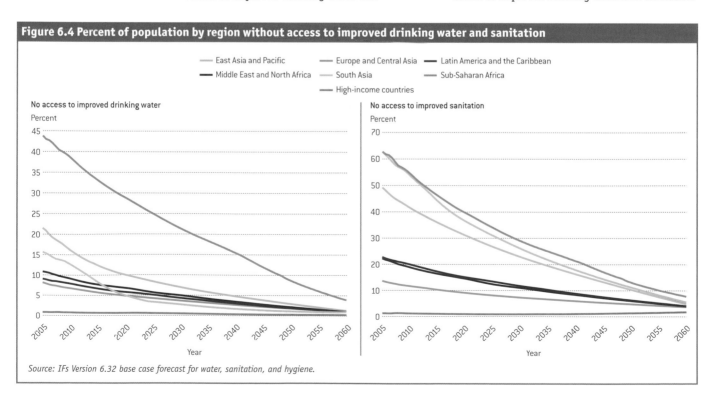

Figure 6.4 Percent of population by region without access to improved drinking water and sanitation

Source: IFs Version 6.32 base case forecast for water, sanitation, and hygiene.

Patterns of Potential Human Progress Volume 3: **Improving Global Health**

and other socio-economic indicators using recent historical data. The key explanatory variables we identified were income per capita, income distribution, education, government expenditures on health, and the rural share of population.[7]

Figure 6.4 presents the results for our base case scenario. At the global level, we forecast less of an improvement than the earlier WHO estimates for 2030, with the percentage of population without access to improved water and sanitation being 10 percent and 27 percent, respectively. Figure 6.4 also highlights significant differences across regions at the present time, with sub-Saharan Africa lagging furthest behind, particularly in terms of access to improved sources of water. These differences persist even as all regions improve their access over the scenario period. Finally, the access to improved sanitation tends to lag behind access to improved drinking water.

Improved drinking water and sanitation:
Health effects under alternative scenarios
Of the more than 2.1 million deaths from diarrheal diseases in 2005, 1.7 million occurred among children under five. Given our base case forecast of progress in access to improved drinking water and sanitation, the burden of disease from diarrheal diseases is likely to fall significantly in the future. The number of children under five dying from diarrheal diseases is projected to fall to just over half a million by 2030 and around 130,000 in 2060 in our base case scenario. Sub-Saharan Africa remains the most affected region in terms of both absolute numbers and mortality rates, but even here dramatic improvement is seen, with the probability of a child dying from diarrheal diseases falling from 25 per 1,000 live births in 2005 to only 2.4 per 1,000 live births in 2060.

Still, there is room for action to enhance these improvements by directly addressing the issue of access to improved water and sanitation. In addition to our base case, we considered two alternative scenarios: a fast improvement scenario and a slow improvement scenario. In these cases, the percentages of households without access are gradually adjusted such that they are, respectively, one standard error below or above the base case projections by the year 2030 and remain one standard error below or above the base case forecasts for the remainder

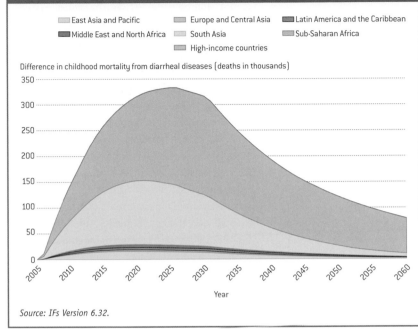

Figure 6.5 Difference in forecasts of child deaths (thousands) from diarrheal diseases between scenarios with slow and fast improvements in access to improved water and sanitation (by region)

Difference in childhood mortality from diarrheal diseases (deaths in thousands)

Legend: East Asia and Pacific · Europe and Central Asia · Latin America and the Caribbean · Middle East and North Africa · South Asia · Sub-Saharan Africa · High-income countries

Source: IFs Version 6.32.

of the period. The standard errors for water and sanitation were taken from estimated cross-sectional relationships, following the logic laid out in Box 5.1.[8] Figure 6.5 presents the differences between these two scenarios in terms of childhood mortality from diarrheal diseases. The effect is most dramatic in the earlier years, when diarrheal diseases are more prevalent in general, with a peak difference of more than 330,000 deaths in the mid-2020s. After this time, the differences between the scenarios decrease as the general decline in diarrheal deaths in both scenarios overtakes the effects of differences in access to improved water and sanitation. The largest differences occur in sub-Saharan African and South Asia, reflecting their dominant share in diarrheal deaths.

Indoor air pollution
People spend much of their time indoors. While shelters provide some protection against air pollution from the outside, there are also numerous sources of air pollution inside buildings. Examples include inter alia the structures themselves, furnishings, cleaning products, fuels used for heating and cooking, certain behaviors such as smoking, and sources from the underlying soil such as radon.

In a fast (as compared to slow) improvement scenario, as many as 330,000 additional annual deaths of children might be averted in the mid-2020s.

These result in exposures to numerous air pollutants that can exceed those from outdoor air pollution by orders of magnitude (Desai, Mehta, and Smith 2004; Smith, Mehta, and Maeusezahl-Feuz 2004; Zhang, Bi, and Hiller 2007). The health effects of many of these pollutants, particularly of newer chemicals, are not currently well understood, but they have been significant enough to introduce a new term in the health lexicon—"sick building syndrome" (Zhang and Smith 2003).

WHO (2009a) provided estimates of the burden of disease from indoor air pollution for three disease outcomes—acute respiratory infections (ARI) for children under five, chronic obstructive pulmonary disease (COPD) for adults over 30, and trachea, bronchus, and lung cancers for adults over 30.[9] Lacking detailed data on actual exposure to indoor air pollution, WHO researchers used estimates of solid fuel use in the household, adjusted for ventilation, as a proxy. Notably, they did not include exposure from tobacco smoke or the use of synthetic chemicals (Zhang and Smith 2003).

While recognizing these limitations, WHO (2009a) estimated that in 2004 indoor air pollution was responsible for a minimum of 1.9 million deaths and 40.4 million DALYs (see again Table 6.1). In some countries, indoor air pollution accounted for nearly 10 percent of all deaths and DALYs.[10] COPD and ARI made up 54 and 44 percent of these deaths, respectively; because it affects children, however, ARI dominated DALYs—75 percent versus 24 percent for COPD. Cancers presented a much smaller burden of disease. ARI is fairly evenly split among boys and girls (52 percent versus 48 percent of both deaths and DALYs in 2004), but COPD and cancers tend to affect women more than men (60 percent of deaths and 56 percent of DALYs in 2004). Separately, Rehfuess, Mehta, and Prüss-Üstün (2006) estimated that indoor air pollution is responsible for 40 percent of global deaths from COPD among women, independent of the effects of smoking; for men, it is responsible for around 10 percent (women have greater exposure because they do most of the cooking). Finally, Figure 6.3 illustrated that the burden of disease attributable to indoor air pollution generally falls with income levels, in line with a decline in solid fuel use in the home.

We adapted the methodology described in Desai, Mehta, and Smith (2004) and Smith, Mehta, and Maeusezahl-Feuz (2004) to estimate the effects of solid fuel use on ARI for children under five and COPD for adults over 30. We have not included cancers as their contribution to the burden of disease from this risk factor is quite small compared to those of ARI and COPD. Given our disease categories, we use respiratory infections and respiratory diseases as proxies for ARI and COPD, respectively.[11]

Drivers and forecasts of solid fuel use for heating and cooking

Historical values on solid fuel use for heating and cooking are available from WHO[12] and as part of the data for the Millennium Development Goal Indicators data set,[13] and Smith, Mehta, and Maeusezahl-Feuz (2004) and Rehfuess, Mehta, and Prüss-Üstün (2006) provided estimates of ventilation. In general, there is a relative paucity of these data, at least at a globally consistent level. And we were unable to find any projections of solid fuel use for heating and cooking. Smith, Mehta, and Maeusezahl-Feuz (2004) and Rehfuess, Mehta, and Prüss-Üstün (2006) described formulations they have used to estimate solid fuel use for countries for which they had no data. We were unable to adopt these directly, because either they did not provide sufficient detail or they included explanatory factors that are not currently in IFs.

Lacking an existing formulation, we estimated a cross-sectional relationship between the use of solid fuels for heating and cooking and other socio-economic indicators using recent historical data. The key explanatory variables we identified were income per capita, income distribution, and education.[14]

Figure 6.6 presents current and future estimates of solid fuel use for our base case scenario. We did not assume any changes in the ventilation coefficients over time in this scenario. The data show significant differences across regions. As with unsafe water and sanitation, the greatest exposure is in sub-Saharan Africa, where more than 80 percent of the population currently uses solid fuels as a primary household energy source. South Asia and East Asia and Pacific also exhibit high levels of solid fuel use, but it should be noted that in China, which dominates the East Asia and Pacific region, there is extensive use of cleaner stoves and improved ventilation, which results in less exposure to indoor air pollution (Smith, Mehta, and Maeusezahl-Feuz 2004). The levels fall over time in the base case, but we forecast that even in 2060 more than 30 percent of the population in sub-Saharan Africa and more than 10 percent in South Asia will still use solid fuel.

Indoor air pollution: Health effects under alternative scenarios

As we did with unsafe water, sanitation, and hygiene, we explore three scenarios in order to understand the effect of indoor air pollution on future health. These include the base case scenario, a fast improvement scenario, and a slow improvement scenario. In these latter two cases, the percentage of households using solid fuels are gradually adjusted such that they are, respectively, one standard error below or above the base case projections by the year 2030 and then remain one standard error below or above the evolving base case projections for the remainder of the period. The standard errors for solid fuel use were taken from estimated cross-sectional relationships, following the logic laid out in Box 5.1.[15] Please note that these differences can be interpreted as a combination of differences in reductions in solid fuel use and improvements in ventilation through such actions as the increased use of improved cook stoves.

The story for respiratory infections among children under five is very similar to that for diarrheal diseases discussed in the previous section. In the base case, total global deaths fall from just under 1.8 million in 2005 to around 590,000 in 2030 and 158,000 in 2060. Most of these deaths occur in sub-Saharan Africa and South Asia, with these two regions accounting for over 85 percent of the deaths in 2005 and over 90 percent in 2060. A comparison of the slow and fast improvement scenarios (Figure 6.7) shows a peak difference on the order of 225,000 deaths in the early 2020s. As with diarrheal diseases, the size of this difference in terms of number of deaths decreases in later years as the overall level of mortality from respiratory infections among children declines. Even so, there are still over 50,000 more deaths in the slow improvement scenario in 2060.

The story for respiratory diseases among adults over 30 is somewhat more complicated. This is

in large part because the size of the adult, and particularly the elderly, population is projected to grow significantly between now and mid-century. In our base case scenario, global mortality from respiratory diseases among adults over 30 rises

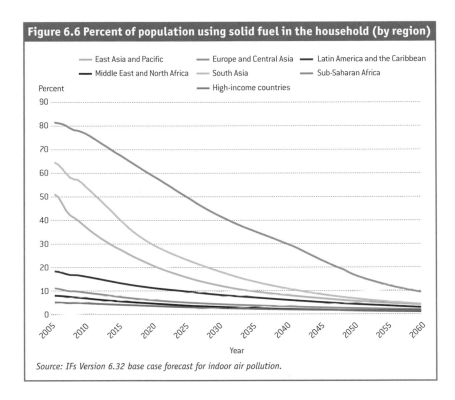

Figure 6.6 Percent of population using solid fuel in the household (by region)

Source: IFs Version 6.32 base case forecast for indoor air pollution.

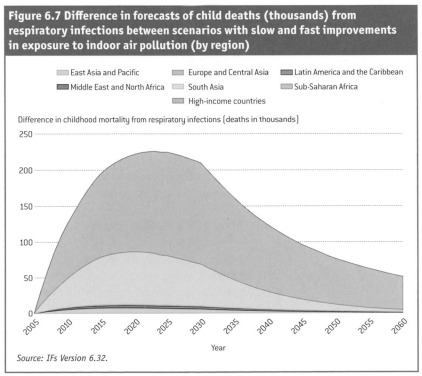

Figure 6.7 Difference in forecasts of child deaths (thousands) from respiratory infections between scenarios with slow and fast improvements in exposure to indoor air pollution (by region)

Source: IFs Version 6.32.

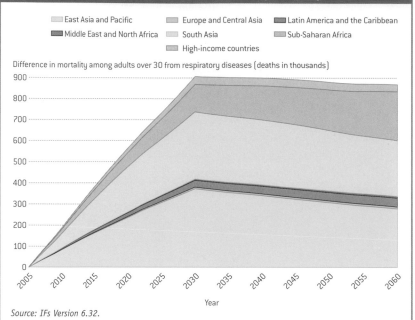

Figure 6.8 Difference in forecasts of deaths (thousands) in adults over 30 from respiratory diseases between scenarios with slow and fast improvements in exposure to indoor air pollution (by region)

East Asia and Pacific   Europe and Central Asia   Latin America and the Caribbean
Middle East and North Africa   South Asia   Sub-Saharan Africa
High-income countries

Difference in mortality among adults over 30 from respiratory diseases (deaths in thousands)

Year

Source: IFs Version 6.32.

from around 3.4 million in 2005 to almost 7 million in 2030 and over 14 million in 2060. In addition, the population attributable fraction (PAF) of indoor air pollution on respiratory diseases among adults over 30 is somewhat larger than on respiratory infections of children. Thus, we have a larger PAF operating on a much larger base over time. Figure 6.8, which shows the difference in mortality between the slow and fast improvement scenarios, reflects this. The difference peaks around 2030, when it exceeds 915,000 deaths, after which time it declines only slowly, still maintaining a level over 875,000 in 2060. Also, while a few regions still dominate the results, the effects are spread more evenly across regions, reflecting the broader distribution of respiratory diseases among adults in general.

Urban outdoor air pollution

At the start of this chapter, we noted the smog episodes in Donora, Pennsylvania, and in London as key events that stimulated the modern environmental movement. Although many countries have worked to improve their air quality over the past several decades, air pollution continues to be a significant health threat, particularly in rapidly growing urban areas in developing countries. Furthermore,

recent studies point to significant adverse health effects even at the relatively low concentrations of urban areas in developed countries (Cohen et al. 2004; Krewski et al. 2009; Pope and Dockery 2006).

WHO (2009a) estimated that urban outdoor air pollution was responsible for at least 1.1 million deaths and 8.7 million DALYs in 2004 (see again Table 6.1). These estimates only considered urban areas with populations over 100,000 and national capitals. More notably, they only considered the effect of particulate matter, even though other air pollutants, specifically ground-level ozone, are also known to have significant health effects (Cohen et al. 2004). Unlike some of the other risk factors considered in this chapter, the poorest countries do not dominate the disease burden from outdoor air pollution. Instead, it is those countries that are in the middle stages of development (see again Figure 6.3). This is in line with Smith and Ezzati's (2005) description of outdoor air pollution as a "community" risk.

For our analysis, we followed the general procedure laid out by Cohen et al. (2004) and by Ostro (2004) for WHO.[16] This narrowed our focus to particulate matter, and we look at those particulates with a diameter of 2.5 micrometers or less ($PM_{2.5}$). Furthermore, we concentrate on the effects on cardiopulmonary diseases for persons over 30. As a proxy for cardiopulmonary diseases, we use the sum of respiratory infections and respiratory diseases plus one half of cardiovascular diseases.[17]

Drivers and forecasts of urban air quality

Local economic activity, particularly through pollution from industry, electricity generation, and transportation, is the primary driver of urban air quality. At the same time, local topography and meteorologic patterns strongly influence it, as is epitomized by the Los Angeles basin, where the mountains that border the region on the east act to impede the movement of air masses. Most countries have implemented policies to try to improve urban air quality due to its known health effects. Many large urban areas monitor air quality, including particulate matter concentrations.

In recent years, the Global Model of Ambient Particulates (GMAPS) (Pandey et al. 2006) and the Global Urban Air quality Model (GUAM)

(Bakkes and Bosch 2008) have been developed to fill data gaps in PM$_{10}$ levels in world cities using demographic, geographic, meteorologic, and emissions data.[18] We cannot use such models for forecasting within IFs, however, because of their data requirements and the local scale at which they operate. Fortunately, the World Bank has used the more detailed data to develop national estimates of population-weighted annual average PM$_{10}$ concentrations in residential areas of urban centers, which they provide as part of their World Development Indicators. Using these data, we were able to estimate a relationship between the PM$_{10}$ values and key socio-economic variables, including income per capita, income distribution, education, government health expenditures, and a time trend reflecting general technological progress.[19] We then used the regional factors provided by Cohen et al. (2004) and by Ostro (2004) to convert PM$_{10}$ concentrations to PM$_{2.5}$ concentrations in different regions.

Figure 6.9 presents current estimates and future forecasts of population-weighted annual average PM$_{2.5}$ concentrations from our base case scenario. Unlike access to improved water and sanitation and the use of solid fuels, the greatest current risk exposure is not in sub-Saharan Africa, but rather in South Asia, Middle East and North Africa, and East Asia and Pacific. By the end of our time horizon, however, the levels in these four regions are similar, as the latter see more rapid declines. Nonetheless, they remain significantly above the levels in Europe and Central Asia, Latin America and the Caribbean, and the high-income countries.

Urban outdoor air pollution: Health effects under alternative scenarios

Again, we explore three scenarios in order to understand the effect of outdoor air pollution on future health. These include our base case scenario, a fast improvement scenario, and a slow improvement scenario. In the latter cases, the concentrations of PM$_{2.5}$ are gradually adjusted such that they are, respectively, one standard error below or above the base case projections (see Figure 6.9) by the year 2030 and remain one standard error below or above the base case projections for the remainder of the period. The standard errors were taken from estimated cross-sectional relationships listed in the previous section, following the logic laid out in Box 5.1.[20]

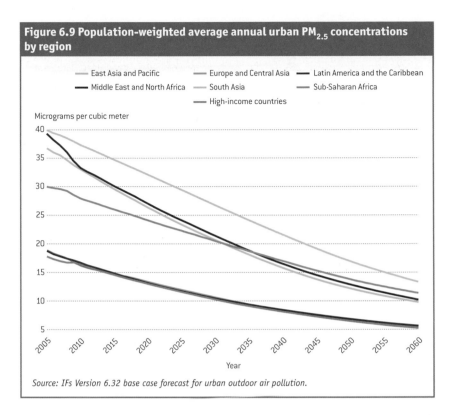

Figure 6.9 Population-weighted average annual urban PM$_{2.5}$ concentrations by region

Legend: East Asia and Pacific — Europe and Central Asia — Latin America and the Caribbean — Middle East and North Africa — South Asia — Sub-Saharan Africa — High-income countries

Microgram per cubic meter

Year

Source: IFs Version 6.32 base case forecast for urban outdoor air pollution.

As noted in our exploration of indoor air pollution, the size of the adult (particularly the elderly) population is projected to grow significantly between now and mid-century. Furthermore, as we have defined cardiopulmonary diseases to include respiratory infections, cardiovascular diseases, and chronic respiratory diseases, the number of persons affected is quite large. In our base case, the global mortality among adults over 30 from cardiopulmonary diseases rises from over 12 million in 2005 to over 20 million in 2030 and over 33 million in 2060. Only a small share of these are attributable to outdoor air pollution (see again Table 6.1), but given this large base, the impacts of different trajectories can be significant. Figure 6.10 shows the difference between slow and fast improvements in urban air quality, rising to a peak of over 2.6 million deaths around 2030 and still hovering close to 2 million deaths in 2060.

The Organisation for Economic Co-operation and Development has also projected changes in the health impacts of urban air pollution between the years 2000 and 2030 (OECD 2008). The OECD projections were based on methods described in Cohen et al. (2004) and Ostro (2004) to include the effects not only

● *WHO estimated that outdoor air pollution from particulate matter caused at least 1.1 million deaths and 8.7 million DALYs in urban areas in 2004.* ●

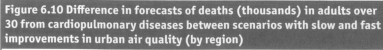

Figure 6.10 Difference in forecasts of deaths (thousands) in adults over 30 from cardiopulmonary diseases between scenarios with slow and fast improvements in urban air quality (by region)

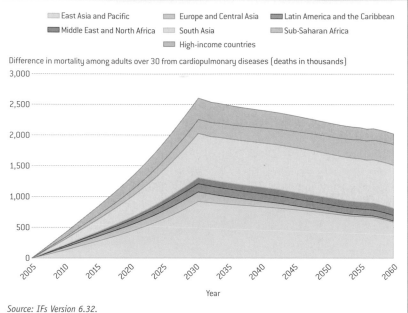

Legend:
- East Asia and Pacific
- Middle East and North Africa
- High-income countries
- Europe and Central Asia
- South Asia
- Latin America and the Caribbean
- Sub-Saharan Africa

Difference in mortality among adults over 30 from cardiopulmonary diseases (deaths in thousands)

(Y-axis: 0, 500, 1,000, 1,500, 2,000, 2,500, 3,000)
(X-axis, Year: 2005, 2010, 2015, 2020, 2025, 2030, 2035, 2040, 2045, 2050, 2055, 2060)

Source: IFs Version 6.32.

> ● Our base case forecast is for decline in particulate matter in all regions; even so outdoor air pollution contributes significantly to adult cardiopulmonary deaths. ●

of particulate matter but also ground-level ozone (Bakkes and Bosch 2008). As with WHO's estimates of the current burden of disease, these projections were only for urban areas with populations greater than 100,000 as of the year 2000. Table 6.2 presents the results from OECD's baseline scenario, which assumed continuation of current trends in such factors as pollutant emissions. If we assume that the PAF for cardiopulmonary diseases remains

around 5 percent (see Table 6.1), then just over 1 million of the 20 million deaths in 2030 due to cardiopulmonary diseases in the IFs base case can be attributed to outdoor air pollution in that year. This is significantly lower than the OECD's estimate of 2.8 million deaths, reflecting a more rapid reduction in urban air pollution in the IFs base case.

We note other items of interest in the OECD's analysis. With respect to exposures to particulate matter, acute respiratory infections for children under five are projected to decline, but lung cancers and cardiopulmonary diseases in adults are projected to increase significantly. Continued increases in particulate emissions combined with continued population growth and urbanization in developing countries primarily drive these changes. The results for ground-level ozone are, if anything, more striking, with projected mortality increasing sixfold and the total burden of disease tenfold. These projected increases are more evenly spread across the globe as less improvement is forecast in ground-level ozone concentrations in developed countries than for particulate matter concentrations.

Climate change

Climate change epitomizes the third phase of the environmental risk transition presented by Smith and Ezzati (2005). Both climate change and its health impacts are extremely complex phenomena: the drivers of a changing climate have accelerated as countries develop; climate change operates on a global scale; there is a

Table 6.2 Global projections of health impacts of urban air pollution in the baseline scenario of the OECD environmental outlook to 2030

	Deaths		DALYs	
	2000	2030	2000	2030
Particulate matter				
Acute respiratory infections, children under five	33,879	24,548	1,202,201	860,839
Lung cancer, adults over 30	70,432	312,593	656,814	2,672,792
Cardiopulmonary disease, adults over 30	853,963	2,779,769	7,714,354	21,829,460
Total	958,273	3,116,910	9,573,369	25,363,090
Ground-level ozone				
All diseases, adults over 30	40,292	252,313	339,093	3,349,122

Note: Projections are only for urban areas with populations greater than 100,000 in 2000.

Source: Compiled from data in OECD (2008).

lengthy time delay between the drivers of the risk and the subsequent health effects; the health impacts are varied and reflect complex pathways; there is a significant potential for low-probability, high-consequence events.

The potential health impacts of climate change
Although the potential impacts of climate change on human health received attention almost from the start of the debate on climate change (Weihe and University Hospital 1979), the first comprehensive review of them did not appear until 1996 (McMichael et al. 1996). Since then they have received increasing attention as both the evidence of a changing climate and the understanding of the links between climate change and human health have become more established.[21] Climate change has been characterized as a "silent crisis" that is already affecting global health today (Global Humanitarian Forum 2009), as the "biggest global health threat of the 21st century" (Costello et al. 2009), and, due to the disparity between those who have contributed most to the risk and those who will suffer the most from its effects, as a "growing ethical crisis" (Patz et al. 2007).

We and other analysts face many challenges in our efforts to identify and quantify the present

health effects of a changing climate, let alone to understand and forecast future effects. The challenges to identifying and quantifying present effects include an incomplete understanding of many disease mechanisms and a lack of reliable data, particularly from developing countries. Together, the challenges pose problems for conceptualizing models, applying them to multiple regions, validating the results, and addressing uncertainty (Ebi 2008; Ebi and Kovats 2007; Martens, Rotmans, and Rothman 2002; Tamerius et al. 2007). In any attempt to forecast future impacts, to these challenges we can add the uncertainties surrounding our ability to project changes in the climate at the appropriate spatial and temporal scales, as well as the demographic, social, technological, economic, and other environmental responses that together will determine the ultimate health effects of a changing climate.

Figure 6.11, modified from McMichael et al. (2004: 1549), illustrates the range and complexity of the pathways by which climate change may affect human health, as well as the significance of moderating influences and adaptation measures. We show health outcomes in a final box in the figure, organized by the three major disease cause-groups used by both

▬ Compared to a slower improvement scenario, faster improvement in urban air quality might avert over 2.6 million adult deaths around 2030. ▬

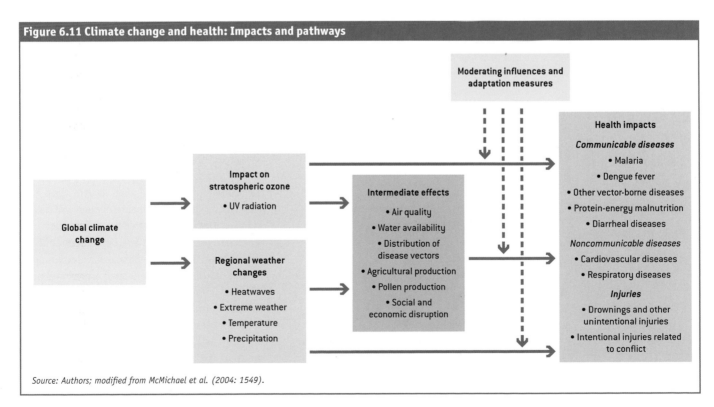

Figure 6.11 Climate change and health: Impacts and pathways

Source: Authors; modified from McMichael et al. (2004: 1549).

WHO and IFs (as well as others). Alternatively, Ebi (2008: 1) grouped impacts into three categories based on their relationship to the changing climate: impacts relatively directly related to climate variability; impacts resulting from environmental changes that occur in response to climate variability and change; and impacts resulting from consequences of climate-induced economic dislocation and environmental decline (e.g., undernutrition due to prolonged drought).

Researchers have focused primarily on heat and cold stress and weather-related disasters in their exploration of the direct health effects of a changing climate. Kovats and Hajat (2008) and Gosling et al. (2009) reviewed much of the recent literature on heat and cold stress, human health, and climate change; much of this work received additional attention following recent heat waves, most notably that in 2003 in Europe. Among the issues the reviews address are the precise nature of the relationships between heat and cold stress and human health, the expected net effect of heat and cold stress in a future climate, the interaction between heat stress and air pollution, human adaptability, and mortality displacement (the idea that persons who die from heat and cold stress would have died shortly afterward irrespective of the extreme temperatures). The population group of most concern is the elderly and, to a somewhat lesser extent, adults with chronic diseases and children. In addition, studies focus on urban areas, both because of the heat island effect whereby cities tend to be warmer than their surroundings and because of the trend toward continued urbanization in much of the world. The health outcomes occur mostly in the form of cardiovascular and respiratory diseases. In general, both reviews reached the following conclusions: increasing mortality from additional heat stress is likely to far exceed decreasing mortality from reduced cold stress at a global level; there is very little evidence of mortality displacement in extreme heat waves; and although there is some evidence of synergistic effects between temperature and air pollution, the effect of temperature alone remains significant even when the effects of air pollution are controlled. Finally, both reviews pointed to the role that public and

private health measures, including providing access to air-conditioned and heated facilities, can play in mediating the effects of warmer and colder temperatures.

Some weather-related disasters—for example, coastal and inland floods, landslides, and windstorms—are clearly related to climate. In recent years, these have been increasing at a rate that significantly exceeds the changing incidence of other natural disasters (Global Humanitarian Forum 2009). Campbell-Lendrum and Woodruff (2007) pointed to the potential for increasingly variable weather, including more intense storms and sea level rise, to increase future mortality. The Global Humanitarian Forum (2009) estimated that presently 40 percent of the impact of weather-related disasters can be attributed to climate change, and that this will rise to 50 percent by 2030.

Vector-borne and water-borne diseases stand out in terms of impacts resulting from environmental changes that occur in response to climate variability and change. Insect, rodent, and other intermediate hosts (generally referred to as vectors) carry malaria and many other diseases.[22] Tamerius et al. (2007) noted that climate is a key determinant of the spatial and temporal variations of both the vectors and the underlying disease-causing agents (viruses, bacteria, protozoa, and helminths), as well as their behavior and potency (e.g., biting rates and incubation periods). At the same time, climate is only one factor in the complex relationship between these organisms and the natural environment. Human actions, ranging from the use of bed nets to deliberate modifications of the landscape (in order to reduce vector populations) to traditional and modern medications, further mediate the ultimate effects on human health. Most researchers agree that climate change will have significant effects on vector-borne diseases, at least in terms of their spatial and temporal distribution; however, debate remains around the net effect of climate change on mortality and morbidity from these diseases.[23]

Climate factors also strongly influence the life cycles of, and human exposure to, many pathogens transmitted through contaminated food and water (Campbell-Lendrum and Woodruff 2007; Lipp, Huq, and Colwell 2002; Lloyd, Kovats, and Armstrong

2007; Tamerius et al. 2007).[24] The resulting diseases include cryptosporidiosis and cholera, as well as diarrheal diseases more generally. Although a range of climate variables, including atmospheric temperature, sea surface temperature, sea surface height, precipitation, and floods are implicated in the occurrence of the diseases associated with these pathogens, most studies to date have focused on the impacts of temperature.

Among the impacts resulting from consequences of climate-induced economic dislocation and environmental decline, food production and resulting levels of malnutrition have received significant attention from researchers and the general public.[25] Climate change is expected to have adverse impacts on food security (Schmidhuber and Tubiello 2007). The Intergovernmental Panel on Climate Change has stated that, whereas moderate warming may increase crop and pasture yields in mid- and high-latitude regions, even slight warming will lead to decreases at lower latitudes, particularly in drier regions (Easterling et al. 2007). The increasing level of atmospheric carbon dioxide, which drives much of the climate change, may ameliorate these declines somewhat, but the most recent evidence indicates that its ameliorating effect on crops is likely to be much less than previously estimated (Leakey et al. 2009; Long et al. 2006). Farmers will certainly try to adapt to the changing conditions, but adaptation is likely to be limited by the availability of key resources, such as arable land and water, which will also face stresses from a changing climate (Cline 2007; Easterling et al. 2007).[26] Factors other than climate obviously affect global food production, and in turn, factors beyond total food availability, including food prices, incomes, and other health conditions, affect levels of undernutrition. Still, the net effect of climate change on global food production, even if it is only slower growth rather than absolute decline, will make it more difficult for individual countries and the world as a whole to address the issue of undernutrition.

In Table 6.1, we noted that WHO has estimated that approximately 141,000 deaths and 5.4 million DALYs were attributable to climate change in the year 2004.[27] While the results represented only a small share of the total burden of disease, it is important to note that they reflected the effects of climate change over a relatively short period, as the baseline climate year used in the analysis was 1990 (McMichael et al. 2004). In addition, WHO considered only a subset of the possible health effects of climate change (Kovats, Campbell-Lendrum, and Matthies 2005; Patz et al. 2005; Zhang, Bi, and Hiller 2007).

Table 6.3 breaks these estimates down by disease, region, and age. The message that these numbers convey is that, at the present time, children in poor countries bear almost the entire health burden from global climate change. Furthermore, the dominant impacted diseases are all affected by undernutrition, indicating that the majority of the current effect of climate change is due to its impact on agricultural yields and the subsequent availability of food.

Climate change: Health effects under alternative scenarios

Efforts have been made to explore the potential human health effects of future global climate change. These efforts have included both structural approaches, which explicitly

■ At the present time, children in poor countries bear almost the entire health burden from global climate change. ■

Table 6.3 Burden of disease (deaths and DALYs) due to global climate change by disease category, region, and age (2004)

	Deaths	DALYs	By Age	Deaths	DALYs
By Disease and Injury Category					
Diarrheal diseases	45.9%	40.2%	0-4	85.2%	87.3%
Malaria	19.1%	19.3%	5-14	4.4%	5.6%
Lower respiratory infections	11.8%	11.0%	15-29	1.8%	3.0%
Measles	4.4%	4.0%	30-44	2.0%	2.1%
Pertussis	3.9%	3.9%	45-59	2.0%	1.2%
Protein-energy malnutrition	3.5%	8.8%	60-69	1.5%	0.5%
30 others	11.3%	12.8%	70-79	1.5%	0.2%
			80+	1.6%	0.1%
By Region					
East Asia and Pacific	4.9%	5.4%			
Europe and Central Asia	0.5%	0.5%			
Latin America and Caribbean	1.2%	1.5%			
Middle East and North Africa	3.0%	3.2%			
South Asia	46.4%	48.0%			
Sub-Saharan Africa	43.8%	41.2%			
High-income countries	0.1%	0.2%			

Source: Computed from WHO data on burden of disease by risk factor, disease, or injury cause by age and sex at the regional level (see http://www.who.int/healthinfo/global_burden_disease/risk_factors/en/index.html).

represent biological and social processes, and statistical approaches, which use statistical relationships between climatic and social variables and specific impacts. In either case, they also require projections of future climate and social variables. To date, most studies have focused on a single impact. Even those that have looked at multiple impacts have generally not done so in an integrated fashion beyond assuming a common climate scenario (McMichael and Campbell-Lendrum et al. 2003; Global Humanitarian Forum 2009). Ebi (2008) laid out an agenda for the development of models to quantitatively estimate the potential health effects of climate change in an integrated fashion, noting the challenges faced, the limited progress to date, and the opportunities for advancement in this area. The TARGETS (Rotmans and de Vries 1997) and MIASMA (Martens 1998) models were early attempts to do so. Hilderink and Lucas (2008) and Pitcher, Ebi, and Brenkert (2008) present more recent efforts in this area.

For this volume, we have limited our quantitative analysis to the potential effects of a changing climate on crop production, with ensuing impacts on food availability and undernutrition. As with the more general analysis of undernutrition described in Chapter 4, the health outcomes of interest are mortality and morbidity from all communicable diseases for children under five. Thus, we examine only one of the potential effects of climate change, but it is the one that many estimate to be having the greatest effect currently and also expect to have the largest effect in the future (Global Humanitarian Forum 2009).

Using the IFs model, we analyze these impacts in the context of a fully integrated social, economic, and environmental structure. Our analysis begins with our base case forecast of the atmospheric concentration of carbon dioxide, driven by land use changes and emissions of carbon dioxide from fossil fuel use. We compute global temperature change from the atmospheric carbon concentration. From global temperature change we derive national-level changes in temperature and precipitation, using data compiled for the MAGICC/SCENGEN climate model (Wigley 2008). Building on detailed work by Cline (2007) and Rosenzweig and Iglesias (2006), we estimate

the impact of national-level changes in temperature and precipitation and changes in the atmospheric concentration of carbon dioxide on crop yields. And we estimate levels of childhood undernutrition in a relationship with calorie availability that is responsive to crop production.[28]

In order to understand the effect of a changing climate, we consider three scenarios: (1) a "no climate change impact" scenario; (2) the base case, which includes the full effects of changing climate on crop production (the effects of change in temperature and precipitation as well as carbon fertilization); and (3) a "no CO_2 fertilization" case in which we shut off only the fertilization effect. We include the latter case because significant debate continues over the level of amelioration CO_2 provides for the otherwise negative effect of climate change on crop production. And in fact, most studies looking at the effect of climate change on agriculture present results with and without a CO_2 fertilization effect.

The changes in climate are basically identical in all three scenarios as the feedbacks from differences in crop production back to the drivers of climate change are fairly minimal. The atmospheric concentration of CO_2 increases from approximately 380 parts per million (ppm) to 450 ppm in 2030 and 550 ppm in 2060. This results in increases in global average surface temperature of 0.75°C and 1.6°C from 2005 to 2030 and 2060, respectively, forecasts that are within the range of most projections (IPCC 2007). At regional levels, by 2060 the temperature increases range from 1.9°C to 2.6°C[29] and changes in annual precipitation range from a decrease of 17.9 percent to an increase of 12.9 percent.

Before we look at the global impact of climate change, it is useful to see how the dynamics of the IFs system modify the initial effect. Figure 6.12 traces out how this occurs, using Nigeria in 2060 as an example. Starting at the left side of this figure, the bars labeled "Climate yield effect" show that the changing climate implies that yields per hectare would be more than 9 percent lower than would otherwise be the case; the decline would actually be closer to 15 percent if it were not for the modeled direct fertilization effect of CO_2. Because of other adjustments in the model (e.g., in capital investments in agriculture), the actual difference in "Yield per hectare" between the scenarios is slightly less. Total production falls less than the yield per hectare, implying an expansion in the area devoted to crops, driven in part by the rise in crop prices. There is more than a 25 percent increase in crop prices in the scenario where no CO_2 fertilization effect is included vis-à-vis an approximately 5 percent increase where it is. Declines in available calories per capita in both cases result in an increased share of undernourished children (approximately 2 and nearly 8 percent in the two scenarios). Finally, there is a more than 1 percent increase in mortality from communicable diseases other than HIV/AIDS for children under five in the scenario with CO_2 fertilization and an increase of over 3 percent when there is no CO_2 fertilization effect. In either case, this is less than might have been expected from the direct effect of climate change on crop yield.

In examining individual countries, we find also that there can be dramatic spikes in mortality in specific years. These occur in countries with very low food reserves, where the changing climate can lead to food shortages when they would not occur otherwise. While this result makes sense, and highlights one of the benefits of using an integrated model, we do not wish to claim that we are able to predict such specific events. Therefore, in Figure 6.13 we present a 10-year moving average of the projected effect of climate change on mortality from communicable diseases other than HIV/AIDS among children under five over time. This allows us to see the more general pattern of the effect. The measures are the forecast differences between the "no climate change" scenario and the scenario without carbon fertilization.

The reader, as were we, at first may be struck by the fairly small size of the effect, peaking at just over 70,000 additional deaths of children under five years of age around 2050. Upon reflection, though, this should not be surprising. Given the significant decline in undernutrition and the total number of children dying from communicable diseases other than HIV/AIDS in our base case scenario, even significant percentage changes due to climate result in fairly small changes in

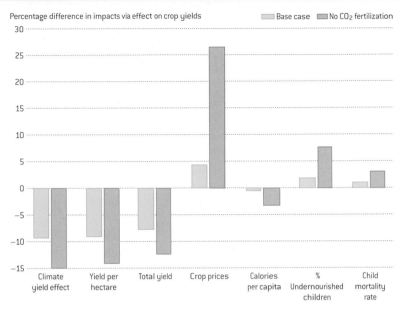

Figure 6.12 Climate change impacts via effects on crop yields in Nigeria: Base case and "no CO_2 fertilization" scenario compared to "no climate change impact" scenario (percentage differences in 2060)

Percentage difference in impacts via effect on crop yields

Base case / No CO_2 fertilization

Note: The "no climate change impact" scenario (not shown) is the reference case for this figure; the IFs base case has full climate change impact (from temperature, precipitation, and CO_2 fertilization effects); the more negative "no CO_2 fertilization" scenario has the often-negative impacts of climate change (from temperature and precipitation change) but not the generally positive impact of CO_2 fertilization.

Source: IFs Version 6.32.

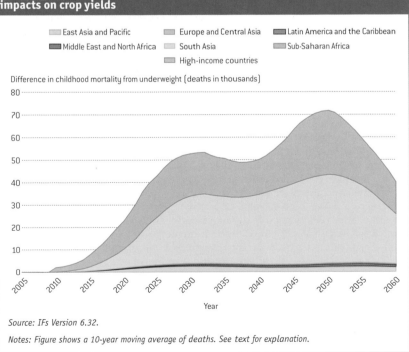

Figure 6.13 Difference in forecasts of deaths (thousands) of children under five from communicable diseases other than HIV/AIDS due to climate change impacts on crop yields

East Asia and Pacific / Europe and Central Asia / Latin America and the Caribbean / Middle East and North Africa / South Asia / Sub-Saharan Africa / High-income countries

Difference in childhood mortality from underweight (deaths in thousands)

Year

Source: IFs Version 6.32.

Notes: Figure shows a 10-year moving average of deaths. See text for explanation.

absolute numbers. We explore this further in Box 6.1. Over time, we see a steady rise until around 2030, followed by a small decline and then a further increase until around 2050, when the number of deaths begins to decline to just over 40,000 in 2060. Recalling that the total number of children dying from communicable diseases other than HIV/AIDS is much smaller by this later period (nearly 6 million in 2020 versus fewer than 1.5 million in 2060 in the base case), the additional deaths related to climate change in 2060 represent a significantly larger share. Finally, it is not surprising that the largest effects occur in sub-Saharan Africa and South Asia, which have the largest absolute numbers of deaths related to these diseases.

Comparing and Combining Analyses of Proximate Risk Factors

This chapter and the previous one have considered the health impacts of eight different risk factors and have explored the

implications of alternative scenarios with respect to each one. However, the discussion of individual risk factors leaves two related questions unanswered.

First, how do interventions across risk factors compare in their possible effects on future health? With respect to each factor other than climate change, we structured somewhat more favorable and less favorable scenarios around the base case, scenarios that take into account the variation in risk factor levels that countries have recently demonstrated relative to a cross-sectional relationship with GDP per capita. In each instance, we have phased in changes to risk factors over aggressive (but hopefully reasonable) periods of 25 years. For climate change, the more optimistic scenario assumed no impact on crop yields from a changing climate, and the more pessimistic scenario included the effects of a changing climate but excluded the potentially positive direct effects from carbon dioxide fertilization. This general uniformity of approach allows us to consider comparative implications for morbidity and mortality. However, at this point we caution against using the analysis across proximate risks as a strong basis for policy analysis, particularly since we have not considered the costs of interventions necessary to shift paths.

The second question addresses the possible implications of combining risk factor interventions. Methodologically, such combination raises many questions, as we identify below. Nonetheless, most societies target multiple proximate risks in order to improve health, making the question an important one. Moreover, combined risk analysis will set the stage for a broader scenario analysis to which Chapter 7 and especially Chapter 8 will return.

Comparative risk analysis

Table 6.4 presents the total difference between the optimistic and pessimistic (or favorable and unfavorable) scenarios in our forecasts of global deaths, years of life lost (YLLs), and disability-adjusted life years for the period 2005–2060 for each risk factor discussed in this and the previous chapter. These values show that actions directed at the individual proximate risk factors have the potential to prevent tens of millions of global deaths and several billion

---

Box 6.1 Understanding different forecasts of climate change impact on health

Nelson et al (2009: vii) stated "By 2050, the decline in calorie availability will increase child malnutrition by 20 percent relative to a world with no climate change." Their more detailed results indicated increases of 16 percent when CO_2 fertilization is considered and 23 percent when it is not. These are significantly larger than our estimates for the same year—a 2 percent increase when CO_2 fertilization is considered and a 9 percent increase when it is not. The differences are even more dramatic in absolute terms—an additional 28 million malnourished children versus "only" an additional 1 to 3 million. This is because, in their estimates of future malnutrition, they only considered changes in calories available per capita as a result of climate, assuming no changes as a result of any of their other explanatory variables—life expectancy, maternal education, and clean water access. Therefore, they applied their percentage increases in malnutrition due to climate change to a much larger base level of malnourished children in the future than we forecast (113 million versus 49 million).

When Nelson et al. included adaptive investments in agriculture, however, their estimates of increased malnutrition fell to 3–4 percent when no CO_2 fertilization effects were included (they do not present results for a case with ameliorating CO_2 fertilization effects). We compared yields per hectare, total production, and food prices between the studies and found comparable results at the global level. Where the studies differ is in forecasts of per capita calorie availability. Our analysis indicates an average increase in developing countries of approximately 16 percent between 2000 and 2050 without climate change and still 12.5 percent with climate change (no CO_2 fertilization effect). Their results indicate an increase of only 7 percent without climate change and a decrease of 10 percent with climate change (no CO_2 fertilization effect). Even with adaptive investments, they only see an increase of 3 percent with climate change (results only presented for a case without CO_2 fertilization effects).

This comparison illustrates in part the complexity and broad range of uncertainty associated with efforts to forecast the future health effects of a changing climate. Even where studies agree on basic changes in climate and the direct impact on factors such as crop yield, the ultimate effects on health will very much depend on our understanding of how these are mediated by other socio-economic factors.

YLLs and DALYs. Because of the different age groups that specific risks most affect, and the different disability weights for specific diseases, the relative impact of some risk factors changes somewhat across the different measures.

Again, these results, while indicative, should not necessarily be seen as a basis on which to set priorities. For example, although we attempted to tie the more optimistic scenarios to what appear to be possible changes in the proximate drivers (based on cross-sectional analysis), our efforts were somewhat crude. And we used a blunt instrument by applying uniform changes to all countries. Further, we made no attempt to consider the costs of such changes in the course of proximate drivers. Finally, to the extent that investments to reduce exposure to these proximate risks may affect other determinants of health, such as growth in average income or education levels, there will be secondary effects (potentially both positive and negative) for society to consider. Despite all these caveats, this analysis does give us some general sense of the potential that attention to different risk factors offers.

Combined risk analysis: WHO and World Bank approach

Recent major reports from the World Bank's Disease Control Priorities Project (Lopez et al. 2006a) and WHO (Ezzati et al. 2004a; WHO 2009a) have gone beyond the analysis and comparison of individual risks to consider also the implications of simultaneously reducing multiple risk factors to theoretical minimum levels. Their theoretical minimums assumed zero exposure when that was theoretically possible (for example, with respect to smoking); when zero exposure was not theoretically possible (e.g., body mass index), the lowest levels observed in some population were used as the theoretical minimums.

Because many diseases involve more than one risk factor, and the reduction or elimination of any one factor can prevent the disease in significant numbers of (but seldom all) people, the combined effect of hypothetically eliminating many risk factors simultaneously is generally less than the calculated sum of the effects of eliminating individual risks. For example, based on an

Table 6.4 Cumulative differences in global forecasts of deaths, YLLs, and DALYs between less and more favorable scenarios of individual proximate risk factors (2005–2060)

Risk factor	Cumulative deaths (millions)	Cumulative YLLs (millions)	Cumulative DALYs (millions)
Undernutrition	70	2,254	2,855
Obesity	68	1,054	1,064
Smoking	31	258	272
Road traffic accidents	107	2,712	3,248
Unsafe WSH	53	1,696	2,103
Indoor air pollution	22	471	649
Outdoor air pollution	87	1,033	1,167
Climate change	1	67	123

Source: IFs Version 6.32

analysis that assumed immediate reduction of risks to theoretical minimum levels, WHO estimated that

> of all infectious and parasitic child deaths . . . , 35% can be attributed to underweight; 26% to unsafe water, hygiene and sanitation; and 15% to smoke from indoor use of solid fuels. The joint effect of all three of these risk factors is, however, 46%. Similarly, 45% of cardiovascular deaths among those older than 30 years can be attributed to raised blood pressure, 16% to raised cholesterol and 13% to raised blood glucose, yet the estimated combined effect of these three risks is about 48% of cardiovascular diseases. (2009a: 28)

In WHO's most recent report on health risks, researchers attributed 25 percent of deaths globally to the five leading risk factors (in order of impact: high blood pressure; tobacco use; high blood glucose; physical inactivity; and overweight and obesity), 33 percent to the ten leading factors (adding, again in order of impact: high cholesterol; unsafe sex; alcohol use; childhood underweight; and indoor smoke from solid fuels), and 44 percent to all 24 proximate risk factors in its analysis set (WHO 2009a: 30, Table 7). Looking across all regions of the world and all risk factors in the CRA set, they concluded

■ *Even with our quite basic approach, it is clear that attention to proximate health risks could prevent tens of millions of global deaths and several billion YLLs and DALYs.* ■

■ A simulated near-immediate shift to theoretical minimum risk levels across our eight risk factors allows us to explore the magnitude of their current health impacts. ■

Had these 24 risks not existed, life expectancy would have been on average almost a decade longer in 2004 for the entire global population . . . . Low and middle income countries have much more to gain than the richest countries: for example, life expectancy would have grown by nearly 13 years in the African Region, but by less than 6 years in the high-income countries. The five leading risks alone shortened life expectancy by about 9 years in Africa in 2004. (WHO 2009a: 29 and 31)

Combined risk analysis: The IFs approach

We similarly conducted an analysis of the combined impacts of simultaneous rapid reduction of multiple risk factors in IFs in comparison with the IFs base case. To do this, we created a model intervention in which we reduced the eight risk factors currently covered in IFs to their theoretical minimum levels between 2005 and 2010.[30] It is important to emphasize that such analysis goes well beyond the favorable risk factor interventions in Chapters 5 and 6. For instance, it requires the complete elimination of undernutrition, smoking, unsafe water and sanitation, and the indoor use of solid fuels in just five years. Neither WHO nor we assume that such elimination of risk factors is possible; the purpose of such analysis is to explore the contemporary health impact of individual and/ or multiple risk factors.

We should quickly caution the reader that in addition to its focus on a limited set of risk factors, our combined analysis of multiple

risks has very significant weaknesses, and two in particular. First, our formulations do not account for all of the overlapping or interacting impacts of risk reductions (we do account for some of the largest ones, such as that between malnutrition and water and sanitation); not doing so leads to summing of some of the impacts and biases our joint risk analysis toward overestimation of the impacts of combined reductions in risks. Second, and less important, for simplicity and sharpness of analysis, our formulations link risk factors only to age categories of populations that are most at risk, such as linking undernutrition only to children under five years of age and cardiovascular diseases only to adults over 30 years of age; this slightly biases both individual and joint risk analysis toward underestimation of the impacts of reduction of risks. The two problems, albeit opposite in direction, obviously do not cancel each other out.

Nonetheless, Table 6.5 shows the joint risk analysis of the eight proximate risks currently represented in IFs and suggests some interesting insights. Overall, the near-immediate reduction in deaths, a total of 19 percent in 2010, is less than the 25 percent that WHO attributes to the five leading global factors alone. The most important reason is that we include only two of the top five risk factors in our analysis (tobacco use and overweight and obesity), albeit in conjunction with our other risk factors. Second, as mentioned above, our formulations tie risk reduction only to the age categories at greatest risk (see again Table 2.1). Also highly important is the very long delay within IFs (and the real world) in the impact of smoking on cardiovascular diseases. That is, even if the world were able immediately to reduce the risk factor to zero, reductions in deaths would appear only very slowly. By 2020, the effects of having eliminated all smoking by 2010 are very apparent in our modeled reduction in noncommunicable diseases. In contrast, the WHO analysis introduced the assumption that the entire population immediately consisted of lifelong nonsmokers.

Another striking result apparent in Table 6.5 is that the impact of the movement of risks to theoretical minimums tends to erode over time, especially with respect to deaths from communicable diseases. In our base case,

Table 6.5 Global reduction in deaths between 2010 and 2060 by disease group with near-immediate shift to theoretical minimum risk levels					
	2010	2040	2060	Cumulative reduction	
	Percent	Percent	Percent	Percent	Million
Communicable diseases	35.6	19.5	7.9	23.4	131.6
Noncommunicable diseases	11.2	13.0	3.1	7.6	242.0
Injuries	24.8	28.0	20.6	25.1	103.5
Total	19.1	15.2	5.1	11.4	477.1

Note: Percentages are relative to the base case.

Source: IFs Version 6.32 minimum risk scenario

communicable diseases already decrease rapidly over time, so the incremental leverage of near-immediate reductions of their proximate drivers to theoretical minimums relative to the base case erodes over time.

The very sizable impact of risk reduction in injuries is still another interesting result of the analysis. In IFs this stems largely from hypothetical movement to zero traffic deaths in the near-immediate reduction scenario. The modeled cumulative death reduction in this category is significant, especially relative to injuries as a cause of death in 2005, and suggests a considerable and growing potential for leverage from interventions to enhance road traffic safety. One implication of the analysis is that a world that planned ahead to reduce deaths would begin now to put additional attention not only on smoking (with its lags in health payoffs) but also on road traffic accidents with their growing rather than shrinking base. To date the CRA framework (see again Table 2.1) has not included road traffic accidents in its analyses; given the potential leverage of interventions it almost certainly should.

Another important factor is that in our analysis, which incorporates forward linkages (as we will discuss further in Chapter 7), reduced deaths in the near term become additional or delayed deaths in the longer term, resulting not only in an aging population that will die of other causes but also in a population that is considerably larger overall (more than 400 million larger in 2060).

To put combined risk analysis into the broader context of this volume, we emphasize dynamic analysis throughout. Across Chapters 5 and 6 we have stressed that proximate drivers are not likely to move rapidly away from the trajectories of the base case forecast, either in negative directions from neglect and bad policy or in positive directions with concerted positive interventions and behavioral changes. Nor are societies likely to succeed in moving risk factors to their theoretical minimums; we chose instead to use one standard deviation as a more likely representation of aggressive action.

The overall orientation of our analysis, therefore, is not static consideration of counterfactuals but rather dynamic analysis related to possible interventions or alternative futures. If we turn from the near-immediate movement of proximate drivers to theoretical minimum levels (as represented in the discussion of CRA results and the IFs results of Table 6.5) to a combination of aggressive but phased-in human action on these eight major drivers as discussed throughout Chapters 5 and 6, we might avert approximately 203 million deaths over the horizon through 2060 and avoid about 4.2 billion discounted years of life loss. This is somewhat less than half of the total with more static analysis and is, we would argue, a more policy-relevant figure.

Conclusion

This chapter has illustrated that analyses cannot ignore the environment in efforts to forecast and, more importantly, to influence future levels of population health. The reduction in infectious and communicable diseases, such as diarrheal and respiratory infections seen in the early stages of the epidemiologic transition, is very much a function of efforts to reduce traditional environmental risk factors such as the lack of access to clean water and sanitation and indoor air pollution. The extent to which currently developing countries will complete this phase of the transition will depend largely on how they are able to address these risk factors. At the same time, continued development has introduced other environmental risk factors, including community risk factors, such as outdoor air pollution and the introduction of man-made chemicals into the work place and wider environment. Further, global risk factors, such as global climate change and stratospheric ozone depletion, are now beginning to have a clear and growing impact on health. Thus, we need to see environmental policy as a key element of health policy.

Even as concern is great and growing in many quarters, tremendous uncertainty remains around the myriad potential health effects of environmental risk factors, particularly in the case of the more modern risk factors. This makes estimating and projecting the quantitative level of these effects both a necessary and a challenging task. The challenge is perhaps most starkly reflected in the limited set of analyses presented in this chapter. We excluded many of the most significant and

● *More dynamic analysis of changes in risks can provide more policy-relevant insights with respect to possible interventions.* ●

growing concerns about environmental drivers of human health in the future, particularly in developed countries.

Regardless of uncertainties and the absence of much-needed analysis, the evidence strongly indicates that the environment has played, and will continue to play, a significant role in human health. Moreover, the exposure to environmental risks differs substantially across countries at similar levels of development as defined by traditional measures such as average income. Because health outcomes reflect these differences, there appears to be very considerable potential for improved health from policies that reduce environmental risks.

This chapter also returned to the broader analysis of proximate drivers, comparing the health implications of the environmental risks analyzed in this chapter with those of the risks that Chapter 5 explored, and considering the implications of combined risk reduction. Although comparative risk analysis suffers from the great differences in various risk factors' character and susceptibility to reduction, we have attempted to create as much comparability as we could. We find that all of the eight risks are important, but that there are clear variations in the impact of alternative assumptions. For instance, the morbidity and mortality associated with climate change over

our horizon is perhaps less great than many would expect (which is not to downplay its growing importance over time). And we find that risks and opportunities around traffic accident deaths are probably more significant than many would anticipate. In fact, across our horizon they exceed those associated with undernutrition, an appropriately primary focus of much current policy. The reality, however, is that income growth is likely to reduce the base impact of undernutrition significantly by 2050, while that same growth will raise the impact of road traffic accidents, especially in lower- and middle-income countries.

Finally, we considered the proximate risks in combination. In spite of the fact that multiple risks are often complicit in any death or disability, and that reduction of multiple risks will therefore save fewer lives than the sum of reductions across them individually, we found that the combined impact of multiple risk reduction is truly huge. At the same time, however, we returned to the importance of undertaking dynamic analysis of health futures for such combined analysis. Such analysis should also ideally take into account the forward linkages of health interventions and the broader contexts of change and uncertainty in which they are made. Those are the topics of Chapters 7 and 8.

1   The range of international efforts reflects significant increase in international attention to questions of health and the environment in recent years. The Millennium Ecosystem Assessment and Fourth Assessment Report of the Intergovernmental Panel on Climate Change (Confalonieri et al. 2007; Corvalán et al. 2005; MA and WHO 2005) paid particular attention to the potential health effects of environmental change. More recently, researchers and policymakers have launched a number of international efforts that focus on the relationships between the environment and human health and the means by which to address problems in this area. Among these are the Earth System Science Partnership's joint project on Global Environmental Change and Human Health (Confalonieri and McMichael 2007), the International Council for Science's Planning Group on Health and Wellbeing in the Urban Environment (ICSU 2007), and the Health and Environment Linkages Initiative of the World Health Organization and the United Nations Environment Programme (WHO and UNEP 2008). Because of children's particular vulnerability, there are also specific efforts focusing on children's health and the environment (CEC 2006; Gordon, Mackay, and Rehfuess 2004). Finally, in an extension of its work on the Global Burden of Disease and building on earlier efforts and the Comparative Risk Assessment, WHO has established a program on quantifying the environmental burden of disease (Prüss-Üstün and Corvalán 2006; Smith, Corvalán, and Kjellström 1999).

2 Huynen (2008: 84) defines the contextual level as consisting of "the macro-level conditions that form the context in which the distal and proximal factors operate and develop." With respect to the environment, she refers to general ecological settings, including climate.

3 Reports in this series can be found at http://www.who.int/quantifying_ehimpacts/national/en/index.html.

4 For further information on this work, see http://www.who.int/quantifying_ehimpacts/en/.

5 The additional data on their website include estimates at the regional level by risk factor, disease, or injury cause, and age and sex (see http://www.who.int/healthinfo/global_burden_disease/risk_factors/en/index.html), and country profiles of the environmental burden of disease (see http://www.who.int/quantifying_ehimpacts/national/countryprofile/intro/en/index.html). Most of the historical data presented in this chapter are taken directly from, or derived from, these data.

6 Health outcomes and risk factors included are: all diarrheal diseases from lack of access to an improved drinking water source and improved sanitation facilities; acute respiratory infections (children under age five); chronic obstructive pulmonary disease (adults over 30 years); lung cancer (adults over 30 years) from the use of solid fuels in the house; and respiratory infections and diseases, lung cancer, and selected cardiovascular diseases from the exposure to fine suspended particles of less than 10 microns in diameter in cities with more than 100,000 inhabitants and in national capitals.

7 Details of this analysis are provided in the technical documentation of the IFs health model (Hughes et al. 2010) available at www.ifs.du.edu.

8 Details of this analysis are provided in the IFs health forecasting technical document available at www.ifs.du.edu.

9 Indoor air pollution was also considered to be a potentially significant risk factor for other health impacts—specifically, asthma, cataracts, perinatal effects, and tuberculosis—for which a lack of sufficient data precluded estimates (Desai, Mehta, and Smith 2004; Smith, Mehta, and Maeusezahl-Feuz 2004).

10 From data publically available from WHO. The specific spreadsheets used were "Estimated deaths and DALYS attributable to selected environmental risk factors" (http://www.who.int/entity/quantifying_ehimpacts/countryprofilesebd2004.xls) and "Estimated deaths and DALYs by cause and WHO member state"(http://www.who.int/entity/healthinfo/global_burden_disease/gbddeathdalycountryestimates2004.xls).

11 In 2004, ARI and COPD accounted for 98 percent and 75 percent of global deaths from respiratory infections and respiratory diseases, respectively (calculated from disease and injury regional estimates, available at http://www.who.int/healthinfo/global_burden_disease/estimates_regional/en/index.html).

12 See http://www.who.int/entity/quantifying_ehimpacts/countryprofilesebd2004.xls.

13 See http://mdgs.un.org/unsd/mdg/Data.aspx.

14 Details of this analysis are provided in the IFs health forecasting technical document available at www.ifs.du.edu.

15 Details of this analysis are provided in the IFs health forecasting technical document available at www.ifs.du.edu.

16 Various other studies have provided concentration-response functions for ozone and particulate matter and a range of health outcomes (Bakkes and Bosch 2008; Cohen et al. 2004; Jerrett et al. 2009; Ostro 2004; Pope and Dockery 2006). In addition, the U.S. Environmental Protection Agency has developed an Environmental Benefits Mapping and Analysis Program (http://www.epa.gov/air/benmap/index.html), which uses many of these relationships.

17 The specific diseases defined as cardiopulmonary in Cohen et al. (2004) are asthma, cerebrovascular disease, chronic obstructive pulmonary disease, hypertensive heart disease, inflammatory heart diseases, ischaemic heart disease, other respiratory diseases, upper respiratory infections, lower respiratory infections, and otitis media. Using our disease categories, at a global level in 2004, mortality from these diseases accounted for 99, 51, and 100 percent of mortality from respiratory infections, cardiovascular diseases, and respiratory diseases, respectively (calculated from disease and injury regional estimates, available at http://www.who.int/healthinfo/global_burden_disease/estimates_regional/en/index.html).

18 The latter has also been used to estimate future levels of air quality as part of the OECD's Environmental Outlook to 2030 (OECD 2008).

19 Details of this analysis are provided in the IFs health forecasting technical document available at www.ifs.du.edu.

20 Details of this analysis are provided in the IFs health forecasting technical document available at www.ifs.du.edu.

21 Recent summary reviews of climate change and its current and potential effects on human health include: Comrie 2007; Confalonieri et al. 2007; Costello et al. 2009; Haines et al. 2006; Haines and Patz 2004; McMichael, Woodruff, and Hales 2006; Patz et al. 2005; Patz et al. 2007; and Zhang, Bi, and Hiller 2007. WHO's Comparative Risk Assessment (McMichael et al. 2004) and Environmental Burden of Disease work (Campbell-Lendrum and Woodruff 2007) identified climate change as a key risk factor. Climate change was a primary focus of the 2008 Annual Review of Public Health, and WHO devoted the 2008 World Health Day to climate change (WHO 2008b). It is a key focus of the Global Humanitarian Forum (2009). Numerous other studies have considered specific health effects, and Confalonieri et al. (2007) reviewed recent studies that provided quantitative projections of climate change impacts on specific health outcomes. These focused on malaria, dengue fever, and other infectious diseases; heat- and cold-related mortality; and health effects related to urban air quality, particularly tropospheric ozone.

22 Among the other diseases are bubonic plague; chikungunya; dengue fever; hantavirus; Lassa fever; leishmaniasis; Lyme disease; lymphatic filariasis; lyssavirus; onchocerciasis (river blindness); schistosomiasis; tick-borne encephalitis; and West Nile virus.

23 See, for example, the recent forum in *Ecology* (volume 90, issue 4, 2009) stimulated by Lafferty (2009).

24 For example, Calicivirus, Campylobacter, Cryptosporidium, Escherichia coli, Giardia, Rotavirus, Salmonella, Shigella, and Vibrio cholerae (Campbell-Lendrum and Woodruff 2007; Tamerius et al. 2007).

25 Even the discussions on climate-induced conflict and associated mortality—for example, in Dyer (2008) and Campbell et al. (2007)—tend to point back to changes in food production as the key driving force behind the conflict.

26 Other ways in which climate change may influence food production include its effect on pests and pathogens, ultraviolet radiation, ground-level ozone, weather extremes, and water quality, which will impact freshwater and marine fisheries (Brander 2007; Easterling et al. 2007; Gregory et al. 2009; Tubiello et al. 2007).

27 This is an update of the analysis of WHO's Global Burden of Disease and Comparative Risk Assessment projects (McMichael and Campbell-Lendrum et al. 2003). We were able to trace almost every global estimate, in all studies that we found, back to this work. The Global Humanitarian Forum (2009) was the one exception, and even there most of the estimation methods used were the same. Epstein and Mills (2005) provide an interesting integrative analysis covering a number of diseases, but their projections are primarily qualitative. Confalonieri et al. (2007) list 16 national/regional health impact assessments of climate change published between the third and fourth IPCC assessments, not including a more recent study by the United States (Gamble et al. 2008). Of these, McMichael and Woodruff et al.'s (2003) study for Australasia has had, perhaps, the most significant impact. For additional results and results presented using different regional or gender breakdowns from the original WHO study, see Ezzati et al. 2002; Patz et al. 2005; and WHO 2002.

28 Climate change may also affect access to improved water and sanitation, which is also one of the explanatory variables for childhood undernutrition. IFs does not currently try to capture this effect.

29 The reason that the forecasted global temperature change falls below the forecasted range for the regions is that the former also includes temperature changes over the oceans, which, in general, warm more slowly than land surfaces.

30 The assumption of reductions over a five-year period was necessitated by the dynamic nature of our model. Our five-year hypothetical phase-in period is in distinction from the WHO 2009 study (WHO 2009a) in which reductions to theoretical minimums all occurred simultaneously and as if at a single point in time.

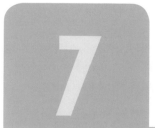

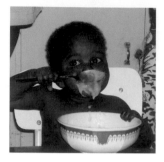

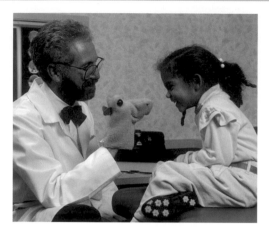

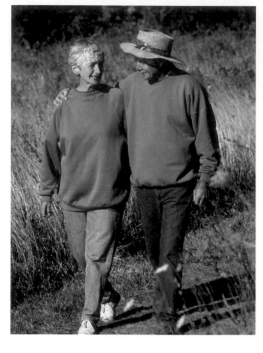

Forward Linkages

A long and healthy life is fundamentally important in and of itself as a central priority for human development. This priority justifies large expenditures on health, regardless of the contributions of such expenditures or changes in health to other aspects of human development, including economic growth.

Nonetheless, policy decisions involve trade-offs. We therefore have every reason to investigate the broader implications of changes in health in order to better understand the relationships between improvements in health and improvements in the general human condition. The International Futures (IFs) health model, embedded in the larger IFs modeling system, offers a tool with which to explore the long-term implications of health status for other outcomes in human welfare and security, what this volume often refers to as forward linkages. There is an ongoing debate surrounding the benefits of health for development, which IFs cannot resolve. However, it is our hope that by exploring how potential investments,

achievements, and setbacks in health might alter societal and global trajectories we may contribute positively to the continuing conversation.

All discussions of the forward linkages from health share the assumption that an individual in better health will experience greater productivity, a relationship that microeconomic evidence (Behrman 1996) strongly supports. Yet until recently, many have concluded that the interaction of healthier individuals in a structurally unchanged economy would remain insignificant at the macroeconomic level—in other words, the view that relative position might change but not overall economic progress. More recently, models of forward linkages have been enhanced by more detailed measurement and specification of microeconomic pathways to macroeconomic impacts, as well as by a better understanding of the behavioral and political pathways by which health can affect development very generally. Our discussion begins with the effects of health on the economy.

From Health to Growth
A core controversy

The most historically significant model of forward linkages comes from the neoclassical school of economics, in which the ratio of capital to labor determines worker productivity and therefore strongly shapes economic growth. According to this model, all else being equal, if the stock of capital remains unchanged, improvements in health—by reducing mortality and driving up population growth—will reduce the capital/labor ratio, reduce productivity, and reduce growth in per capita income (Acemoglu and Johnson 2007; Weil 2007).[1] Looking at the same phenomenon from a different perspective, a number of historical studies have tied the industrial takeoff of Europe, Britain in particular, to reduced resource pressures resulting from the great plagues of the 14th and 15th centuries (see Young 2005). By extension, many suggest that the HIV/AIDS epidemic, while a tragedy in terms of individual human suffering, will result in increased per capita GDP growth and productivity (Young 2005).

Many have questioned the neoclassical approach for ignoring the health benefits experienced by the living, for assuming that capital will remain constant in the face of changes in health, and for implying that lower mortality will necessarily lead to population growth. In fact, a growing consensus is emerging around a limited but significant role of health as a stimulus to growth. This consensus draws on Sen's support-led model of human development (Dreze and Sen 1989; Sen 1999b). It also follows from Becker's theory of human capital, which introduced a number of microeconomic behavioral changes in the allocation of capital resulting from improved health and survival, including increased public and private investments in children's education, increased life-course savings rates, and reduced fertility (Becker 1962). Fogel's theory of technophysio evolution integrates these disparate threads, noting how the gradual accumulation of micro-level biological and behavioral improvements can eventually lead to the wholesale restructuring of society around the productive capabilities and behaviors of long-lived, healthy populations (Fogel 2004a; Fogel and Costa 1997). Placed within the broader dynamics of a highly globalized economy, healthier societies might

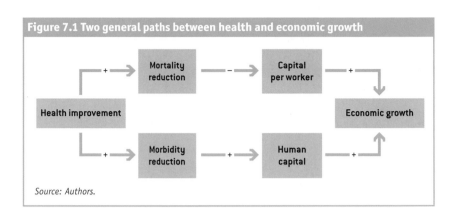

Figure 7.1 Two general paths between health and economic growth

Source: Authors.

also attract external investment flows. Taken together, these threads point to a virtuous or synergistic cycle of development and productivity for which health is a necessary, if not sufficient, precursor.[2] Historically, Fogel (1994) attributed one-third of the economic growth in England between 1790 and 1980 to improvements in health and nutrition, and Arora (2001) attributed 30 to 40 percent of developed-country growth from the 1870s to the 1990s to improvements in health. In contrast to the neoclassical approach, then, these theories would suggest that the HIV/AIDS epidemic could pose grave threats to economic productivity.

The two perspectives on the relationship between health and growth are, of course, not mutually exclusive; Figure 7.1 sketches the main elements of both, showing the negative relationship between health and growth above and the positive one below. We seek in this chapter to elaborate the many important paths linking health and broader human development (not simply economic growth) and to consider with the help of the IFs system the complex feedback systems that those paths create.

Empirical analysis

A quick review of cross-national regression studies of health and economic growth illustrates the limitations and opportunities of modeling forward linkages. Bloom, Canning, and Sevilla (2004) conducted a review of 12 regression-based studies. Of these, 11 found a positive effect of life expectancy on growth, but the size of the effects ranged considerably, from a 0.15 percent increase in GDP growth associated with a five-year improvement in life expectancy (Bloom et al. 1999) to a 0.58 percent increase (Barro and Lee 1994).[3]

> A growing consensus is emerging around a limited but significant role of health as a stimulus to economic growth.

Acemoglu and Johnson (2007) conducted a careful, cross-national regression analysis of the impact of health improvements on economic growth in the post–World War II era, a period of epidemiologic transition in much of the developing world. The authors looked separately at changing population, total economic growth, and growth per capita in order to separate out the effect of health on total GDP and the effect of increased population in diminishing per capita trends. The authors found positive but not very significant effects of health on total GDP, increasing over time. Nonetheless, population growth swamped these growth effects, resulting, if anything, in a decline in GDP per capita. Countries with improved health did experience reductions in fertility, but they were insufficient to counteract the effects of population growth on per capita income.

The Acemoglu and Johnson paper offered two notes of caution with respect to the potential impacts and equilibrium dynamics of future health interventions:

> First . . . the international epidemiological transition was a unique event, and perhaps similar changes in life expectancy today would not lead to an increase in population and the impact on GDP per capita may be more positive. Second, the diseases that take many lives in the poorer parts of the world today are not the same ones as those 60 years ago; most notably HIV/AIDS is a major killer today but was not so in 1940. Many of the diseases we focus on had serious impacts on children (with the notable exception of tuberculosis), whereas HIV/AIDS affects individuals at the peak of their labor productivity and could have a larger negative impact on growth. (2007: 975–976)

The authors also noted that in today's increasingly globalized markets for labor, capital, and trade, poor countries may be better able to leverage improved health into economic growth. Thus, the neoclassical assumption of constant capital in the face of improved health

(and population size) may now be less binding.

Nevertheless, the literature points to a gap between the value we ascribe to health, our expectations for the impacts of health, and empirical results with respect to the impact of improved health on growth. Theorists, policymakers, and academics continue to search for ways to circumvent what one paper refers to as a "repugnant conclusion"— essentially that mortality may be good for development (Grimm and Harttgen 2008). One simple solution involves incorporating the perceived losses associated with mortality, or the benefits of longevity, into a measure of human development (Sen 1998). A number of papers have opted to measure health impacts with a "full income" approach, which incorporates the value of statistical life lost due to premature death (Becker, Philipson, and Soares 2005; Bloom, Canning, and Jamison 2004); another alternative is to move away from income-dominated approaches to those such as the Human Development Index (HDI) that focus more directly on human well-being. While such approaches neatly resolve any questions regarding the general value of health investments, they do so by avoiding specification of the actual forward linkages that could nonetheless shape the fates of societies. We wish to explore those further.

Decomposing the pathways between health and growth

An increasingly popular alternative to aggregate statistical analysis involves the development of general equilibrium models and forecasts that incorporate existing "stylized facts" from the empirical literature, in particular some powerful relationships replicated in population-based and cross-national analysis. A general equilibrium model approach generally represents the interaction of profit-seeking producers and welfare-maximizing households in equilibrating markets for labor as well as goods and services. These models have produced three important benefits. First, theoretical analysis can identify the relative importance of particular forward linkages and the conditions under which health improvements could lead to improved or diminished growth.[4] Second, empirical forecasts can help identify the health contributions underlying historical growth trajectories or counterfactual growth scenarios (Abegunde et al. 2007; Weil 2007). Finally, analysts can use historical forecasts to reconstruct the likely health contribution to past growth, adding valuable depth to growth regression results (Bloom, Canning, and Sevilla 2004; Gyimah-Brempong and Wilson 2004; Shastry and Weil 2003).

Needless to say, like more aggregate and less elaborate approaches, such approaches produce similarly divergent estimates of the impact of health on economic outcomes. Nonetheless, a rapidly growing micro-level empirical literature, a substantial number of equilibrium studies, and a smaller number of cross-national regressions have produced a general consensus on the more significant pathways linking health to growth (see Figure 7.2 to see some of those as they relate to the three elements of most production functions, namely, capital, labor, and productivity). In analysis with IFs, we focus on multifactor productivity, the output per unit of labor and capital in combination. In the next section, we proceed to discuss pathways, following in particular the models employed by Ashraf, Lester, and Weil (2008) and Weil (2007).

Ideally, an exploration of health and economic growth via such an elaborated set of paths should not restrict itself to the representation of general equilibrium in economics. It should link the economic model to a population model that endogenously adjusts fertility and, therefore, to the trajectory of population growth in light of changes in income per capita that result from improved health. The approach should also consider the implications of improved health for societal expenditures on health and, in turn, the implications of potential savings in those expenditures for shifting money to education or other uses—in fact, the implications of changes in total government spending for the crowding out or facilitation of savings and investment in the economy. Even better would be embedding the economic model inside a social accounting matrix (SAM) that represents the financial transfers among households, firms, and governments. The IFs modeling system does tie an equilibrium-seeking economic model to a full population model and does embed it in a SAM framework that assures balances of

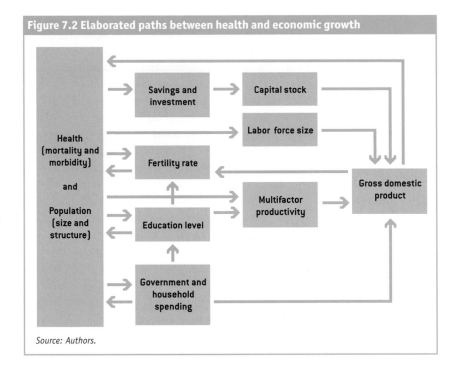

Figure 7.2 Elaborated paths between health and economic growth

Source: Authors.

financial flows. The discussion of the various possible paths below will outline also the IFs approach to representation of them.[5]

The Paths of Forward Linkages from Health to Economic Growth

Following the structure of linkages between health and economic growth that Figure 7.2 laid out, we will look in turn, and in different order for ease of presentation, at the impact of health (morbidity and mortality) on economic growth via labor, productivity, and capital. After identifying some of the important literature and arguments with respect to each linkage, we in turn sketch the approach represented in IFs.

Health and labor

The forward effects of health on economic growth via population and labor force size and structure work through changes in mortality and fertility. These changes have both automatic or "mechanical" components and behavioral components. We consider first the mechanical components.

To the extent that health improvements lead to improved survival, they lead—at least in the short run until fertility adjusts downward—to an automatic increase in population size and in the total labor supply (see Figure 7.3), with potentially positive consequences for economic

Health connects with economic outcomes through impacts on all three elements of most production functions: capital stocks, labor, and productivity.

growth. However, as discussed earlier, not all impacts of the increase in population size are necessarily positive for health and economic outcomes. If capital stock is held constant in the face of increased population and labor supply, the increased population would lead to a reduced amount of capital per population or per worker, reflected in greater competition for jobs or agricultural plots. In addition to capital dilution, mortality reductions among infants lead to an increased youth dependency ratio (before they result in a larger labor force), with possible short-run burdens on nutritional and educational resources for children.

On the other hand, if mortality is rising there is a direct mechanical effect that lowers fertility through the death of women who are or would be mothers. Furthermore, the morbidity associated with diseases such as HIV/AIDS might reduce the rate of childbearing among the living, through increased levels of sterility, through women being too weak to bear children, through fears of transmitting HIV/AIDS to children through the mother-to-child transmission or breastfeeding pathway, and through fears of sexual intercourse due to the risk of HIV/AIDS (Glynn et al. 2000; Gray et al. 1998).

Going beyond the simple mechanical implications of mortality for population and labor supply, we also must consider the behavioral effect of mortality on fertility via its implications for family formation strategies.

In classical demographic transition theory, declining mortality is the cause of declining fertility; high mortality causes parents not only to replace those children who already died but also to have a much larger number of children to insure against the future death of multiple children (Coale 1986; Eckstein, Mira, and Wolpin 1999; Galloway, Lee, and Hammel 1998; Preston 1978; Wolpin 1997). Modern demographic transitions display a strong correlation over time between mortality decline and fertility decline. Such a fertility decline not only mitigates the population increase effect noted above, it leads to a so-called *demographic dividend*, in which a final, large cohort of young children is followed by an increasingly small number of siblings, generating improved welfare outcomes for all siblings and serendipitous dependency ratios as these large, healthy cohorts move into prime age (Bloom, Canning, and Graham 2003).

Becker's (1962) theory of human capital implies another pathway by which parents who value child success, whether for evolutionary reasons or to ensure old-age support, engage in a quality-quantity trade-off, preferring to have fewer, well-educated, and healthy children rather than a large number of children with little investment in each. Previous research attributed the quality-quantity trade-off to increasing returns to human capital (via economic development) and decreased costs of human capital investment, typically through reductions in the price of schooling (Bloom, Canning, and Chan 2006; Galor and Moav 2002; Galor and Weil 1999; 2000). More recent work has incorporated decreases in the cost of health investment (for instance through child health and nutrition programs) in promoting this trade-off, suggesting a pathway from mortality (or at least morbidity) reductions to fertility reductions (Behrman 1996).

The result of the interactions of the mechanical and behavioral linkages between overall mortality and fertility is a generally positive relationship (higher mortality and fertility are linked). Yet the patterns can be complex, as in the case of HIV/AIDS (see Box 7.1)

Turning to the forecasting of this volume, the IFs demographic model captures the mechanical or accounting effects of mortality on population (see the solid paths in Figure 7.3).

> ▬ *Changes in mortality have both mechanical and behavioral impacts on population size and structure, including the absolute and relative size of the labor force.* ▬

Figure 7.3 Pathways linking health and demography

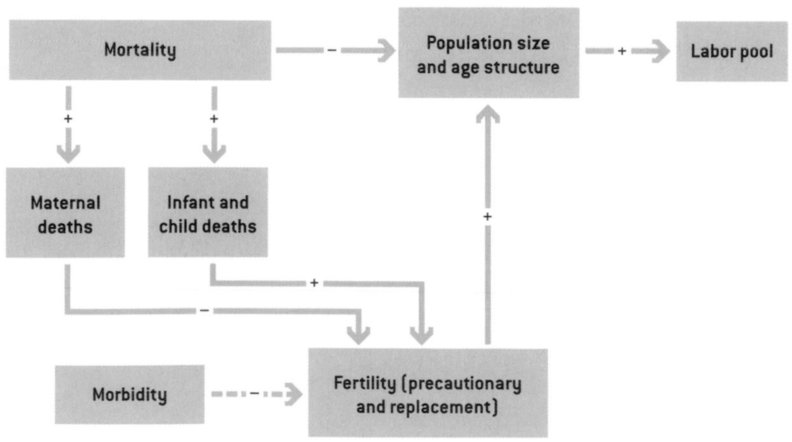

Note: Relationships shown with dashed lines (morbidity to fertility in this figure) are not explicitly represented in the IFs model.

Source: Authors.

A key pathway passes from mortality through adult age population to labor supply (including aging-related lags).[6] Similarly, IFs captures the mechanical effect of mortality on fertility through the death of women of childbearing age.

The most important non-mechanical linkage is almost certainly the relationship between child mortality and fertility, and IFs represents this also. As discussed earlier, couples may increase their fertility in the face of children's deaths both to replace those children and to have extra children against the perceived risk of future child mortality. GDP per capita drove the earliest formulations in IFs for forecasting fertility because that relationship is very strong. We subsequently replaced the more distal formulation using GDP per capita with driving variables closer to human agency, namely, the log of educational level of those age 15 and older (neither the education of women alone nor the education of those 15–24 works as well) and the percentage of the population who use modern contraception. Adding the rate of infant mortality boosted the overall adjusted R-squared to 0.81.[7] Child mortality did not work quite as well.

Health and productivity

The scientific literature recognizes that health is a form of human capital (Sen 1987), and we know that health in early life has profound implications for health later in life. Health affects the ability to acquire further human capital through processes of cognitive development and educational attainment and

the application of that attainment in productive work. Figure 7.4 sketches the linkages of particular interest to us.

Immediate effects of disability on productivity
A discussion of health and productivity begins with the effects of current disability on work attendance, employment, and productivity at work. Chapter 2 noted that it is possible to assign a disability weight to measure disability on a scale of severity ranging from full health (equal to 0) to death (equal to 1, a complete loss). Similarly, we can characterize worker productivity on a relative scale between "no loss of productivity" (equaling 0) and "full loss

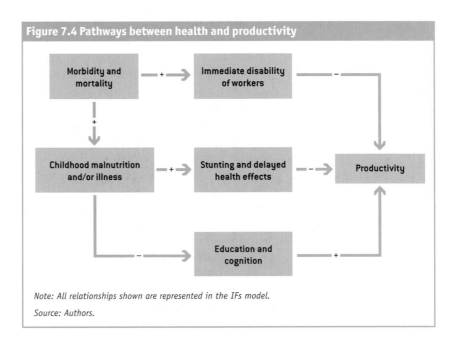

Figure 7.4 Pathways between health and productivity

Note: All relationships shown are represented in the IFs model.
Source: Authors.

of productivity" (equaling 1). This suggests the potential of using the disability weights that the Global Burden of Disease (GBD) project developed as proxies for the concurrent loss of productivity (Abegunde et al. 2007; Ashraf, Lester, and Weil 2008).

Some concerns arise immediately, however. First, problems often attend generalization from the micro to the macro level. The temporary loss of a worker could be filled by colleagues or through overtime labor, and the lost wages could be paid to another worker. Yet as a societal disease burden accumulates, particularly in the prime ages, it may become increasingly difficult to replace workers. A good illustration of this possibility is reflected in the earliest antiretroviral treatment campaigns in sub-Saharan Africa, which were instituted not by governments but by major employers, such as AngloAmerican Mining and Coca Cola, who recognized that the potential death or disability of multiple workers on the same shift or in the same job could lead to a wholesale loss of production (Rosen et al. 2003).

The use of disability weights to get at the relationship between morbidity and productivity raises a particular concern since they are intended to capture a great deal more than productivity—including pain, suffering, and financial burden. Yet many of these variations may average out as long as disability weights capture a proportionate element of lost productivity across diseases. A fairly substantial literature assesses the costs in terms of absenteeism, unemployment, and on-the-job productivity for many of the world's leading causes of disability, including cardiovascular diseases, diabetes, obesity, and even HIV/AIDS.[8] But such estimates only cover a moderate proportion of all disability, and mostly only for rich countries, which could either experience less substantial losses due to better treatment and accommodations for the disabled, or more substantial losses due to higher levels of survival among individuals experiencing severe morbidity.

Delayed effects of disability on productivity
A bigger set of concerns revolves around the effect of health not merely on current productivity but also on the accumulation of work-related human capital over the life course, whether referring to

seniority, job training, or education itself (see the second path in Figure 7.4). With regard to seniority and job-specific training, the disability weights may also capture these effects, because the panelists assigned to estimate disability weights considered duration in their calculations. One study of the economic impacts of chronic disease used disability-adjusted life years (DALYs), which immediately account for the full loss due to disability and death at the time of illness (Abegunde et al. 2007). Yet this approach may dramatically overstate the losses associated with a particular disease by counting all DALYs lost up to the standard age (80 for men, 85 for women) as lost years of productivity when many of those years are typically ones of retirement and dependency (Mathers et al. 2002).[9]

While it is relatively straightforward to estimate the productivity costs associated with concurrent morbidity, it is a bigger challenge to address throughout the life course the cumulative effects of health, many of which transcend a particular disease. Perhaps the most important arena of health impacts research, both in terms of the volume of microeconomic knowledge and the macroeconomic significance, lies in the study of life-course effects of health in early life. Specifically, we now understand that health and nutrition early in life—in the womb, as a newborn, through the early years of childhood, and even in adolescence—can have measurable and macro-economically significant effects on levels of cognitive performance, on levels of education attained, and on the occurrence of disease and mortality in adulthood. These impacts are intimately connected to one another through processes of human skeletal, metabolic, and immunological development. The nexus of developmental delay and resulting life-long compromise in health status also ties together nutritional and health pathways through a pathological synergy: undernutrition creates vulnerability to disease, which leads to further undernutrition. This synergy results in what is frequently referred to as "stunting," often measured by the proxy of achieved height, which makes an appropriate focal point for our discussion.

Paleontologists and developmental biologists have long been aware of a relationship between achieved height and outcomes such as immunological strength and cognition.

Grantham-McGregor et al. (2007) constructed a rough estimate of 200 million stunted children in the world and assessed the implications for life-course development. They arrived at this figure first by estimating the percentage of children who are stunted. They found a substantial rate of stunting in all developing regions, 28 percent of all children, or more than 150 million out of the 550 million children in those countries. They found especially high rates in sub-Saharan Africa (37 percent) and the highest rates in South Asia (39 percent), even though the latter region has lower rates of poverty than the former.

To supplement their stunting estimates (and to capture better the more extreme level of deprivation in sub-Saharan Africa), they estimated the number of children in poverty who were not officially recorded as stunted, and incorporated these children into an estimate of children who are potentially stunted. In summarizing the existing literature on stunting and poverty, the authors estimated lost years of schooling of 0.91 for stunted children, 0.71 for impoverished children, and 2.15 years for children who are both impoverished and stunted. They further noted evidence of a deficit due to stunting in the rate of learning per completed year of schooling. When they combined this evidence with known relationships between schooling, cognition, and earnings, the authors calculated that children who are stunted are losing about 22.2 percent of their future adult earnings, while those who are stunted and poor are losing 30.1 percent.

For example, the work leading up to Fogel's theory of technophysio evolution brought widespread attention to the relationship between height, health, and productivity (Fogel 1994; 2004b; Fogel and Costa 1997). Fogel's historical study of the health system records of U.S. Army veterans from 1848 to 1920 demonstrated a strong relationship between the study subjects' heights and rates of morbidity and mortality due to a range of medical conditions as well as productivity. Subsequent to Fogel's work, numerous historical, micro-level, and cross-national studies have validated the relationship of height to conditions of childhood and the effects of height on outcomes later in life.[10] (See Box 7.2 for information on the extent of stunting globally.)

Macro analysis of health and productivity
So far in this section, we have been trying to learn from the micro literature and to consider how that might aid in forecasting. A significant macro literature also explores the relationship between health and productivity. That literature generally relies on cross-sectional data, often with panels across time so as to introduce longitudinal analysis. The good news is that the literature most often finds a positive relationship between measures of health and economic growth. For instance, Barro and Sala-i-Martin (1998: 432) found that an increase in life expectancy by one standard deviation, which they calculated to be 13 years in the 1965–1975 period, raised economic growth by 1.4 percent per year. Updated analysis (Barro and Sala-i-Martin 2003: 525) found a slightly lower growth impact (1.1 percent) from the reciprocal of life expectancy. Bloom, Canning, and Sevilla (2001: 5 and 16) found that a rise of one year in life expectancy raised output by 1–4 percent.[11]

Jamison, Lau, and Wang (2005: ii) used a "meta-production function" approach around a Cobb-Douglas function to explore a wide range of factors that drive multifactor productivity (MFP) and concluded that health improvements had accounted for 11 percent of economic growth in 53 countries over the 1965–1990 period (compared to 14 percent from education and 67 percent from expansion of capital stocks). Similarly, Weil (2007: Abstract) found that the fraction of cross-country variance in income explained by variation in health ranged from 8 to 20 percent, depending on the measure of health (he moved away from life expectancy to alternative measures such as average height, body mass, adult survival age, and age of menarche).

Health and productivity in IFs
The approach IFs uses to represent changes in multifactor productivity as a function of multiple drivers, including elements of human and social capital, combines a meta-production function with an elasticity-like approach (see Hughes 2005). We compare values of driving forces (such as completed years of formal education by adults, spending on education, or stunting levels) with the "expected" value for those variables given the development level of the country (using GDP per capita at PPP as a proxy for development). Improvements or deterioration in drivers relative to the initial variations from expected levels determine changes in productivity attributed to that variable.

> ■ *Macroeconomic studies most often find a positive relationship between measures of health and economic growth.* ■

The long-standing approach in IFs to the impact of investments and improvements in health and education on productivity has been to draw on macroeconomic statistical studies from the cross-sectional/panel literature, many of which go to great length to control for other variables likely to affect the relationship. To operationalize education, we have used completed years of education at age 15 or older (we could have used 25 and older as in the GBD formulations, but 15- to 25-year-olds also often work) and education spending as a percentage of GDP. For health, we have used life expectancy and health spending as a percentage of GDP. Volume 2 of this series (see Dickson, Hughes, and Irfan 2010: Chapter 8) documented the approach with respect to education.

While maintaining the more aggregate relationships of life expectancy and health spending to multifactor productivity as options in the background, this volume's analysis disaggregated the relationships consistent with the above literature discussion (see Figure 7.4). We initialize adult stunting in a long-term lagged relationship (using a moving average of 25 years)[12] with child undernutrition and forecast it as a function of both undernutrition and child mortality as a proxy for morbidity. Initial values in 2005 range up to about 55 percent for India and Bangladesh and even over 80 percent for Somalia; in the base case these generally but not universally decrease.[13]

To this undernutrition-based stunting term we add one related to child morbidity (using change in mortality as a proxy for change in morbidity). We follow the analysis of country-age-specific variations in height by Bozzoli, Deaton, and Quintana-Domeque (2009), which predicts average height for a cohort of women as a function of "pre-adult mortality," or an estimated probability of dying between ages 0 and 14, dependent upon their year of birth.[14] We compare the reduction related to actual mortality with that related to an expected mortality rate from a cross-sectional relationship of mortality with income (thereby controlling for the effect of expected undernutrition in the first term). We lag the childhood mortality effect on adult height with a 25-year moving average. Using a somewhat comparable series of values from the USAID's Demographic and Health Surveys (DHS), we found that a 1 centimeter increase in height

corresponded to a 2 percentage-point decrease in the percentage of adults who are stunted, and we adjust the stunting computation from undernutrition accordingly. In forecasts, changes in the relationship between stunting rates and those expected at changing development levels add to or reduce the human capital contribution to productivity.[15]

Childhood undernutrition and related stunting do not give rise to all disability in working years; much also comes from disabilities arising during the working years. The IFs approach adds another term to the growth of economic productivity that reflects the changing difference between expected and forecasted values of disability incurred in the working lifetime. For the expected value, we used contemporary data on the world average years of living with disability across a global worker's lifetime—in 2005 that value was 0.097 (poor mental health is the biggest disability source and accounts for 0.025 years).[16] For the forecasted value, IFs calculates millions of years of living with disability that can be associated with mortality rates specific to the working-age population (see the discussion around Table 3.2 of the changing relationship over time between mortality and morbidity).[17] Because mental health disability rates tend to be quite constant, and because mental health is a large element of working-age disability, forecasts of disability exhibit considerable stability over time.

The fact that the literature describes the relationship between health and educational attainment in many different ways complicates the representation of a relationship in IFs between health and educational attainment and on to productivity (see again Figure 7.4). For instance, Baldacci et al. (2004: 25–26) found that a 1 point increase in spending on health as a percentage of GDP would increase the net school enrollment rate at the primary level in developing countries by about 2 percentage points. In the IFs model, however, GDP per capita is the principal driver of demand for education in the model and for public spending on education, as well as for spending on health. Thus, there was already an implicit relationship between health spending and enrollment.

Other literature focuses on the relationship between stunting and educational attainment (see Grantham-McGregor et al. 2007); we have already discussed, however, a direct path from stunting to productivity and wish to avoid duplicate representation of impacts. More directly relevant to a path from health to educational attainment, Soares (2006: 72) found in cross-sectional analysis that 10 years of additional life expectancy add 0.7 years to the average years of education attained. And Ashraf, Lester, and Weil (2008: 10) built on other work concerning seven sub-Saharan African countries to conclude that 20 years of additional life expectancy add 0.386 average years of education. We used this analysis to support our relationship between life expectancy (as a proxy for morbidity, including that of children) to productivity via increased education.[18]

Health and capital stocks

Even the fairly substantial individual-level gains in human capital and productivity that the previous section ascribed to improved health would have limited impact on macroeconomic change if concomitant increases in population size were to result in a diminished capital/labor ratio. For health to generate substantial positive development impacts, we ought also to observe increases in the stock and allocation of financial and physical capital available per person. To this point, we have discussed the role that health-related demographic change can play in changing the size of the labor force (which

also affects the capital/labor ratio, potentially perversely in the case of mortality reductions). And we have considered how improved health and human capital can increase productivity. Now we turn to the extent to which health can impact the availability of capital, the third major factor of production and therefore potential route of connection between health and changes in economic growth (see again Figure 7.2)

Figure 7.5 sketches the primary paths between health (morbidity and mortality) and capital stock. Most capital stock consists of buildings and machinery for producing goods and services; some representations may include land also, but most treat land separately and largely as a constant (although land developed for crop production or grazing can, in fact, be highly variable). Most immediately, investment increases capital stock and depreciation reduces it. Although there is certainly some impact of morbidity and mortality on the rate of depreciation of both built physical and natural capital, the relationship may not be substantial, and we do not understand it well enough to model it. Turning our focus to the paths that affect investment, the two major ones run though health spending, which can crowd out savings and investment in capital stocks, and through the age structure of societies, which affects the savings rate. We explore each in turn.

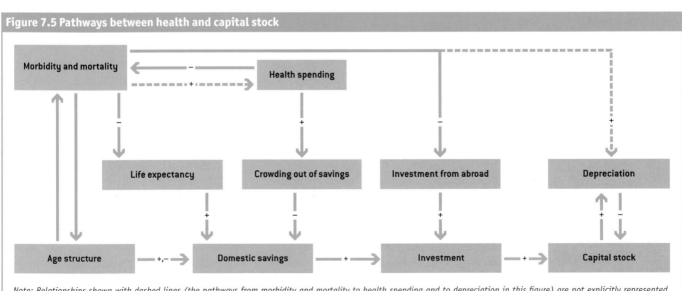

Figure 7.5 Pathways between health and capital stock

Note: Relationships shown with dashed lines (the pathways from morbidity and mortality to health spending and to depreciation in this figure) are not explicitly represented in the IFs model.

Source: Authors.

Health expenditures: Competition with savings

Health spending, by both households and governments, competes with other spending and with savings. It can crowd out other uses of income, reducing domestic savings and investment (Aísa and Pueyo 2004; 2006; Goldman et al. 2004; Tabata 2005). This is a fundamentally important path via which societal commitments to health affect capital stock. The path is, of course, a major concern for high-income societies now facing growing pressures for health spending from aging populations.

In thinking more generally, however, about the impact of health expenditures on growth, at least two other issues demand consideration. The first is the forecasting of health expenditures as a result of changing morbidity patterns associated in part with changing age structures. The impact of aging on health expenditures will depend significantly on whether extra years of life are healthy or unhealthy and also on the relative costs of both good health and ill-health at older ages versus younger ages (Payne et al. 2007). In general, of course, the old demand more health care than the young. The key question is how much more they demand. Even as prevalence of some diseases increases due to greater survivorship, reductions in the average severity of disease may be so great as to reduce the overall burden of morbidity (Crimmins 2004; Mathers et al. 2004).

The second issue that complicates thinking about the implications of health spending for economic growth involves the path of health spending back to mortality and morbidity (the upper left corner of Figure 7.5). In the process of (hopefully) reducing mortality and morbidity, health expenditures also have potential positive impacts on economic growth, via the path from morbidity to productivity that we discussed earlier in association with Figure 7.4 and via the impact of changed mortality on age structure and life cycle–related savings (to which we return later). One important aspect of the issue is that not all health spending is equal in its impact on morbidity and mortality. Ideally, health expenditures are investments in better current and future health with associated productivity enhancement. Unfortunately, some health expenditures may primarily add to financial burdens of individuals and governments (Aísa and Pueyo 2004; Bhattacharya and Qiao

2007; Ehrlich and Chuma 1990; Grossman 1972; Tabata 2005), thereby crowding out savings without significant reductions in morbidity and mortality that could provide offsetting productivity gains.

Two prominent examples merit particular consideration. First, expenditures on the treatment of HIV/AIDS, which are much higher than the costs of preventing it, may reduce the societal disease burden (and potentially prevent further transmission), but they are also incredibly costly and may pose an especially great drain on consumption in more productive sectors, on investment in other social sectors, and on savings rates (Azomahou, Diene, and Soete 2009; Boucekkine, Diene, and Azomahou 2007; Freire 2002). The second example returns to the costs of health care for the elderly in developed and developing countries alike (Goldman et al. 2004; Rannan-Eliya and Wijesinghe 2006; Seshamani and Gray 2004; Shang and Goldman 2008; Stearns and Norton 2004). Rapidly growing elderly cohorts can place increasing burdens on savings and productivity as they cash out their private savings and then turn to public safety nets for health care and pension funds over long periods of retirement (Preston 1984). In pre-modern societies a retired person consumes very few resources in the absence of any savings mechanism or many resources to consume. Modern medical technologies and public health insurance programs, however, allow elders to more than make up for reduced consumption in other sectors through the consumption of health care resources, particularly in the final years of life (Seshamani and Gray 2004). As a result, most of today's developed countries have seen relatively unchecked increases in the percentage of GDP devoted to health expenditures (Goldman et al. 2004). Far more than pension systems, old-age health expenditures could pose a potential impediment to economic growth (Aísa and Pueyo 2004; Tabata 2005).

Longevity, the incentive to save, and the supply of investment

On the other hand, increased longevity (whether as a result of greater health spending or other forces) may create an incentive to save more.[19] Individuals who can expect to live an uncertain number of years past the typical age of retirement (in contrast to ancestors who most often died in prime age or shortly thereafter) may begin preparing to pay for that additional longevity (Hurd, McFadden, and Gan 1998; Tsai, Chu, and Chung 2000), while those with a low likelihood of surviving will value future wealth accumulation less (Ben-Porath 1967).

Any increments in the savings rate of individuals planning for retirement are temporary, of course, and will reverse as retirees draw on accumulations (Ando and Modigliani 1963; Higgins 1998; Kelley and Schmidt 1996; Mason 1988; Willis 1982). At a societal level we can therefore expect that a dramatic increase in longevity should lead first to a rise and then to a fall in savings rates (Ando and Modigliani 1963).[20] For example, a World Bank study concluded that:

> An increase in the young age dependency ratio of 3.5 percentage points leads to about a 1 percentage point decline in private saving; an increase in the old age dependency ratio has a negative savings effect more than twice as large. (1999: 4)

The societal supply of savings and investment will also depend on the availability of viable savings mechanisms and the returns to savings, each of which health also affects. With respect to the returns to savings in a market economy, productivity of the economy drives in substantial part the rate of return on savings. To the extent that health drives up productivity through the pathways outlined earlier, this will increase the overall rate of return on investments, adding a further stimulus to savings rates. With respect to viable savings mechanisms, investment in physical capital is not always the only or best alternative, especially in low-income societies. In populations where families form the principal basis of education financing and old-age support, for instance, increasing returns to children's education, driven by labor market improvements and better health, can encourage rapid parental investment in children's education and job market opportunities.[21]

The same logic that we apply to internal rates of savings and investment can be applied to external capital flows. If increased productivity and reduced labor market uncertainty increase the profitability of business enterprises, then the flow of foreign direct investment (FDI) would increase and capital markets would receive greater liquidity. Thus, good and improving health tends to increase the inflows of foreign investment (Jamison 2006: 8).

Health and capital stock in IFs

The IFs modeling system treats capital stock dynamically over time, investing in it and allowing it to depreciate (see again Figure 7.5). Investment is responsive to both domestic savings and foreign flows. Thus, the necessary elements for considering the impact of morbidity and mortality, via paths such as those across health spending and age structure, are part of the economic model's core structure. In addition, as described earlier, the IFs model uses a social accounting matrix (SAM) structure. Thus, the flow of funds into health spending automatically competes with other consumption uses and with savings and investment. In addition, health spending does affect mortality (Chapter 3 discussed the linkage back to communicable diseases of children).

For the analyses of this volume we have also added paths that link morbidity and mortality to domestic savings. That important linkage has two elements. The most fundamental one, via the age structure of the population, represents the understanding of life-cycle dynamics in income, consumption, and savings. The cycle for income is fairly clear-cut with a peak in the middle-to-latter periods of the working years. Workers set aside some portion of income as savings and that portion, too, tends to peak in the middle and late period of working years. The second fundamental element is that both the horizon of life expectancy and the average income level can have an impact on the portion set aside for savings and the degree to which it rises and then falls. That is, the life-cycle "bulge" of savings may be earlier and/or flatter in developing countries.

We implemented the relationships within IFs in accord with that understanding. The IFs economic model generates total income and the household consumption portion of income. Relying on analyses of selected countries undertaken by Fernández-Villaverde and Krueger (2007) and Deaton and Paxson (2000), we developed vectors

For the analyses of this volume we have added paths that link morbidity and mortality to domestic savings and to foreign direct investment flows.

(across five-year age categories) based on general stylized patterns of the savings life cycle to represent more and less developed countries. In forecasting we use the pattern for less developed countries when life expectancy falls below 40 years, use that for more developed countries when life expectancy exceeds 80 years, and interpolate in between for all other countries.

Another important piece in the logic of Figure 7.5 is the potential for morbidity to force up health spending (and to a generally lesser degree for near-mortality to do the same, especially in cases such as the massive late-life health interventions that occur in the United States). Currently in IFs, health expenditures as a portion of GDP are linked to income (generally rising), with some protection of country-specific variations around the curve, such as the high level of U.S. spending. Our search for health-outcome variables (such as morbidity rates) that could supplement, if not replace, income in explaining/forecasting health expenditures has not been productive. We have found, however, that some political economy variables appear to affect health expenditures.[22] This analysis suggests the somewhat provocative conclusion that political-economic variables may be more important in determining health spending than are morbidity and mortality patterns, but we have not incorporated such a relationship into IFs.[23]

Finally, the path linking health to foreign direct investment is potentially quite important. Alsan, Bloom, and Canning (2006: 613) report that one additional year of life expectancy boosts FDI inflows by 9 percent, controlling for other variables. We have implemented that relationship in IFs.[24]

Exploring Forward Linkages
In the remainder of this chapter, we explore how widely varying health forecasts might affect other elements of the human development system. Specifically and somewhat arbitrarily, but consistently with the wide uncertainty around health futures, we explore the implications of increases or decreases of 30 percent in disease-specific mortality rates relative to the base case, phased in through 2060 (and these changes in mortality pass through to associated changes in morbidity rates as discussed in Chapter 3).[25] This type of "brute force" intervention or model run, lacking the

subtlety of exploration of individual alternative assumptions about proximate drivers in the last two chapters or the sophistication of integrated scenario intervention in the coming chapter, allows us to explore the broader implications of health changes very directly.

Reductions in communicable diseases affect primarily infants and children (although AIDS affects adults heavily), and reductions in noncommunicable diseases affect the elderly especially. The age profile of impact from injuries differs from both, affecting working adults in particular. Given these patterns and significant variation in regional disease burdens, the implications of our interventions will differ across regions.

The three major paths from health (and demographics more generally) to economic growth, which the first half of this chapter detailed, can usefully frame discussion of the impact of alternative health forecasts. Therefore, we look first at the interventions themselves, and at their aggregate demographic and economic impacts, before turning to exploration of the three more specific paths of economic impact of alternative health forecasts via labor supply, productivity, and capital stock.

The interventions
Figure 7.6 shows the total global mortality profiles in 2060 of the high and low mortality interventions (30 percent higher and lower than the base case, respectively). The pattern between the two scenarios shows little difference until about 50 years of age, reinforcing what we saw in Chapter 4— namely, that chronic disease patterns (which predominantly affect older adults) will most likely dominate the global "story" with respect to mortality by mid-century.

Especially in terms of years of life lost, and especially in sub-Saharan Africa and South Asia, the mortality story today has two clear story lines, that of infant and child mortality and that of chronic disease. At 91 per 1,000 in sub-Saharan Africa and 61 per 1,000 in South Asia, infant mortality continues to loom horrendously large. But in 2060 those numbers could well, even in the high mortality case, be nearer 24 and 8 per 1,000, with even the higher figure close to that of upper-middle-income countries today, thereby fundamentally completing a transition from numbers that were near 160 as recently as 1960.

The year 2060 is, of course, quite distant. In the nearer-term horizon of 2030 to 2040, a probable temporal focal range as the world community moves attention beyond the Millennium Development Goals, communicable diseases will continue to claim a large number of lives, especially of infants and children. Figure 7.7 shows us more about that transition in cause-groups. It moves below the global level, distinguishing explicitly between low- and high-income countries, using sub-Saharan African countries as a proxy for the former (as we did in Chapter 4). Although the range of uncertainty is clearly large, probably even larger than that of the figure, it appears likely that by 2060 the burden of disease in sub-Saharan Africa will be either roughly equally divided between communicable and noncommunicable diseases or tilted toward the noncommunicable diseases.

The aggregate demographic and economic effects of the interventions

Before turning to the paths of each specific forward linkage from health, it is useful to consider the aggregate impact that might arise from the modeled variation in future

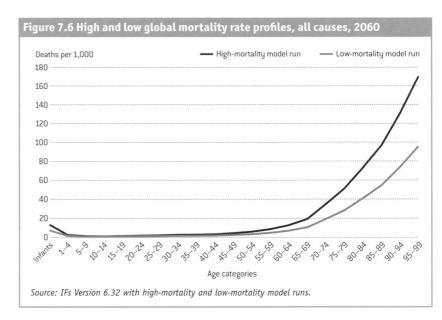

Source: IFs Version 6.32 with high-mortality and low-mortality model runs.

mortality and associated morbidity rates. The range of mortality rates chosen for this analysis may not appear terribly large across the two interventions (30 percent above and below the base case, phased in through 2060). Yet by 2060 life expectancy varies by about eight years between the two interventions in sub-Saharan Africa and by about six years in high-income countries.

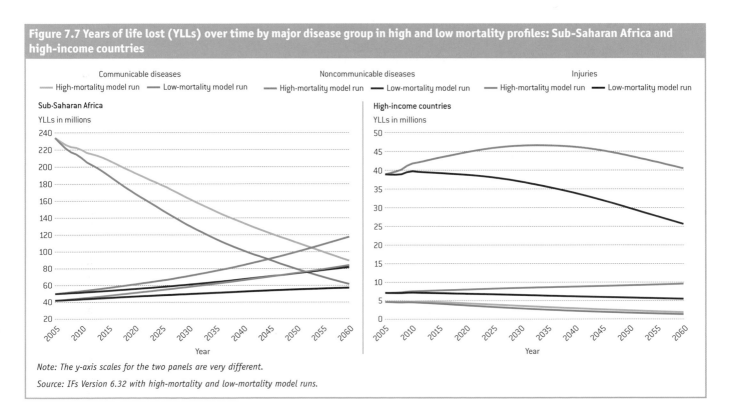

Note: The y-axis scales for the two panels are very different.

Source: IFs Version 6.32 with high-mortality and low-mortality model runs.

The demographic consequences of such variation in assumptions about mortality and resultant life expectancy are significant. Figure 7.8 shows the global population results, extending the horizon to 2100 so as to indicate also the full impact across the century. The difference grows to a global population variation of about 1 billion people. Most of that outcome is a mechanical result of the differences in mortality rates. All else equal, an extension of global life expectancy by nearly 10 percent translates into a population about that same amount larger, once it plays out over a period of average life expectancy. (In contrast, high mortality affects population not just directly but also in many indirect ways, including the reinforcing secondary reduction of population via the death of potential parents.)

As Figure 7.3 and the discussion around it indicated, there is a relationship between life expectancy increase and fertility decrease that could offset some of the increase in population size that would mechanically result from life expectancy increase alone. Yet there is a lag in that counteracting effect, long enough that movement from high mortality to low mortality does significantly increase population overall throughout this period. This has been, of course, the pattern of the epidemiologic transition in developing countries since World War II—

significant drops in mortality followed only later by drops in fertility. Thus, it should be no surprise that an acceleration of the completion of that transition would exhibit the same result.

Turning to the economic impact of different mortality trajectories, Figure 7.9 suggests that, rather than high mortality leading to more capital and other resources per capita and therefore to higher average income (the simple neoclassical story of the relationship between population and growth), the low mortality intervention generates somewhat higher GDP over time for the world as a whole (about 16 percent higher by 2060) and for all regions. The boost to GDP is potentially greatest in Europe and Central Asia (26 percent) and least for East Asia and Pacific (4 percent), with sub-Saharan Africa in the middle (18 percent). Taking into account the higher population of the low morality case, however, reduces the global gain in GDP per capita to 8 percent by 2060 and that of sub-Saharan Africa to 11 percent. GDP per capita in East Asia and Pacific is actually 4 percent lower with the low mortality intervention than in the high mortality one. Although a reasonable hypothesis for that result might be that China already has a potential problem with a rapidly aging population that low mortality would actually exacerbate, we turn below to the various paths by which mortality affects economic growth and drill down for explanations of these patterns.

First, however, it is important to emphasize that the great gap shown in Figure 7.8 between the size of the global population under the high and low mortality interventions, which considerably reduces the economic impact of the lower mortality case (the GDP per capita affect of Figure 7.9), is by no means a certain outcome of reduced mortality. The international community mobilized family planning programs very rapidly in the 1950s and 1960s to address the surges in population that followed the post–World War II drops in mortality. We may be underestimating the potential for similar accelerations of fertility decline in the low mortality case. Therefore, we have explored a variation on that case with a modestly more rapid but still historically reasonable fertility decline, one that still leads to a higher population than in the high mortality case but only marginally higher. Specific to regions, the

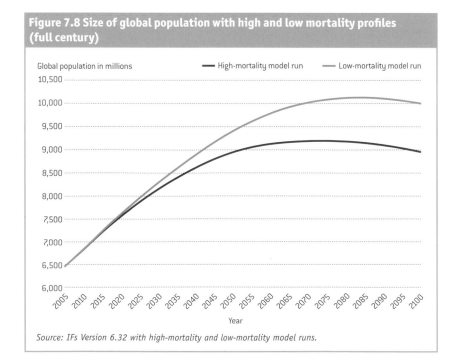

Figure 7.8 Size of global population with high and low mortality profiles (full century)

Global population in millions

— High-mortality model run   — Low-mortality model run

Year

Source: IFs Version 6.32 with high-mortality and low-mortality model runs.

variation has the greatest impact on sub-Saharan Africa (reducing the total fertility rate there by about 0.5 points relative to the low mortality case). Subsequent discussion will return to the impact of this and other *counterfactuals* (by which we mean variations) relative to the assumptions of the low morality intervention.

Exploring paths between health and growth: Demographics and labor supply

The earlier discussion identified three paths that link changes in mortality and morbidity to economic growth: via demographics (especially labor supply); via multifactor productivity; and via capital stock. While we have just seen (Figure 7.9) that in the aggregate the low mortality scenario has a modestly positive impact on economic growth, the impacts across the three paths are varied and, in fact, are not all in the same direction. We consider each in turn, beginning with labor supply (see again Figure 7.3).

Although demand for labor has its own critical importance, the portion of total population that falls into the typical years of a working career shapes the labor supply of societies. When that working-age demographic segment is relatively large, as when population growth rates and young dependent population portions decline, a society experiences a demographic dividend. By some estimates (Bloom and Canning 2004: 22), such a dividend can explain as much as one-third of the rapid growth of East Asian countries in recent decades. Although the dividend is poised for rapid and accelerating decline, about 70 percent of the population of East Asia was of working age as recently as 2005.

Thus the demographic patterns of Figure 7.10—both the overall patterns and the variations across interventions—are significant. High-income countries benefitted substantially from having about 67 percent of their total population of working age at the beginning of the 21st century, while South Asia and Latin America and the Caribbean had about 62–64 percent and sub-Saharan Africa had just 54 percent. However, whereas the share of the population at working age in high-income countries is decreasing under both the high mortality and the low mortality interventions (and will be soon in East Asia and Pacific), the

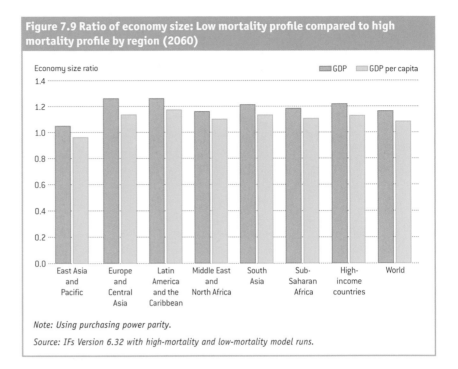

Figure 7.9 Ratio of economy size: Low mortality profile compared to high mortality profile by region (2060)

Economy size ratio

Legend: GDP ■ GDP per capita

Note: Using purchasing power parity.

Source: IFs Version 6.32 with high-mortality and low-mortality model runs.

shares in sub-Saharan Africa will rise sharply throughout our forecast horizon under both mortality assumptions, as will those in South Asia before beginning to decline in about 2040.

Given fundamentally different starting points and trajectories, the impacts of the mortality pattern changes would be quite different across regions. In the high-income countries, low mortality would accelerate the decline in the proportional share of the labor force by increasing the share of elderly in the population, thereby tending (in terms of labor force implications alone—we return later to savings rates) to create some drag on economic growth. With a lag, the same is true for South Asia. In contrast, the impact of lower mortality on the labor force population share in sub-Saharan Africa would largely wash out—it appears that the continent can look forward to an almost inevitable long-term increase in the working-age population (although growth in the population over 65 would accelerate with lower mortality, it is still not likely to exceed 10 percent by 2060). In fact, in the low population variant (from a faster rate of fertility decline) of the low mortality case, the share of working population grows even more rapidly, reaching 68 percent by 2060 (the low population variant affects South Asia and high-income countries relatively little).

The global gain in GDP per capita with low mortality is about 8 percent by 2060, but highly variable by region (East Asia and Pacific actually declines).

Various supplemental interventions (such as additional fertility reduction or increased crop yields) could boost the positive impact of lower mortality.

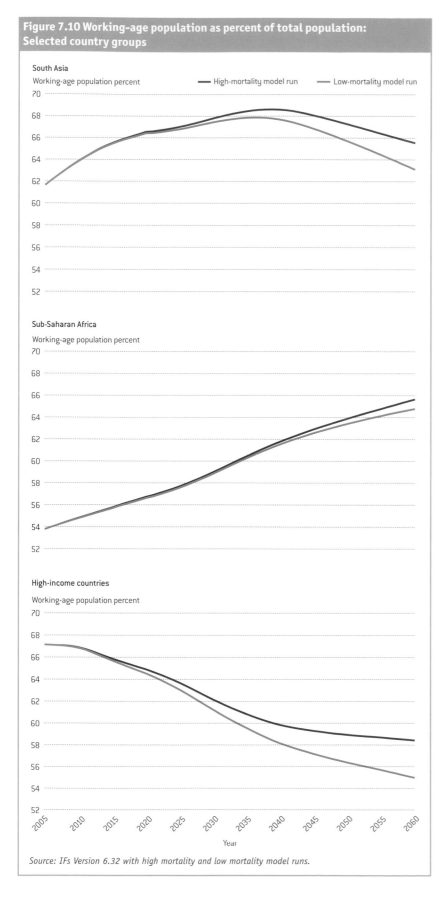

Figure 7.10 Working-age population as percent of total population: Selected country groups

South Asia

Working-age population percent

High-mortality model run — Low-mortality model run

70
68
66
64
62
60
58
56
54
52

Sub-Saharan Africa

Working-age population percent

70
68
66
64
62
60
58
56
54
52

High-income countries

Working-age population percent

70
68
66
64
62
60
58
56
54
52

2005 2010 2015 2020 2025 2030 2035 2040 2045 2050 2055 2060

Year

Source: IFs Version 6.32 with high mortality and low mortality model runs.

Overall, on this dimension the low mortality intervention contributes negatively to long-term economic growth in most of the world (with a time lag of course) by reducing the productive labor force relative to the dependent population, particularly the older population. The effects are most pronounced in the middle- and higher-income countries of the world, where the mortality reduction most immediately increases life expectancy of post-working-age people. The exception would be sub-Saharan Africa, were it able to couple mortality reduction with accelerated fertility reduction; the region has plenty of "working room" to do that.

Age structures have socio-political as well as economic consequences. For example, populations heavy with young men have traditionally been less stable socially and politically. From 1970 to 1999, countries in which 60 percent of the population was less than 30 years of age experienced 80 percent of all civil conflicts.[26] Demographers define *youth bulge* in various ways but direct much attention to the portion of 15- to 29-year-olds in a population and to values above 40 percent (Cincotta, Engelman, and Anastasion 2003). The percentage within that age category in two of the least stable areas of sub-Saharan Africa, the middle or central region and the eastern region, now exceeds 50 percent, and although near peak values in both regions, will remain high for many years even in the low mortality intervention. But better health, through its secondary impact on fertility rates, would bring down the bulges more quickly. Given the devastating impact that domestic conflict often has on economies, and the cycles of broad socio-political failure it sets up (Collier 2007), this important path should augment the discussion that Figure 7.3 framed. The absence in IFs of linkages from youth bulge to conflict and on to economic growth will cause us to somewhat underestimate the economic contribution of improved health via demographics.

Exploring paths between health and growth: Productivity

Earlier discussion (see Figure 7.4) traced multiple paths by which mortality and morbidity can affect multifactor productivity, including a direct path via disability of workers and more indirect paths via stunting and delayed health effects related to undernutrition and via education and cognition. Because of the close association between mortality and morbidity, reductions in mortality rates more often than not reduce morbidity of those in the work force (although generally not in direct proportion; see again Table 3.2). Figure 7.11 shows the significant differences in worker years of morbidity between the high and low mortality cases, showing both sub-Saharan Africa and high-income countries. The difference between the scenarios is considerably greater for sub-Saharan Africa because of its relatively higher burden of communicable diseases. Lower mortality associated with communicable diseases reduces society-wide morbidity to a greater degree than does lower mortality from noncommunicable diseases, in part because communicable diseases strike younger populations and can leave longer morbidity "footprints." Thus, this pathway can contribute increased productivity to lower-income regions such as sub-Saharan Africa.

An additional contribution to productivity from lower mortality is via decreased stunting of the work force, which lags changes in child undernutrition and morbidity by 25 years or so. Figure 7.12 shows that such stunting for sub-Saharan Africa would likely be somewhat lower in the low mortality case. The effect is not great, however—a somewhat counterintuitive result that appears because two forces work against each other. On one side is the direct contribution of better health to both lower mortality and morbidity, and the translation of lower morbidity into greater height and less stunting. On the other side is a perverse effect that lower mortality can have on undernutrition and that does appear in sub-Saharan Africa. In 2060 the low mortality scenario does not significantly change undernutrition in Latin America; it increases rates by about 0.50 percent in sub-Saharan Africa and on a global basis increases rates by about 0.25 percent (and raises total numbers by about 2.5 million). We need to remember that the low mortality scenario adds nearly 1 billion people to the global population by 2100. Were mortality to decline for a single country or region, it would not likely affect the global food market a great deal. Such a large population increase would do so, however, and even in the face of increased labor supply

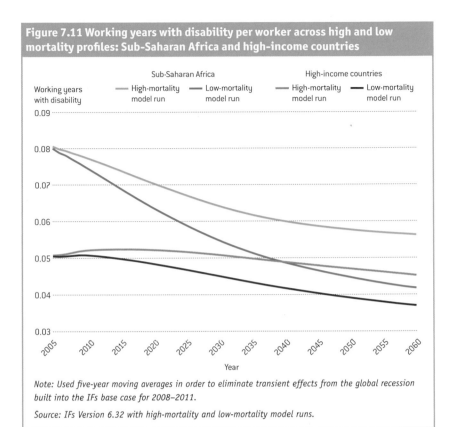

Figure 7.11 Working years with disability per worker across high and low mortality profiles: Sub-Saharan Africa and high-income countries

Note: Used five-year moving averages in order to eliminate transient effects from the global recession built into the IFs base case for 2008–2011.

Source: IFs Version 6.32 with high-mortality and low-mortality model runs.

for production, it is likely that the impacts on global food costs and/or availability would be adverse. Moving analysis of alternative health futures from the local to the global level has important consequences.

Yet it is possible that greater agricultural productivity could accompany a low mortality future, not least because healthy workers could produce more, both through direct labor effects and through more rapid adoption of improved technology. The global community could also more intentionally couple health and agricultural production initiatives around the world. The linkages of morbidity decline to productivity in IFs may underestimate such effects. We therefore created a second variation or counterfactual for the low mortality intervention (in addition to the first one leading to lower fertility) that increases agricultural productivity for the developing countries of the world by an additional 0.4 percent annually through 2060, roughly a 20 percent cumulative increase relative to the low mortality case by 2060. Because it essentially relieves the somewhat Malthusian food restrictions on the higher population of the low mortality case,

Overall, the low mortality intervention reduces the size of the labor force relative to the dependent population and increases especially the older population.

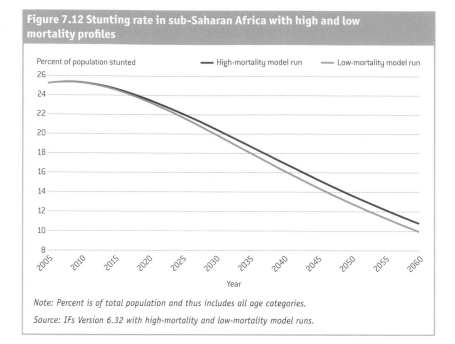

Figure 7.12 Stunting rate in sub-Saharan Africa with high and low mortality profiles

Percent of population stunted — High-mortality model run — Low-mortality model run

Note: Percent is of total population and thus includes all age categories.

Source: IFs Version 6.32 with high-mortality and low-mortality model runs.

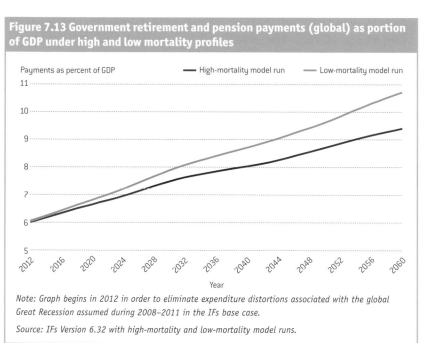

Figure 7.13 Government retirement and pension payments (global) as portion of GDP under high and low mortality profiles

Payments as percent of GDP — High-mortality model run — Low-mortality model run

Note: Graph begins in 2012 in order to eliminate expenditure distortions associated with the global Great Recession assumed during 2008–2011 in the IFs base case.

Source: IFs Version 6.32 with high-mortality and low-mortality model runs.

it further reduces stunting for regions like sub-Saharan Africa. Stunting in 2060 would be nearly 1 percent lower across the continent in this case. (We will return later to the economic implications of these modifications for the low mortality case.)

More generally, analysis with IFs shows that there is limited overall difference in the paths of multifactor productivity across the high and low mortality cases. Again, that is

somewhat surprising. Why would that be? The determinants of productivity in the real world, and in the IFs system, are numerous and complex, as we have attempted to describe. And there are trade-offs.

Turning explicitly to social trade-offs, the larger and older global populations in the low mortality intervention require the direction of additional resources to those populations, including old-age security and pension spending (see Figure 7.13). On a global basis, the low mortality scenario could require 1.3 percent of GDP more for such purposes than would the high mortality scenario. That additional increment of spending appears roughly comparable across regions at currently different levels of economic development. This increased spending on the elderly would divert some potential funding from all other government expenditure categories, including education, and the IFs forecast for education expenditures is therefore lower. Moreover, at least in the short and mid-terms, until fertility patterns adjusted, lower mortality would mean larger student-age populations, especially in regions with current high communicable disease burdens, thereby diluting educational expenditures per student. And the absence in IFs of a linkage from aging to higher health care spending means that our analysis probably actually underestimates somewhat the diversion of expenditures from education.

Proposals for boosting spending on health with the expectation of economic return to help pay the costs of such increases (see, for example, Commission on Macroeconomics and Health 2001) often recommend that external resources augment locally generated ones. This analysis suggests one good argument in support of that recommendation, namely, the need to protect other and complimentary investments in human capital.

For that reason we created a third (and final) counterfactual for the low mortality case, one in which the global community helps relieve the constraint of these trade-offs by increasing foreign aid. We were not so rash as to posit that major aid-giving countries would move transfers to the long-requested 0.7 percent of GDP, but we did move them to 0.5 percent, leaving countries already above that level unchanged. (As before, we will return later to the economic implications of our variations for the low mortality case.) We ultimately find that global multifactor productivity rises negligibly in the low mortality scenario in the early years relative to the high mortality scenario, and that by 2060 the high mortality scenario actually produces annually higher gains of about 0.1 percentage points, with the advantage returning marginally to low mortality by the end of the century. The temporal pattern reflects demographic ones, with some immediate benefit from lower disability of working-age populations, offset in the mid-range by growing proportions of the elderly, and reaching a new equilibrium in the long run.

Overall, the two mortality interventions make surprisingly little difference for multifactor productivity. The fact that our basic scenario targeted only mortality is important in that outcome, because incremental population gains with low mortality pose a number of challenges for productivity. Although fertility adjusts, it does so slowly. As our counterfactuals suggest, scenario variations that simultaneously target fertility, that place additional emphasis on agricultural productivity, or that benefit from additional outside resources, have more positive impacts on productivity. In the discussion of Figure 7.14 near the end of this chapter we return to analysis of those impacts.

Exploring paths between health and growth: Savings and capital

The third general linkage between health and economic growth works through capital stock, and Figure 7.5 elaborated its more specific paths. Those paths include the potential crowding out of savings by spending on health, the higher savings of populations with longer life expectancy, and the greater attractiveness with respect to foreign direct investment of economies with healthier and more productive populations. Collectively, those paths in analysis with IFs lead to higher capital stock by 2060 across all regions (especially high-income countries) in the low mortality intervention than in the high mortality intervention (see Table 7.1). To put the numbers for 2060 in context, the capital stock per worker in high-income countries in 2005 was $120,000.

Table 7.1 suggests three somewhat surprising and perhaps counterintuitive results. First and most fundamentally, simplified analysis with a neoclassical framework might suggest that the lower mortality and associated higher population would dilute capital and lead to smaller values per person. Why then does Table 7.1 suggest the opposite outcome? It does so first because it focuses on capital per worker, not per person. Because those who expect to live longer beyond retirement age will generally save more in preparation for it, savings for the society as a whole will normally rise with greater longevity, pushing up capital per worker. Second, although those who live past retirement will draw on their savings, life-cycle pattern analysis suggests that many will save more than they subsequently draw out, passing the excess to the next generations. Finally, positive effects and higher growth compound over time, producing quite large gains even from relatively small increments.

> ■ The association of mortality and morbidity, other things being equal, means reductions in mortality rates translate into a healthier and more productive work force. ■

> ■ On the other hand, the 1 billion more people in the low mortality case put pressure on the global food supply and could result in some increase in undernutrition. ■

> ■ The low mortality case requires additional spending on behalf of the larger and older global population, redirecting some public resources from other human development. ■

Table 7.1 Capital stock per worker (thousands of dollars) by region under high and low mortality profiles (2060)	High-mortality model run	Low-mortality model run
East Asia and Pacific	162.5	168.9
Europe and Central Asia	66.4	117.9
Latin America and the Caribbean	64.4	116.3
Middle East and North Africa	51.8	78.4
South Asia	38.8	58.5
Sub-Saharan Africa	13.9	18.1
High-income countries	284.7	477.7
World	**90.0**	**124.8**

Source: IFs Version 6.32 with high-mortality and low-mortality model runs.

Second, it may be somewhat surprising that there is such a large difference between the two scenarios for high-income countries. The explanation lies in the fact that for such societies most of the additional longevity is that of post-retirement-age populations and requires higher savings for an extended retirement period. Again, some increased savings may prove to be an excess safety cushion and may pass to subsequent generations. But even if they do not, the interim higher savings boost the total for the economy and per worker.

A third possible surprise from Table 7.1 is that the forecast for capital per worker in East Asia and Pacific countries is only marginally different between the high and low mortality model runs. The reason is that savings and gross capital formation as a portion of GDP in that region are already exceptionally high; additional longevity results in a draw-down of lifelong savings by the elderly that roughly balances the relatively small impetus for still higher savings levels.

Although it would not necessarily increase global totals of capital stock, movement of capital stock to regions with improved health (e.g., via foreign direct investments) should also improve overall productivity of the system. Our analysis suggests that FDI flows into sub-Saharan Africa could be higher by as much as 1 percent of GDP in the low mortality scenario.

Conclusions concerning the three paths between health and economic growth

We have obviously not undertaken here a cost-benefit analysis of investment in health.[27] Some individual interventions, such as the use of insecticide-soaked bed nets and the provision of micronutrients, have such a low cost and high health return that there can be no doubt of a large and quite fast return in terms of human well-being. Many other interventions, however, and unfortunately even the expenditures that governments make on health care systems, have very uncertain returns with respect to health outcomes. Instead of systematic cost-benefit analysis, we have shown that there are positive returns in the aggregate to investments in better health.

Of the three major paths from reduced mortality and morbidity to economic growth, rise in capital stock from higher savings for

older age appears to have the greatest potential for boosting economic growth. With respect to the labor path, decreased childhood mortality provides a direct boost to labor force size, but decreases in noncommunicable diseases can cause rapid increases in the post-retirement populations. The net result for most regions (with sub-Saharan Africa being a partial exception) is an overall decrease in the working-age population as a share of the total population. With respect to the productivity path, increased spending on pensions and other expenses associated with aging populations may squeeze productivity gains from health and education that roughly offset the economic advantages of reduced stunting of workers and adult incidence of disability. (We should not forget that this improved health would mean that people had a better quality of life overall, even if GDP per capita did not increase.)

We should not assume that even the path via capital stock is rock-solid with respect to gains from lower morbidity or that there is completely convincing evidence that lower mortality will boost economic growth in the long run. The higher savings rate as a percent of GDP associated with the low mortality intervention narrows beyond 2060, in part because the continually aging population eventually draws on accumulated savings (and our omission from the analysis of direct use of savings by the elderly for health spending may also lead to some upward bias in the conclusion that low mortality has economic benefit). Even with the savings effect, the economic growth advantage of the low mortality scenario overall erodes somewhat for all regions between the middle and the end of the century.

In short, our conclusion is that lower mortality does not, as some analyses would suggest, actually reduce GDP per capita, but that its contribution to higher levels of GDP per capita is likely to be more modest than still other studies conclude. We also recognize, of course, that many of the paths we have represented remain contested; also, although we have provided a fairly rich treatment of the subject, we have not explored all possible paths.

Even with all appropriate caveats, this analysis still suggests the potential for real contributions of health improvements to economic growth and income levels. Figure 7.9 showed a 16 percent rise in global GDP and an 8 percent increase in GDP per capita between the high and low mortality cases. And this discussion has emphasized the potential that additional levers have to complement the impact of health improvements, commenting specifically on fertility reduction, agricultural yield improvement, and increases in foreign assistance.

Figure 7.14 contrasts not only the low mortality intervention again with the high mortality case but also the three "augmented" low mortality interventions with the high mortality case. Finally, it compares a combined case (the low mortality intervention with all augmentations) with the high mortality case. The impact of these additional interventions would be felt most strongly in sub-Saharan Africa and Latin America and the Caribbean. Effective fertility reduction (coming on the tail of a more rapid mortality decline) would boost the relative increase in future GDP per capita from 11 to 21 percent in sub-Saharan Africa and from 17 to 18 percent in Latin America and the Caribbean. Improvements in crop yield and fiscal balance sheets (with higher financial aid) generate less relative increase in GDP per capita for sub-Saharan Africa than does fertility reduction, but the three together could boost the region's GDP per capita in the low mortality scenario 28 percent above that of the high mortality scenario.

Not surprisingly, a final conclusion must be that there is no simple relationship between improved health and economic performance. It depends on the balance of mortality causes within a region, on the underlying demographic and economic structures of the region, and on the policies with which health interventions might be combined. The good news, nonetheless, is that there seems to be clear potential for positive micro- and macroeconomic impacts of reductions in mortality.

Returning to the intrinsic benefits of health

Even if reduced mortality (without supplemental policy interventions) may not greatly boost GDP per capita, we all know it to have large intrinsic value, and it is important to return to that foundational reality. Increased life expectancy is arguably the highest human value, most especially when it comes also with improved

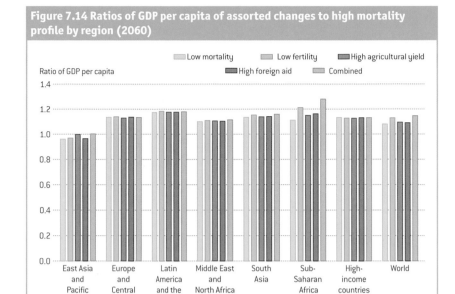

Figure 7.14 Ratios of GDP per capita of assorted changes to high mortality profile by region (2060)

Legend: Low mortality · Low fertility · High agricultural yield · High foreign aid · Combined

Ratio of GDP per capita

Notes: Using purchasing power parity; low fertility, high agricultural yield, and high foreign aid variations are each combined individually with the low mortality assumption until the final category, which combines all variations together with low-mortality.

Source: IFs Version 6.32 with high mortality, low mortality, and low-mortality variations.

quality of life, as the disability forecasting formulations of the Global Burden of Disease analysis (and therefore our own) suggest is generally the case. If we were to add the value of extra and often healthier years of life to income per capita, thereby moving toward a "full income" assessment that accounts for the monetary value of longevity gains, our analysis would obviously support a very large investment in improved health (Becker, Philipson, and Soares 2005).

As a step in that direction, Figure 7.15 shows the difference in the Human Development Index[28] values to which high and low mortality assumptions give rise for sub-Saharan Africa and South Asia. By mid-century the HDI for both regions is about 5 percentage points higher in the lower mortality case. The figure almost certainly underestimates the benefits of lower mortality and morbidity for the Human Development Index because our analysis does not directly pass through the impact of reduced morbidity to educational achievement.[29]

Conclusion

At the individual level, no one questions the benefits of improved health. Good things at the individual level do not always scale, however, to

Augmenting the low mortality case with variations in fertility, foreign aid, and crop yield boosts the economic returns to low mortality alone, especially in sub-Saharan Africa.

The low mortality case boosts values on the Human Development Index for developing regions.

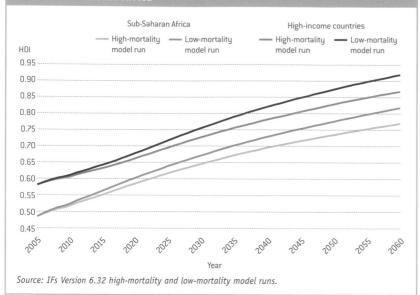

Figure 7.15 Human development index (HDI) across mortality profiles: South Asia and sub-Saharan Africa

Sub-Saharan Africa
High-mortality model run — Low-mortality model run

High-income countries
High-mortality model run — Low-mortality model run

HDI

Year

Source: IFs Version 6.32 high-mortality and low-mortality model runs.

● *Across many paths of relationship, the positive impacts of improved health on economic outcomes outweigh the negative effects.* ●

good things at the aggregate level. In the case of the (over)use of common property resources, such as tuna from the ocean or timber from tropical forests, scaling ultimately produces bad things; in the case of connections to the internet and contributions to human knowledge, scaling has at least the possibility of producing good things.

With respect to health, there may be a mixture of scaling effects. Overall, our analysis of health and economic growth suggests that the positive impacts of improved health on economic outcomes outweigh the negative effects, and

that when we add the intrinsic value of health, the return to improved health is sharply positive at both micro and macro levels.

It is again important to emphasize, however, that not all implications of health for economic growth and social well-being more generally are unambiguously positive. We did not even consider, for instance, the impact on the environment of more and richer people. A comparison of the environmental footprints of the citizens of North America and the European Union with sub-Saharan Africa, two groupings having roughly the same population, would most likely suggest that creating healthier and richer people, as well as more of them, could have decidedly mixed aggregate implications.

There is little forecasting of the potential broader economic and social effects of different health futures. Given the number of paths that this chapter identified and explored, that may not be surprising—the causal picture is very complicated and this discussion has needed to push analytic frontiers. Even while pushing the limits of analysis of health's broader impacts (and we hope making a contribution by doing so), we began and concluded by emphasizing the great uncertainty of analysis around health futures. That reiteration takes us to the next chapter, devoting attention specifically to uncertainty.

1   Solow's extension of the Harrod-Domar version of the neoclassical model added an exogenous and generally constant technological change term. That extension allows labor productivity to grow without increase in capital. Yet improvements in health or other human capital do not affect production with that extension. Endogenous growth theory and its representations, like that in IFs, break that limitation and move beyond the traditional neoclassical form.

2   See Bloom, Canning, and Jamison 2004; Bloom and Sachs 1998; Commission on Macroeconomics and Health 2001; Gallup and Sachs 2001; Lorentzen, McMillan, and Wacziarg 2008.

3   Barro (1996) found the effect of life expectancy on economic growth to be larger than the effect of education. Another study looked at the effects of adult survival rate and found positive overall returns but lower returns at higher levels of GDP per capita (Bhargava et al. 2001). Another modeled diminishing returns to life expectancy by using a square term, finding small effects for the average country but

quite large effects for those with the lowest life expectancy (Sachs and Warner 1997). Jamison, Lau, and Wang (2005) found that improvements in health accounted for about 10 percent of all economic growth in a sample of 50 countries between 1965 and 1990. Age- or disease-specific studies have found increased growth associated with reductions in the occurrence of malaria (Bleakley and Lange 2009; Gallup and Sachs 2001; Gallup, Sachs, and Mellinger 1999; Sachs and Malaney 2002), HIV/AIDS (Ainsworth and Over 1994; Cuddington 1993; Dixon, McDonald, and Roberts 2001; Over 1992), and cardiovascular diseases (Suhrcke et al. 2006; Suhrcke and Urban 2006).

4   See Aïsa and Pueyo 2004; Ashraf, Lester, and Weil 2008; Azomahou, Diene, and Soete 2009; Boucekkine, Diene, and Azomahou 2007; 2008; Cervellati and Sunde 2007; Chakraborty, Papageorgiou, and Pérez-Sebastián 2005; DeLeire and Manning 2004; Gollin and Zimmermann 2007; Kalemli-Ozcan 2002; Strulik 2004; van Zon and Muysken 2001.

5   For full documentation of IFs, see its help system and project documents on the website.

6   IFs also includes income-based formulations for changing the female participation rate in the labor force.

7   The function is thus Total Fertility Rate = 3.8812 + 0.0217 * Infant Mortality – 0.8327 * ln(Adult Education) – 0.00948 * Percent using Modern Contraception. Even though the GBD used years of education for those 25 and older, we used years of education for those 15 and older for two reasons: (1) women between the ages of 15 and 25 bear many children and (2) the statistical relationship was as strong as for those older than 25.

8   See Alavinia and Burdorf 2008; Arndt 2006; Arndt and Wobst 2002; DeLeire and Manning 2004; Jusot et al. 2008; Stewart 2001; Thirumurthy, Zivin, and Goldstein 2008; Tunceli et al. 2005; van de Mheen et al. 1999.

9 With good prevalence data for a wide range of diseases (such data are not currently available), it would be possible to allow burdens to accumulate by increasing the disability weight associated with a disease as cohorts experiencing a morbidity burden progress through the age pyramid. For example, given a disability weight for a chronic disease of 0.3, we could compound that disability weight by a certain percentage for each additional year with the disease. This increasingly large disability weight would of course be applied to the standard age-specific productivity/earnings profile, so that compounded productivity losses for a 50-year-old versus a 40-year-old would be set against the relatively higher wages of the average 50-year-old. Similarly, impact of the disability effect would be diminished as cohorts moved towards the lower earnings and productivity of the retirement ages.

10 See the following resources for evidence on the effects of height on earnings: Hoddinott et al. 2008; Schultz 2002; 2005; Thomas and Frankenberg 2002; and Thomas and Strauss 1997. With respect to the relationship of height and adult health, see Blackwell, Hayward, and Crimmins 2001; and Crimmins and Finch 2006. For experimental and quasi-experimental evidence on the long-term determinants and consequences of height, see Alderman et al. 2001; Alderman, Hoddinott, and Kinsey 2006; Almond, Chay, and Lee 2005; Barham 2009; Cutler and Miller 2005; Hoddinott et al. 2008; and Miguel and Kremer 2004. For historical and cross-national perspectives, see Deaton 2007; and Steckel 1995. For evidence on the effects of early life conditions on achieved height, see Bozzoli, Deaton, and Quintana-Domeque 2009; Scrimshaw 2003; and Stephensen 1999. For next-generation effects on cognitive skills of women, see Behrman et al. 2009.

11 Focusing on health spending, Baldacci et al. (2004: 25–27) analyzed 120 countries from 1975 to 2000 and concluded that spending an additional 1 percent of GDP on health raises growth in annual GDP per capita by 0.5 percent, as well as reducing under-five child mortality by 0.6 percentage points.

12 The lag is the difference from the midpoint of childhood (7.5) to the midpoint of adulthood (32.5).

13 Global data on stunting among adults appear nearly nonexistent. UNICEF (2009: 5) suggests that under-five stunting exceeds that of undernutrition (200 million versus 130 million) and that stunting is nearly irreversible with aging; these facts suggest very high percentages of stunting among global adults, concentrated in Africa and Asia.

14 That function is HEIGHT (NOW) = -0.06746 * PREADLTMORT + 0.00014 * PREADLTMORT2 (where PRADLTMORT is pre-adult mortality per 1,000). The study uses only women because the Demographic and Health Surveys, which interview just women, provide the only reasonable multi-country height series for poor countries. The analysis actually measures not pre-adult mortality but infant mortality and then uses model life tables to transform that into pre-adult mortality.

15 To parameterize this relationship, we analyzed the extent of deviations in stunting levels of countries from the function and found that it seldom exceeds 10 percent. In the most extreme cases it can reach 40 percent. We assigned a parameter value of -0.025, which means that, in the extreme cases, stunting might be costing close to 1 percent in annual economic growth.

16 Dividing disability years for the working population by the population age 15–65 generates worker-specific lifetime rates in 2005 that range from around 0.20–0.27 at the top end of the range (Afghanistan, Cambodia, Montenegro, Puerto Rico, Timor-Leste, and other [mostly African] countries) to 0.05–0.06 at the bottom end (Algeria, Cape Verde, Japan, Kuwait, UAE, and other [mostly rich] countries).

17 Assigning a parameter to the relationship between changes in forecasted disability levels relative to expected ones and productivity is problematic, and we set it at -0.5. That means that the initial implicit impact of the YLD rate on MFP for Timor-Leste at 0.278 million years of disability per million workers (relative to a world average of 0.097) would be a drag of -0.09 percentage points of growth per year. Japan at 0.055 would be gaining a boost of 0.02 percent in productivity and growth. In reality, we should use a disability weight instead of YLD, because the latter is a cumulative lifetime measure rather than an annual incidence measure (i.e., it incorporates not just this year's morbidity but all subsequent morbidity for those afflicted in a current year). Yet the disability weight and YLD will essentially change in parallel, meaning that the difference between them is largely a scaling factor, already captured by the parameter assigned in the linkage to productivity.

18 We associated each year of incremental life expectancy with a value of 0.035 years of education for those 15 years of age and older (thus, in essence, using education years as a proxy for quality as well as quantity of educational attainment).

19 See Deaton and Paxson 1994; and Lee, Mason, and Miller 2000 for single-country results; see Bloom, Canning, and Graham 2003; and Lorentzen, McMillan, and Wacziarg 2008 for cross-country results.

20 A number of recent equilibrium simulation experiments have found that we can only explain longitudinal variations in growth, particularly those for today's developed nations, if we incorporate relationships between longevity and increased savings rates (Aísa and Pueyo 2004; Bloom, Canning, and Graham 2003; Boucekkine, Diene, and Azomahou 2007; 2008; Lorentzen, McMillan, and Wacziarg 2008; Soares 2005).

21 In such societies, the survival risks imposed by HIV/AIDS could, however, drive down both the incentives to save for capital investment and the incentives to invest savings in children. Prime-age adults may save less if they anticipate their own premature mortality. Those anticipating a long life for themselves, and thus needing retirement savings, may doubt the reliability of their children as a source of old-age support, thereby discouraging intergenerational investments. This may push savings into alternative investments, such as land, or simply reduce savings significantly overall.

22 For instance, adding the Fraser Institute's measure of economic freedom (focused on free use of property; see www.freetheworld.com) raises the cross-sectional variation explained by GDP per capita (32 percent) by 15 percentage points. The t-value is not significant; the sign is interestingly negative in spite of the United States being highly free and high spending. The Freedom House measure of civil and political liberties (www.

freedomhouse.org) does almost as well, and Polity's (www.systemicpeace.org) democracy measure adds 16 percentage points with strong significance. The Polity democracy measure and economic freedom together take the R-squared from 0.32 with GDP per capita alone to an impressive 0.60 (the sign on economic freedom remains negative and the t-value approaches 2).

23 There is also no linkage between health and capital depreciation in IFs; as discussed earlier, that pathway is not very certain.

24 The representation of FDI in IFs captures the accumulation over time of FDI inflows and outflows in stocks. In addition, the stocks set up their own dynamics, including the tendency for stocks to reinforce flows. For that reason, we have set the base case parameter for the impact of each year of life expectancy on FDI flows to 0.05 (5 percent), lower than the estimate of Alsan, Bloom, and Canning (2006).

25 This is not an extreme range of intervention assumptions. The report of the Commission on Social Determinants of Health (CSDH 2008: 197) called for a 95 percent reduction in under-five mortality rates between 2000 and 2040. In sub-Saharan Africa the 30 percent reduction relative to the base accomplishes only a 70 percent decline in 2040 relative to 2005 and produces a mortality rate that is only 50 percent lower than the high intervention.

26 See the analysis by Population Action International at http://www.cfr.org/publication/13093/.

27 The Patterns of Potential Human Progress volume *Advancing Global Education* (Dickson, Hughes, and Irfan 2010) did undertake such an analysis with respect to education because the costs of educating children at different levels are relatively easier to quantify and compare against the return. That study found that the break-even point with respect to contribution of more spending on education to economic growth could be two or more decades in the future, depending on the country and region, but that the return continued to grow over the long term. That is a result quite different from the one suggested by this chapter.

28 The HDI is a composite measure of several human development factors—namely, income, literacy, education, and life expectancy. It was developed by the United Nations Development Programme (UNDP) in 1990 under the guidance of Mahbub ul Haq. The UNDP updates the HDI for all countries each year in the annual UNDP Human Development Report.

29 We do represent the probable education-related contribution of morbidity reduction to multifactor productivity but do not show it in educational attainment.

8

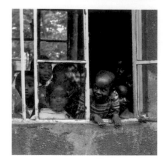

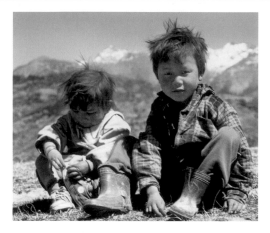

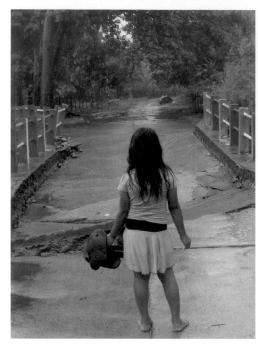

Broadening and Integrating Our Perspective

■ *Our base case tells a story of continued progress for system leaders and convergence toward their health conditions by other countries.* ■

This volume has gradually elaborated a story about possible long-term global health futures. The central thrust of our story has been one of continued human progress in meeting the challenges to living longer and healthier lives. Those challenges are many. The burden of communicable diseases globally, and especially in the developing world, remains heavy, greatly exacerbated by the surge of HIV/AIDS and the persistence and even resurgence of killers such as malaria. Progress against the burden of noncommunicable diseases has produced many additional and generally healthier years of later life, although the progress sometimes seems painfully slow. Nonetheless, most of humanity has experienced a steady path forward, and our story for the coming 50 years has quite consistently anticipated continued positive movement on two dimensions: continued progress in health for system leaders and convergence toward their conditions by other countries around the world.

How confident are we in that story, especially as we look out 50 years? It is quite possible that our base case forecast, built in substantial part on the foundation of past trends, could dramatically overstate or understate the pace of health progress that the world will actually experience in the coming years.

Past chapters have addressed our uncertainty—and our leverage—in a number of specifically targeted ways, such as exploring the impact of changes in individual distal and proximate drivers. Building on that earlier analysis, this chapter steps back, returning our perspective also to the broader and more integrative framing uncertainties that Chapters 1 and 2 introduced—namely, those that surround the biological context of health outcomes and the scope and nature of human activity affecting health. With respect to the biological context, Chapter 2 sketched the significant debate concerning the ultimate potential of the human genome to support significantly longer life expectancies and therefore a continuation of the rate of advance in life spans of those countries at the leading edge. Within the biological context we also recognize, of course, the potential for mutational change in pathogens that could overwhelm even our best efforts to limit that change and contain its effects. There are many wild cards on this dimension.

Regarding human activity, Chapter 2 introduced three super-distal drivers or driver categories that frame our core model of interactions between distal drivers, proximate drivers, and health outcomes (see again Figure 2.4 and the discussion surrounding it). The first of those is technological change, which the distal-driver model includes implicitly within its time term, but only as a constant exogenous element. We must consider the possibility that technological advance could accelerate significantly because of remarkable insights from genetic analysis (for example), as well as the possibility that (in part in interaction with biological constraints) it might slow in its ability to advance frontiers against disease.

The second super-distal driver is the natural environmental context beyond human biology. Human activity directed intentionally or unintentionally at changing the natural environment and the human relationship with it has had both positive and negative implications for human health. In fact, even the same actions, such as spraying with DDT to kill mosquitoes, have often had both. What we now have come to understand is that at least one such unintentional change, that of global warming, could have quite dramatic implications for health in the longer run, albeit most significantly beyond our current forecasting horizon.

The third super-distal category contains human activity that shapes what we might term the social environment of human health. Global initiatives, national policy efforts, actions of nongovernmental organizations (including corporations), and behavior of subpopulations and individuals collectively shape factors as disparate as the pace of HIV/AIDS transmission, the level of obesity, and the rate of vehicle accidents. Human activity with respect to the social environment could be broad, deep, and well organized—it could also be underfunded, scattered in focus, and badly managed.

Intervening chapters have partially explored these super-distal categories in the process

of analysis of distal and proximate drivers. In considering alternative assumptions about distal drivers, for example, Chapter 4 began to explore the implications of alternative assumptions concerning technological change. Chapter 5 considered the potential power of several proximate drivers, substantially linked to the social environment, to produce alternative futures. Chapter 6 extended consideration further to some of the changes in the natural environment that we know to be adding to our uncertainty. And Chapter 7 then addressed the derivative uncertainty concerning forward linkages from health to demographic and economic patterns; positive and negative feedback loops across economic and social change also can affect the long-term dynamics of health futures.

In Figure 8.1 we step back to suggest how these driving forces of health might interact with biological context and human activity to give rise to four very different global health futures.[1] Good human biological prospects and strong and positive human activity could create a future that combines Luck and Enlightenment. Should biological prospects prove less accommodating than we would hope, we could still aggressively and thoughtfully continue within that constraint a Steady Slog toward better health futures and continued convergence of health outcomes toward a maximum standard. Although it seems perverse that we would be so foolish as not to take advantage of a favorable biological context,

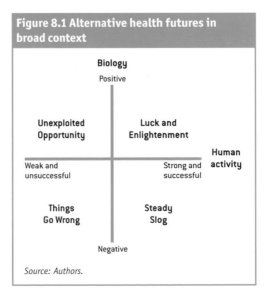

Figure 8.1 Alternative health futures in broad context

Source: Authors.

■ How confident are we in the story our base case tells? ■

■ To explore that question, we look at our forecasts relative to axes of uncertainty concerning the biological context of health and the super-distal human drivers of health. ■

one can in fact imagine a future of Unexploited Opportunity, especially in selected countries and regions, one major consequence of which might be further divergence in health outcomes between nations. And, unfortunately, it is quite possible also to imagine a future in which rising resistance to our current armory of drugs and other treatment modalities, and/or the emergence of new threats, is accompanied by a failure of global and state-level governance to respond well to the setback or new challenge. In this future, a future in which Things Go Wrong, progress in health would greatly slow or potentially even reverse.

This chapter will address two primary questions. First, where in the universe of possible health futures of Figure 8.1 does the base case forecast of this volume appear to sit? We cannot assume that the forecasts already provided (see especially Chapter 4) sit at the origin of that figure and that alternative movement into each quadrant of the figure is equally likely. It could be, for instance, that our forecasts already implicitly assume Luck and Enlightenment and that the downside risk relative to our base case is much greater than the upside potential. Second, what is the extent of uncertainty around our base case? We may be particularly interested in knowing something about the magnitude of downside risks.

How Might We Characterize Our Base Forecasts?

Two critical dimensions of variation in forecasts of health futures are (1) the rate of advance in mortality and morbidity reduction at the leading edge of human health, and (2) the extent of variation in those rates across countries and subpopulations within countries. Together, for example, rates of leaders and distributional patterns of followers determine the global average life expectancy. Before assessing the character of our forecasts (looking, in turn, at communicable and noncommunicable diseases), we consider the historical patterns.

Historical patterns as a reference point

The historical trend of recent decades has been very considerable improvement in levels of health across most societies, as well as considerable convergence between rich and poor countries. Going back somewhat further, Figure 1.4 (see also Table 4.1) showed that since the mid- to late 1700s the life expectancy of the world's longest-lived societies has continued to rise. These life expectancy gains resulted from a mix of improvements in the frontiers of the human life span and an increasing proportion of people who actually reach a higher, more typical life span (an increase that began in the currently rich countries and is still gradually spreading across the world).

For long-lived populations, longevity experts often summarize the practical human life span as being four standard deviations above the mean life span, or the life span that the longest-lived one in every 15,000 people experiences. It would be easy to assume that random genetic variation accounts for such incredible longevity, but this value has, in fact, increased consistently over time in many developed countries. For example, we see this in Figure 8.2, which charts both gains in the life-span frontier and gains in average life spans for Sweden since 1860. With respect to the recorded life-span frontier, the life span of the top one in every 10,000 people went from just above 100 years in 1860 to nearly 110 years at present. Similar patterns characterize gains in the top 1,000th of the population, the top 1 percent, and the top 5 percent. While the improvement in survival to 110 reflects sustained improvements in age-specific mortality at advanced ages, better

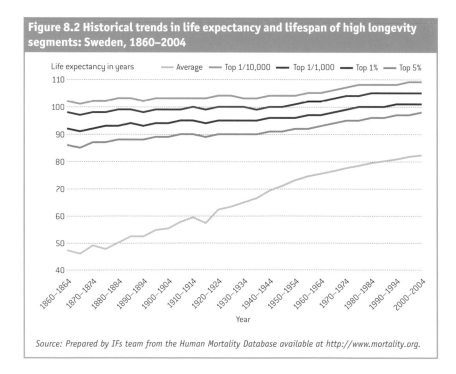

Figure 8.2 Historical trends in life expectancy and lifespan of high longevity segments: Sweden, 1860–2004

Life expectancy in years — Average — Top 1/10,000 — Top 1/1,000 — Top 1% — Top 5%

Year

Source: Prepared by IFs team from the Human Mortality Database available at http://www.mortality.org.

survival at younger ages accounts by far for the bulk of the average increase of life expectancy in Sweden during this period.

Historical change in life expectancy in Sweden has exhibited the process often referred to as *rectangularization* (discussed in Chapter 4), with the shape of the survival curve becoming more like a rectangle in which most people live to a certain (typically older) age and then die within relatively few years of one another. Rectangularization characterizes most historical life expectancy improvements in high-income countries and most current improvements in poor countries. While the failure to reach a typical life span clearly reflects some random variation in physical fitness, today's high-income societies display incredibly high probabilities of survival to age 60 or even 70 before a rapid increase in mortality. Societies achieved these historical improvements in survival through improvements in living standards and technology and also through a wide range of efforts to improve the governance and delivery of public health, hygiene, and medical services to broader segments of the population.

Given the long-term convergence of average life expectancy toward leading life expectancy within countries like Sweden and the generalization of the phenomenon of rectangularization around the world, it is not surprising that life expectancies have also been converging globally. In the early post–World War II and post–African independence period (that is, through the 1950s, 1960s, and 1970s), the average life expectancy of countries around the world rose more rapidly than did those of high-income countries. Figure 8.3 shows how, in particular, lower-middle-income and low-income countries significantly narrowed the gap in life expectancy between themselves and the high-income countries (which have also experienced convergence among themselves).

Yet the convergence pattern between developing and high-income countries has been by no means steady. As Chapter 4 noted (see also Figure 4.7, which shows mortality patterns for all World Bank regional groupings separately), the so-called Great Leap Forward in China disrupted life expectancy so much that we have omitted from Figure 8.3 the low values of 1960–1965 for lower-middle-income countries. This episode in China's history illustrates well how the human

activity dimension can be extremely disruptive to advances in health. More relevant to the issue of broad long-term global convergence, the developing economies as a whole largely ceased closing the gap with the high-income countries in about 1990, at which time the mostly low-income sub-Saharan countries began to diverge because of AIDS deaths. Thus, disruption related to the biological dimension substantially changed the global pattern of convergence in life expectancy. Yet the experience of even upper-middle-income countries (including Brazil, Mexico, Russia, South Africa, and Turkey) suggests that convergence may not always occur—as a group they have shown little or none since the 1960s. The major lesson of Figure 8.3 is that we should not take for granted the convergence that our forecasts demonstrate.

Given these historical patterns in which important dimensions of uncertainty in the global system have given rise to complicated paths around an overall trend improvement, let us turn more directly to the issue of how the base case forecasts of International Futures (IFs) appear to fit in the uncertainty space of Figure 8.1. We separately consider communicable and noncommunicable diseases; because accidents and injuries constitute a relatively small proportion of the global mortality and disability burden we do not include them in this discussion.

> ● *History tells us that we cannot take for granted the convergence that our forecasts project; paths around overall trend improvement are complicated.* ●

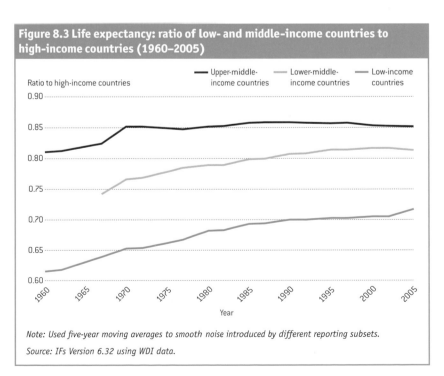

Figure 8.3 Life expectancy: ratio of low- and middle-income countries to high-income countries (1960–2005)

Note: Used five-year moving averages to smooth noise introduced by different reporting subsets.
Source: IFs Version 6.32 using WDI data.

Communicable disease futures

Our base case forecast for communicable diseases (CDs) is on the whole more optimistic than our noncommunicable disease (NCD) forecasts. We essentially forecast the neutralization, if not the near elimination, of CDs, including HIV/AIDS, in most countries by the year 2060 (see again Chapter 4). Even such a positive forecast may be realistic, rather than optimistic, if the evidence supports the plausibility of such a trend. Does it?

Supporting the positive CD forecast is the reality that technologies already exist to treat almost every CD and that most high- and middle-income countries have applied them to great effect. One could argue that these favorable baseline technological conditions thus support placement of a very aggressive base case at the origin of Figure 8.1, leaving room for still greater technological improvements. We can, in fact, imagine a few potential technological advancements that would sufficiently reduce the costs or political barriers to disease prevention and mitigation so as to further accelerate CD reduction in even the world's most challenging environments. The two most relevant diseases in this regard are also the target of the most substantial investments in new technologies: HIV/AIDS and malaria. We argue, however, that the base case forecast, by predicting the elimination of most existing CDs through the effects of the income and time drivers, already incorporates a very high level of technological efficacy and is, in fact, optimistic. Optimistic forecasts do not well incorporate downside risks; for this and other reasons forecasting is subject to a well-known "optimism bias" (Armstrong 2001; Coates 2004).

One great source of uncertainty in our CD forecasts relates to disease governance at the global and national levels. The second half of the 20th century showed that countries could achieve very large CD reductions, even in the absence of economic advance, through the use of antibiotics, vaccination, and chemical spraying of infectious disease vectors in poor countries (Davis 1956; Easterlin 1999; Kremer 2002; Soares 2005). These improvements were the result not merely of technology but also of efforts to transfer technology, fund its delivery, and provide technical support, all carried out through the intergovernmental framework embodied in the World Health Organization

(Cutler, Deaton, and Lleras-Muney 2006; Mosley 1984; Preston 1975; 1980; 1996).[2] While continued progress in the fight against communicable diseases will certainly depend on the pace of new technologies, much of the progress will be determined by our ability to cooperate to address the proximate drivers of disease in poor countries.

Current global efforts at disease surveillance, control, and eradication all hold tremendous promise. As mentioned earlier, the new set of International Health Regulations (IHRs) now mandates active global reporting and surveillance of outbreaks of many communicable diseases. Global nongovernmental organizations and aid agencies are effectively targeting specific killers such as HIV/AIDS, malaria, and tuberculosis, and continue in efforts to eradicate a number of other diseases, most notably polio. And recent evidence points to impressive reductions in childhood mortality and even progress against HIV/AIDS. The magnitude and innovation of these efforts suggest that our present environment is indeed one of better-than-average CD governance, at least in comparison to the immediate post–Cold War era. While our forecasts do not incorporate these efforts explicitly, our base case forecasts of continued rapid decline of CDs suggest (and perhaps require) that these governance efforts will persist and succeed.

On the other hand, history tells us that such governance is not guaranteed. The experience of the post–World War II epidemiologic transition offers an example of the exhaustion and gradual dismantling of CD control regimes, events that if they were to occur again could create a global setting in which communicable diseases would not further abate or might reemerge. In addition, the disease-specific programs of earlier eras left many countries with little health system infrastructure to address recurrent, endemic, or challenging new disease risks. In fact, a number of the world's most politically and economically challenged nations saw limited progress against even easily preventable diseases.

Turning to the present and the future, there are a number of challenges to effective global health governance. Many analysts point to the fragility of the new IHRs, which create tremendous obligations for poor nations but offer little financial support and few incentives for cooperation. And many argue that satisfaction with short-term successes or exhaustion with diminishing achievements could lead to a pullback of government, multilateral, and nonprofit financial support for further CD reductions. A continuing global economic crisis or a restructuring of global political alignments could contribute to this disruption of support (as was seen at the end of the Cold War).

The list of what could go wrong relative to the potential for human action (and its interaction with the biological environment) is very long. We have seen it go wrong before. At the end of World War II, the global community believed that it had the tools to beat back malaria and many other communicable diseases. Mass production of chloroquine was possible; DDT had proven effective in control of mosquitoes; and antibiotics were available for use around the world. The World Health Organization came into being in 1948 with a mandate to use such tools, and a global malaria eradication program rolled out in the 1950s and 1960s. In fact, 24 countries that eliminated malaria in that era remain malaria-free (Smith and Tatem 2009: 11). Yet progress slowed as resistance (biological and environmental) to DDT developed and donor fatigue appeared, and malaria bounced back strongly in much of the world. Yet it was not just known diseases that disrupted plans and much early success in reducing deaths from communicable diseases. The official recognition of the AIDS epidemic in 1981 preceded at least 20 years of spreading health catastrophe around the world—we still cannot be certain that the global peak of deaths is behind us. The epidemic of cholera in Zimbabwe under Mugabe is still another example. We can no longer doubt the ability of additional diseases, such as avian flu, to wreak havoc in our forecasts and our lives, and for poor human choices to contribute significantly to that outcome.

Noncommunicable disease futures

The world has experienced relatively uninterrupted historical progress in longevity extension on the one hand, alongside heightened worries about the growing burden of NCD risk factors on the other. The resulting tension is in part responsible for the tremendous variation between optimistic and pessimistic longevity forecasts for the world's longest-lived population (see again Chapter 2, especially Box 2.3). Plausible forecasts for the year 2100 range from about 87 years, essentially unchanged from today's female population of Japan, to 105 years. The IFs base case forecast anticipates the life expectancy of females in the longest-lived society (still forecast to be Japan) to be 95.4 years in 2100, slightly below the mid-point of that range. Looking out just to mid-century, the IFs forecast of 91.3 years for Japanese females in 2050 is consistent with the United Nations Population Division's projection of 91.0 years for that year.[3] Our cause-specific forecasts (see again Chapter 4) naturally imply a deceleration of longevity progress as causes of death currently in rapid decline (e.g., cardiovascular diseases) are gradually replaced by causes that we forecast will decline less rapidly (e.g., diabetes).[4] Overall, we forecast much more modest decline for NCDs than for CDs.

Our reading of the considerable evidence on NCD-related risk factors such as obesity, smoking, alcohol abuse, and environmental factors suggests a reasonable case for a slow pace of NCD progress for most countries, particularly middle-income ones, perhaps even below those of our base case forecast. On the other hand, technologies may emerge to mitigate these risk factors (e.g., an anti-obesity pill).

Most probably, effective progress against NCDs for most countries—iin particular, the closing of their gap with the longest-lived countries—will require considerable behavioral change efforts on a national and global scale. While rates of smoking have declined in many high-income countries, they remain high and even rising in many low- and middle-income countries that have not yet felt the full effects of earlier smoking on disease levels. Further progress against smoking-related deaths will depend on effective national programs. Progress may also depend on the Global Framework Convention on Tobacco Control and other multilateral treaties governing the export and sale of tobacco products.

Similar concerns pertain to obesity, alcohol use, and other health risk factors. For example, as lower-income populations grow increasingly wealthy, sedentary, and connected to global commodity chains, including fast foods and other calorie-dense foods, the possibility increases for a truly global obesity epidemic.

Is our base case forecast of a much more modest decline in NCDs too pessimistic?

Further concern arises from a growing burden of environmental risk factors, such as pollution, which may increase the risk of certain cancers. In each of these cases we can imagine a considerable downside uncertainty, as well as some upside arising from the potential for transformative treaties or social movements against chronic disease risk factors.

The current template for concern about the trajectory of NCDs lies in the Russian Federation, where recent sharp increases in chronic diseases and violent mortality among men have occurred (Men et al. 2003; Shkolnikov, McKee, and Leon 2001). Analysts generally attribute this mortality spike to increases in behavioral risk factors (e.g., alcohol abuse, smoking, and consumption of rich foods), stimulated in part by Russia's recent political situation, socioeconomic uncertainty, and environmental contamination (Leon et al. 2007; Zaridze et al. 2009). While Russia offers an extreme example of rising behavioral risks, we can point also to rising levels of obesity in many developed countries, a flattening of NCD mortality improvements in many parts of the United States, and a skyrocketing incidence of diabetes in India to support the pessimistic scenario (Cooper et al. 2000; Murray et al. 2006; Ramachandran et al. 2008; Rogers et al. 2007).

Above and beyond any increase in behavioral risks, at least some populations of countries currently undergoing epidemiologic transition may experience an elevated predisposition to NCDs. For example, a growing body of evidence suggests that the genetic, nutritional, and immunological histories of many populations in transition (e.g., South Asians) make them uniquely vulnerable to NCDs (Barker 1998; Barker et al. 1989; Barker and Osmond 1986; Finch and Crimmins 2004; Hales and Barker 1992). The co-occurrence of CD and NCD may also create negative synergies, for instance, in the possible tendency toward chronic disease among elders affected by the HIV epidemic (Hosegood et al. 2007). While some of these forces are "merely" transitional and were experienced by today's post-transition societies with only limited negative impact, the possibility remains that this scenario will play out differently in today's transition societies. If indeed—as evidence suggests is possible (McKeigue, Shah, and Marmot 1991; Mohan et al. 2007)—some populations have a

genetic predisposition to heightened chronic disease risk, a number of currently emerging countries could face tremendous operational challenges in scaling up treatment and prevention of chronic diseases compared to, say, the United States or Great Britain in the 1950s. On the other hand, while the potential for such downside possibilities derives from compelling evidence, we should also once again look to past examples of human mortality progress outstripping even our most optimistic expectations, as in the case of mortality reductions from cardiovascular diseases in the United States in the 1960s.

Overall, the relatively slow progress of life expectancy in leading countries makes the base case forecasts of NCD appear pessimistic on the biological dimension. In contrast, the relatively significant convergence of mortality rates across global income levels makes it appear relatively optimistic on the human activity dimension, especially in light of this recitation of challenges to rapid progress.

Summary characterization and adjustment of the base case

In light of the discussion above, Figure 8.4 summarizes our perception of the positioning of our base case forecasts for NCDs and CDs. We conclude that our base case CD forecasts are relatively optimistic on both dimensions, while our base case NCD forecasts are relatively optimistic on the human activity dimension but pessimistic on the biological dimension.

Adjustment to the base case in order to "correct" it for these subjectively assessed deviations from the most likely path forward is inevitably arbitrary.[5] We have done so, quite conservatively, by bending the curves of the base case in two primary ways.

First, we have slowed down the rates of reduction in communicable diseases globally (the developing countries experience the greater impact). For instance, in the unadjusted base case, total global malaria deaths decline by 50 percent between 2005 and 2025 (this is even in the face of a growing global population). The adjusted base case pushes that point of reduction out to 2038. With respect to AIDS deaths, the point of 50 percent reduction in the adjusted base case moves from 2041 to 2060, and in the case of other communicable diseases the year slips from 2036 to 2044.

Second, we have accelerated the time factor of mortality reduction in the Global Burden of Disease (GBD) formulations, increasing it proportionately more for higher-income countries. The reason for this intervention was implicitly to relax the biological constraint for NCDs. The GBD formulations and our reproduction of them do not include any explicit representation of the biological constraint. The biological constraint and technology interact closely, however, and an acceleration of technological advance for NCDs is effectively equivalent to assuming a lesser constraint and therefore more leverage from technology. Although the time factor also affects CDs in high-income countries, the rates of those are so low that this adjustment strongly targets NCDs, the diseases of the old, and therefore the point at which relaxed biological constraints would appear. We focus on the high-income countries because (1) we do not want this "biological constraint relaxation" to affect the CDs of the developing countries; and (2) we assume that the lower-income countries have less economic and technological potential for taking advantage of relaxed biological constraints. These adjustments are obviously not normatively based; they seek to better project the path we appear to be on, as suggested by the earlier historical discussion.

Figure 8.5 shows the implications for mortality probabilities of adjusting the base case. In spite of quite dramatic declines relative to 2005 in both the base case and the adjusted base, child mortality is anticipated in 2060 to be somewhat higher nearly everywhere in the forecasts of the adjusted base case. In sub-Saharan Africa child mortality still drops very considerably by 2060 (in 2005, 146 of 1,000 children in sub-Saharan Africa died before their fifth birthdays), but 45 per 1,000 in the adjusted base case is more than one-third higher than in the unadjusted base.

Similarly, adult mortality in sub-Saharan Africa (the probability of a 15-year-old dying before reaching age 60) is somewhat more than 10 percent higher in the adjusted base case. For other regions the changes in adult mortality are mostly relatively minor increases.

Looking at older adults, however, the mortality pattern reverses, and most regions show small decreases relative to the unadjusted base case.

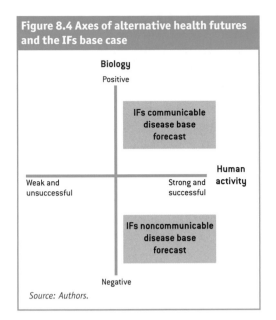

Figure 8.4 Axes of alternative health futures and the IFs base case

Biology
Positive

IFs communicable disease base forecast

Human activity

Weak and unsuccessful

Strong and successful

IFs noncommunicable disease base forecast

Negative

Source: Authors.

■ Based on these conclusions, we adjusted the base case to slow the rate of decline in CDs. ■

For high-income countries, the adjustments for noncommunicable diseases prove especially significant. In fact, because of the mortality declines for high-income older adults in the adjusted base (as rectangularization of the J-curve pushes deaths into still older years), life expectancy in richer countries increases by about two years relative to the unadjusted base case. Overall, life expectancy for high-income countries rises by about nine years between 2005 and 2060, and is more consistent than was the base case with the longer-term historical pattern of increase. Illustratively, Japanese women reach a life expectancy of 95 years in 2059, nearly three years longer than in the unadjusted base.

One of the important consequences of these seemingly relatively modest changes to mortality probabilities in the adjusted base case, however, is that the goals of the Commission on Social Determinants of Health (CSDH 2008) appear even less likely to be met than in our base case forecasts. With the exception of South Asia in the base case, even by 2060 the rates of child mortality reductions in *both* scenarios fall short of the 90 percent called for by CSDH between 2000 and 2040. And only sub-Saharan Africa meets by 2060 the 2040 goal for a 50 percent reduction in adult mortality (it meets it in the 2040–2050 decade in both scenarios).

In addition, the chances for narrowing the gap in life expectancy between the populations of the longest-lived third of countries and the shortest-lived third to 10 years by 2040 are

■ We made a second adjustment based on our conclusions— namely, we accelerated the effect of technology in reducing NCDs as income rises. ■

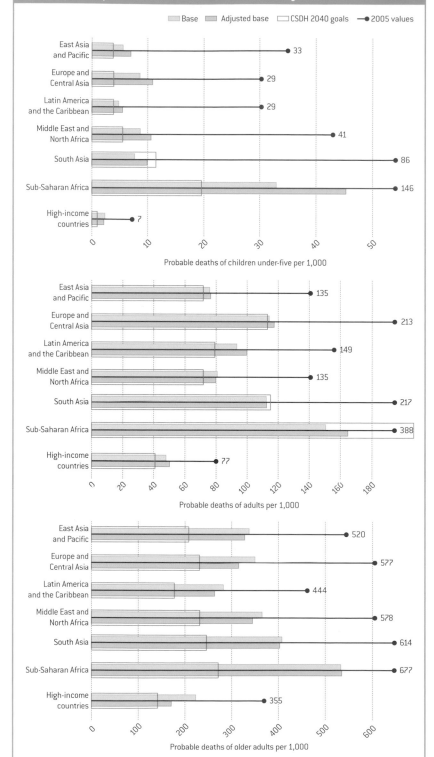

Figure 8.5 Comparison of mortality probabilities (expressed as probable deaths per 1,000) for 2060 in the base case and the adjusted base case

Legend: Base | Adjusted base | CSDH 2040 goals | 2005 values

Probable deaths of children under-five per 1,000

Region	2005 value
East Asia and Pacific	33
Europe and Central Asia	29
Latin America and the Caribbean	29
Middle East and North Africa	41
South Asia	86
Sub-Saharan Africa	146
High-income countries	7

Probable deaths of adults per 1,000

Region	2005 value
East Asia and Pacific	135
Europe and Central Asia	213
Latin America and the Caribbean	149
Middle East and North Africa	135
South Asia	217
Sub-Saharan Africa	388
High-income countries	77

Probable deaths of older adults per 1,000

Region	2005 value
East Asia and Pacific	520
Europe and Central Asia	577
Latin America and the Caribbean	444
Middle East and North Africa	578
South Asia	614
Sub-Saharan Africa	677
High-income countries	355

Note: Mortality probability is that of death before reaching end of age range (0–4 for child mortality; 15–59 for adult mortality; 60–79 for older adult mortality). "CSDH 2040 goals" refers to the mortality reduction goals of the Commission on Social Determinants of Health (2008).

Source: IFs Version 6.32.

further reduced with the adjusted base case. Even in the unadjusted base case, the gap remains at 12 years in 2040, and in the adjusted base case it falls only to 15 years. In fact, our forecast in the adjusted base case is that the gap will still be 13 years even in 2060.

The first question framing this chapter concerned the positioning of the base case within the likely range of longer-term futures with respect to global health. All in all, it appears reasonably well situated within the space of uncertainty that we have identified, but we have adjusted it modestly so as to capture somewhat slower likely progress with respect to communicable diseases and somewhat faster progress with respect to noncommunicable diseases. These corrections reconcile our base case somewhat more soundly with historical experience and our judgment of the likely trajectory, thereby establishing a foundation for discussion of the uncertainty space more generally.

Alternative Health Futures: Integrated Scenario Analysis

This volume has repeatedly emphasized the complexity of interaction among proximate, distal, and super-distal factors in the shaping of health futures. As difficult as it may be, a consideration of the long-term future of health should step back and at least speculate on the breadth of variation in alternative possible health futures across such factors in interaction. To help in doing so we structure and present the two most different alternatives framed by the dimensions of technology/biology and human activity, those that Figure 8.1 labeled Luck and Enlightenment and Things Go Wrong (hereafter often referred to as L&E and TGW, respectively).

In the analysis we take advantage of the full hybrid health modeling system unfolded in this volume. The adjusted base case reflects the combination of (1) the distal-driver formulations of the GBD project (with some extensions and adjustments discussed in Chapter 3); (2) the proximate-driver specifications (built into the base case along with the distal-driver formulations); (3) the backward and forward linkages of the health model to demographics, economics, environmental representations, and other elements of the IFs modeling system (also in the base case); and (4) the adjustments to the base case parameters discussed above.

Building the scenarios

The scenarios differ in a number of aspects from the adjusted base case and from one another (Box 8.1 summarizes the scenarios of this chapter). One is with respect to the interaction of technology and biology—the biology of the human genome may provide the headroom for health advances, but technology is needed to take advantage of it; or biological limits or evolution may retard or even reverse health advances (as in the case of pathogen mutation), making technology much less effective. In the L&E scenario we increased the rate of growth in the technological element of the distal-driver set by half (as in the framing scenario analysis of Chapter 4). In TGW we decreased it by half.

A second difference between the scenarios reflects different futures with respect to proximate risk factors. As discussed near the end of Chapter 6, we have explored combined packages of risk factor variations. We built a package of aggressive but reasonable proximate risk factor improvements relative to the adjusted base case into the L&E scenario and a largely symmetrical package of slowing proximate risk factor improvements or actual deteriorations into the TGW scenario.

On these first two elements the two scenarios are mostly symmetrical. Other elements are more uniquely tailored to the scenarios. One asymmetrical element is of special importance to L&E. We have emphasized that proximate drivers (especially our limited set of eight drivers) do not fully represent the human action dimension of our uncertainty space. To help understand this, look again at Figure 2.5. That representation of the relationship between GDP per capita (as a proxy for income) and life expectancy shows a number of outliers.

> ● The adjustments to the base case somewhat accelerate progress against disease in leading countries and slow it in others, retarding the convergence process. ●

> ● We can use the full IFs system to compare two very different scenarios on top of our adjusted base: "Luck and Enlightenment" (L&E) and "Things Go Wrong" (TGW). ●

> ● L&E and TGW differ with respect to advance in technology and in the rate of proximate risk factor improvements. ●

Box 8.1 Summary of Luck and Enlightenment and Things Go Wrong scenarios

Differences of the adjusted base case from the base case (see Box 4.1)

- Technological advance accelerates proportionally to income in high-income countries (a maximum of 50 percent for countries at $40,000 per capita and higher)
- Advances against HIV infections are 40 percent slower for all countries
- Advances against AIDS deaths are 75 percent slower for all countries
- Mortality from diarrhea, respiratory infections, and other noncommunicable diseases is 40 percent higher in 55 years, with the percentage rising linearly over time
- Mortality from malaria is 150 percent higher in 70 years, with the percentage rising linearly over time

Differences of the Luck and Enlightenment scenario from the adjusted base case

- All proximate-driver interventions move to the values of the favorable scenarios of Chapters 5 and 6
- Technological advance accelerates by 50 percent for the portion of the population five years of age and above in all countries with GDP per capita above $3,000, and for children under five in all countries coded as "0" (mainly high-income countries) in the GBD formulations
- Technological advance accelerates by 50 percent for everyone five years of age or older in all countries with GDP per capita below $3,000, and for children under five in all countries coded as "5" in the GBD formulations (primarily countries in the Middle East and North Africa)

- Mortality for countries that initially have higher mortality than anticipated on the basis of distal drivers converges to anticipated levels over 55 years

Differences of the Things Go Wrong scenario from the adjusted base case

- All proximate-driver interventions move to the values of the unfavorable scenarios of Chapters 5 and 6
- Technological advance decelerates by 50 percent for people five years of age and above in all countries with GDP per capita above $3,000, and for children under five in all countries coded as "0" in the GBD formulations
- Technological advance decelerates by 50 percent for everyone five years of age or older in all countries with GDP per capita below $3,000 and for children under five in countries coded as "5" in the GBD formulations
- Advances against HIV infections are 50 percent slower for all countries
- Advances against AIDS deaths are 40 percent slower for all countries
- Multifactor productivity growth in technology leader (United States) declines 1.0 percent in absolute terms
- Multifactor productivity additive term declines 1.5 percent in China and 0.5 percent in sub-Saharan Africa, South Asia, and Latin America and the Caribbean

---

Although some countries sit somewhat above the curve in Figure 2.5 (for instance, Cuba), many sit significantly below the curve (including some of the AIDS-afflicted countries such as South Africa and Botswana).

The Russian Federation is among the countries with life expectancy considerably below the level we would expect based on income, illustrating some of the potential for health improvements relating to human action that lies deeper than the proximate and even the distal drivers (falling more clearly into the social environment category of the super-distal drivers). After the fall of communism, life expectancy also fell. Although immediately tied to factors such as a rise in alcohol abuse, deeper roots include the tremendous disruption of life for many adults, often previously at the peak of their careers, and major changes in the health care system. Russia and other countries that currently have significantly poorer health conditions than we would expect based on their distal drivers (notably income and education) are perhaps quite likely to experience convergence toward the expected values in the coming years. Along with changes in proximate-driver patterns, we have built such upward health outcome convergence to expected patterns into the L&E scenario, phasing in the convergence across our 2060 forecast horizon.

Other asymmetrical elements particularly affect TGW. A substantial share of the dramatic gains in life expectancy in our base forecast is driven by expected health improvements related to continued economic growth in rich and poor nations alike. It is at least possible, however, that the Great Recession (2008–2011 in the IFs base case) could ultimately morph into an interruption of globalization processes with significantly slowing economic growth prospects, especially for developing countries. There is, of course, an infinite set of possible unfoldings of such a scenario. Most versions would include a slowing of annual multifactor productivity growth in technologically leading countries, with transmission of that slowing around the world (we have posited a significant 1 percent reduction). Most would also include a somewhat related additional slowing of growth in developing countries (we have posited an additional reduction of growth in China by

1.5 percent annually and reductions elsewhere of 0.5 percent).

To this point we have introduced no direct change in assumptions about the biological context. We know, however, that both malaria and AIDS have surprised us before and that other communicable diseases, including dengue fever, could adversely surprise us again. There are an uncountable number of wild cards that could make our global health futures much worse. The earlier discussion of communicable disease risks and resultant adjustments to the base case elaborated some of the downside risk and noted the common optimism bias of forecasting.

Rather than speculate, however, about many specific possible scenario elements, most of which would involve worse trajectories with respect to communicable diseases, we explicitly introduce only some relatively modest further slowing of recovery from the HIV/AIDS epidemic (the scenario's slower economic growth implicitly carries with it assumptions of broader but non-specific setbacks in the advance against CDs). All in all, TGW is far from a worst-case scenario.

Contrasting Luck and Enlightenment versus Things Go Wrong

The differences between the two scenarios are huge in their aggregate global implications. The global difference in annual deaths grows in Things Go Wrong to 34 million more by 2060 than in Luck and Enlightenment. Based on death rates, the gap would be still larger were it applied to identical populations. However, the global populations of the two scenarios diverge markedly, to just over 10 billion in L&E and just over 9 billion in TGW (compared to an adjusted base case value of 9.4 billion).

In 2060, the large majority (a total of 800 million people) of the additional population in L&E compared to TGW are 65 and older. The global population between 15 and 65 in L&E is only 236 million greater than that in TGW, and the population under 15 is actually 39 million higher in TGW because higher fertility rates more than offset higher child death rates. Overall, the global dependency ratio (elderly plus children as a percentage of total population) is nearly 4 percent higher in L&E relative to the 37 percent rate in TGW (the percentage of those 65 and older is 6 percent higher in L&E).

These aggregate demographic implications of the global push for the elements of the L&E scenario are only now becoming widely recognized and explored—until very recently most attention in demography and health to alternative global population futures has focused on alternative assumptions concerning fertility rates. And interestingly, the aggregate demographic differences between L&E and the adjusted base case exceed those between TGW and the adjusted base. One reason is that the poorer health futures of TGW largely mean more deaths for children from communicable diseases with some offsetting upward adjustments in fertility (a negative or controlling feedback loop). In contrast, better health futures with longer-lived adults and seniors would not necessarily lead to an offsetting reduction in fertility; in fact, greater survival and better health of adults in their child-bearing years could increase fertility and further increase population in a positive feedback loop.

Even more, the economic implications of such different health futures are not well understood. It is important to emphasize, for instance, that one should not presume that any negative affect from the very large number of additional seniors would dominate the economic impact. The balance of economic consequences of the extra 236 million working-aged adults and the 800 million people aged 65 and older is not obvious on the surface (and would vary considerably by region). Many of those additional working-age people would likely have extra years of life due to a reduction in child or young adult mortality and might potentially look forward to most or all of a 40-year or more working and savings life. Among other aspects of the two scenarios, the economic difference is one that we wish to explore.

Disease burden patterns across alternative health futures

Although the scenarios differ very significantly with respect to health futures, they also demonstrate one very fundamental and important similarity, the ongoing global shift from communicable to noncommunicable disease burdens. Figure 8.6 shows the strength of that steady march, even in the face of quite widely varying assumptions. In 2005, communicable diseases accounted globally for 32 percent of deaths and 55 percent of years of life lost (YLLs). In neither scenario nor the adjusted base case do communicable diseases in 2060 account for more than 12 percent of deaths or 31 percent of YLLs. Even in Things Go Wrong, YLLs from NCDs exceed those from CDs by about 2031.

Within the general context of this steady shift to NCDs, however, there are major differences between the scenarios. In L&E, for example, the portion of global deaths from CDs drops to about 4 percent in 2060, only slightly more than a third of the level in TGW. Figure 8.7 shows the differences in death patterns across the scenarios

● There are 1 billion more people in L&E in 2060, and a large majority of them are 65 and older. ●

● In both scenarios, despite their quite widely varying assumptions, we see an ongoing global shift from CDs to NCDs. ●

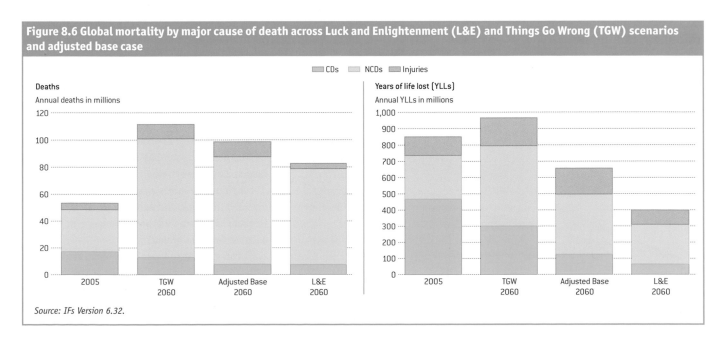

Figure 8.6 Global mortality by major cause of death across Luck and Enlightenment (L&E) and Things Go Wrong (TGW) scenarios and adjusted base case

Source: IFs Version 6.32.

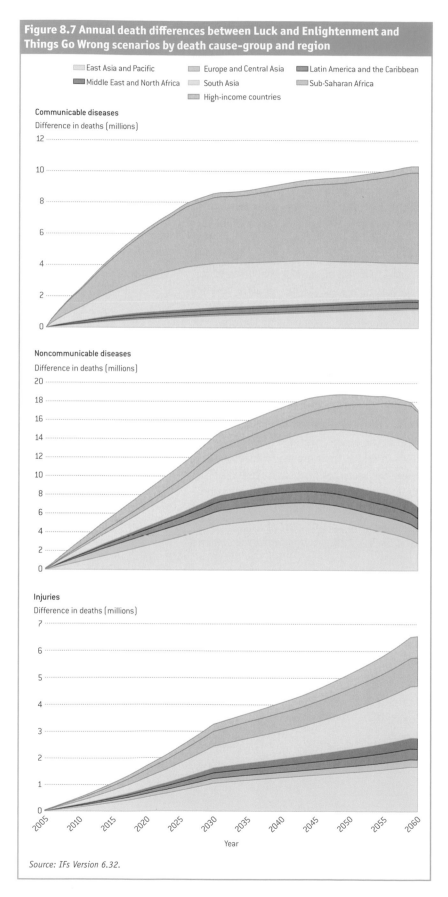

Figure 8.7 Annual death differences between Luck and Enlightenment and Things Go Wrong scenarios by death cause-group and region

Legend:
- East Asia and Pacific
- Middle East and North Africa
- Europe and Central Asia
- South Asia
- High-income countries
- Latin America and the Caribbean
- Sub-Saharan Africa

Communicable diseases
Difference in deaths (millions)

Noncommunicable diseases
Difference in deaths (millions)

Injuries
Difference in deaths (millions)

Year

Source: IFs Version 6.32.

by major disease groups and by region. Those differences represent a combination of changing mortality rates (to which we will return) and the dynamic demographic patterns that the scenarios set in motion.

Deaths are consistently higher everywhere and in every cause-group in the Things Go Wrong scenario. For instance, the global difference in annual deaths between the two scenarios for communicable diseases grows to about 10 million deaths per year and plateaus at that level. The largest differences in deaths from communicable diseases between the scenarios are in sub-Saharan Africa, followed by South Asia—not surprising because those regions now suffer the greatest numbers of such deaths. These two regions have a huge stake in maintaining and accelerating progress against communicable diseases.

The greatest difference in number of annual deaths between the two scenarios is, however, from NCDs, and it grows globally to almost 19 million before beginning a slow decline. Declines in differences in deaths from NCDs ultimately appear for two reasons: (1) the TGW scenario ultimately yields some decrease in death rates from NCDs; (2) although L&E postpones deaths relative to TGW, the resultant and substantially increased elderly population does ultimately die. Through 2030, East Asia and Pacific countries and South Asian countries dominate the cross-scenario variation in death numbers by virtue of their huge regional population numbers. After 2030, the differences between the scenarios begin to erode for East Asia and Pacific countries as well as for high- and upper-middle-income regions more generally. In contrast, the differences between the two scenarios continue to grow for South Asia and especially for sub-Saharan Africa. Again, one primary insight from these patterns is that, roughly over the next generation, sub-Saharan and other low-income countries have an especially great stake in continued progress against communicable diseases, but that thereafter the importance to them of chronic disease advances will also become very prominent.

Turning again to years of life lost, the difference between CDs and NCDs in health differentials of the two scenarios is much smaller than Figure 8.7 might suggest, because the average CD-related death is at a much younger age. Through 2060, the cumulative difference between scenarios in global YLLs approximates 11 billion for communicable diseases versus about 8 billion for chronic ones. The cause-group with the smallest difference in deaths across scenarios is injuries, just as it is today by far the smallest category of absolute deaths. The growth in the difference between the two scenarios over time is steady, however, and that result may be counterintuitive. Like other "counterintuitive" results, however, understanding the larger dynamics of the system makes it clearer—many of the forces that create health improvement in the Luck and Enlightenment scenario have the least impact on injuries. Thus, when people do not die prematurely from other causes, the deaths attributable to injuries will rise. The difference between scenarios in annual global deaths grows steadily through 2060, reaching 6.6 million (about two-thirds the level of those from communicable diseases) and the cumulative difference in global YLLs reaches 3 billion. South Asian and East Asia and Pacific countries have the highest number of absolute lives at stake with respect to controlling the growth of injuries, but all regions exhibit steadily rising differences between the two scenarios.

It is obvious that the regional differences across the two scenarios are tied strongly to income levels (although the burden of tropical diseases in sub-Saharan Africa in particular has a strong geographic characteristic as well). By income level, the major break-point of scenario difference separates low-income countries from lower-middle-income countries (see Figure 8.3). For low-income countries, Things Go Wrong really means that *things go very wrong*, with an actual increase in child deaths in coming years and a huge gap, exceeding 3 million child deaths annually for most of the forecast horizon, between the patterns of that scenario and Luck and Enlightenment. For lower-middle-income countries, the World Bank category that includes China and India, the spread in total deaths is also large, exceeding 2 million for many years, but even TGW shows some significant, steady improvement. The difference in child deaths across scenarios becomes progressively smaller as income levels increase.

Drilling down further into comparison of the two scenarios, Figure 8.9 shows the child, adult, and older adult mortality probabilities.

The relative differences in probabilities are very large across all regions and mortality levels, with the mortality probabilities in the two scenarios varying quite often by a factor of two or even more. Relative differences are especially great for infant mortality, and those for sub-Saharan Africa and South Asia stand out. The level of absolute variation in adult and older adult mortality probability is also striking, however, particularly again for sub-Saharan Africa and South Asia. In the case of sub-Saharan Africa, the scope of the HIV/AIDS epidemic is so sweeping and the likelihood of some progress so great that the probability of adult mortality falls from 388 per 1,000 to 219 per 1,000 even under TGW; in L&E it falls much further, to 105 per 1,000. In South Asia and in Europe and Central Asia, where NCDs largely drive adult mortality, the two scenarios differ dramatically in the rate of progress over the next 50 years. In South Asia for instance, adult mortality probability in 2005 was 217 per 1,000. In the L&E scenario, South Asia's adult mortality rate plunges to 64 per 1,000, comparable to today's high-income societies, whereas in TGW the rate only falls to 165 per 1,000.

The gap between the outcomes in the two scenarios is so large that they significantly affect the likelihood of meeting goals such as

■ Deaths are consistently higher everywhere and in every cause-group in the TGW scenario; the biggest differences are in NCDs. ■

■ For low-income countries, TGW really means that things go very wrong, resulting in annual increases in child deaths until about 2025. ■

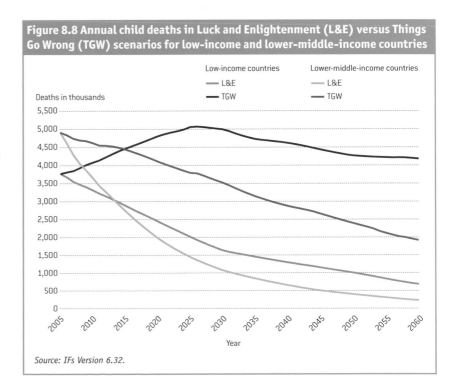

Figure 8.8 Annual child deaths in Luck and Enlightenment (L&E) versus Things Go Wrong (TGW) scenarios for low-income and lower-middle-income countries

Source: IFs Version 6.32.

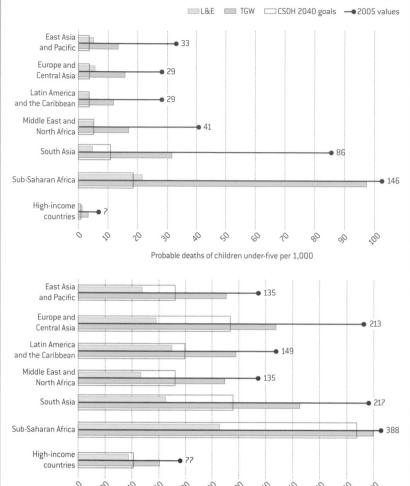

Figure 8.9 Comparison of mortality probabilities for 2060 in Luck and Enlightenment (L&E) and Things Go Wrong (TGW) by region

Legend: L&E   TGW   CSDH 2040 goals   —●— 2005 values

Probable deaths of children under-five per 1,000

East Asia and Pacific — 33
Europe and Central Asia — 29
Latin America and the Caribbean — 29
Middle East and North Africa — 41
South Asia — 86
Sub-Saharan Africa — 146
High-income countries — 7

Probable deaths of adults per 1,000

East Asia and Pacific — 135
Europe and Central Asia — 213
Latin America and the Caribbean — 149
Middle East and North Africa — 135
South Asia — 217
Sub-Saharan Africa — 388
High-income countries — 77

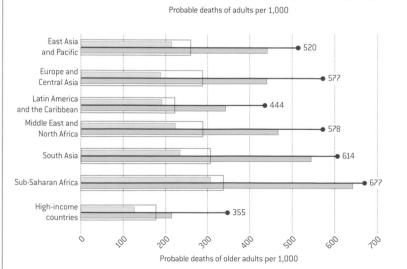

Probable deaths of older adults per 1,000

East Asia and Pacific — 520
Europe and Central Asia — 577
Latin America and the Caribbean — 444
Middle East and North Africa — 578
South Asia — 614
Sub-Saharan Africa — 677
High-income countries — 355

Note: Mortality probability is shown as the number of probable deaths per 1,000 before reaching end of age range (0–4 for child mortality; 15–59 for adult mortality; 60–79 for older adult mortality).

Source: IFs Version 6.32.

those of the Commission on Social Determinants of Health. If something even close to TGW came to pass, child and adult mortality rate reduction goals for 2040 would not be met even by 2060 almost anywhere. If something close to L&E came to pass, most goals would be met by 2060, and many even by 2040. For instance, only Latin America and the Caribbean and high-income country regions would fail to meet the CSDH goal of reducing adult mortality probability by 50 percent by 2040. Those failures would be largely because of the lack of "headroom" for upper-middle- and high-income countries, as it is difficult to cut already low mortality rates in half. In something of a reversal, if the 50 percent target is applied also to older adults, only high-income countries and Europe and Central Asia meet the goal by 2040 in L&E, although most regions other than sub-Saharan Africa are close. The major problem with respect to the CSDH goals is the target of 90 percent reduction in child mortality. We find in our analysis that no region will meet such a goal by 2040, even in Luck and Enlightenment.

The summary implications for life expectancy
Throughout this chapter we have given special attention to the extent of health progress by global system leaders and the convergence toward their conditions by other countries around the world. Figure 8.10 uses life expectancy as a summary measure to compare those two aspects of global health futures in the Luck and Enlightenment and Things Go Wrong scenarios, also providing historical data for context. We would certainly expect future trajectories for life expectancy to lie closer to the middle of the ones that the scenarios bracket (as does our adjusted base case), but the forecasts for the scenarios do not appear impossible. Further, although the range of uncertainty indicated for high-income countries is considerable (a difference of six years of life expectancy in 2060), the stakes are obviously considerably higher for developing regions. The differences are 17 years for sub-Saharan Africa and 16 years for South Asia.

In L&E there is very considerable convergence of those two developing regions toward high-income countries. Sub-Saharan Africa's life expectancy climbs from 65 percent of that in high-income countries to 87 percent (the gap falls to 12 years). South Asia's life expectancy moves to only five years less than that in high-income countries, a remarkable potential convergence. In TGW, however, the convergence is much less. Sub-Saharan Africa's life expectancy rises to only 74 percent of that in high-income countries, and South Asia's moves only from 80 percent to 83 percent. Figure 8.3 earlier sketched the rather complex historical patterns of convergence globally across World Bank groupings of countries by economy classifications. In TGW there is almost no convergence of upper-middle-income and lower-middle-income country groupings to life expectancies of high-income countries and only modest convergence of low-income countries as a whole (remember that low-income countries benefit from slow but quite steady reductions in communicable disease burdens even in TGW).

The regional stories cannot, of course, convey the rich diversity of situations across individual countries. There are more than 50 countries whose life expectancies in 2060 vary by 15 years or more between the two scenarios, a variation that at its maximum reaches 31 years. The countries that stand to benefit the most in life expectancy from L&E are those whose life expectancy trajectories have been held down by a variety of socio-political factors, both domestic and international. The countries at the top of the list include Afghanistan, Angola, Central African Republic, Chad, Democratic Republic of Congo, Republic of Congo, Equatorial Guinea, Gabon, Ghana, Rwanda, Somalia, and Tajikistan. Russia is also high on the list (the members of the BRICs grouping vary greatly, with China and Brazil showing much less difference across the two scenarios than India and Russia). As discussed earlier, countries that have unusually poor levels of health and life expectancy relative to income and education levels (as many of these countries do) are perhaps likely to converge upward over time, and we built such convergence into L&E. Still, as in TGW, the forces that have suppressed their life expectancies may either continue to exert a hold on these countries or even reach out to affect still other countries.

As we indicated earlier, even in the TGW scenario health conditions improve around much of the world over the next half century. Life expectancy globally climbs from 69 in 2005 to 73 in 2060, and in sub-Saharan Africa it rises from

52 to 63. Although certainly not impossible, it appears highly improbable that the now several-centuries-long pattern of relatively steady improvement in global health would suddenly slow as much as in TGW. That said, however, and even considering implications for the fiscal and physical environments of hundreds of millions of additional seniors, humanity has a tremendous stake in pressing very hard to bring about some version of Luck and Enlightenment, with its global life expectancy approaching 87 years in 2060. The prospect of very significant global longevity improvements implied by L&E carries obvious implications for policy and planning with respect to population, aging, and labor markets, and so we return at last to look at the generally benign and moderately positive implications of this scenario for economic growth.

The economic consequences of alternative health futures

Chapter 7 analyzed a pair of "brute force" interventions with respect to health futures so as to explore the economic consequences of more- and less-healthy global futures. It concluded that healthier futures would bring at least marginal economic advantages, not negative consequences. Thus, it should not be surprising that L&E with respect to health could

> *If something even close to TGW came to pass, child and adult mortality rate reduction goals for 2040 would not be met even by 2060 almost anywhere.*

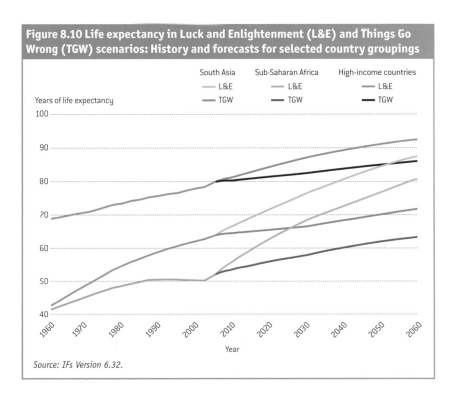

Figure 8.10 Life expectancy in Luck and Enlightenment (L&E) and Things Go Wrong (TGW) scenarios: History and forecasts for selected country groupings

Source: IFs Version 6.32.

provide positive economic returns relative to the adjusted base case (TGW incorporates substantial exogenous economic slowing and is therefore incomparable with respect to the economic consequences of health).

Figure 8.11 suggests the potential magnitude of the positive impact from L&E by showing the ratios of GDP per capita of the L&E scenario to the adjusted base case. Unlike some of the analysis of Chapter 7, neither the scenario nor figure includes any variations or counterfactuals, such as accelerated fertility reduction or greater attention to food production.

In all regions except East Asia and Pacific, the L&E scenario increases per capita GDP relative to the adjusted base case. As Chapter 7 explained, the different result in East Asia and Pacific flows from the large number of older adults (and of the elderly who are beyond the 60–79 age range) that China will experience relative to its working-age population in coming years—most of the reduced mortality for the region occurs in those age categories and intensifies the fiscal pressures the elderly will likely place on the society. The same phenomenon appears to a lesser degree in high-income countries, leading to an absence of economic difference between the two scenarios.

In sharp contrast, South Asia would benefit most from the L&E scenario, followed by sub-Saharan Africa and Middle East and North Africa.

The swing in GDP per capita for South Asia between the two scenarios reaches 37 percent in 2060 in spite of the increased population in L&E. As in Chapter 7, South Asia's relative gains stem from the imminent arrival of its demographic dividend cohorts into prime working ages, and the larger numbers of relatively healthier new workers bring considerable benefit. Sub-Saharan Africa would experience about a 22 percent swing in GDP by 2060, while Middle East and North Africa would gain about 15 percent.

The economic boost of the L&E scenario is near or past its peak for most regions and the world as a whole by 2060. Given ongoing relative aging of populations in that scenario, and continued, century-long rise after 2040 in dependency ratios for all regions except sub-Saharan Africa, the economic gains decline somewhat thereafter. While the lag structure of forward linkages means that countries with relatively younger populations would still experience somewhat greater relative benefit from L&E after 2060, even sub-Saharan Africa as a whole is near its peak relative economic gains from the scenario by 2065. As discussed in Chapter 7, simultaneous attention to other aspects of development, including fertility reduction and food production (and therefore nutrition of larger populations) could further enhance the gains shown for L&E by itself—the incremental gain for sub-Saharan Africa would be especially great, moving the 22 percent improvement in GDP per capita from health alone to 36 percent.

Conclusion

Forecasting human health through the middle of the century is subject to huge uncertainty. To a considerable degree this entire volume has been an effort to explore the extent of that uncertainty and to consider the factors that may shape alternative futures, especially human action. The considerations of key distal drivers in Chapter 4 and of selected proximate drivers in Chapters 5 and 6 provided some of the building blocks, as did the discussions of super-distal drivers and the exploration of forward linkages in Chapter 7. This chapter has brought a number of those elements together into an integrated analysis of better and less-good futures. We have been particularly interested in the combined opportunities and risks around different aspects of human activity because that activity, in

Figure 8.11 GDP per capita (PPP) ratios in 2060 of the Luck and Enlightenment scenario to the adjusted base case

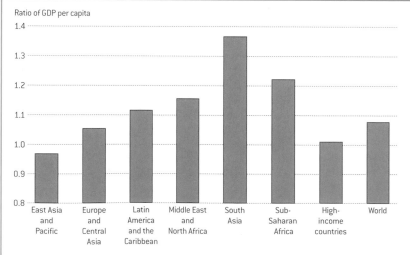

Note: We do not compare Things Go Wrong because it included exogenous assumptions of slowing economic growth; economic growth in the scenarios of the figure is fully endogenous.

Source: IFs Version 6.32.

interaction with biological systems, frames the choices we have. Forecasters of health futures will almost certainly devote increasing attention to the impact of proximate, distal, and super-distal risk factors singly and in combination; by going beyond past efforts, we have hopefully contributed to that development.

The base case forecasts of earlier chapters, rooted in substantial part in distal-driver formulations developed by the Global Burden of Disease project, appear to us to build in expectations of a continued and relatively high level of human activity directed at creating better futures. In the case of communicable disease burden reduction, they also appear quite optimistic. The rather limited time horizon of the historical database on which we must all build our forecasting formulations in part explains such optimism. We have stretched forecasting with such formulations to and beyond the limits for which they were intended. Thus, it appears to us that there is greater downside risk than upside potential relative to such forecasts of communicable disease futures, even with the anticipated high levels of human effort. Hence, we began by reconsidering our base case for communicable diseases and adjusting it. In contrast, however, the basic distal formulations for noncommunicable disease appear implicitly to build in overly strong biological constraints with respect to continued progress; we relaxed those somewhat in our base case adjustment.

This chapter also developed and explored a Luck and Enlightenment scenario relative to a Things Go Wrong scenario. The analysis suggests several conclusions. The first is the very broad range of health futures that may be possible, especially in middle- and low-income countries. A second is that the swing in focus of attention from communicable diseases to noncommunicable diseases and injuries will very likely move within our forecast horizon quite rapidly through middle-income countries and even into low-income countries. Another is that success of the type represented by the Luck and Enlightenment category could have a significant unintended consequence in terms of the expansion of global population, especially the elderly; it should nonetheless modestly enhance economic growth. Finally and most fundamentally, the analysis suggests strongly the great health-enhancing leverage of our human activity. We can exercise that leverage with proximate drivers and advances in technology. We can also do it through improvement of conditions (convergence toward more normal values) of poorly performing societies that may benefit from socio-political change (such as reduction in domestic conflict) and from the efforts of the global health governance system. Efforts within a broad range of systems have very considerable influence over health outcomes. By 2060, several years of life expectancy (in fact, well above a decade on average across our more extreme scenarios) for each of more than 9 billion people depend significantly on those efforts.

Global GDP per capita in 2060 would be 8 percent higher with L&E than in the adjusted base case; for South Asia the difference would be 37 percent.

---

1 See Huynen (2008: 115–149) for a very useful analysis of the way in which various global scenario sets have treated (or not well treated) health futures and for her own set of health scenarios. Her Age of Emerging Infectious Diseases has much in common with Things Go Wrong. We might place her Age of Medical Technology (which she draws from Martens 2002) near the top of our vertical axis, because it presumes an accommodating biological context. And her Age of Sustained Health overlaps much with our Luck and Enlightenment, both building on positive human activity with respect to the natural and social environments and making clear that subscenarios build on each of these subdimensions. Finally, her Age of Chronic Diseases, focusing on non-Western countries, recognizes that technological ability to address chronic diseases might not transfer smoothly to developing countries, leaving them in a situation of Steady Slog. Throughout, she places much weight on the future character of globalization processes as a driver of different futures.

2 Following from the role of international cooperation in driving earlier survival improvements, some have attempted to attribute mortality reversals to the macroeconomic restructuring of the 1990s (McMichael and Beaglehole 2000; Stuckler, King, and Basu 2008; and Stuckler, King, and McKee 2009).

3 The two projects arrive at these similar numbers using very different methods. The UN bases its forecast on extrapolation of trends in all-cause mortality by age, an approach that would yield considerably higher life expectancy outcomes if they did not model a deceleration of longevity progress. The UN does not offer high-variant longevity forecasts in which this deceleration is turned off, but others do so and arrive at a best-practice life expectancy of around 97 years.

4 The use of logarithmic formulations in the GBD project's distal formulations also mechanically drives saturation effects within each death cause.

5 The specific adjustments in the model's ".sce" file moved hltechshift to 1.5 (from 0) to introduce faster technological advance for high income countries and chronic disease (the faster technological advance becomes proportionately greater with higher GDP per capita); on the communicable side, changes reduced the annual advance in technology on HIV/AIDS by roughly 40 percent and gradually (over 60 years) increased the rates of mortality from all other communicable diseases by 40 percent relative to the base case.

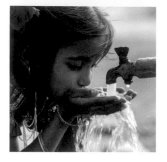

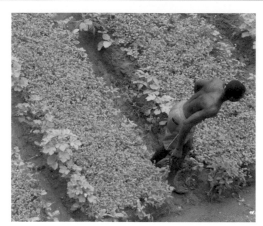

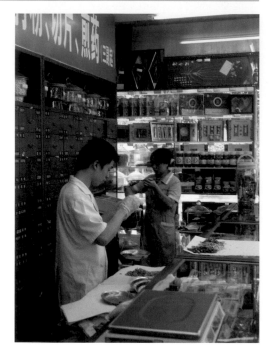

The Future of Global Health

Given the importance of health to all individuals and societies, surprisingly few previous volumes have looked extensively at the future of global health. We have aimed to make contributions on two fronts. The first is to improve our tools for thinking about alternative global health futures. The second, interacting with the first, is to use that enhanced toolkit to explore where patterns of change in human health might be taking us, to consider how much leverage we might have to improve health around the world relative to those patterns, and to think about how more rapid improvement in health might interact with broader human development.

Expanding Capability for Health Forecasting

Although forecasting of human population size and characteristics routinely extends to mid-century, and often to the end of the century or beyond, forecasting of health has for the most part not looked beyond 2030, and has been relatively rare in general. As in other volumes in this series on the Patterns of Potential Human Progress, we look out a half century, and we have targeted 2060 in most of this volume's analysis. There is little doubt that the global community will continue to set goals for health, and that insights gained from longer horizons can inform that process.

More generally, governments at all levels need to understand the size of their prospective future populations, their age patterns, and their likely health conditions. Limited information is available to most countries concerning prospective health (both risks to health and opportunities for improving health) of their populations. The tables that accompany this volume, and the public availability of the International Futures (IFs) system for further analysis, help fill that hole for 183 countries, as well as for the many groupings that build on them.

Societies not only want to understand the possible future health of citizens, they want to know how to improve it. Although our forecasting tool and analysis are at a high level of aggregation, we have explored several sets of important drivers of change in health, in part so as to expand our understanding of human leverage. We began with the distal drivers (income, education, and time/technology) of the World Health Organization's Global Burden of Disease project. That was possible only because of that project's generosity in providing us with its data and modeling formulations. We expanded our model and exploration to include some of the more immediate or proximate risks to human health, again building on work from the World Health Organization (WHO) and its Comparative Risk Assessment project, creating what we have termed "an integrated, hybrid model." We further expanded our conceptualization of the drivers of health to include super-distal factors, such as change in natural and social environments.

As important as it is, health is only one part of the larger human development system, and understanding the linkages between health and other elements of that system is critical as a foundation for forecasting health futures. As super-distal, distal, and proximate drivers shape changes in health, so health changes in turn affect demographic and economic systems in particular, and all of human development more generally. Integrating our health model within the broader IFs modeling system has been another key element of our effort to build a stronger forecasting tool. That integration allowed us to analyze in some detail the implications of health for economic growth and to develop and explore scenarios that sketch very different health futures than our base case forecast.

We hope and expect that integrative analysis of health and the broader human development system will be able to build on and go beyond our efforts (including further use of the IFs system for analysis of both base case and many alternative scenarios). Our modeling and analysis represent only one milestone in collective efforts to conduct integrative, policy-relevant forecasting of global health futures. We invite readers to explore potential applications of the International Futures platform in their own efforts (the full system is available at www.ifs.du.edu).

Understanding the Future of Global Health

Over at least four decades, social and medical scientists have mapped the broad outlines of a nested and overlapping set of global health transitions, elaborating them with increasing detail. Most societies have moved through or are moving through multiple stages in a broadly encompassing demographic/epidemiologic transition (see Chapter 1). In the process, most are moving also through a general risk factor transition (see Chapter 5) and even more specific risk transitions such as that for environmental factors (see Chapter 6). While noting the inherent danger of assuming that these transitions will inevitably take place at all, or that they must unfold in a particular fashion, we do find that the most likely path forward for global health involves a continuation of these transitions for most countries (and a resumption for some whose progress has been stalled or reversed), with mostly positive consequences for other dimensions of human development. The next 50 years will, of course, offer up many surprises; it will require much hard work to remain on the current, mostly optimistic path.

With these caveats in mind, this volume has provided a great deal of information concerning the current and prospective future movement of developing countries across geographic regions, and all countries across economy classifications, through these transitions. One of the central forecasts of the volume is that progress against communicable diseases will likely continue at a quite rapid pace. In our base case forecast, the battle against communicable diseases will largely be won by the end of our primary forecast horizon in 2060. Sometime between 2040 and 2050 the annual global deaths attributable to communicable diseases will very likely fall below 10 percent of those from noncommunicable diseases (from about 50 percent now), and will also fall below the numbers due to injuries. Within this global pattern there are variations by country and by region; we have traced the patterns by region within the volume, and present them for individual countries in the end tables at the back of this volume. Our forecast of continued quite rapid decline of communicable diseases has broad demographic ramifications.

Understanding the linkages between health and other elements of the larger human development system is critical to improving the human condition.

Our modeling and analysis represent only one milestone in collective efforts to conduct integrative, policy-relevant forecasting of global health futures.

The next 50 years will offer up many surprises; it will require much hard work to remain on the current, mostly optimistic path..

Since communicable diseases mainly strike the young, the reduction's early impact will be a demographic dividend. Over the longer run it will add to the challenges of old age dependency and chronic diseases.

Another important implication is that the effort to reduce specific risk factors that affect the earlier stages of the risk transition will have special importance in the window of time through about mid-century, by which time the world will have largely passed through those earlier stages and the character of dominant risks will have shifted significantly. We have seen that risk factors as different as undernutrition; unsafe water, sanitation, and hygiene; and indoor air pollution each tend to contribute to between 1 and 2 million deaths annually, most of those falling among the roughly 16 million deaths from communicable diseases (and most among the roughly 9 million deaths of children under five years of age). By mid-century, the total deaths from communicable diseases could fall to about half that level (with child deaths falling below 2 million by 2060), largely because of the extensive attacks mounted on such risk factors and on key diseases such as AIDS and malaria. The speed of progress in this period is literally a matter of life and death, and of reduced morbidity burden and better life-course health, for many tens of millions.

As the world as a whole increasingly moves through and beyond the receding pandemic stage of the broad epidemiologic transition, other risk factors will become steadily even more important, including overweight, smoking, road traffic accidents, and outdoor air pollution. While deaths from communicable diseases will likely decline by 50 percent toward mid-century, those from both noncommunicable diseases and injuries will probably each more than double. Again, there are broad ramifications. The lag effects associated with many risk factors predisposing people to chronic diseases means that anticipation of their future impacts becomes even more important. Changing patterns will also increasingly direct our attention to middle-income countries where such risks are often growing most rapidly, and to working-age and older adults, whom they affect the most. Nearly 15 million working-age adults die

globally each year now from all causes, and we anticipate that number will not decrease significantly by mid-century.

In Chapter 6 we considered the complicated interactions linking varying risk factors to one another and to specific health outcomes. Our ability to track and model these connections at the country level lags far behind our ability to model individual risks. Nevertheless, we have traced in this volume the generalized process of transition in both communicable and noncommunicable diseases and associated risk factors, again by region in the text and by country in the accompanying tables.

Epidemiologic, demographic, and proximate risk transitions play out within the larger human development process. The embedding of our integrated, hybrid health model in the larger set of models of the IFs system has allowed us to explore broad systemic linkages. It facilitated our consideration of super-distal factors, such as change in the natural environment via global warming. We found, for example, that the impact through 2060 of changes in temperature and precipitation on undernutrition and attributable childhood mortality was not as great as some analyses conclude, in large part because we forecast significant decline in undernutrition levels by mid-century (driven most fundamentally by increasing incomes) even as climate change effects intensify. Similarly, we were able to enrich forecasts of other risk factors including body mass index, smoking, and indoor/outdoor air pollution, so as to deepen our understanding of their interaction with the larger epidemiologic transition. All such factors have distinct geographic and temporal footprints (see again Chapters 5 and 6).

Our integration of health forecasting with that of broader human development systems has had other benefits. We were able (see especially Chapters 7 and 8) to link changing mortality outcomes to fertility within the population model so as to see their aggregate impact (and to have that impact on population then re-enter and close the loop with the health model). We found the effects of improved health on population growth to be substantial, with large-scale health interventions potentially increasing global population by hundreds of millions of people. These effects have positive implications but also give rise to concerns. Many in this increased population would initially be part of "demographic dividend" cohorts (that is, working-age adults rather than dependent populations), driving nations to development. Yet these positive effects would be limited without accompanying declines in fertility, a finding that supports efforts to connect family planning activities with health initiatives. Moreover, large and increasing numbers of these survivors would already be elderly or eventually reach old age, increasing dependency ratios for retired populations.

In looking at the connections between health and broader human development systems, we also tackled the contentious issue of the implications of improvement in health outcomes for economic performance. Building on past analyses that have teased apart the positive and negative consequences of health, we have incorporated these pathways into our integrated IFs modeling system (Chapter 7). While many analysts have raised concerns that population increases of the scale noted in the preceding paragraph could lower economic well-being, we find a significant, albeit modest, net positive impact of health improvements on per capita GDP. We see little evidence of a potential Malthusian trap in which health improvements merely lead to overpopulation and reduced growth, as demonstrated by the substantially more positive returns to health for sub-Saharan Africa and South Asia than for other regions. The economic returns to health improvements, however, would be further enhanced not only by family planning activities but also by add-on investments in agriculture and nutrition. Finally, the less beneficial impact of mortality reductions on high-income societies and East Asia (dominated by China) points once again to the costs of old age dependency; yet even here we find that mortality reductions are largely neutral to growth, not negative.

Throughout the volume, the issue of uncertainty in forecasting arose again and again. Somewhat belying the rather simple description above of the major transition stages and their implications for mortality and morbidity patterns, scenario analysis suggests quite broad confidence intervals around the base case forecast (see Chapter 8). Moreover, our analysis could by no means even identify, much less address, all sources of systemic risk or uncertainty (as well as weaknesses in our forecasting specifications). In the environmental arena, for instance, it is quite possible that through 2060, overuse of fossil groundwater could prove a more significant factor in constraining food production and slowing or stopping reduction in undernutrition than will global warming, and we did not explore that issue. Although Chapter 8 noted the possibility of extremely negative wild-card events around infectious diseases, we were not able to explore them meaningfully. Not least, in the face of great uncertainties around the longevity potential of the human genome (and our ability to modify it), some stages of the ongoing epidemiologic transition have barely been conceptualized. Given the larger confidence intervals around mortality in low- and middle-income countries, our scenarios illustrate the uncertainty not merely in overall global health but also in the pace at which the majority of the world's population can potentially achieve the levels of health currently attained by only a small number of societies.

Although we have substantial confidence in the methods by which we arrived at our generally optimistic conclusions, we remain cognizant not only of the high level of uncertainty just noted but also of the tendency for long-term, macro-level forecasts such as ours to obscure the conditions of individuals who will actually live throughout this forecast horizon. Even our most optimistic scenarios will see millions of lives lost or wasted to poor health, both along the way and still in 2060. Most of our readers would probably endorse the ambitious cross-societal goals of the WHO Commission on Social Determinants of Health, but even our optimistic forecast will see us fall well short of some of its goals. Our ability to assess the local or global value of governance interventions that might allow us to achieve these goals—such as tobacco control treaties, the scale-up of cost-effective health systems in poor countries, or truly collaborative infectious disease control regimes—remains preciously thin. Finally, we reiterate that broad trajectories of transition and improvement in poor and rich countries alike obscure the significance of health

The integration of health forecasting with that of other global systems provides insights, including the size of net economic gains that health improvements bring.

Much uncertainty surrounds both the pace of health advance in system leaders and the speed of convergence or catch-up by other countries.

Global health forecasting will continue to improve, and those improvements should in turn help us improve health itself.

differentials within societies. IFs is not able to address explicitly the continued exclusion of many disadvantaged group members (women, minorities, indigenous populations, those in rural areas and slums) from improvements that may be observed at the societal level. Future forecasting must pay increasingly close attention to the within-society health issues and goals that were also a focus of the Commission on Social Determinants of Health.

The development and presentation of this new global health forecast do leave us completely certain of two things. First, health will remain fundamentally important in efforts to enhance human development. Second, our collective desire and ability to anticipate possible health futures, and thereby to shape better ones, will continue to develop.

Appendix: Countries in IFs by World Bank Developing Region and Country Economy Classification

East Asia and Pacific Developing Countries

Cambodia (low-income)	Micronesia, Fed. Sts. (lower-middle-income)	Timor-Leste (lower-middle-income)
China (lower-middle-income)	Mongolia (lower-middle-income)	Tonga (lower-middle-income)
Fiji (upper-middle-income)	Myanmar (low-income)	Vanuatu (lower-middle-income)
Indonesia (lower-middle-income)	Papua New Guinea (lower-middle-income)	Vietnam (low-income)
Korea, Dem. Rep. (low-income)	Philippines (lower-middle-income)	
Lao PDR (low-income)	Solomon Islands (lower-middle-income)	
Malaysia (upper-middle-income)	Thailand (lower-middle-income)	

Europe and Central Asia Developing Countries

Albania (lower-middle-income)	Kyrgyz Republic (low-income)	Russian Federation (upper-middle-income)
Armenia (lower-middle-income)	Latvia (upper-middle-income)	Serbia (upper-middle-income)
Azerbaijan (lower-middle-income)	Lithuania (upper-middle-income)	Tajikistan (low-income)
Belarus (upper-middle-income)	Macedonia, FYR (upper-middle-income)	Turkey (upper-middle-income)
Bosnia and Herzegovina (upper-middle-income)	Moldova (lower-middle-income)	Turkmenistan (lower-middle-income)
Bulgaria (upper-middle-income)	Montenegro (upper-middle-income)	Ukraine (lower-middle-income)
Georgia (lower-middle-income)	Poland (upper-middle-income)	Uzbekistan (low-income)
Kazakhstan (upper-middle-income)	Romania (upper-middle-income)	

Latin America and the Caribbean Developing Countries

Argentina (upper-middle-income)	Ecuador (lower-middle-income)	Nicaragua (lower-middle-income)
Belize (lower-middle-income)	El Salvador (lower-middle-income)	Panama (upper-middle-income)
Bolivia (lower-middle-income)	Grenada (upper-middle-income)	Paraguay (lower-middle-income)
Brazil (upper-middle-income)	Guatemala (lower-middle-income)	Peru (upper-middle-income)
Chile (upper-middle-income)	Guyana (lower-middle-income)	St. Lucia (upper-middle-income)
Colombia (upper-middle-income)	Haiti (low-income)	St. Vincent and the Grenadines (upper-middle-income)
Costa Rica (upper-middle-income)	Honduras (lower-middle-income)	Suriname (upper-middle-income)
Cuba (upper-middle-income)	Jamaica (upper-middle-income)	Uruguay (upper-middle-income)
Dominican Republic (upper-middle-income)	Mexico (upper-middle-income)	Venezuela, RB (upper-middle-income)

Middle East and North Africa Developing Countries

Algeria (upper-middle-income)	Jordan (lower-middle-income)	Syrian Arab Republic (lower-middle-income)
Djibouti (lower-middle-income)	Lebanon (upper-middle-income)	Tunisia (lower-middle-income)
Egypt, Arab Rep. (lower-middle-income)	Libya (upper-middle-income)	Yemen, Rep. (low-income)
Iran, Islamic Rep. (lower-middle-income)	Morocco (lower-middle-income)	
Iraq (lower-middle-income)	Palestine (lower-middle-income)*	

South Asia Developing Countries

Afghanistan (low-income)	India (lower-middle-income)	Pakistan (lower-middle-income)
Bangladesh (low-income)	Maldives (lower-middle-income)	Sri Lanka (lower-middle-income)
Bhutan (lower-middle-income)	Nepal (low-income)	

Sub-Saharan Africa Developing Countries

Angola (lower-middle-income)	Gabon (upper-middle-income)	Niger (low-income)
Benin (low-income)	Gambia, The (low-income)	Nigeria (lower-middle-income)
Botswana (upper-middle-income)	Ghana (low-income)	Rwanda (low-income)
Burkina Faso (low-income)	Guinea (low-income)	São Tomé and Príncipe (lower-middle-income)
Burundi (low-income)	Guinea-Bissau (low-income)	Senegal (low-income)
Cameroon (lower-middle-income)	Kenya (low-income)	Sierra Leone (low-income)
Cape Verde (lower-middle-income)	Lesotho (lower-middle-income)	Somalia (low-income)
Central African Republic (low-income)	Liberia (low-income)	South Africa (upper-middle-income)
Chad (low-income)	Madagascar (low-income)	Sudan (lower-middle-income)
Comoros (low-income)	Malawi (low-income)	Swaziland (lower-middle-income)
Congo, Dem. Rep. (low-income)	Mali (low-income)	Tanzania (low-income)
Congo, Rep. (lower-middle-income)	Mauritania (low-income)	Togo (low-income)
Côte d'Ivoire (lower-middle-income)	Mauritius (low-income)	Uganda (low-income)
Eritrea (low-income)	Mozambique (low-income)	Zambia (low-income)
Ethiopia (low-income)	Namibia (upper-middle-income)	Zimbabwe (low-income)

High-income countries

Australia	Czech Republic	Iceland	Netherlands	Slovenia
Austria	Denmark	Ireland	New Zealand	Spain
Bahamas, The	Equatorial Guinea	Israel	Norway	Sweden
Bahrain	Estonia	Italy	Oman	Switzerland
Barbados	Finland	Japan	Portugal	Trinidad and Tobago
Belgium	France	Korea, Rep.	Puerto Rico	United Arab Emirates
Brunei Darussalam	Germany	Kuwait	Qatar	United Kingdom
Canada	Greece	Liechtenstein	Saudi Arabia	United States
Croatia	Hong Kong	Luxembourg	Singapore	
Cyprus	Hungary	Malta	Slovak Republic	

* In IFs but not included in World Bank listings

Bibliography

Abegunde, Dele O., Colin D. Mathers, Taghreed Adam, Monica Ortegon, and Kathleen Strong. 2007. "The Burden and Costs of Chronic Diseases in Low-Income and Middle-Income Countries." *Lancet* 370(9603): 1929–1938. doi:10.1016/S0140-6736(07)61696-1.

Acemoglu, Daron, and Simon Johnson. 2007. "Disease and Development: The Effect of Life Expectancy on Economic Growth." *Journal of Political Economy* 115(6): 925–985.

Adams, John G. U. 1987. "Smeed's Law: Some Further Thoughts." *Traffic Engineering and Control* 28(2): 70–73.

Aginam, Obijiofor. 2002. "International Law and Communicable Diseases." *Bulletin of the World Health Organization* 80(12): 946–951.

Ahluwalia, Montek S., Nicholas Carter, and Hollis Chenery. 1979. "Growth and Poverty in Developing Countries." *Journal of Development Economics* 6(2): 299–341.

Ainsworth, Martha, and Mead Over. 1994. "AIDS and African Development." *World Bank Research Observer* 9(2): 203–240.

Aísa, Rosa, and Fernando Pueyo. 2004. "Endogenous Longevity, Health and Economic Growth: A Slow Growth for a Longer Life?" *Economics Bulletin* 9(3): 1–10.

———. 2006. "Government Health Spending and Growth in a Model of Endogenous Longevity." *Economics Letters* 90(2): 249–253. doi:10.1016/j.econlet.2005.08.003.

Alavinia, Seyed M., and Alex Burdorf. 2008. "Unemployment and Retirement and Ill-Health: A Cross-Sectional Analysis Across European Countries." *International Archives of Occupational and Environmental Health* 82(1): 39–45.

Alderman, Harold, Jere R. Behrman, Victor Lavy, and Rekha Menon. 2001. "Child Health and School Enrollment: A Longitudinal Analysis." *Journal of Human Resources* 36(1): 185–205.

Alderman, Harold, John Hoddinott, and Bill Kinsey. 2006. "Long Term Consequences of Early Childhood Malnutrition." *Oxford Economic Papers* 58(3): 450–474.

Almond, Douglas, Kenneth Y. Chay, and David S. Lee. 2005. "The Costs of Low Birth Weight." *Quarterly Journal of Economics* 120(3): 1031–1083. doi:10.1162/003355305774268228.

Alsan, Marcella, David E. Bloom, and David Canning. 2006. "The Effect of Population Health on Foreign Direct Investment Inflows to Low- and Middle-Income Countries." *World Development* 34(4): 613–630. doi:10.1016/j.worlddev.2005.09.006.

Anand, Sudhir, and Kara Hanson. 1997. "Disability-Adjusted Life Years: A Critical Review." *Journal of Health Economics* 16(6): 685–702. doi:10.1016/S0167-6296(97)00005-2.

Anand, Sudhir, and Martin Ravallion. 1993. "Human Development in Poor Countries: On the Role of Private Incomes and Public Services." *Journal of Economic Perspectives* 7(1): 133–150.

Ando, Albert, and Franco Modigliani. 1963. "The 'Life Cycle' Hypothesis of Saving: Aggregate Implications and Tests." *American Economic Review* 53(1): 55–84.

Armstrong, J. Scott. 2001. *Principles of Forecasting: A Handbook for Researchers and Practitioners*. Boston: Kluwer Academic Publishers.

Arndt, Channing. 2006. "HIV/AIDS, Human Capital, and Economic Growth Prospects for Mozambique." *Journal of Policy Modeling* 28(5): 477–489.

Arndt, Channing, and Peter Wobst. 2002. "HIV/AIDS and Labor Markets in Tanzania." Trade and Macroeconomics Division Discussion Paper no. 102. Trade and Macroeconomics Division, International Food Policy Research Institute, Washington, DC.

Arnesen, Trude, and Lydia Kapiriri. 2004. "Can the Value Choices in DALYs Influence Global Priority-Setting?" *Health Policy* 70(2): 137–149. doi:10.1016/j.healthpol.2003.08.004.

Arnesen, Trude, and Erik Nord. 1999. "The Value of DALY Life: Problems with Ethics and Validity of Disability Adjusted Life Years." *British Medical Journal* 319(7222): 1423–1425.

Arora, Suchit. 2001. "Health, Human Productivity, and Long-Term Economic Growth." *Journal of Economic History* 61(3): 699–749.

Ashraf, Quamrul H., Ashley Lester, and David N. Weil. 2008. "When Does Improving Health Raise GDP?" NBER Working Paper no. 14449. National Bureau of Economic Research, Cambridge, MA.

Azomahou, Theophile T., Bity Diene, and Luc Soete. 2009. "The Role of Consumption and the Financing of Health Investment under Epidemic Shocks." Maastricht Economic and Social Research and Training Center on Innovation and Technology Working Paper series no. 2009-006. United Nations University, Maastricht, Netherlands.

Bakkes, Jan A., and Peter R. Bosch, eds. 2008. *Background Report to the OECD Environmental Outlook to 2030: Overviews, Details, and Methodology of Model-Based Analysis*. Bilthoven, Netherlands: Netherlands Environmental Assessment Agency.

Baldacci, Emmanuele, Benedict Clements, Sanjeev Gupta, and Oiang Cui. 2004. "Social Spending, Human Capital, and Growth in Developing Countries: Implications for Achieving the MDGs." IMF Working Paper WP/04/217. International Monetary Fund, Washington, DC.

Barham, Tania. 2009. "Effects of Family Planning and Child Health Interventions on Adolescent Cognitive Functioning: Evidence from Matlab in Bangladesh." Institute of Behavioral Science Working Paper series. University of Colorado, Boulder.

Barker, David J. P. 1998. *Mothers, Babies and Disease in Later Life*. Edinburgh: Churchill Livingstone.

Barker, David J. P., and Clive Osmond. 1986. "Infant Mortality, Childhood Nutrition, and Ischaemic Heart Disease in England and Wales." *Lancet* 327(8489): 1077–1081. doi:10.1016/S0140-6736(86)91340-1.

Barker, J. P., C. Osmond, P. D. Winter, B. Margetts, and S. J. Simmonds. 1989. "Weight in Infancy and Death from Ischaemic Heart Disease." *Lancet* 334(8663): 577–580. doi:10.1016/S0140-6736(89)90710-1.

Barro, Robert J. 1996. "Health and Economic Growth." Pan American Health Organization Program on Public Policy and Health, Division of Health and Human Development, Washington, DC.

Barro, Robert J., and Jong-Wha Lee. 1994. "Sources of Economic Growth." *Carnegie-Rochester Conference Series on Public Policy* 40:1–46. doi:10.1016/0167-2231(94)90002-7.

———. 1996. "International Measures of Schooling Years and Schooling Quality." *American Economic Review* 86(2): 218–223.

———. 2000. "International Data on Educational Attainment: Updates and Implications." NBER Working Paper no. 7911. National Bureau of Economic Research, Cambridge, MA.

———. 2001. "International Data on Educational Attainment: Updates and Implications." *Oxford Economic Papers* 53(3): 541–563.

Barro, Robert J., and Xavier Sala-i-Martin. 1998. *Economic Growth*. Cambridge: Massachusetts Institute of Technology Press.

———. 2003. *Economic Growth*, 2nd ed. Cambridge: Massachusetts Institute of Technology Press.

Becker, Gary. 1962. "Investment in Human Capital: A Theoretical Analysis." *Journal of Political Economy* 70(5): 9–49.

Becker, Gary S., Tomas J. Philipson, and Rodrigo R. Soares. 2005. "The Quantity and Quality of Life and the Evolution of World Inequality." *American Economic Review* 95(1): 277–291.

Behrman, Jere R. 1996. "The Impact of Health and Nutrition on Education." *World Bank Research Observer* 11(1): 23–37.

Behrman, Jere R., Maria Cecilia Calderon, Samuel Preston, John Hoddinott, Reynaldo Martorell, and Aryeh D. Stein. 2009. "Nutritional Supplementation of Girls Influences the Growth of Their Children: Prospective Study in Guatemala." *American Journal of Clinical Nutrition* 90(5): 1372–1379.

Ben-Porath, Yoram. 1967. "The Production of Human Capital and the Life Cycle of Earnings." *Journal of Political Economy* 75(4): 352–365.

Berkman, Lisa F., Thomas Glass, Ian Brissette, and Teresa E. Seeman. 2000. "From Social Integration to Health: Durkheim in the New Millennium." *Social Science and Medicine* 51(6): 843–857. doi:10.1016/S0277-9536(00)00065-4.

Besley, Timothy, and Masayuki Kudamatsu. 2006. "Health and Democracy." *American Economic Review* 96(2): 313–318.

Bettcher, Douglas W., Derek Yach, and G. Emmanuel Guindon. 2000. "Global Trade and Health: Key Linkages and Future Challenges." *Bulletin of the World Health Organization* 78(4): 521–534.

Bhargava, Alok, Dean T. Jamison, Lawrence J. Lau, and Christopher J. L. Murray. 2001. "Modeling the Effects of Health on Economic Growth." *Journal of Health Economics* 20(3): 423–440. doi:10.1016/S0167-6296(01)00073-X.

Bhattacharya, Joydeep, and Xue Qiao. 2007. "Public and Private Expenditures on Health in a Growth Model." *Journal of Economic Dynamics and Control* 31(8): 2519–2535.

Bidani, Benu, and Martin Ravallion. 1997. "Decomposing Social Indicators Using Distributional Data." *Journal of Econometrics* 77(1): 125–139. doi:10.1016/S0304-4076(95)01809-3.

Black, Robert E., Lindsay H. Allen, Zulfiqar A. Bhutta, Laura E. Caulfield, Mercedes de Onis, Majid Ezzati, Colin D. Mathers, and Juan Rivera. 2008. "Maternal and Child Undernutrition: Global and Regional Exposures and Health Consequences." *Lancet* 371(9608): 243–260. doi:10.1016/S0140-6736(07)61690-0.

Black, Robert E., Saul S. Morris, and Jennifer Bryce. 2003. "Where and Why Are 10 Million Children Dying Every Year?" *Lancet* 361(9376): 2226–2234. doi:10.1016/S0140-6736(03)13779-8.

Blackwell, Debra L., Mark D. Hayward, and Eileen M. Crimmins. 2001. "Does Childhood Health Affect Chronic Morbidity in Later Life?" *Social Science and Medicine* 52(8): 1269–1284. doi:10.1016/S0277-9536(00)00230-6.

Bleakley, Hoyt, and Fabian Lange. 2009. "Chronic Disease Burden and the Interaction of Education, Fertility, and Growth." *Review of Economics and Statistics* 91(1): 52–65. doi:10.1162/rest.91.1.52.

Bloom, David E., and David Canning. 2004. "Global Demographic Change: Dimensions and Economic Significance." NBER Working Paper no. W10817. National Bureau of Economic Research, Cambridge, MA.

Bloom, David E., David Canning, and Kevin Chan. 2006. "Higher Education and Economic Development in Africa." Study Commissioned by the World Bank. Human Development Sector, Africa Region, Washington, DC.

Bloom, David E., David Canning, David K. Evans, Bryan S. Graham, Patrick Lynch, and Erin E. Murphy. 1999. *Population Change and Human Development in Latin America*. Background study for the Inter-American Development Bank. Cambridge, MA: Harvard Institute for International Development.

Bloom, David E., David Canning, and Bryan Graham. 2003. "Longevity and Life-Cycle Savings." *Scandinavian Journal of Economics* 105(3): 319–338.

Bloom, David E., David Canning, and Dean T. Jamison. 2004. "Health, Wealth, and Welfare." *Finance and Development* 41(1): 10–15.

Bloom, David E., David Canning, and Jaypee Sevilla. 2001. "The Effect of Health on Economic Growth: Theory and Evidence." NBER Working Paper no. W8587. National Bureau of Economic Research, Cambridge, MA.

———. 2004. "The Effect of Health on Economic Growth: A Production Function Approach." *World Development* 32(1): 1–13. doi:10.1016/j.worlddev.2003.07.002.

Bloom, David E., and Jeffrey D. Sachs. 1998. "Geography, Demography and Economic Growth in Africa." *Brookings Papers on Economic Activity* 2: 207–295.

Blössner, Monika, and Mercedes de Onis. 2005. *Malnutrition: Quantifying the Health Impact at National and Local Levels*. Environmental Burden of Disease Series, no 12. Geneva: World Health Organization.

Boehmer, Ulrike, and John B. Williamson. 1996. "The Impact of Women's Status on Infant Mortality Rate: A Cross-National Analysis." *Social Indicators Research* 37(3): 333–360.

Bokhari, Farasat A. S., Yunwei Gai, and Pablo Gottret. 2007. "Government Health Expenditures and Health Outcomes." *Health Economics* 16(3): 257–273. doi:10.1002/hec.1157.

Bongaarts, John. 2005. "Long-Range Trends in Adult Mortality: Models and Projection Methods." *Demography* 42(1): 23–49.

———. 2006. "How Long Will We Live?" *Population and Development Review* 32(4): 605–628.

Boucekkine, Raouf, Bity Diene, and Theophile Azomahou. 2007. "On the Relationship Between Longevity and Development." *International Journal of Ecology and Development* 6: 31–50.

———. 2008. "Growth Economics of Epidemics: A Review of the Theory." *Mathematical Population Studies* 15(1): 1–26.

Bozzoli, Carlos, Angus Deaton, and Climent Quintana-Domeque. 2009. "Adult Height and Childhood Disease." *Demography* 46(4): 647–669.

Brander, Keith M. 2007. "Global Fish Production and Climate Change." *Proceedings of the National Academy of Sciences* 104(50): 19709–19714.

Brundtland, Gro Harlem. 2004. "The Globalization of Health." *Whitehead Journal of Diplomacy and International Relations* 4(2): 7–12.

Bryce, Jennifer, Shams el Arifeen, George Pariyo, Claudio F. Lanata, Davidson Gwatkin, and Jean-Pierre Habicht. 2003. "Reducing Child Mortality: Can Public Health Deliver?" *Lancet* 362(9378): 159–164. doi:10.1016/S0140-6736(03)13870-6.

Caballero, Benjamin. 2007. "The Global Epidemic of Obesity: An Overview." *Epidemiology Review* 29(1): 1–5. doi:10.1093/epirev/mxm012.

Caldwell, John C. 1986. "Routes to Low Mortality in Poor Countries." *Population and Development Review* 12(2): 171–220.

Campbell, Kurt M., Jay Gulledge, J. R. McNeill, John Podesta, Peter Ogden, Leon Fuerth, R. J. Woolsey, Alexander T. Lennon, Julianne Smith, and Richard Weitz. 2007. "The Age of Consequences: The Foreign Policy and National Security Implications of Global Climate Change." Center for Strategic and International Studies and Center for a New American Security, Washington, DC.

Campbell-Lendrum, Diarmid, and Rosalie Woodruff. 2007. *Climate Change*. Geneva: World Health Organization.

Cantor, David, and Carsten Timmermann. 2005. "Lung Cancer." In Jordan Goodman, ed., *Tobacco in History and Culture: An Encyclopedia*, vol. 1. Detroit: Charles Scribner's Sons, 320–326.

Carey, James R. 2003. *Longevity: The Biology and Demography of Life Span*. Princeton, NJ: Princeton University Press.

Carey, James R., and Debra S. Judge. 2001. "Life Span Extension in Humans Is Self-Reinforcing: A General Theory of Longevity." *Population and Development Review* 27(3): 411–436.

Carnes, Bruce A., and S. Jay Olshansky. 2007. "A Realist View of Aging, Mortality, and Future Longevity." *Population and Development Review* 33(2): 367–381. doi:10.1111/j.1728-4457.2007.00172.x.

Carson, Rachel. 1962. *Silent Spring*. Boston: Houghton Mifflin.

Cassels, Susan. 2006. "Overweight in the Pacific: Links Between Foreign Dependence, Global Food Trade, and Obesity in the Federated States of Micronesia." *Globalization and Health* 2(1): 10. doi:10.1186/1744-8603-2-10.

Centers for Disease Control and Prevention (CDC) and The Merck Company Foundation. 2007. *The State of Aging and Health in America 2007*. Whitehouse Station, NJ: The Merck Company Foundation.

Cervellati, Matteo, and Uwe Sunde. 2007. "Human Capital, Mortality and Fertility: A Unified Theory of the Economic and Demographic Transition." Discussion Paper no. 2905. Institute for the Study of Labor (IZA), Bonn, Germany.

Chakraborty, Shankha, Chris Papageorgiou, and Fidel Pérez-Sebastián. 2005. "Diseases and Development." Louisiana State University, Department of Economics Working Paper no. 2005-12.

Cincotta, Richard P., Robert Engelman, and Daniele Anastasion. 2003. "The Security Demographic: Population and Civil Conflict After the Cold War." Population Action International, Washington, DC.

Cline, William R. 2007. *Global Warming and Agriculture: Impact Estimates by Country*. Washington, DC: Peterson Institute for International Economics.

Coale, Ansley J. 1986. "The Decline of Fertility in Europe Since the Eighteenth Century as a Chapter in Demographic History." In Ansley J. Coale and Susan C. Watkins, eds., *The Decline of Fertility in Europe: The Revised Proceedings of a Conference on the Princeton European Fertility Project*. Princeton, NJ: Princeton University Press.

Coale, Ansley J., and Paul Demeny. 1983. *Regional Model Life Tables and Stable Populations*. New York: Academic Press.

Coates, Joseph. 2004. "Coming to Grips with the Future." *Research-Technology Management* 47(5): 23–32.

Cohen, Aaron J., H. Ross Anderson, Bart Ostro, Kiran Dev Pandey, Michal Krzyzanowski, Nino Künzli, Kersten Gutschmidt, Arden Pope III, Isabelle Romieu, Jonathan M. Samet, and Kirk R. Smith. 2004. "Urban Air Pollution." In Majid Ezzati, Alan D. Lopez, Anthony Rodgers, and Christopher J. L. Murray, eds., *Comparative Quantification of Health Risks: Global and Regional Burden of Disease Attributable to Selected Major Risk Factors*. Geneva: World Health Organization, 1353–1434.

Collier, Paul. 2007. *The Bottom Billion*. Oxford, UK: Oxford University Press.

Commission for Environmental Cooperation (CEC). 2006. *Children's Health and the Environment in North America: A First Report on Available Indicators and Measures*. Montreal: Commission for Environmental Cooperation.

Commission on Macroeconomics and Health (CMH). 2001. *Macroeconomics and Health: Investing in Health for Economic Development*. Geneva, Switzerland: World Health Organization.

Commission on Social Determinants of Health (CSDH). 2008. *Closing the Gap in a Generation: Health Equity Through Action on the Social Determinants of Health*. Geneva: World Health Organization.

Comrie, Andrew. 2007. "Climate Change and Human Health." *Geography Compass* 1(3): 325–339.

Confalonieri, Ulisses, and Anthony McMichael, eds., 2007. "Global Environmental Change and Human Health: Science Plan and Implementation Strategy." ESSP Report no. 4. Earth System Science Partnership, Paris.

Confalonieri, Ulisses, Bettina Menne, Rais Sakhtar, Kristie L. Ebi, Maria Hauengue, R. Sari Kovats, Boris Revich, and Alistair Woodward. 2007. "Human Health." In Martin L. Parry, Osvaldo F. Canzianin, Jean P. Palutikof, Paul J. van der Linden, and Clair E. Hanson, eds., *Climate Change 2007: Impacts, Adaptation and Vulnerability. Contribution of Working Group II to the Fourth Assessment Report of the Intergovernmental Panel on Climate Change*. Cambridge, UK: Cambridge University Press, 391–431.

Cooper, Richard, Jeffrey Cutler, Patrice Desvigne-Nickens, Stephen P. Fortmann, Lawrence Friedman, Richard Havlik, Gary Hogelin, John Marler, Paul McGovern, Gregory Morosco, Lori Mosca, Thomas Pearson, Jeremiah Stamler, Daniel Stryer, and Thomas Thom. 2000. "Trends and Disparities in Coronary Heart Disease, Stroke, and Other Cardiovascular Diseases in the United States: Findings of the National Conference on Cardiovascular Disease Prevention." *Circulation* 102(25): 3137–3147.

Corvalán, Carlos, and Diarmid Campbell-Lendrum. 2005. "Focusing on the Future Through the Looking Glass: Building Scenarios of Health and Environment." *EcoHealth* 2(1): 22–25.

Corvalán, Carlos, Simon Hales, Alistair Woodward, Diarmid Campbell-Lendrum, Kristie L. Ebi, Fernando Dias de Ávila-Pires, and Colin L. Soskolne. 2005. "Consequences and Options for Human Health." In Millennium Ecosystem Assessment, ed., *Ecosystems and Human Well-being: Policy Responses*, vol 3. Washington, DC: Island Press, 467–486.

Costello, Anthony, Mustafa Abbas, Adriana Allen, Sarah Ball, Sarah Bell, Richard Bellamy, Sharon Friel, Nora Groce, Anne Johnson, Maria Kett, Maria Lee, Caren Levy, Mark Maslin, David McCoy, Bill McGuire, Hugh Montgomery, David Napier, Christina Pagel, Jinesh Patel, José Antonio Puppim de Oliveira, Nanneke Redclift, Hannah Rees, Daniel Rogger, Joanne Scott, Judith Stephenson, John Twigg, Jonathan Wolff, and Craig Patterson. 2009. "Managing the Health Effects of Climate Change: Lancet and University College London Institute for Global Health Commission." *Lancet* 373(9676): 1693–1733. doi:10.1016/S0140-6736(09)60935-1.

Cox, D. R. 1959. "The Analysis of Exponentially Distributed Life-Times with Two Types of Failure." *Journal of the Royal Statistical Society. Series B (Methodological)* 21(2): 411–421.

Crimmins, Eileen M. 2004. "Trends in the Health of the Elderly." *Annual Review of Public Health* 25(1): 79–98. doi:10.1146/annurev.publhealth.25.102802.124401.

Crimmins, Eileen M., and Caleb E. Finch. 2006. "Infection, Inflammation, Height, and Longevity." *Proceedings of the National Academy of Sciences of the United States of America* 103(2): 498–503.

Cuddington, John T. 1993. "Modeling the Macroeconomic Effects of AIDS, with an Application to Tanzania." *World Bank Economic Review* 7(2): 173–189.

Cutler, David, Angus Deaton, and Adriana Lleras-Muney. 2006. "The Determinants of Mortality." *Journal of Economic Perspectives* 20(3): 97–120.

Cutler, David, and Grant Miller. 2005. "The Role of Public Health Improvements in Health Advances: The Twentieth-Century United States." *Demography* 42(1): 1–22.

Daily, Gretchen C., and Paul R. Ehrlich. 1996. "Impacts of Development and Global Change on the Epidemiological Environment." *Environment and Development Economics* 1(3): 311–346.

Danaei, Goodarz, Eric L. Ding, Dariush Mozaffarian, Ben Taylor, Jürgen Rehm, Christopher J. L. Murray, and Majid Ezzati. 2009. "The Preventable Causes of Death in the United States: Comparative Risk Assessment of Dietary, Lifestyle, and Metabolic Risk Factors." *PLoS Med* 6(4): 1–23, e1000058.

Dargay, Joyce, Dermot Gately, and Martin Sommer. 2007. "Vehicle Ownership and Income Growth, Worldwide: 1960–2030." *Energy Journal* 28(4): 163–190.

Davis, Devra Lee. 2002. *When Smoke Ran like Water: Tales of Environmental Deception and the Battle Against Pollution*. New York: Basic Books.

Davis, Kingsley. 1956. "The Amazing Decline of Mortality in Underdeveloped Areas." *American Economic Review* 46(2): 305–318.

Deaton, Angus. 2002. "Policy Implications of the Gradient of Health and Wealth." *Health Affairs* 21(2): 13–30. doi:10.1377/hlthaff.21.2.13.

———. 2003. "Health, Inequality, and Economic Development." *Journal of Economic Literature* 41(1): 113–158.

———. 2007. "Height, Health, and Development." *Proceedings of the National Academy of Sciences* 104(33): 13232–13237.

Deaton, Angus, and Christina H. Paxson. 1994. "Saving, Growth, and Aging in Taiwan." In David A. Wise, ed., *Studies in the Economics of Aging*. Chicago: National Bureau of Economic Research and University of Chicago Press, 331–357.

———. 2000. "Growth and Saving Among Individuals and Households." *Review of Economics and Statistics* 82(2): 212–225.

de la Croix, David, and Clara Delavallade. 2009. "Growth, Public Investment and Corruption with Failing Institutions." *Economics of Governance* 10(3): 187–219. doi:10.1007/s10101-008-0057-4.

DeLeire, Thomas, and Willard Manning. 2004. "Labor Market Costs of Illness: Prevalence Matters." *Health Economics* 13(3): 239–250.

Desai, Manish A., Sumi Mehta, and Kirk R. Smith. 2004. *Indoor Smoke from Solid Fuels*. Environmental Burden of Disease series, no. 4. Geneva: World Health Organization.

de Waal, Alex. 2002. "Modeling the Governance Implications of the HIV/AIDS Pandemic in Africa: First Thoughts." AIDS and Governance Discussion Paper no. 2. Justice Africa, London, UK.

Diamanti-Kandarakis, Evanthia, Jean-Pierre Bourguignon, Linda C. Giudice, Russ Hauser, Gail S. Prins, Ana M. Soto, R. Thomas Zoeller, and Andrea C. Gore. 2009. "Endocrine-Disrupting Chemicals: An Endocrine Society Scientific Statement." *Endocrine Reviews* 30(4): 293–342.

Dickson, Janet R., Barry B. Hughes, and Mohammod T. Irfan. 2010. *Advancing Global Education*. vol. 2, Patterns of Potential Human Progress series. Boulder, CO, and New Delhi, India: Paradigm Publishers and Oxford University Press.

Dixon, Simon, Scott McDonald, and Jennifer Roberts. 2001. "AIDS and Economic Growth in Africa: A Panel Data Analysis." *Journal of International Development* 13(4): 411–426.

Doll, Richard. 1998. "Uncovering the Effects of Smoking: Historical Perspective." *Statistical Methods in Medical Research* 7(2): 87–117. doi:10.1177/096228029800700202.

———. 2004. "Evolution of Knowledge of the Smoking Epidemic." In Peter Boyle, Nigel Gray, Jack Henningfield, John Seffrin, and Witold Zatonski, eds., *Tobacco and Public Health: Science and Policy*. Oxford, UK: Oxford University Press.

Doll, Richard, Richard Peto, Jillian Boreham, and Isabelle Sutherland. 2004. "Mortality in Relation to Smoking: 50 Years' Observations on Male British Doctors." *British Medical Journal* 328(7455): 1519–1528. doi:10.1136/bmj.38142.554479.AE.

Doyle, Cathal, and Preeti Patel. 2008. "Civil Society Organisations and Global Health Initiatives: Problems of Legitimacy." *Social Science and Medicine* 66(9): 1928–1938. doi:10.1016/j.socscimed.2007.12.029.

Dreze, Jean, and Amartya Sen. 1989. *Hunger and Public Action*. Oxford, UK: Clarendon Press.

Dyer, Gwynne. 2008. *Climate Wars*. Toronto: Random House.

Easterlin, Richard A. 1999. "How Beneficent Is the Market? A Look at the Modern History of Mortality." *European Review of Economic History* 3(3): 257–294. doi:10.1017/S1361491699000131.

Easterling, William E., Pramod K. Aggarwal, Punsalmaa Batima, Keith M. Brander, Lin Erda, S. Mark Howden, Andrei Kirilenko, John Morton, Jean-François Guégan, Josef Schmidhuber, and Francesco N. Tubiello. 2007. "Food, Fibre and Forest Products." In Martin L. Parry, Osvaldo F. Canzianin, Jean P. Palutikof, Paul J. van der Linden, and Clair E. Hanson, eds., *Climate Change 2007: Impacts, Adaptation and Vulnerability. Contribution of Working Group II to the Fourth Assessment Report of the Intergovernmental Panel on Climate Change*. Cambridge, UK: Cambridge University Press, 273–313.

Ebi, Kristie L. 2008. "Healthy People 2100: Modeling Population Health Impacts of Climate Change." *Climatic Change* 88(1): 5–19.

Ebi, Kristie L., and R. Sari Kovats. 2007. "Developments in Health Models for Integrated Assessments." In Michael E. Schlesinger, Harron S. Kheshgi, Joel Smith, Francisco C. de la Chesnaye, John M. Reilly, Tom Wilson, and Charles Kolstad, eds., *Human-Induced Climate Change: An Interdisciplinary Assessment*. Cambridge, UK: Cambridge University Press, 135–146.

Eckstein, Zvi, Pedro Mira, and Kenneth I. Wolpin. 1999. "A Quantitative Analysis of Swedish Fertility Dynamics: 1751–1990." *Review of Economic Dynamics* 2(1): 137–165. doi:10.1006/redy.1998.0041.

Ehrlich, Isaac, and Hiroyuki Chuma. 1990. "A Model of the Demand for Longevity and the Value of Life Extension." *Journal of Political Economy* 98(4): 761–782.

Ehrlich, Isaac, and Francis T. Lui. 1991. "Intergenerational Trade, Longevity, and Economic Growth." *Journal of Political Economy* 99(5): 1029–1059.

Elinder, Liselotte Schäfer. 2005. "Obesity, Hunger, and Agriculture: The Damaging Role of Subsidies." *British Medical Journal* 331(7528): 1333–1336. doi:10.1136/bmj.331.7528.1333.

Epstein, Paul R., and Evan Mills, eds. 2005. *Climate Change Futures: Health, Ecological and Economic Dimensions*. Cambridge, MA: Center for Health and the Global Environment, Harvard Medical School.

Ezzati, Majid, Ari B. Friedman, Sandeep C. Kulkarni, and Christopher J. L. Murray. 2008. "The Reversal of Fortunes: Trends in County Mortality and Cross-County Mortality Disparities in the United States." *PLoS Med* 5(4): 0557–0568.

Ezzati, Majid, and Alan D. Lopez. 2004. "Smoking and Oral Tobacco Use." In Majid Ezzati, Alan D. Lopez, Anthony Rodgers, and Christopher J. L. Murray, eds., *Comparative Quantification of Health Risks: Global and Regional Burden of Disease Attributable to Selected Major Risk Factors*. Geneva: World Health Organization, 883–957.

Ezzati, Majid, Alan D. Lopez, Anthony Rodgers, and Christopher J. L. Murray, eds. 2004a. *Comparative Quantification of Health Risks: Global and Regional Burden of Disease Attributable to Selected Major Risk Factors*. Geneva: World Health Organization.

———. 2004b. "Preface." In Majid Ezzati, Alan D. Lopez, Anthony Rodgers, and Christopher J. L. Murray, eds., *Comparative Quantification of Health Risks: Global and Regional Burden of Disease Attributable to Selected Major Risk Factors*. Geneva: World Health Organization, xix–xxiv.

Ezzati, Majid, Alan D. Lopez, Anthony Rodgers, Stephen Vander Hoorn, and Christopher J. L. Murray. 2002. "Selected Major Risk Factors and Global and Regional Burden of Disease." *Lancet* 360(9343): 1347–1360.

Ezzati, Majid, Stephen Vander Hoorn, Alan D. Lopez, Goodarz Danaei, Colin D. Mathers, and Christopher J. L. Murray. 2006. "Comparative Quantification of Mortality and Burden of Disease Attributable to Selected Risk Factors." In Alan D. Lopez, Colin D. Mathers, Majid Ezzati, Dean T. Jamison, and Christopher J. L. Murray, eds., *Global Burden of Disease and Risk Factors*. New York and Washington, DC: Oxford University Press and World Bank, 241–396.

Fauci, Anthony S. 2001. "Infectious Diseases: Considerations for the 21st Century." *Clinical Infectious Diseases* 32(5): 675–685.

Fernández-Villaverde, Jesús, and Dirk Krueger. 2007. "Consumption over the Life Cycle: Facts from Consumer Expenditure Survey Data." *Review of Economics and Statistics* 89(3): 552–565.

Fewtrell, Lorna, Annette Prüss-Üstün, Robert Bos, Fiona Gore, and Jamie Bartram. 2007. *Water, Sanitation and Hygiene*. Geneva: World Health Organization.

Fidler, David. 2008/2009. "After the Revolution: Global Health Politics in a Time of Economic Crisis and Threatening Future Trends." *Global Health Governance* 2(2): 1–21.

Filmer, Deon, Jeffrey S. Hammer, and Lant H. Pritchett. 2000. "Weak Links in the Chain: A Diagnosis of Health Policy in Poor Countries." *World Bank Research Observer* 15(2): 199–224.

———. 2002. "Weak Links in the Chain II: A Prescription for Health Policy in Poor Countries." *World Bank Research Observer* 17(1): 47–66.

Filmer, Deon, and Lant Pritchett. 1999. "The Impact of Public Spending on Health: Does Money Matter?" *Social Science and Medicine* 49(10): 1309–1323.

Finch, Caleb, and Eileen M. Crimmins. 2004. "Inflammatory Exposure and Historical Changes in Human Life-Spans." *Science* 305(5691): 1736–1739.

Fishman, Steven M., Laura E. Caulfield, Mercedes de Onis, Monika Blössner, Adnan A. Hyder, Luke Mullany, and Robert E. Black. 2004. "Childhood and Maternal Underweight." In Majid Ezzati, Alan D. Lopez, Anthony Rodgers, and Christopher J. L. Murray, eds., *Comparative Quantification of Health Risks: Global and Regional Burden of Disease Attributable to Selected Major Risk Factors*. Geneva: World Health Organization, 39–161.

Flegg, A. T. 1982. "Inequality of Income, Illiteracy and Medical Care as Determinants of Infant Mortality in Underdeveloped Countries." *Population Studies* 36(3): 441–458.

Fogel, Robert W. 1994. "Economic Growth, Population Theory, and Physiology: The Bearing of Long-Term Processes on the Making of Economic Policy." *American Economic Review* 84(3): 369–395.

———. 2004a. *The Escape from Hunger and Premature Death, 1700–2100*. Cambridge, UK: Cambridge University Press.

———. 2004b. "Health, Nutrition, and Economic Growth." *Economic Development and Cultural Change* 52(3): 643–658.

Fogel, Robert W., and Dora L. Costa. 1997. "A Theory of Technophysio Evolution, with Some Implications for Forecasting Population, Health Care Costs, and Pension Costs." *Demography* 34(1): 49–66.

Food and Agricultural Organization (FAO). 2003. *Projections of Tobacco Production, Consumption and Trade to the Year 2010*. Rome: Food and Agricultural Organization of the United Nations.

———. 2006. *World Agriculture: Towards 2030/2050 (Interim Report)*. Rome: Global Perspectives Studies Unit, Food and Agricultural Organization of the United Nations.

———. 2008. *The State of Food Insecurity in the World 2008*. Rome: Food and Agricultural Organization of the United Nations.

Franco, Álvaro, Carlos Álvarez-Dardet, and Mária Teresa Ruiz. 2004. "Effect of Democracy on Health: Ecological Study." *British Medical Journal* 329(7480): 1421–1423.

Freire, Sandra. 2002. "The Impact of HIV/AIDS on Saving Behavior in South Africa." University Paris I. Sorbonne, France.

Frey, R. Scott, and Carolyn Field. 2000. "The Determinants of Infant Mortality in the Less Developed Countries: A Cross-National Test of Five Theories." *Social Indicators Research* 52(3): 215–234.

Fries, Brant E., John N. Morris, Kimberly A. Skarupski, Caroline S. Blaum, Andrzej Galecki, Fred Bookstein, and Miel Ribbe. 2000. "Accelerated Dysfunction Among the Very Oldest-Old in Nursing Homes." *Journal of Gerontology: MEDICAL SCIENCES* 55A(6): M336–M341.

Fries, James F. 1980. "Aging, Natural Death, and the Compression of Morbidity." *New England Journal of Medicine* 303(3): 130–135.

Galloway, Patrick R., Ronald D. Lee, and Eugene A. Hammel. 1998. "Infant Mortality and the Fertility Transition: Macro Evidence from Europe and New Findings from Prussia." In Barney Cohen and Mark R. Montgomery, eds., *From Death to Birth: Mortality Decline and Reproductive Change*. Washington, DC: National Academy Press, 182–226.

Gallup, John Luke, and Jeffrey D. Sachs. 2001. "The Economic Burden of Malaria." *American Journal of Tropical Medicine and Hygiene* 64(1, 2 Supplement): 85–96.

Gallup, John Luke, Jeffrey D. Sachs, and Andrew D. Mellinger. 1999. "Geography and Economic Development." *International Regional Science Review* 22(2): 179–232. doi:10.1177/016001799761012334.

Galor, Oded, and Omer Moav. 2002. "Natural Selection and the Origin of Economic Growth." *Quarterly Journal of Economics* 117(4): 1133–1191.

Galor, Oded, and David N. Weil. 1999. "From Malthusian Stagnation to Modern Growth." *American Economic Review* 89(2): 150–154.

———. 2000. "Population, Technology, and Growth: From Malthusian Stagnation to the Demographic Transition and Beyond." *American Economic Review* 90(4): 806–828.

Gamble, Janet L., Kristie L. Ebi, Anne E. Grambsch, Frances G. Sussman, and Thomas J. Wilbanks. 2008. *Analyses of the Effects of Global Change on Human Health and Welfare and Human Systems. A Report by the U.S. Climate Change Science Program and the Subcommittee on Global Change Research*. Washington, DC: U.S. Environmental Protection Agency.

Garrett, Laurie. 2007. "The Challenge of Global Health." *Foreign Affairs* 86(1): 14–38.

Gauri, Varun, and Peyvand Khaleghian. 2002. "Immunization in Developing Countries: Its Political and Organizational Determinants." *World Development* 30(12): 2109–2132.

Gaziano, Thomas A., K. Srinath Reddy, Fred Paccaud, Susan Horton, and Vivek Chaturvedi. 2006. "Cardiovascular Disease." In Dean T. Jamison, Joel T. Breman, Anthony R. Measham, George Alleyne, Mariam Claeson, David B. Evans, Prabhat Jha, Anne Mills, and Philip Musgrove, eds., *Disease Control Priorities in Developing Countries*, 2nd ed. New York and Washington, DC: Oxford University Press and World Bank, 645–662.

Global Humanitarian Forum. 2009. *Human Impact Report: Climate Change—The Anatomy of a Silent Crisis*. Geneva: Global Humanitarian Forum.

Glynn, Judity R., Anne Buvé, Michel Caraël, Maina Kahindo, Isaac B. Macauley, Rosemary M. Musonda, Eva Jungmann, Francis Tembo, and Leopold Zekeng. 2000. "Decreased Fertility Among HIV-1-Infected Women Attending Antenatal Clinics in Three African Cities." *Journal of Acquired Immune Deficiency Syndromes* 25(4): 345–352.

Goldman, Dana P., Paul G. Shekelle, Jayanta Bhattacharya, Michael Hurd, Geoffrey F. Joyce, Darius N. Lakdawalla, Dawn H. Matsui, Sydne J. Newberry, Constantijn W. A. Panis, and Baoping Shang. 2004. "Health Status and Medical Treatment of the Future Elderly: Final Report." RAND Corporation, Santa Monica, CA.

Goldman, Lee, and E. Francis Cook. 1984. "The Decline in Ischemic Heart Disease Mortality Rates: An Analysis of the Comparative Effects of Medical Interventions and Changes in Lifestyle." *Annals of Internal Medicine* 101(6): 825–836. doi:10.1059/0003-4819-101-6-825.

Gollin, Douglas, and Christian Zimmermann. 2007. "Malaria: Disease Impacts and Long-Run Income Differences." Discussion Paper no. 2997. Institute for the Study of Labor (IZA), Bonn, Germany.

Gompertz, Benjamin. 1825. "On the Nature of the Function Expressive of the Law of Human Mortality, and on a New Mode of Determining the Value of Life Contingencies." *Philosophical Transactions of the Royal Society of London* 115: 513–583.

Goodman, Jordan. 1993. *Tobacco in History: The Cultures of Dependence*. London and New York: Routledge.

Gordon, Bruce, Richard Mackay, and Eva Rehfuess. 2004. *Inheriting the World: The Atlas of Children's Health and the Environment*. Geneva: World Health Organization.

Gordon, Theodore J., and Olaf Helmer-Hirschberg. 1964. "Report on a Long-Range Forecasting Study." RAND Paper P-2982. RAND Corporation, Santa Monica, CA.

Gosling, Simon, Jason Lowe, Glenn McGregor, Mark Pelling, and Bruce Malamud. 2009. "Associations Between Elevated Atmospheric Temperature and Human Mortality: A Critical Review of the Literature." *Climatic Change* 92(3): 299–341.

Grantham-McGregor, Sally, Yin Bun Cheung, Santiago Cueto, Paul Glewwe, Linda Richter, Barbara Strupp, and the International Child Development Steering Group. 2007. "Child Development in Developing Countries 1: Developmental Potential in the First 5 Years for Children in Developing Countries." *Lancet* 369(9555): 60–70.

Graunt, John. 1662. "Natural and Political Observations Mentioned in a Following Index, and Made upon the Bills of Mortality." London. Republished with a foreword by B. Benjamin in the *Journal of the Institute of Actuaries*, vol. 90 (1964):1–61.

Gray, Ronald H., Maria J. Wawer, David Serwadda, Nelson Sewankambo, Chuanjun Li, Frederick Wabwire-Mangen, Lynn Paxton, Noah Kiwanuka, Godfrey Kigozi, Joseph Konde-Lule, Thomas C. Quinn, Charlotte A. Gaydos, and Denise McNairn. 1998. "Population-Based Study of Fertility in Women with HIV-1 Infection in Uganda." *Lancet* 351(9096): 98–103.

Gregory, Peter J., Scott N. Johnson, Adrian C. Newton, and John S. I. Ingram. 2009. "Integrating Pests and Pathogens into the Climate Change/Food Security Debate." *Journal of Experimental Botany* 60(10): 2827–2838.

Grimm, Michael, and Kenneth Harttgen. 2008. "Longer Life, Higher Welfare?" *Oxford Economic Papers* 60(2): 193–211.

Grossman, Michael. 1972. "On the Concept of Health Capital and the Demand for Health." *Journal of Political Economy* 80(2): 223–255.

Gupta, Sanjeev, Marjin Verhoeven, and Erwin R. Tiongson. 2002. "The Effectiveness of Government Spending on Education and Health Care in Developing and Transition Economies." *European Journal of Political Economy* 18(4): 717–737.

Gyimah-Brempong, Kwabena, and Mark Wilson. 2004. "Health, Human Capital and Economic Growth in Sub-Saharan African and OECD Countries." *Quarterly Review of Economics and Finance* 44(2): 296–320. doi:10.1016/j.qref.2003.07.002.

Haines, Andy, R. Sari Kovats, Diarmid Campbell-Lendrum, and Carlos Corvalán. 2006. "Climate Change and Human Health: Impacts, Vulnerability, and Mitigation." *Lancet* 367(9528): 2101–2109.

Haines, Andy, and Jonathan A. Patz. 2004. "Health Effects of Climate Change." *Journal of the American Medical Association* 291(1): 99–103. doi:10.1001/jama.291.1.99.

Hales, C. Nicholas, and David J. P. Barker. 1992. "Type 2 (non-Insulin-Dependent) Diabetes Mellitus: The Thrifty Phenotype Hypothesis." *Diabetologia* 35(7): 595–601.

Harris, Jeffrey E. 1980. "Patterns of Cigarette Smoking." In Department of Health, Education, and Welfare (DHEW), ed., *Health Consequences of Smoking for Women: A Report of the Surgeon General*. Washington, DC: U.S. Department of Health and Human Services, 15–42.

Hayflick, Leonard. 1996. *How and Why We Age*. New York: Ballantine Books.

Henderson, Donald. 1998. "Smallpox Eradication—A Cold War Victory." *World Health Forum* 19: 113–119.

Higgins, Matthew. 1998. "Demography, National Savings, and International Capital Flows." *International Economic Review* 39(2): 343–369.

Hilderink, Henk, and Paul Lucas. 2008. "Towards a Global Integrated Sustainability Model: GISMO 1.0 status report." PBL Report 550025002. Netherlands Environmental Assessment Agency (PBL), Bilthoven, Netherlands.

Hilderink, Henk, Paul Lucas, J. W. Hoekstra, and L. W. Niessen. Forthcoming. "The Future of Global Environmental Health: An Integrated Modelling Approach." Netherlands Environmental Assessment Agency (PBL), Bilthoven, Netherlands.

Hilderink, Henk, Paul Lucas, and Marcel Kok. 2009. *Beyond 2015: Long-Term Development and the Millennium Development Goals*. Bilthoven, Netherlands: Netherlands Environmental Assessment Agency (PBL).

Hill, James O. 2006. "Understanding and Addressing the Epidemic of Obesity: An Energy Balance Perspective." *Endocrine Review* 27(7): 750–761. doi:10.1210/er.2006-0032.

Hill, M. Anne, and Elizabeth M. King. 1992. "Women's Education in the Third World: An Overview." In Elizabeth M. King and M. Anne Hill, eds., *Women's Education in Developing Countries: Barriers, Benefits and Policy*. Baltimore: Johns Hopkins University Press, 1–50.

Hoddinott, John, John A. Maluccio, Jere R. Behrman, Rafael Flores, and Reynaldo Martorell. 2008. "Effect of a Nutrition Intervention During Early Childhood on Economic Productivity in Guatemalan Adults." *Lancet* 371(9610): 411–416.

Homer, Jack B., and Gary B. Hirsch. 2006. "System Dynamics Modeling for Public Health: Background and Opportunities." *American Journal of Public Health* 96(3): 452–458.

Homer, Jack B., Andrew Jones, Don Seville, Joyce Essien, Bobby Milstein, and Dara Murphy. 2004. "The CDC's Diabetes Systems Modeling Project: Developing a New Tool for Chronic Disease Prevention and Control." Paper delivered at the 22nd International Conference of the System Dynamics Society, Oxford, England, July 25–29.

Hosegood, Victoria, Eleanor Preston-Whyte, Joanna Busza, Sindile Moitse, and Ian M. Timaeus. 2007. "Revealing the Full Extent of Households' Experiences of HIV and AIDS in Rural South Africa." *Social Science and Medicine* 65(6): 1249–1259. doi:10.1016/j.socscimed.2007.05.002.

Hughes, Barry B. 2004a. "The Base Case of International Futures (IFs): Comparison with Other Forecasts." Pardee Center for International Futures Working Paper prepared for the National Intelligence Council Project 2020 and International Futures (IFs) Project Use, Denver, CO. Available on the IFs website: http://www.ifs.du.edu/documents/reports.aspx.

———. 2004b. "Forecasting the Human Development Index." Pardee Center for International Futures Working Paper, University of Denver, Denver, CO. Available on the IFs website: http://www.ifs.du.edu/documents/reports.aspx.

———. 2005. "Productivity in IFs." Pardee Center for International Futures Working Paper, University of Denver, Denver, CO. Available on the IFs website: http://www.ifs.du.edu/documents/reports.aspx.

Hughes, Barry B., and Evan E. Hillebrand. 2006. *Exploring and Shaping International Futures*. Boulder, CO: Paradigm Publishers.

Hughes, Barry B., Mohammod T. Irfan, Haider Khan, Krishna Kumar, Dale S. Rothman, and José R. Solórzano. 2009. *Reducing Global Poverty*. vol. 1, Patterns of Potential Human Progress series. Boulder, CO, and New Delhi, India: Paradigm Publishers and Oxford University Press.

Hughes, Barry B., Randall Kuhn, Cecilia M. Peterson, Dale S. Rothman, and José R. Solórzano. 2010. "Forecasting Global Health in IFs: Technical Documentation." IFs Working Paper, Denver, CO. Available on the IFs website: http://www.ifs.du.edu/documents/reports.aspx.

Hunink, Maria G. M., Lee Goldman, Anna N. A. Tosteson, Murray A. Mittleman, Paula A. Goldman, Lawrence W. Williams, Joel Tsevat, and Milton C. Weinstein. 1997. "The Recent Decline in Mortality from Coronary Heart Disease, 1980–1990: The Effect of Secular Trends in Risk Factors and Treatment." *Journal of the American Medical Association* 277(7): 535–542.

Hurd, Michael, Daniel McFadden, and Li Gan. 1998. "Subjective Survival Curves and Life Cycle Behavior." In David Wise, ed., *Inquiries in the Economics of Aging*. Chicago: University of Chicago Press, 259–305.

Huynen, Maud M. T. E. 2008. *Future Health in a Globalising World*. Netherlands: Maastricht University International Centre for Integrated Assessment and Sustainable Development.

International Council for Science (ICSU). 2007. "Towards a Systems Analysis Approach to Health and Wellbeing in the Changing Urban Environment: Report of a CSPR ad hoc Scoping Group on Human Health." Final Draft Report. International Council for Science, Paris.

Intergovernmental Panel on Climate Change (IPCC). 2007. *Climate Change 2007: Synthesis Report*. Geneva, Switzerland: Intergovernmental Panel on Climate Change.

James, W. Philip T., Rachel Jackson-Leach, Cliona Ni Mhurchu, Eleni Kalamara, Maryam Shayeghi, Neville J. Rigby, Chizuru Nishida, and Anthony Rodgers. 2004. "Overweight and Obesity (High Body Mass Index)." In Majid Ezzati, Alan D. Lopez, Anthony Rodgers, and Christopher J. L. Murray, eds., *Comparative Quantification of Health Risks: Global and Regional Burden of Disease Attributable to Selected Major Risk Factors*. Geneva: World Health Organization, 497–596.

Jamison, Dean T. 1996. "Global Burden of Disease and Injury Series Foreword." In Christopher J. L. Murray and Alan D. Lopez, eds., *Global Burden of Disease: A Comprehensive Assessment of Mortality and Disability from Diseases, Injuries and Risk Factors in 1990 and Projected to 2020*. Cambridge, MA: Harvard University Press, xv–xxiii.

———. 2006. "Investing in Health." In Dean T. Jamison, Joel G. Breman, Anthony R. Measham, George Alleyne, Mariam Claeson, David B. Evans, Prabhat Jha, Anne Mills, and Philip Musgrove, eds., *Disease Control Priorities in Developing Countries*, 2nd ed. New York and Washington, DC: Oxford University Press and World Bank.

Jamison, Dean T., Joel G. Breman, Anthony R. Measham, George Alleyne, Mariam Claeson, David B. Evans, Prabhat Jha, Anne Mills, and Philip Musgrove, eds. 2006. *Disease Control Priorities in Developing Countries*, 2nd ed. New York and Washington, DC: Oxford University Press and World Bank.

Jamison, Dean T., Lawrence J. Lau, and Jia Wang. 2005. "Health's Contribution to Economic Growth in an Environment of Partially Endogenous Technical Progress." In Guillem López-Casanovas, Berta Rivera, and Luis Currais, eds., *Health and Economic Growth: Findings and Policy Implications*. Cambridge: Massachusetts Institute of Technology Press, 67–94.

Jamison, Dean T., Anthony R. Measham, W. Henry Mosley, and José Luis Bobadilla, eds. 1993. *Disease Control Priorities in Developing Countries*. New York: Oxford University Press.

Jamison, Dean T., Jia Wang, Kenneth Hill, and Juan Luis Londoño. 1996. "Income, Mortality and Fertility in Latin America: Country Level Performance, 1960–90." *Revista de Analisis Economico* 11(2): 219–261.

Jerrett, Michael, Richard T. Burnett, C. Arden Pope III, Kazuhiko Ito, George Thurston, Daniel Krewski, Yuanli Shi, Eugenia Calle, and Michael Thun. 2009. "Long-Term Ozone Exposure and Mortality." *New England Journal of Medicine* 360(11): 1085–1095.

Jha, Prabhat, and Frank J. Chaloupka, eds. 2000. *Tobacco Control in Developing Countries*. Oxford Medical Publications. Oxford, UK: Oxford University Press.

Jones, Kate E., Nikkita G. Patel, Marc A. Levy, Adam Storeygard, Deborah Balk, John L. Gittleman, and Peter Daszak. 2008. "Global Trends in Emerging Infectious Diseases." *Nature* 451(7181) (2): 990–993. doi:10.1038/nature06536.

Jusot, F., M. Khlat, T. Rochereau, and C. Serme. 2008. "Job Loss from Poor Health, Smoking and Obesity: A National Prospective Survey in France." *Journal of Epidemiology and Community Health* 62(4): 332–337. doi:10.1136/jech.2007.060772.

Kalbfleisch, John D., and Ross L. Prentice. 2002. *The Statistical Analysis of Failure Time Data*, 2nd ed. Hoboken, NJ: John Wiley and Sons.

Kalemli-Ozcan, Sebnem. 2002. "Does the Mortality Decline Promote Economic Growth?" *Journal of Economic Growth* 7(4): 411–439.

———. 2006. "AIDS, 'Reversal' of the Demographic Transition and Economic Development: Evidence from Africa." NBER Working Paper no. W12181. National Bureau of Economic Research, Cambridge, MA.

Kalemli-Ozcan, Sebnem, Harl E. Ryder, and David N. Weil. 2000. "Mortality Decline, Human Capital Investment, and Economic Growth." *Journal of Development Economics* 62(1): 1–23. doi:10.1016/S0304-3878(00)00073-0.

Kaplan, Hillard. 2006. "The Life Course of a Skill-Intensive Foraging Species." *Daedalus* 135(1): 48–57. doi:10.1162/001152606775320960.

Kaufmann, Daniel, Aart Kraay, and Massimo Mastruzzi. 2004. "Governance Matters III: Governance Indicators for 1996, 1998, 2000, and 2002." *World Bank Economic Review* 18(2): 253–287. doi:10.1093/wber/lhh041.

Kawachi, Ichiro, Bruce P. Kennedy, and Kimberly Lochner. 1997. "Long Live Community: Social Capital as Public Health." *American Prospect* 8(35): 56–59.

Kelley, Allen C., and Robert M. Schmidt. 1996. "Saving, Dependency and Development." *Journal of Population Economics* 9(4): 365–386.

Kelly, Christopher, Nora Pashayan, Sreetharan Munisamy, and John W. Powles. 2009. "Mortality Attributable to Excess Adiposity in England and Wales in 2003 and 2015: Explorations with a Spreadsheet Implementation of the Comparative Risk Assessment Methodology." *Population Health Metrics* 7(11): 1–7.

Kerr, J. Austin, ed. 1970. *Building the Health Bridge: Selections from the Works of Fred L. Soper*. Bloomington: Indiana University Press.

Keusch, Gerald T., Olivier Fontaine, Alok Bhargava, Cynthia Boschi-Pinto, Zulfiqar A. Bhutta, Eduardo Gotuzzo, Juan A. Rivera, Jeffrey Chow, Sonbol A. Shahid-Salles, and Ramanan Laxminarayan. 2006. "Diarrheal Diseases." In Dean T. Jamison, Joel G. Breman, Anthony R. Meacham, George Alleyne, Mariam Claeson, David B. Evans, Prabhat Jha, Anne Mills, and Philip Musgrove, eds., *Disease Control Priorities in Developing Countries*, 2nd ed. New York and Washington, DC: Oxford University Press and World Bank, 371–388.

Khaleghian, Peyvand. 2004. "Decentralization and Public Services: The Case of Immunization." *Social Science and Medicine* 59(1): 163–183.

Kopits, Elizabeth, and Maureen Cropper. 2005. "Traffic Fatalities and Economic Growth." *Accident Analysis and Prevention* 37(1): 169–178. doi:10.1016/j.aap.2004.04.006.

Kovats, R. Sari, Diarmid Campbell-Lendrum, and Franziska Matthies. 2005. "Climate Change and Human Health: Estimating Avoidable Deaths and Disease." *Risk Analysis* 25(6): 1409–1418.

Kovats, R. Sari, and Shakoor Hajat. 2008. "Heat Stress and Public Health: A Critical Review." *Annual Review of Public Health* 29(1): 41–55. doi:10.1146/annurev.publhealth.29.020907.090843.

Kremer, Michael. 2002. "Pharmaceuticals and the Developing World." *Journal of Economic Perspectives* 16(4): 67–90.

Krewski, Daniel, Michael Jerrett, Richard T. Burnett, Renjun Ma, Edward Hughes, Yuanli Shi, Michelle C. Turner, C. Arden Pope III, George Thurston, Eugenia E. Calle, and Michael J. Thun. 2009. *Extended Follow-up and Spatial Analysis of the American Cancer Society Study Linking Particulate Air Pollution and Mortality*. Boston: Health Effects Institute.

Kuhn, Randall. 2010. "Routes to Low Mortality in Poor Countries Revisited: A 25-Year Perspective." Working Paper. Josef Korbel School of International Studies, University of Denver, Denver, CO.

Kunitz, Stephen J. 1987. "Explanations and Ideologies of Mortality Patterns." *Population and Development Review* 13(3): 379–408.

Lafferty, Kevin D. 2009. "The Ecology of Climate Change and Infectious Diseases." *Ecology* 90(4): 888–900.

Laxminarayan, Ramanan, Jeffrey Chow, and Sonbol A. Shahid-Salles. 2006. "Intervention Cost-Effectiveness: Overview of Main Messages." In Dean T. Jamison, Joel G. Breman, Anthony R. Measham, George Alleyne, Mariam Claeson, David B. Evans, Prabhat Jha, Anne Mills, and Philip Musgrove, eds., *Disease Control Priorities in Developing Countries*, 2nd ed. New York and Washington, DC: Oxford University Press and World Bank, 35–86.

Leakey, Andrew D. B., Elizabeth A. Ainsworth, Carl J. Bernacchi, Alistair Rogers, Stephen P. Long, and Donald R. Ort. 2009. "Elevated CO_2 Effects on Plant Carbon, Nitrogen, and Water Relations: Six Important Lessons from FACE." *Journal of Experimental Botany* 60(10): 2859–2876.

Lee, H., S. J. Yoon, H. S. Ahn, and O. R. Moon. 2007. "Estimation of Potential Health Gains from Reducing Multiple Risk Factors of Stroke in Korea." *Public Health* 121(10): 774–780. doi:10.1016/j.puhe.2007.03.002.

Lee, Ronald, Andrew Mason, and Timothy Miller. 2000. "Life Cycle Saving and the Demographic Transition: The Case of Taiwan." *Population and Development Review* 26(Supplement): 194–219.

Lena, Hugh F., and Bruce London. 1993. "The Political and Economic Determinants of Health Outcomes: A Cross-National Analysis." *International Journal of Health Services: Planning, Administration, Evaluation* 23(3): 585–602.

Leon, David A., Lyudmila Saburova, Susannah Tomkins, Evgueny Andreev, Nikolay Kiryanov, Martin McKee, and Vladimir M. Shkolnikov. 2007. "Hazardous Alcohol Drinking and Premature Mortality in Russia: A Population Based Case-Control Study." *Lancet* 369(9578): 2001–2009. doi:10.1016/S0140-6736(07)60941-6.

Lipp, Erin K., Anwar Huq, and Rita R. Colwell. 2002. "Effects of Global Climate on Infectious Disease: The Cholera Model." *Clinical Microbiology Reviews* 15(4): 757–770.

Lloyd, Simon J., R. Sari Kovats, and Ben G. Armstrong. 2007. "Global Diarrhoea Morbidity, Weather and Climate." *Climate Research* 34(2): 119–127.

Long, Stephen P., Elizabeth A. Ainsworth, Andrew D. B. Leakey, Josef Nösberger, and Donald R. Ort. 2006. "Food for Thought: Lower-Than-Expected Crop Yield Stimulation with Rising CO_2 Concentrations." *Science* 312(5782): 1918–1921.

Lopez, Alan D., Neil E. Collishaw, and Tapani Piha. 1994. "A Descriptive Model of the Cigarette Epidemic in Developed Countries." *Tobacco Control* 3(3): 242–247.

Lopez, Alan D., Colin D. Mathers, Majid Ezzati, Dean T. Jamison, and Christopher J. L. Murray, eds. 2006a. *Global Burden of Disease and Risk Factors*. New York and Washington, DC: Oxford University Press and World Bank.

———. 2006b. "Measuring the Global Burden of Disease and Risk Factors, 1990–2001." In Alan D. Lopez, Colin D. Mathers, Majid Ezzati, Dean T. Jamison, and Christopher J. L. Murray, eds., *Global Burden of Disease and Risk Factors*. New York and Washington, DC: Oxford University Press and World Bank, 1–13.

Lorentzen, Peter, John McMillan, and Romain Wacziarg. 2008. "Death and Development." *Journal of Economic Growth* 13(2): 81–124.

Lutz, Wolfgang, Warren C. Sanderson, and Sergei Scherbov, eds. 2004. *The End of World Population Growth in the 21st Century: New Challenges for Human Capital Formation and Sustainable Development*. London and Sterling, VA: Earthscan.

———. "The Coming Acceleration of Global Population Ageing." *Nature* 451(7179): 716–719.

Lutz, Wolfgang, and Sergei Scherbov. 2008. "Exploratory Extension of IIASA's World Population Projections: Scenarios to 2300." Interim Report IR-08-022. International Institute for Applied Systems Analysis, Laxenburg, Austria.

Magnusson, R. S. 2009. "Rethinking Global Health Challenges: Towards a 'Global Compact' for Reducing the Burden of Chronic Disease." *Public Health* 123(3): 265–274.

Mahapatra, Prasanta, Kenji Shibuya, Alan D. Lopez, Francesca Coullare, Francis C. Notzon, Chalapati Rao, and Simon Szreter. 2007. "Civil Registration Systems and Vital Statistics: Successes and Missed Opportunities." *Lancet* 370(9599):

1653–1663. doi:10.1016/S0140-6736(07)61308-7.

Martens, W. J. M. Pim. 1998. *Health and Climate Change: Modelling the Impacts of Global Warming and Ozone Depletion*. London: Earthscan.

———. 2002. "Health Transitions in a Globalising World: Towards More Disease or Sustained Health?" *Futures* 34(7): 635–648. doi:10.1016/S0016-3287(02)00005-8.

Martens, W. J. M. Pim, Jan Rotmans, and Dale S. Rothman. 2002. "Integrated Assessment Modelling of Human Health Impacts." In W. J. M. Pim Martens and Anthony J. McMichael, eds., *Environmental Change, Climate and Health: Issues and Research Methods*. Cambridge, UK: Earthscan, 197–225.

Martinez, José L. 2009. "The Role of Natural Environments in the Evolution of Resistance Traits in Pathogenic Bacteria." *Proceedings of the Royal Society B: Biological Sciences* 276(1667): 2521–2530. doi:10.1098/rspb.2009.0320.

Mason, Andrew. 1988. "Saving, Economic Growth, and Demographic Change." *Population and Development Review* 14(1): 113–144.

Mathers, Colin D., Christina Bernard, Kim Moesgaard Iburg, Mie Inoue, Doris Ma Fat, Kenji Shibuya, Claudia Stein, Niels Tomijima, and Hongyi Xu. 2003. "Global Burden of Disease in 2002: Data Sources, Methods and Results." Global Programme on Evidence for Health Policy Discussion Paper no. 54. World Health Organization, Geneva.

Mathers, Colin D., Majid Ezzati, Alan D. Lopez, Christopher J. L. Murray, and Anthony Rodgers. 2002. "Causal Decomposition of Summary Measures of Population and Health." In Christopher J. L. Murray, J. Salomon, Colin D. Mathers, and Alan D. Lopez, eds., *Summary Measures of Population Health: Concepts, Ethics, Measurement, and Applications*. Geneva: World Health Organization, 273–290.

Mathers, Colin D., Doris Ma Fat, Mie Inoue, Chalapati Rao, and Alan D. Lopez. 2005. "Counting the Dead and What They Died From: An Assessment of the Global Status of Cause of Death Data." *Bulletin of the World Health Organization* 83(3): 171–177.

Mathers, Colin D., Kim Iburg, Joshua Salomon, Ajay Tandon, Somnath Chatterji, Bedirhan Ustun, and Christopher J. L. Murray. 2004. "Global Patterns of Healthy Life Expectancy in the Year 2002." *BMC Public Health* 4(66). doi:10.1186/1471-2458-4-66.

Mathers, Colin D., and Dejan Loncar. n.d. "New Projections of Global Mortality and Burden of Disease from 2002 to 2030." Protocol S1 Technical Appendix to Mathers and Loncar 2006.

———. 2005. "Updated Projections of Global Mortality and Burden of Disease, 2002–2030: Data Sources, Methods and Results." Evidence and Information for Policy Working Paper. World Health Organization, Geneva.

———. 2006. "Projections of Global Mortality and Burden of Disease from 2002 to 2030." *PLoS Med* 3(11): 2011–2030. doi:10.1371/journal.pmed.0030442.

Mathers, Colin D., Alan D. Lopez, and Christopher J. L. Murray. 2006. "The Burden of Disease and Mortality by Condition: Data, Methods, and Results for 2001." In Alan D. Lopez, Colin D. Mathers, Majid Ezzati, Dean T. Jamison, and Christopher J. L. Murray, eds., *Global Burden of Disease and Risk Factors*. New York and Washington, DC: Oxford University Press and World Bank, 45–240.

McGee, Daniel L, and the Diverse Populations Collaboration (DPC). 2005. "Body Mass Index and Mortality: A Meta-Analysis Based on Person-Level Data from Twenty-Six Observational Studies." *Annals of Epidemiology* 15(2): 87–97.

McKeigue, P., B. Shah, and M. G. Marmot.

1991. "Relation of Central Obesity and Insulin Resistance with High Diabetes Prevalence and Cardiovascular Risk in South Asians." *Lancet* 337(8738): 382–386. doi:10.1016/0140-6736(91)91164-P.

McKeown, Thomas. 1976. *The Modern Rise of Population*. New York: Academic Press.

McKeown, Thomas, and R. G. Record. 1962. "Reasons for the Decline of Mortality in England and Wales during the Nineteenth Century." *Population Studies* 16(2): 94–122.

McMichael, Anthony J. 2000. "The Urban Environment and Health in a World of Increasing Globalization: Issues for Developing Countries." *Bulletin of the World Health Organization* 78(9): 1117–1126.

———. 2001. *Human Frontiers, Environments and Disease: Past Patterns, Uncertain Futures*. Cambridge, UK: Cambridge University Press.

McMichael, Anthony J., and Robert Beaglehole. 2000. "The Changing Global Context of Public Health." *Lancet* 356(9228): 495–499.

McMichael, Anthony J., Diarmid H. Campbell-Lendrum, Carlos F. Corvalán, Kristi L. Ebi, A. K. Githeko, Joel D. Scheraga, and Alistair Woodward. 2003. *Climate Change and Human Health: Risks and Responses*. Geneva: World Health Organization.

McMichael, Anthony J., Diarmid Campbell-Lendrum, R. Sari Kovats, Sally Edwards, Paul Wilkinson, Theresa Wilson, Robert Nicholls, Simon Hales, Frank Tanser, David Le Sueur, Michael Schlesinger, and Natasha Andronova. 2004. "Global Climate Change." In Majid Ezzati, Alan D. Lopez, Anthony Rodgers, and Christopher J. L. Murray, eds., *Comparative Quantification of Health Risks: Global and Regional Burden of Disease Attributable to Selected Major Risk Factors*. Geneva: World Health Organization, 1543–1650.

McMichael, Anthony J., Andrew Haines, Rudi Slooff, and R. Sari Kovats, eds. 1996. *Climate Change and Human Health: An Assessment Prepared by a Task Group on Behalf of the World Health Organization, the World Meteorological Organization and the United Nations Environment Programme*. Geneva: World Health Organization.

McMichael, Anthony J., Rosalie E. Woodruff, and Simon Hales. 2006. "Climate Change and Human Health: Present and Future Risks." *Lancet* 367(9513): 859–869. doi:10.1016/S0140-6736(06)68079-3.

McMichael, Anthony J., Rosalie Woodruff, Peter Whetton, Kevin Hennessy, Neville Nicholls, Simon Hales, Alistair Woodward, and Tord Kjellström. 2003. *Human Health and Climate Change in Oceania: A Risk Assessment*. Canberra: Commonwealth Department of Health and Aging.

Mellor, Jennifer M., and Jeffrey Milyo. 2001. "Income, Inequality and Health." *Journal of Health Politics, Policy and Law* 20(1): 151–155.

Men, Tamara, Paul Brennan, Paolo Boffetta, and David Zaridze. 2003. "Russian Mortality Trends for 1991–2001: Analysis by Cause and Region." *British Medical Journal* 327(7421): 964–969. doi:10.1136/bmj.327.7421.964.

Miguel, Edward, and Michael Kremer. 2004. "Worms: Identifying Impacts on Education and Health in the Presence of Treatment Externalities." *Econometrica* 72(1): 159–217.

Millennium Ecosystem Assessment (MA), and World Health Organization (WHO). 2005. *Ecosystems and Human Well-Being: Health Synthesis*. Geneva: Millennium Ecosystem Assessment and World Health Organization.

Mohan, V., S. Sandeep, R. Deepa, B. Shah, and C. Varghese. 2007. "Epidemiology of Type 2 Diabetes: Indian Scenario." *Indian Journal of Medical Research* 125(3): 217–230.

Morrow, Richard H., and J. H. Bryant. 1995. "Health Policy Approaches to Measuring and Valuing Human Life: Conceptual and Ethical Issues." *American Journal of Public Health* 85(10): 1356–1360. doi:10.2105/AJPH.85.10.1356.

Mosca, C. L., J. A. Marshall, G. K. Grunwald, M. A. Cornier, and J. Baxter. 2004. "Insulin Resistance as a Modifier of the Relationship Between Dietary Fat Intake and Weight Gain." *International Journal of Obesity* 28(6): 803–812.

Mosley, W. Henry. 1984. "Child Survival: Research and Policy." *Population and Development Review* 10(Supplement): 3–23.

Mosley, W. Henry, and Lincoln C. Chen. 1984. "An Analytical Framework for the Study of Child Survival in Developing Countries." *Population and Development Review* 10(Supplement): 25–45.

Murray, Christopher J. L. 1996. "Rethinking DALYs." In Christopher J. L. Murray and Alan D. Lopez, eds., *Global Burden of Disease: A Comprehensive Assessment of Mortality and Disability from Diseases, Injuries and Risk Factors in 1990 and Projected to 2020*. Cambridge, MA: Harvard University Press, 1–98.

———. 2007. "Towards Good Practice for Health Statistics: Lessons from the Millennium Development Goal Health Indicators." *Lancet* 369(9564): 862–873. doi:10.1016/S0140-6736(07)60415-2.

Murray, Christopher J. L., Majid Ezzati, Alan D. Lopez, Anthony Rodgers, and Stephen Vander Hoorn. 2004. "Comparative Quantification of Health Risks: Conceptual Framework and Methodological Issues." In Majid Ezzati, Alan D. Lopez, Anthony Rodgers, and Christopher J. L. Murray, eds., *Comparative Quantification of Health Risks: Global and Regional Burden of Disease Attributable to Selected Major Risk Factors*. Geneva: World Health Organization, 1–38.

Murray, Christopher J. L., Sandeep C. Kulkarni, Catherine Michaud, Niels Tomijima, Maria T. Bulzacchelli, Terrell J. Iandiorio, and Majid Ezzati. 2006. "Eight Americas: Investigating Mortality Disparities Across Races, Counties, and Race-Counties in the United States." *PLoS Med* 3(9): e260. doi:10.1371/journal.pmed.0030260.

Murray, Christopher J. L., and Alan D. Lopez. 1996a. "Estimating Causes of Death: New Methods and Global and Regional Applications for 1990." In Christopher J. L. Murray and Alan D. Lopez, eds., *Global Burden of Disease: A Comprehensive Assessment of Mortality and Disability from Diseases, Injuries and Risk Factors in 1990 and Projected to 2020*. Cambridge, MA: Harvard University Press, 118–200.

———, eds. 1996b. *The Global Burden of Disease: A Comprehensive Assessment of Mortality and Disability from Diseases, Injuries, and Risk Factors in 1990 and Projected to 2020*. Cambridge, MA: Harvard University Press.

Musgrove, Philip. 1996. "Public and Private Roles in Health: Theory and Financing Patterns." HNP Discussion Paper no. 29290. World Bank, Washington, DC.

Narayan, K. M. Venkat, Ping Zhang, Alka M. Kanaya, Desmond E. Williams, Michael M. Engelgau, Giuseppina Imperatore, and Ambady Ramachandran. 2006. "Diabetes: The Pandemic and Potential Solutions." In Dean T. Jamison, Joel G. Breman, Anthony R. Measham, George Alleyne, Mariam Claeson, David B. Evans, Prabhat Jha, Anne Mills, and Philip Musgrove, eds., *Disease Control Priorities in Developing Countries*, 2nd ed. New York and Washington, DC: Oxford University Press and World Bank, 591–604.

Nathanson, Constance A. 1996. "Disease Prevention as Social Change: Toward a Theory of Public Health." *Population and Development Review* 22(4): 609–637.

National Research Council. 1999. *Hormonally Active Agents in the Environment*. Washington, DC: National Academy Press.

Navarro, Vicente. 2004. "Inequalities Are Unhealthy." *Monthly Review* 56(2): 26–30.

Navarro, Vincente, and Leiyu Shi. 2001. "The Political Context of Social Inequalities and Health." *Social Science and Medicine* 52: 481–491.

Navia, Patricio, and Thomas D. Zweifel. 2003. "Democracy, Dictatorship, and Infant Mortality Revisited." *Journal of Democracy* 14(3): 90–103.

Nelson, Gerald C., Mark W. Rosegrant, Jawoo Koo, Richard Robertson, Timothy Sulser, Tingju Zhu, Claudia Ringler, Siwa Msangi, Amanda Palazzo, Miroslav Batka, Marilia Magalhaes, Rowena Valmonte-Santos, Mandy Ewing, and David Lee. 2009. *Climate Change Impact on Agriculture and Costs of Adaptation*. Food Policy Report. Washington, DC: International Food Policy Research Institute (IFPRI).

Nixon, John, and Philippe Ulmann. 2006. "The Relationship Between Health Care Expenditure and Health Outcomes: Evidence and Caveats for a Causal Link." *European Journal of Health Economics* 7(1): 7–18. doi:10.1007/s10198-005-0336-8.

Nussbaum, Martha C. 2004. "Women's Education: A Global Challenge." *Signs: Journal of Women in Culture and Society* 29(2): 325–355. doi:10.1086/378571.

Oeppen, Jim, and James W. Vaupel. 2002. "Broken Limits to Life Expectancy." *Science* 296(5570): 1029–1031.

Olshansky, S. Jay, and Bruce A. Carnes. 1994. "Demographic Perspectives on Human Senescence." *Population and Development Review* 20(1): 57–80.

———. 1997. "Ever Since Gompertz." *Demography* 34(1): 1–15.

Olshansky, S. Jay, Bruce A. Carnes, and Jacob Brody. 2002. "A Biodemographic Interpretation of Life Span." *Population and Development Review* 28(3): 501–513.

Omran, Abdel R. 1971. "The Epidemiologic Transition: A Theory of the Epidemiology of Population Change." *Milbank Memorial Fund Quarterly* 49(4): 509–538.

———. 1998. "The Epidemiologic Transition Theory Revisited Thirty Years Later." *World Health Statistics Quarterly* 51(2–4): 99–119.

O'Neill, Brian. 2009. "Preventing Passenger Vehicle Occupant Injuries by Vehicle Design—A Historical Perspective from IIHS." *Traffic Injury Prevention* 10(2): 113. doi:10.1080/15389580802486225.

Organisation for Economic Co-operation and Development (OECD). 2006. *Infrastructure to 2030: Telecom, Land Transport, Water and Electricity*. Paris: Organisation for Economic Co-operation and Development.

———. 2008. *OECD Environmental Outlook to 2030*. Paris: Organisation for Economic Co-operation and Development.

Ostro, Bart. 2004. *Outdoor Air Pollution*. Environmental Burden of Disease series, no. 5. Geneva: World Health Organization.

Over, Mead. 1992. "The Macroeconomic Impact of AIDS in Sub-Saharan Africa." World Bank Working Paper. World Bank, Washington, DC.

Pampel, Fred C., and Vijayan K. Pillai. 1986. "Patterns and Determinants of Infant Mortality in Developed Nations, 1950–1975." *Demography* 23(4): 525–542.

Pandey, Kiran Dev, David Wheeler, Bart Ostro, Uwe Deichmann, Kirk Hamilton, and Katie Bolt. 2006. "Ambient Particulate Matter Concentrations in Residential and Pollution Hotspot Areas of World Cities: New Estimates Based on the Global Model of Ambient Particulates (GMAPS)." World Bank Development Economics Research Group and the Environment Department Working Paper. World Bank, Washington, DC.

Patz, Jonathan A., Diarmid Campbell-Lendrum, Tracey Holloway, and Jonathan A. Foley. 2005. "Impact of Regional Climate Change on Human Health." *Nature* 438: 310–317.

Patz, Jonathan A., Holly Gibbs, Jonathan Foley, Jamesine Rogers, and Kirk Smith. 2007. "Climate Change and Global Health: Quantifying a Growing Ethical Crisis." *EcoHealth* 4(4): 397–405.

Payne, Greg, Audrey Laporte, Raisa Deber, and Peter C. Coyte. 2007. "Counting Backward to Health Care's Future: Using Time-to-Death Modeling to Identify Changes in End-of-Life Morbidity and the Impact of Aging on Health Care Expenditures." *Milbank Quarterly* 85(2): 213–257.

Pelletier, David L. 1994. "The Relationship Between Child Anthropometry and Mortality in Developing Countries: Implications for Policy, Programs and Future Research." *Journal of Nutrition* 124(10): 2047–2081.

Pelletier, David L., Edward A. Frongillo, Jr., and Jean-Pierre Habicht. 1993. "Epidemiologic Evidence for a Potentiating Effect of Malnutrition on Child Mortality." *American Journal of Public Health* 83(8): 1130–1133. doi:10.2105/AJPH.83.8.1130.

Peters, J. C., H. R. Wyatt, W. T. Donahoo, and J. O. Hill. 2002. "From Instinct to Intellect: The Challenge of Maintaining Healthy Weight in the Modern World." *Obesity Reviews* 3(2): 69–74. doi:10.1046/j.1467-789X.2002.00059.x.

Peto, Richard, Jillian Boreham, Alan D. Lopez, Michael Thun, and Clark Heath, Jr. 1992. "Mortality from Tobacco in Developed Countries: Indirect Estimation from National Vital Statistics." *Lancet* 339(8804): 1268–1278. doi:10.1016/0140-6736(92)91600-D.

Pitcher, Hugh, Kristie L. Ebi, and Antoinette Brenkert. 2008. "A Population Health Model for Integrated Assessment Models." *Climatic Change* 88(1): 35–57.

Ploeg, Martine, Katja K. H. Aben, and Lambertus A. Kiemeney. 2009. "The Present and Future Burden of Urinary Bladder Cancer in the World." *World Journal of Urology* 27(3): 289–293. doi:10.1007/s00345-009-0383-3.

Pope III, C. Arden, and Douglas W. Dockery. 2006. "Health Effects of Fine Particulate Air Pollution: Lines That Connect." *Journal of the Air and Waste Management Association* 56(6): 709–742.

Popkin, Barry M. 2002. "An Overview on the Nutrition Transition and Its Health Implications: The Bellagio Meeting." *Public Health Nutrition* 5(1A): 93–103.

Popkin, Barry M., and Colleen M. Doak. 1998. "The Obesity Epidemic Is a Worldwide Phenomenon." *Nutrition Reviews* 56(4): 106–114.

Popkin, Barry M., and P. Gordon-Larsen. 2004. "The Nutrition Transition: Worldwide Obesity Dynamics and Their Determinants." *International Journal of Obesity* 28(S3): S2–S9.

Preston, Samuel H. 1975. "The Changing Relation Between Mortality and Level of Economic Development." *Population Studies* 29(2): 231–248.

———. 1976. *Mortality Patterns in National Populations: With Special Reference to Recorded Causes of Death*. New York: Academic Press.

———, ed. 1978. *The Effects of Infant and Child Mortality on Fertility*. New York: Academic Press.

———. 1980. "Causes and Consequences of Mortality Declines in Less Developed Countries During the Twentieth Century." In R. A. Easterlin, ed., *Population and Economic Change in Developing Countries*. Chicago: University of Chicago Press, 289–360.

———. 1984. "Children and the Elderly: Divergent Paths for America's Dependents." *Demography* 21(4): 435–457.

———. 1996. "Population Studies of Mortality." *Population Studies* 50(3): 525–536.

Pritchett, Lant, and Lawrence H. Summers. 1996. "Wealthier Is Healthier." *Journal of Human Resources* 31(4): 841–868.

Proctor, Robert N. 2001. "Commentary: Schairer and Schöniger's Forgotten Tobacco Epidemiology and the Nazi Quest for Racial Purity." *International Journal of Epidemiology* 30(1): 31–34. doi:10.1093/ije/30.1.31.

Prüss-Üstün, Annette, and Carlos Corvalán. 2006. *Preventing Disease Through Healthy Environments: Towards an Estimate of the Environmental Burden of Disease*. Geneva: World Health Organization.

Prüss-Üstün, Annette, David Kay, Lorna Fewtrell, and Jamie Bartram. 2004. "Unsafe Water, Sanitation and Hygiene." In Majid Ezzati, Alan D. Lopez, Anthony Rodgers, and Christopher J. L. Murray, eds., *Comparative Quantification of Health Risks: Global and Regional Burden of Disease Attributable to Selected Major Risk Factors*. Geneva: World Health Organization, 1321–1352.

Przeworski, Adam, Michael E. Alvarez, José Antonio Cheibub, and Fernando Limongi. 2000. *Democracy and Development: Political Institutions and Well-Being in the World, 1950–1990*. Cambridge, UK: Cambridge University Press.

Rajkumar, Andrew Sunil, and Vinaya Swaroop. 2008. "Public Spending and Outcomes: Does Governance Matter?" *Journal of Development Economics* 86(1): 96–111.

Ramachandran, Ambady, Simon Mary, Annasami Yamuna, Narayanasamy Murugesan, and Chamukuttan Snehalatha. 2008. "High Prevalence of Diabetes and Cardiovascular Risk Factors Associated with Urbanization in India." *Diabetes Care* 31(5): 893–898. doi:10.2337/dc07-1207.

Rannan-Eliya, Ravi P., and Ruki Wijesinghe. 2006. "Global Review of Projecting Health Expenditures for Older Persons in Developing Countries." Center for Health Development. World Health Organization, Geneva.

Rawls, John. 1971. *A Theory of Justice*. Cambridge, MA: Harvard University Press.

Rehfuess, Eva, Sumi Mehta, and Annette Prüss-Üstün. 2006. "Assessing Household Solid Fuel Use: Multiple Implications for the Millennium Development Goals." *Environmental Health Perspectives* 114(3): 373–378.

Richter, Elihu D., Lee S. Friedman, Tamar Berman, and Avraham Rivkind. 2005. "Death and Injury from Motor Vehicle Crashes: A Tale of Two Countries." *American Journal of Preventive Medicine* 29(5): 440–449. doi:10.1016/j.amepre.2005.08.035.

Riley, James C. 2001. *Rising Life Expectancy: A Global History*. Cambridge, UK: Cambridge University Press.

Robine, Jean-Marie, and Jean-Pierre Michel. 2004. "Looking Forward to a General Theory on Population Aging." *Journal of Gerontology: MEDICAL SCIENCES* 59(6): 590–597.

Rockett, I. R. H. 1999. "Population and Health: An Introduction to Epidemiology." *Population Bulletin* 54(4): 3–42.

Rogers, Richard G., Robert McNown, Justin T. Denney, and Steven Doubilet. 2007. "Forecasting U.S. Life Expectancy in an Age of Uncertainty." Paper presented at the Annual Meeting of the Southern Demographic Association, Greenville, S.C., October 11–13.

Rosen, Sydney, Jonathon Simon, Jeffrey R. Vincent, William MacLeod, Matthew Fox, and Donald M. Thea. 2003. "AIDS Is Your Business." *Harvard Business Review* 81(2): 80–87.

Rosenzweig, Cynthia, and Ana Iglesias. 2006. "Potential Impacts of Climate Change on World Food Supply: Data Sets from a Major Crop Modeling Study." Center for International Earth Science Information Network, Columbia University, New York.

Ross, Michael. 2006. "Is Democracy Good for the Poor?" *American Journal of Political Science* 50(4): 860–874.

Rotmans, Jan, and Bert de Vries, eds. 1997. *Perspectives on Global Change: The TARGETS Approach*. Cambridge, UK: Cambridge University Press.

Rudy, Jarrett. 2005. "Cigarettes." In Jordan Goodman, ed., *Tobacco in History and Culture: An Encyclopedia*. Detroit: Charles Scribner's Sons, 144–150.

Ruger, Jennifer Prah. 2007. "Global Health Governance and the World Bank." *Lancet* 370(9597): 1471–1474. doi:10.1016/S0140-6736(07)61619-5.

Ruger, Jennifer Prah, and Derek Yach. Fall 2008/Spring 2009. "The Global Role of the World Health Organization." *Global Health Governance* 2(2): 1–11.

Ruhm, Christopher. 2007. "Current and Future Prevalence of Obesity and Severe Obesity in the United States." NBER Working Paper no. 13181. National Bureau of Economic Research, Cambridge, MA.

Sachs, Jeffrey, and Pia Malaney. 2002. "The Economic and Social Burden of Malaria." *Nature* 415(6872): 680–685.

Sachs, Jeffrey D., and Andrew M. Warner. 1997. "Sources of Slow Growth in African Economies." *Journal of African Economies* 6(3): 335–376.

Schmidhuber, Josef, and Francesco N. Tubiello. 2007. "Global Food Security Under Climate Change." *Proceedings of the National Academy of Sciences* 104(50): 19703–19708.

Schultz, T. Paul. 2002. "Wage Gains Associated with Height as a Form of Health Human Capital." *American Economic Review* 92(2): 349–353.

———. 2005. "Productive Benefits of Health: Evidence from Low-Income Countries." Discussion Paper no. 1462. Institute for the Study of Labor (IZA), Bonn, Germany.

Scrimshaw, Nevin S. 2003. "Historical Concepts of Interactions, Synergism and Antagonism between Nutrition and Infection." *Journal of Nutrition* 133(1): 316S–321S.

Sen, Amartya. 1985. *Commodities and Capabilities*. Amsterdam: North-Holland.

———. 1987. *The Standard of Living*. Cambridge, UK: Cambridge University Press.

———. 1998. "Mortality as an Indicator of Economic Success and Failure." *Economic Journal* 108(446): 1–25.

———. 1999a. *Development as Freedom*. New York: Knopf.

———. 1999b. "Health in Development." *Bulletin of the World Health Organization* 77(8): 619–623.

Seshamani, Meena, and Alastair M. Gray. 2004. "A Longitudinal Study of the Effects of Age and Time to Death on Hospital Costs." *Journal of Health Economics* 23(2): 217–235. doi:10.1016/j.jhealeco.2003.08.004.

Setel, Philip W., Sarah B. Macfarlane, Simon Szreter, Lene Mikkelsen, Prabhat Jha, Susan Stout, and Carla AbouZahr. 2007. "A Scandal of Invisibility: Making Everyone Count by Counting Everyone." *Lancet* 370(9598): 1569–1577. doi:10.1016/S0140-6736(07)61307-5.

Shandra, John M., Jenna Nobles, Bruce London, and John B. Williamson. 2004. "Dependency, Democracy, and Infant Mortality: A Quantitative, Cross-National Analysis of Less Developed Countries." *Social Science and Medicine* 59(2): 321–333.

Shang, Baoping, and Dana Goldman. 2008. "Does Age or Life Expectancy Better Predict Health Care Expenditures?" *Health Economics* 17(4): 487–501. doi:10.1002/hec.1295.

Shastry, Gauri Kartini, and David N. Weil. 2003. "How Much of Cross-Country Income Variation Is Explained by Health?" *Journal of the European Economic Association* 1(2/3): 387–396.

Shen, C. E., and John B. Williamson. 1997. "Child Mortality, Women's Status, Economic Dependency, and State Strength: A Cross-National Study of Less Developed Countries." *Social Forces* 76(2): 667–700.

———. 2001. "Accounting for Cross-National Differences in Infant Mortality Decline (1965–1991) Among Less Developed Countries: Effects of Women's Status, Economic Dependency, and State Strength." *Social Indicators Research* 53(3): 257–288.

Shibuya, Kenji, Mie Inoue, and Alan D. Lopez. 2005. "Statistical Modeling and Projections of Lung Cancer Mortality in Four Industrialized Countries." *International Journal of Cancer* 117(3): 476–485. doi:10.1002/ijc.21078.

Shkolnikov, Vladimir, Martin McKee, and David A. Leon. 2001. "Changes in Life Expectancy in Russia in the Mid-1990s." *Lancet* 357(9260): 917–921. doi:10.1016/S0140-6736(00)04212-4.

Smeed, R. J. 1949. "Some Statistical Aspects of Road Safety Research." *Journal of the Royal Statistical Society* 112(1): 1–24.

Smith, David L., and Andrew J. Tatem. 2009. "This Could Be the Last Time: The Bioeconomics of Eradicating Malaria." *Resources* 173(Fall): 10–12.

Smith, Kirk R. 1990. "The Risk Transition." *International Environmental Affairs* 2(3): 227–251.

———. 1997. "Development, Health, and the Environmental Risk Transition." In Gurinder S. Shahi, Barry S. Levy, Al Binger, Tord Kjellström, and Robert Lawrence, eds., *International Perspectives on Environment, Development, and Health: Toward a Sustainable World*. New York: Springer, 51–62.

———. 2001. "Environment and Health: Issues for the New U.S. Administration." *Environment* 43(4): 34–42.

Smith, Kirk R., Carlos F. Corvalán, and Tord Kjellström. 1999. "How Much Global Ill Health Is Attributable to Environmental Factors?" *Epidemiology* 10(5): 573–584.

Smith, Kirk R., and Majid Ezzati. 2005. "How Environmental Health Risks Change with Development: The Epidemiologic and Environmental Risk Transitions Revisited." *Annual Review of Environment and Resources* 30(1): 291–333. doi:10.1146/annurev.energy.30.050504.144424.

Smith, Kirk R., Sumi Mehta, and Mirjam Maeusezahl-Feuz. 2004. "Indoor Air Pollution from Household Use of Solid Fuels." In Majid Ezzati, Alan D. Lopez, Anthony Rodgers, and Christopher J. L. Murray, eds., *Comparative Quantification of Health Risks: Global and Regional Burden of Disease Attributable to Selected Major Risk Factors*. Geneva: World Health Organization, 1435–1494.

Soares, Rodrigo R. 2005. "Mortality Reductions, Educational Attainment, and Fertility Choice." *American Economic Review* 95(3): 580–601.

———. 2006. "The Effect of Longevity on Schooling and Fertility: Evidence from the Brazilian Demographic and Health Survey." *Journal of Population Economics* 19(1): 71–97.

Sridhar, Devi. 2009. "Post-Accra: Is There Space for Country Ownership in Global Health?" *Third World Quarterly* 30(7): 1363–1377. doi:10.1080/01436590903134981.

Starfield, Barbara, and Leiyu Shi. 2002. "Policy Relevant Determinants of Health: An International Perspective." *Health Policy* 60(3): 201–218. doi:10.1016/S0168-8510(01)00208-1.

Stearns, Sally C., and Edward C. Norton. 2004. "Time to Include Time to Death? The Future of Health Care Expenditure Predictions." *Health Economics* 13(4): 315–327. doi:10.1002/hec.831.

Steckel, Richard H. 1995. "Stature and the Standard of Living." *Journal of Economic Literature* 33(4): 1903–1940.

Stephensen, Charles B. 1999. "Burden of Infection on Growth Failure." *Journal of Nutrition* 129(2): 534.

Stewart, Jennifer M. 2001. "The Impact of Health Status on the Duration of Unemployment Spells and the Implications for Studies of the Impact of Unemployment on Health Status." *Journal of Health Economics* 20(5): 781–796. doi:10.1016/S0167-6296(01)00087-X.

Stover, J., P. Johnson, B. Zaba, M. Zwahlen, F. Dabis, and R. E. Ekpini. 2008. "The Spectrum Projection Package: Improvements in Estimating Mortality, ART Needs, PMTCT Impact and Uncertainty Bounds." *Sexually Transmitted Infections* 84(Supplement 1): i24–i30.

Strulik, Holger. 2004. "Economic Growth and Stagnation with Endogenous Health and Fertility." *Journal of Population Economics* 17(3): 433–453.

Stuckler, David, Lawrence P. King, and Sanjay Basu. 2008. "International Monetary Fund Programs and Tuberculosis Outcomes in Post-Communist Countries." *PLoS Med* 5(7): 1079–1090. doi:10.1371/journal.pmed.0050143.

Stuckler, David, Lawrence P. King, and Martin McKee. 2009. "Mass Privatisation and the Post-Communist Mortality Crisis: A Cross-National Analysis." *Lancet* 373(9661): 399–407. doi:10.1016/S0140-6736(09)60005-2.

Subbarao, K., and Laura Raney. 1995. "Social Gains from Female Education: A Cross-National Study." *Economic Development and Cultural Change* 44(1): 105–128.

Subramanian, S. V., Paolo Belli, and Ichiro Kawachi. 2002. "The Macroeconomic Determinants of Health." *Annual Review of Public Health* 23(1): 287–302. doi:10.1146/annurev.publhealth.23.100901.140540.

Suhrcke, Marc, Martin McKee, David Stuckler, Regina Sauto Arce, Svetla Tsolova, and Jorgen Mortensen. 2006. "The Contribution of Health to the Economy in the European Union." *Public Health* 120(11): 994–1001.

Suhrcke, Marc, and Dieter Urban. 2006. "Are Cardiovascular Diseases Bad for Economic Growth?" CESifo Working Paper no. 1845. CESifo Group, Munich.

Summers, Lawrence H. 1994. *Investing in All the People: Educating Women in Developing Countries*. Washington, DC: World Bank Publications.

Swinburn, B. A., I. Caterson, J. C. Seidell, and W. P. T. James. 2004. "Diet, Nutrition and the Prevention of Excess Weight Gain and Obesity." *Public Health Nutrition* 7(1a): 123–146. doi:10.1079/PHN2003585.

Szreter, Simon. 1997. "Economic Growth, Disruption, Deprivation, Disease, and Death: On the Importance of the Politics of Public Health for Development." *Population and Development Review* 23(4): 693–728.

Tabata, Ken. 2005. "Population Aging, the Costs of Health Care for the Elderly and Growth." *Journal of Macroeconomics* 27(3): 472–493.

Tamerius, James D., Erika K. Wise, Christopher K. Uejio, Amy L. McCoy, and Andrew C. Comrie. 2007. "Climate and Human Health: Synthesizing Environmental Complexity and Uncertainty." *Stochastic Environmental Research and Risk Assessment (SERRA)* 21(5): 601–613.

Tanumihardjo, Sherry A., Cheryl Anderson, Martha Kaufer-Horwitz, Lars Bode, Nancy J. Emenaker, Andrea M. Haqq, Jessie A. Satia, Heidi J. Silver, and Diane D. Stadler. 2007. "Poverty, Obesity, and Malnutrition: An International Perspective Recognizing the Paradox." *Journal of the American Dietetic Association* 107(11): 1966–1972. doi:10.1016/j.jada.2007.08.007.

Thirumurthy, Harsha, Joshua Graft Zivin, and Markus Goldstein. 2008. "The Economic Impact of AIDS Treatment." *Journal of Human Resources* 43(3): 511–552.

Thomas, Duncan, and Elizabeth Frankenberg. 2002. "Health, Nutrition and Prosperity: A Microeconomic Perspective." *Bulletin of the World Health Organization* 80(2): 106–113.

Thomas, Duncan, and John Strauss. 1997. "Health and Wages: Evidence on Men and Women in Urban Brazil." *Journal of Econometrics* 77(1): 159–185.

Thornton, Joseph W., Michael McCally, and Jane Houlihan. 2002. "Biomonitoring of Industrial Pollutants: Health and Policy Implications of the Chemical Body Burden." *Public Health Reports* 117(4): 315–323.

Thun, Michael, and Jane Henley. 2004. "The Great Studies of Smoking and Disease in the Twentieth Century." In Peter Boyle, Nigel Gray, Jack Henningfield, John Seffrin, and Witold Zatonski, eds., *Tobacco and Public Health: Science and Policy*. Oxford, UK: Oxford University Press, 17–36.

Tsai, I-Ju, C. Y. Cyrus Chu, and Ching-Fan Chung. 2000. "Demographic Transition and Household Saving in Taiwan." *Population and Development Review* 26(Supplement): 174–193.

Tubiello, Francesco N., Jeffrey S. Amthor, Kenneth J. Boote, Marcello Donatelli, William Easterling, Gunther Fischer, Roger M. Gifford, Mark Howden, John Reilly, and Cynthia Rosenzweig. 2007. "Crop Response to Elevated CO_2 and World Food Supply: A Comment on 'Food for Thought...' by Long et al., *Science* 312: 1918–1921, 2006." *European Journal of Agronomy* 26(3): 215–223.

Tunceli, Kaan, Cathy J. Bradley, David Nerenz, L. Keoki Williams, Manel Pladevall, and Jennifer Elston Lafata. 2005. "The Impact of Diabetes on Employment and Work Productivity." *Diabetes Care* 28(11): 2662–2667.

UNICEF. 2009. *Tracking Progress on Child and Maternal Nutrition*. New York: UNICEF Division of Communication.

United Nations. 2007. *Human Development Report 2007/2008: Fighting Climate Change—Human Solidarity in a Divided World*. New York: United Nations.

United Nations. 2009. *Millennium Development Goals Report 2008*. New York: United Nations.

United Nations Environment Programme (UNEP). 2007. *Global Environment Outlook: Environment for Development (GEO-4)*. Nairobi: United Nations Environment Programme and Earthprint.

United Nations Population Division (UNPD). 2003. "World Population Prospects: The 2002 Revision, Highlights." Working Paper no. ESA/P/WP 180. United Nations, Department of Economic and Social Affairs, Population Division, New York.

———. 2005. "World Population Prospects: The 2004 Revision, Highlights." Working Paper no. ESA/P/WP 193. United Nations, Department of Economic and Social Affairs, Population Division, New York.

———. 2007. "World Population Prospects: The 2006 Revision, Highlights." Working Paper no. ESA/P/WP 202. United Nations, Department of Economic and Social Affairs, Population Division, New York.

———. 2009a. "World Population Prospects: The 2008 Revision, Highlights." Working Paper no. ESA/P/WP 210. United Nations, Department of Economic and Social Affairs, Population Division, New York.

———. 2009b. World Population Prospects: The 2008 Revision, Population Database. United Nations. http://esa.un.org/unpp/.

United Nations Population Fund (UNFPA). 1999. The State of World Population 1999. New York: United Nations Population Fund.

United States National Intelligence Council (USNIC). 2004. Mapping the Global Future: Report of the National Intelligence Council's 2020 Project. Washington, DC: United States National Intelligence Council.

———. 2008. Global Trends 2025: A Transformed World. Washington, DC: United States National Intelligence Council.

Van de Mheen, H., K. Stronks, C. T. M. Schrijvers, and J. P. Mackenbach. 1999. "The Influence of Adult Ill Health on Occupational Class Mobility and Mobility out of and into Employment in the Netherlands." Social Science and Medicine 49(4): 509–518. doi:10.1016/S0277-9536(99)00140-9.

Van Zon, Adriaan, and Joan Muysken. 2001. "Health and Endogenous Growth." Journal of Health Economics 20(2): 169–185.

Wagstaff, Adam. 2002. "Inequalities in Health in Developing Countries: Swimming Against the Tide?" Policy Research Working Paper 2795. The World Bank Development Research Group, Public Services and Human Development Network, Health, Nutrition, and Population Team. World Bank, Washington, DC.

Wang, Y. Claire, Graham A. Colditz, and Karen M. Kuntz. 2007. "Forecasting the Obesity Epidemic in the Aging U.S. Population." Obesity 15(11): 2855–2865.

Weihe, W. H., and Basel (Switzerland) Biological Central Lab University Hospital. 1979. "Climate, Health and Disease." Proceedings of the World Climate Conference: A Conference of Experts on Climate and Mankind. Geneva: World Meteorological Organization, 313–368.

Weil, David N. 2007. "Accounting for the Effect of Health on Economic Growth." Quarterly Journal of Economics 122(3): 1265–1306.

Wigley, Tom M. L. 2008. MAGICC/SCENGEN 5.3: User Manual (version 2). Boulder, CO: National Center for Atmospheric Research (NCAR). http://www.cgd.ucar.edu/cas/wigley/magicc/UserMan5.3.v2.pdf.

Wilkinson, Richard G. 1996. Unhealthy Societies: The Afflictions of Inequality. London: Routledge.

Wilkinson, Richard G. 2007. "Commentary: The Changing Relation Between Mortality and Income." International Journal of Epidemiology 36(3): 492–494. doi:10.1093/ije/dym077.

Wilkinson, Richard G., and Kate E. Pickett. 2006. "Income Inequality and Population Health: A Review and Explanation of the Evidence." Social Science and Medicine 62(7): 1768–1784. doi:10.1016/j.socscimed.2005.08.036.

Williams, Allan F., and Veronika I. Shabanova. 2003. "Responsibility of Drivers, by Age and Gender, for Motor-Vehicle Crash Deaths." Journal of Safety Research 34(5): 527–531. doi:10.1016/j.jsr.2003.03.001.

Willis, Robert J. 1982. "The Direction of Intergenerational Transfers and Demographic Transition: The Caldwell Hypothesis Reexamined." Population and Development Review 8(Supplement): 207–234.

Wilmoth, John R. 1997. "In Search of Limits." In K. W. Wachter and C. E. Finch, eds., Between Zeus and the Salmon: The Biodemography of Longevity. Washington, DC: National Academy Press, 38–64.

Wolpin, Kenneth I. 1997. "Determinants and Consequences of the Mortality and Health of Infants and Children." In Mark R. Rosenzweig and Oded Stark, eds., Handbook of Population and Family Economics. Amsterdam: Elsevier Science, 483–557.

World Bank. 1993. World Development Report 1993: Investing in Health. New York: Oxford University Press.

———. 1999. "Why Do Savings Rates Vary Across Countries." World Bank Policy and Research Bulletin 10(1): 1–4.

———. 2009. World Development Indicators (on CD). Washington, DC: World Bank.

World Commission on Environment and Development (WCED). 1987. Our Common Future. Oxford, UK: Oxford University Press.

World Health Organization (WHO). 2002. The World Health Report 2002: Reducing Risks, Promoting Healthy Life. Geneva: World Health Organization.

———. 2008a. The Global Burden of Disease: 2004 Update. Geneva: World Health Organization.

———. 2008b. Protecting Health from Climate Change: World Health Day 2008. Geneva: World Health Organization.

———. 2008c. WHO Report on the Global Tobacco Epidemic, 2008: The MPOWER package. Geneva: World Health Organization.

———. 2009a. Global Health Risks: Mortality and Burden of Disease Attributable to Selected Major Risks. Geneva: World Health Organization.

———. 2009b. Global Status Report on Road Safety: Time for Action. Geneva: World Health Organization.

World Health Organization (WHO) and United Nations Children's Fund (UNICEF). 2000. *Global Water Supply and Sanitation Assessment 2000 Report*. Geneva: World Health Organization and United Nations Children's Fund.

———. 2008. *Progress on Drinking Water and Sanitation: Special Focus on Sanitation*. Geneva: World Health Organization and United Nations Children's Fund.

World Health Organization (WHO) and United Nations Environment Programme (UNEP). 2008. *Health Environment: Managing the Linkages for Sustainable Development: A Toolkit for Decision-Makers: Synthesis Report*. Geneva: WHO/UNEP Health and Environment Linkages Initiative.

World Health Organization Global Infobase Team. 2005. *The Surf Report 2. Surveillance of Chronic Disease Risk Factors: Country-Level Data and Comparable Estimates*. Geneva: World Health Organization.

Wrigley, Edward A., and Roger S. Schofield. 1981. *The Population History of England 1541–1871: A Reconstruction*, 1st ed. Cambridge, MA: Harvard University Press.

Yach, Derek, Corinna Hawkes, C. Linn Gould, and Karen J. Hofman. 2004. "The Global Burden of Chronic Diseases: Overcoming Impediments to Prevention and Control." *Journal of the American Medical Association* 291(21): 2616–2622.

Young, Alwyn. 2005. "The Gift of the Dying: The Tragedy of AIDS and the Welfare of Future African Generations." *Quarterly Journal of Economics* 120(2): 423–466.

Zaridze, David, Dimitri Maximovitch, Alexander Lazarev, Vladimir Igitov, Alex Boroda, Jillian Boreham, Peter Boyle, Richard Peto, and Paolo Boffetta. 2009. "Alcohol Poisoning Is a Main Determinant of Recent Mortality Trends in Russia: Evidence from a Detailed Analysis of Mortality Statistics and Autopsies." *International Journal of Epidemiology* 38(1): 143–153. doi:10.1093/ije/dyn160.

Zhang, Junfeng, and Kirk R. Smith. 2003. "Indoor Air Pollution: A Global Health Concern." *British Medical Bulletin* 68(1): 209–225.

Zhang, Ying, Peng Bi, and Janet E. Hiller. 2007. "Climate Change and Disability-Adjusted Life Years." *Journal of Environmental Health* 70(3): 32–36.

Forecast Tables:
Introduction and Glossary

Forecasts (or simulation results) from **International Futures (IFs) are dynamic calculations of the full modeling system, not extrapolations of series, results of isolated multiple regressions, or representations of the forecasts of others. To understand more about the forecasts of IFs and the specific formulations for the variables shown in output tables, see the text of the volume, especially Chapter 3, and the documentation of the model available at http://www.ifs.du.edu.**

Base case forecasts for 183 individual countries over a long period of time appear in the tables at the back of each volume in the Patterns of Potential Human Progress (PPHP) series. Such forecasts are seldom done, and there are good reasons for reluctance to provide them, including:

- Data in any series are seldom available for all countries, particularly for smaller ones or those that have undergone substantial socio-political transitions. IFs separately represents 183 countries and uses estimation procedures to fill data holes as necessary.
- Every country is very much unique. Formulating a large-scale dynamic model to behave reasonably in the face of such complexity is extremely challenging, and structures of the system will never be completely free of poor behavior for many countries, especially under extreme or new circumstances.
- Some variables, such as the future level of democracy, have especially weak bases for forecasting.

Most longer-term global forecasting reduces the severity of these problems in several ways, including reliance on regional aggregations of countries and significantly limiting the forecast horizon. The accompanying tables obviously ignore those practical approaches and simply present the numbers that the model produces. This volume has repeatedly stressed that we should never treat any model results as predictions; we should instead use them for thinking about and exploring possible futures. That is the spirit behind these tables. With continuing development of the modeling system, results will change and presumably improve on average.

The forecast tables are organized by geographic, substantive, and temporal attributes. Geographically, the first of multiple sets begins with global and four continent totals (Africa, the Americas, Asia with Oceania, and Europe), followed by the UN subregional divisions within each of the continents. The subsequent six pages of each set provide IFs base case forecasts for each of the country members of the subregional divisions within the four continents. The countries appear in subregions in descending order based on our forecasts of their populations in 2060.

The multiple sets cover six substantive issue areas. The first provides a variety of population measures, land area, and an overall measure of human development. The remaining sets of forecasting variables are divided into five categories: poverty and standard economic variables, health, education, infrastructure, and governance. These categories correspond to the topics that the PPHP volume series addresses, and forecasts in each category are therefore being developed across volumes. Each of the PPHP volumes is posted online, including the forecast tables, at http://www.ifs.du.edu.

Temporally, each series contains values for 2010, 2035, and 2060, thereby providing a forecast horizon of 50 years. In many cases, an additional column shows the cumulative percentage change forecast from 2010 through 2060. The model is currently initialized in 2005, and it computes annual results recursively from 2005 through the simulation horizon. The model uses actual GDP data through 2008 and International Monetary Fund forecasts of GDP through 2015. Otherwise, all results in years after 2005 are IFs model computations rather than actual values (even when data are available) or the forecasts of others.

To facilitate the reading and interpretation of the tables, the glossary that follows provides both the names of the variables as they appear in the tables and in IFs, along with brief definitional information and the sources of initial conditions. Variables are listed in the order in which they appear in the end tables. Please refer to the list of acronyms that immediately follows the glossary for the full names of organizations and data sources referred to in it.

Variables	IFs Names	Sources and Notes
Population, Land Area, and Human Development Index		
Population	POP	Total number of people within a country. Total initialized from WDI data; IFs also has cohort data on age/sex distribution, fertility, and mortality from UNPD.
Land area in 1,000 sq kilometers	LANDAREA	Total national land area in 1,000 square kilometers. Initialized with data from FAO via WDI. Constant over time.
Land area in 1,000 sq miles	No variable name in model; calculated by converting square kilometers	Total national land area in 1,000 square miles. Constant over time.
Population density per sq kilometer	No variable name in model; calculated from LANDAREA and POP	Population per land area measured in square kilometers.
Population density per sq mile	No variable name in model; calculated by converting density per square kilometer	Population per land area measured in square miles.
Urban population	No variable name in model; calculated from others	Percentage of population living in urban areas. Initialized with WDI data.
Population growth rate	POPR	Annual percentage change. See description of "Population" entry at beginning of glossary.
Total fertility rate	TFR	The average number of children a woman is expected to bear throughout her life. Initialized from WDI data. Forecasts initialized with cohort data on fertility from UNPD.
Population below 15 years of age	POPLE15	The total number of people in this age category, which is generally considered a period of economic dependence on others.
Population 65 years of age and older	POPGT65	The total number of people in this age category, which is generally considered a period of nonparticipation in the labor force.
Youth bulge	YTHBULGE	Although the youth bulge is always an indicator of the portion of the adult or near-adult population that is young, specific definitions vary. In IFs the definition is the population age 15–29 as a percentage of the population 15 and older. A bulge exists when this ratio is above a specified level, such as 50 percent.
Human Development Index	HDI	This corresponds very closely to the Human Development Index of the UNDP (see http://hdr.undp.org), which is an average of three components: long and healthy life; knowledge (literacy and education); and standard of living (GDP/capita). Computed in IFs population model from nearly identical drivers within IFs (see Hughes 2004b for specifics).
HDI with Higher Ceilings	HDI21STFIX	An IFs-specific measure. Computed in IFs population model from driver categories within IFs corresponding to the UNDP's Human Development Index but with maximum values raised to levels that constitute better upper limits for the 21st century (notably, life expectancy of 120 years and GDP per capita of $100,000).

Variables	IFs Names	Sources and Notes
Poverty		
Poverty below $1 per day	INCOMELT1LN	Population living below $1.08 per day at 1993 international prices (purchasing power parity). Initialized from the World Bank's PovcalNet. The forecasting formulation is based on an assumption that income in a country is subject to log-normal distribution and is also responsive to the Gini index of distribution. There are complexities in the conversion of values from 1993 dollars to contemporary currency levels; although changes in the global consumer price index suggest that $1.08 in 1993 dollars would be $1.98 in 2000 dollars and $2.82 in 2005 dollars, the problems converting different countries with different market baskets and inflation patterns preclude such simple translation.
Poverty below $2 per day	INCOMELT2LN	Population living below $2.15 per day at 1993 international prices (purchasing power parity). Initialized from the World Bank's PovcalNet. See immediately preceding description of "Poverty below $1 per day" for further information and interpretation.
Poverty below $5 per day	No variable name in model; calculated from others	Population living below $5.40 per day at 1993 international prices (purchasing power parity). See preceding description on this page of "Poverty below $1 per day" for further information and interpretation. The forecasts of values at income poverty levels above $2 per day do not use survey data for initial conditions, but rather use the log-normal formulation and survey data for $2 per day to estimate initial conditions.
Poverty below $10 per day	No variable name in model; calculated from others	Population living below $10.80 per day at 1993 international prices (purchasing power parity). See preceding descriptions on this page of "Poverty below $1 per day" for general interpretation and "Poverty below $5 per day" for a note on initialization.
Poverty below $20 per day	No variable name in model; calculated from others	Population living below $21.60 per day at 1993 international prices (purchasing power parity). See preceding descriptions on this page of "Poverty below $1 per day" for general interpretation and "Poverty below $5 per day" for a note on initialization.
GDP per capita at PPP	GDPPCP	Gross domestic product at purchasing power parity (using 2000 dollars) divided by total population. GDP is explained in the variable that immediately follows ("Gross domestic product"). OECD defines purchasing power parity as "a price relative which measures the number of units of country B's currency that are needed in country B to purchase the same quantity of an individual good or service as 1 unit of country A's currency will purchase in country A" (http://stats.oecd.org/glossary/detail.asp?ID=2204). In other words, purchasing power parities eliminate price level differences between countries in order to make better comparisons of actual purchasing power.
Gross domestic product	GDP	Gross domestic product is defined as either the sum of value added across all sectors of an economy or as the sum of goods and services delivered to meet final demand of an economy. Initialized from WDI data using 2000 dollars; forecasts use much other data including series from the GTAP.

Health		
Life expectancy at birth	LIFEXP	The average number of years a newborn is expected to live. Initialized from WDI data.
Infant mortality rate	INFMOR	The probability an infant will die before her/his first birthday, expressed as a rate per 1,000 live births. Initialized from WDI data.
Child mortality probability	No variable name in model; calculated using IFs population model	The probability that a child will die before her/his fifth birthday, expressed as a rate per 1,000 live births. Initialized from UNPD data.
Adult mortality probability	No variable name in model; calculated using IFs population model	The probability that a 15-year-old person will die before her/his 60th birthday, expressed as a rate per 1,000 population. Initialized from UNPD data.
Calories per capita	CLPC	Estimate of available calories per day from all sources, measured in kilocalories. Initialized with data originally from the FAO.
Undernourished children	MALNCHP	As defined by WHO (http://www.who.int/healthinfo/statistics/indchildrenstunted/en/), "Percentage of children underweight is the percentage of children under five years who have a weight-for-age below minus two standard deviations of the NCHS/WHO reference median." Individual countries may look at children at ages three, four, or five. Initialized from WDI data using weight-based malnutrition measure.
Adult obesity rate	HLOBESITY	The prevalence of obesity among adults 30 years of age and older, expressed as the percentage who have a body mass index (BMI) of 30 or greater. Initialized using WHO estimates (available at http://apps.who.int/bmi/index.jsp) and forecast based on the historical relationship between obesity and available calories per capita.
Adult smoking rate	HLSMOKING	The prevalence of smoking, expressed as the percentage of the adult population (typically defined by countries as those 15 or 18 and older) who currently smoke tobacco. Initialized with data from WHO and WDI.
HIV Prevalence Rate	HIVRATE	The percentage of the total population infected with HIV. Initialized using data from UNAIDS.

Variables	IFs Names	Sources and Notes
Government spending on health	No variable name in model; calculated as GDSHealth divided by GDP and then multiplied by 100	Government spending on domestic health as a percentage of GDP; initialized with WDI data.
Disability-adjusted life years	HLDALYCommun HLDALYNonCom HLDALYInjuries	Total disability-adjusted life years (DALYs) across a population, expressed as years in millions. DALYs are calculated as the sum of years of life lost (YLLs), which are calculated as deviation from life expectancy, and years lived with disability (YLDs). YLDs initialized from WHO Global Burden of Disease estimates and YLLs initialized from calculations inside IFs. DALYs are shown for the three major categories of disease: communicable diseases (this category also includes all maternal and perinatal diseases); noncommunicable diseases; and injuries.
Years lived with disabilities	HLYLDCommun HLYLDNonCom HLYLDInjuries	Total years lived with disability (YLDs) across a population, expressed as years in millions. Initialized from WHO Global Burden of Disease estimates. YLDs are shown for the three major categories of disease: communicable diseases (this category also includes all maternal and perinatal diseases); noncommunicable diseases; and injuries.
Total annual deaths	DEATHS	Total number of annual deaths in millions. Initialized from UNPD mortality data.
Deaths and age-standardized death rates from communicable diseases	DEATHCAT, AIDS, Diarrhea, Malaria, RespInfec, and OthCommunDis	This variable is expressed with two measures. The first is the total number of annual deaths from communicable diseases (expressed in thousands). The second is a weighted average of age-specific mortality rates per 100,000 people, using a standard population distribution by age from WHO in order to enable comparison of death rates across countries regardless of differences in the age distribution of their populations. Initialized using WHO Global Burden of Disease cause-specific mortality rates for communicable diseases (including also all other causes of maternal and perinatal mortality, including nutritional deficiencies). Separate forecasts are shown for AIDS; diarrheal diseases; malaria; respiratory infections; and a combined category of all other communicable, maternal, and perinatal diseases.
Deaths and age-standardized death rates from noncommunicable diseases	DEATHCAT, CardioVasc, Diabetes, Digestive, MaligNeoPl, MentalHealth, Respiratory Conditions, OtherNonComm	See explanation for deaths and age-standardized mortality rates for communicable diseases. Initialized using WHO Global Burden of Disease cause-specific mortality rates for noncommunicable diseases and conditions. Separate forecasts are shown for cardiovascular diseases, diabetes, digestive diseases, malignant neoplasms, mental health, respiratory conditions, and a combined category of all other noncommunicable diseases.
Deaths and age-standardized death rates from injuries	DEATHCAT, ntInj, TrafficAcc, UnintInj	See explanation for deaths and age-standardized mortality rates for communicable diseases. Initialized using WHO Global Burden of Disease cause-specific mortality rates for injuries. Separate forecasts are shown for road traffic accidents, other unintentional injuries, and intentional injuries.

Education

Literacy	LIT	The basic definition is the ability of adults to read and write, but different countries use very different standards. IFs uses 15 and older as the definition of adult for this variable. Initialized from WDI data.
Years of education, Adults 25+	EDYRSAG25	Average number of years of completed education, presented separately for females and males 25 years of age and older. Initialized from the Barro and Lee data set (Barro and Lee 2001).
Primary education enrollment rate, net	EDPRIENRN	The percentage of the official primary age group enrolled at the primary level. Contrast this with gross enrollment, which includes enrolled students from all age groups but maintains the base of the official age group and can therefore exceed 100 percent. Initialized with UNESCO data.
Lower secondary enrollment rate, gross	EDSECLOWRENRG	All students of any age enrolled at the lower secondary level as a percentage of those of the official age to enroll at that level (see "Primary education enrollment rate, net" earlier in this section of the glossary for the distinction between gross and net enrollment rates). Lower secondary education for most countries is approximately grades 7–9. Initialized with UNESCO data.
Upper secondary enrollment rate, gross	EDSECUPPRENRG	All students of any age enrolled at the upper secondary level as a percentage of those of the official age to enroll at that level (see "Primary education enrollment rate, net" earlier in this section of the glossary for the distinction between gross and net enrollment rates). Upper secondary education for most countries is approximately grades 10–12. Initialized with UNESCO data.
Tertiary enrollment rate, gross	EDTERENRG	All students of any age enrolled at the tertiary or post-secondary degree level as a percentage of those of the official age (frequently considered to be 18–21) to enroll at the tertiary level. Initialized with UNESCO data.
Knowledge Society Index	KNOWSOC	Adapted from the technological connectivity subindex of the A. T. Kearney Globalization Index (see "Globalization Index" entry at end of this glossary). Supplemented in IFs with ties to R&D spending and tertiary graduation rate (see Hughes 2005 Part 2 for specification).

Variables	IFs Names	Sources and Notes
Infrastructure: Health-Related		
Water safety	WATSAFE	Percentage of population without access to piped water on premises, public taps or standpipes, tube wells or boreholes, protected dug wells, protected springs, or rainwater collection. Initialized with data from WHO and UNICEF.
Sanitation	SANITATION	Percentage of population without access to personal (as opposed to shared or public) sanitation facilities that ensure hygienic separation of human excreta from human contact. Initialized with data from WHO and UNICEF.
Household use of solid fuels	ENSOLFUEL	Percentage of population using solid fuels for household cooking and/or open heating; used in IFs as measure of indoor air pollution. Initialized with data from WHO.
Urban residential outdoor air pollution	ENVPM2PT5	Micrograms of particulate matter with a diameter of 2.5 micrometers or less per cubic centimeter; used in IFs to measure level of urban outdoor air pollution, expressed as an annual average. Initialized in IFs by converting World Bank data on PM_{10} concentrations based on regional factors associated with the PM_{10} concentrations.
Infrastructure: Resource-Related		
Water use per capita	WATUSEPC	Annual water withdrawals (all uses) divided by population. Initialized with data from FAO via Earth Trends from the WRI. Formulation in IFs is very basic and does not include feedback from water supply constraints.
Crop yield	YL	Annual agricultural crop production of all kinds divided by land area devoted to crop production, measured as metric tons per hectare. Initialized with production and land data originating with UN FAO.
Energy demand per capita	ENDEM divided by POP	The units of energy consumed per capita expressed as equivalent barrels of oil. Initialized using energy data from British Petroleum and OECD and population data from WDI. A technology parameter heavily influences forecasts.
Electricity use	INFRAELEC	Defined as kilowatt hours per capita per year. Initialized from WDI data. Formulations for this and other infrastructure variables in IFs are very simple at this stage.
Annual carbon emissions	CARANN	Releases to the atmosphere of carbon from human activity (burning fossil fuels or deforestation) in billion tons or gigatons (1,000 million). Computed in IFs without initialization from a data source.
Infrastructure: Transportation		
Road density	INFRAROAD	Defined as the total kilometers of road (both paved and unpaved) per 1,000 hectares. Initialized from WDI data.
Cars, Buses, and Freight Vehicles	VEHICFLPC	Total number of cars, buses, and freight vehicles per capita, expressed as a rate per 1,000 population. Does not include motor scooters or other two-wheeled vehicles. Initialized with International Road Federation World Road Statistics via WDI.
Infrastructure: Communication		
Mobile phone usage	ICTMOBIL	Percentage of population with access to mobile phones; can exceed 100 percent because of multiple phones per individual. Initialized from ITU data.
Internet usage	INFRANET	The percentage of the population with Internet access. Initialized from ITU data.
Broadband usage	ICTBROAD	Percentage of population with access to broadband. Initialized from ITU data.
Infrastructure: Other		
R&D expenditures	Not directly available in model; calculated as RANDDEXP over GDP	The OECD defines research and development to cover basic research, applied research, and experimental development; expenditures can be private or public. Initialized from OECD and WDI data and expressed here as a percentage of GDP.

Governance		
Freedom House Index (inverted)	FREEDOM	This variable is based on, and initialized with data from, the annual surveys conducted by Freedom House and published in the Freedom in the World series. The surveys measure freedom—defined as the opportunity to act spontaneously in a variety of fields outside the control of the government and other centers of potential domination—in terms of political rights and civil liberties. The category of political rights combines three subcategories (electoral process, political pluralism and participation, and functioning of government) and the civil liberties category combines four subcategories (freedom of expression and beliefs, associational and organizational rights, rule of law, and personal autonomy and individual rights). Countries are assigned a separate score on each of the two major categories; scoring runs from 1 to 7, with 1 indicating "most free" and 7 indicating "least free" (see www.freedomhouse.org). In IFs, the two scores are added and the valence is reversed, resulting in composite country-level freedom scores that can range from 2 to 14 with higher numbers being more free.

Variables	IFs Names	Sources and Notes
Polity Democracy Index	DEMOCPOLITY	This variable is based on, and initialized from, Polity Project data (see http://www.systemicpeace. org/polity/polity4.htm). The index or "Polity Score" measures a spectrum of governance structures from fully institutionalized autocracies through mixed authority regimes ("anocracies") to fully institutionalized democracies. The Polity Project expresses polity scores on a 21-point scale ranging from -10 (hereditary monarch) to +10 (consolidated democracy). Adapted in IFs as the Polity measure of democracy minus the Polity measure of autocracy plus 10.
Economic Freedom Index	ECONFREE	This variable is based on an index developed by the Fraser Institute and initialized with data from its annual Economic Freedom of the World (EFW) series. The definition of economic freedom includes personal choice, voluntary exchange coordinated by markets, freedom to enter and compete in markets, and protection of persons and their property from aggression by others. The EFW index utilizes data from external sources (e.g., the International Monetary Fund, the World Bank, and the World Economic Forum) and includes 42 variables across the following five components: size of government; legal structure and security of property rights; access to sound money; freedom to trade internationally; and regulation of credit, labor, and business. Each component is rated on a scale from 0 to 10 based on the underlying country-level data, with higher ratings indicating greater economic freedom. The final country-level rating also ranges from 0 to 10 and is determined by averaging its component ratings (see www.freetheworld.com).
Government Corruption Perceptions Index	GOVCORRUPT	This variable is based on, and initialized with data from, Transparency International's Corruption Perceptions Index (TI-CPI). Broadly speaking, corruption is defined as the misuse of public power for private benefit. The TI-CPI's purpose is the country-level assessment of the perceived extent of public and political sector corruption as indicated by the frequency and/or the size of corrupt transactions (e.g., bribes). The TI-CPI is an aggregate indicator: it draws on 13 different sources (none of which covers all countries) that share this common purpose. Evaluative assessments are made by country experts (both residents and non-residents) and by business leaders. Individual ratings of ranks are combined through a standardization process into a country-level composite score that ranges from 1 to 10, with higher values representing less corruption (see www.transparency.org).
Economic Integration Index	ECONINTEG	The Economic Integration Index in IFs is adapted from the economic integration component of the FOREIGN POLICY Globalization Index (developed by the international management consulting group A. T. Kearney) and is initialized with values from the broader IFs database (primarily WDI and the United Nations Conference on Trade and Development's World Investment Report). The index combines measures of a country's trade and foreign direct investment inflows and outflows in relation to its GDP (e.g., relative to its capacity to participate rather than to the absolute size of its participation). Values run from 0 to 100, with higher values representing greater economic integration. See Hughes 2005 for IFs specification.
Globalization Index	GLOBALIZ	The Globalization Index in IFs is adapted from the FOREIGN POLICY Globalization Index developed by the international management consulting group A. T. Kearney. A. T. Kearney's index is a composite of four sub-indices: economic integration, personal contact, technological connectivity, and political engagement. In IFs, economic integration is measured by trade (exports) and foreign direct investment (inflows of capital), while personal contact is represented by telephone infrastructure and worker remittances (net) relative to GDP. Technological connectivity is represented by an electronic network infrastructure measure, and political engagement is calculated from the sum of foreign aid expenditures or receipts as a portion of GDP relative to the global average. See Hughes 2005 for expanded specification of the components of the index in IFs. The index is initialized with data from the broader IFs database.

Data Source Organization Abbreviations

FAO: Food and Agriculture Organization of the United Nations

GTAP: Global Trade and Analysis Project

ITU: International Telecommunications Union

OECD: Organisation for Economic Co-operation and Development

NCHS: National Center for Health Statistics

UNAIDS: United Nations Program on AIDS

UNDP: United Nations Development Programme

UNESCO: United Nations Educational, Scientific and Cultural Organization

UNICEF: United Nations Children's Fund

UNPD: United Nations Population Division

WDI: World Development Indicators (World Bank)

WHO: World Health Organization

WRI: World Resource Institute

Forecast Tables: Maps of Continents and Subregions

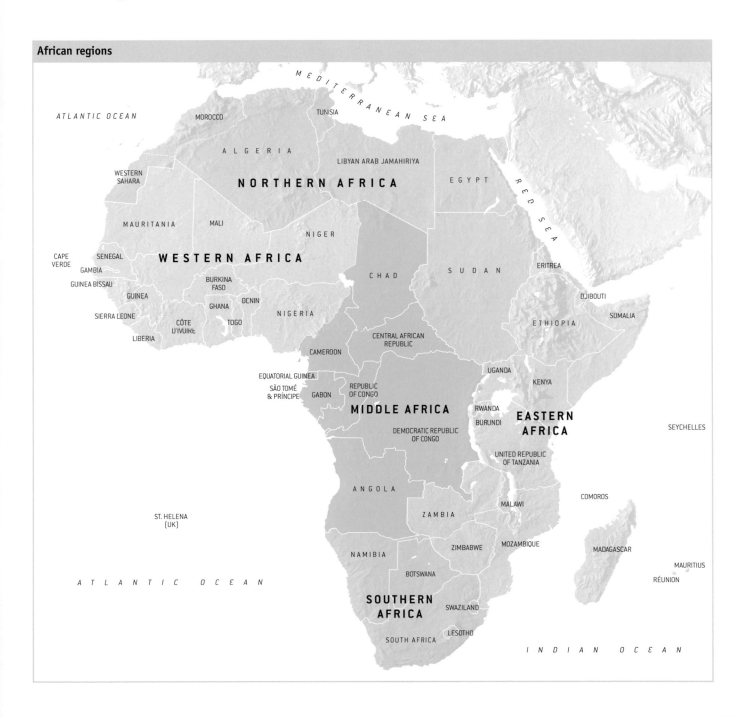

African regions

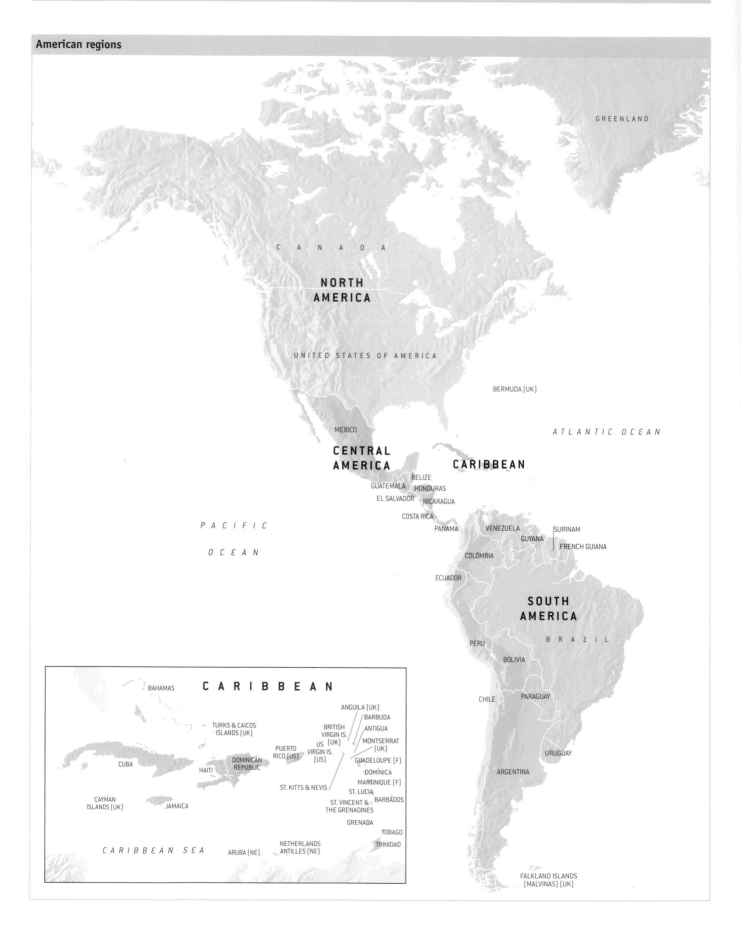

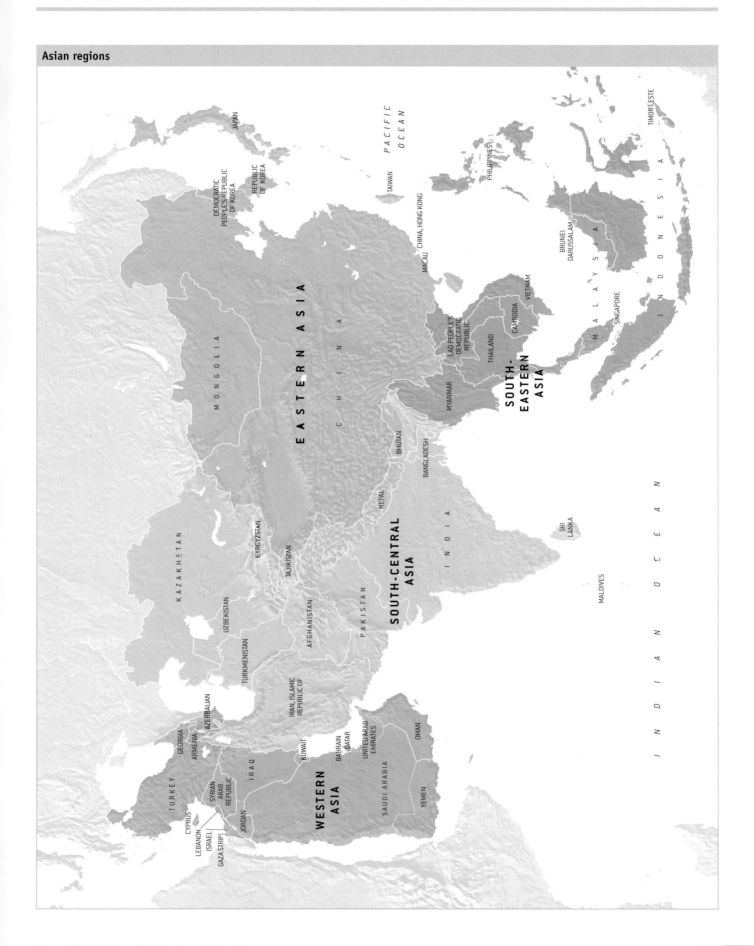

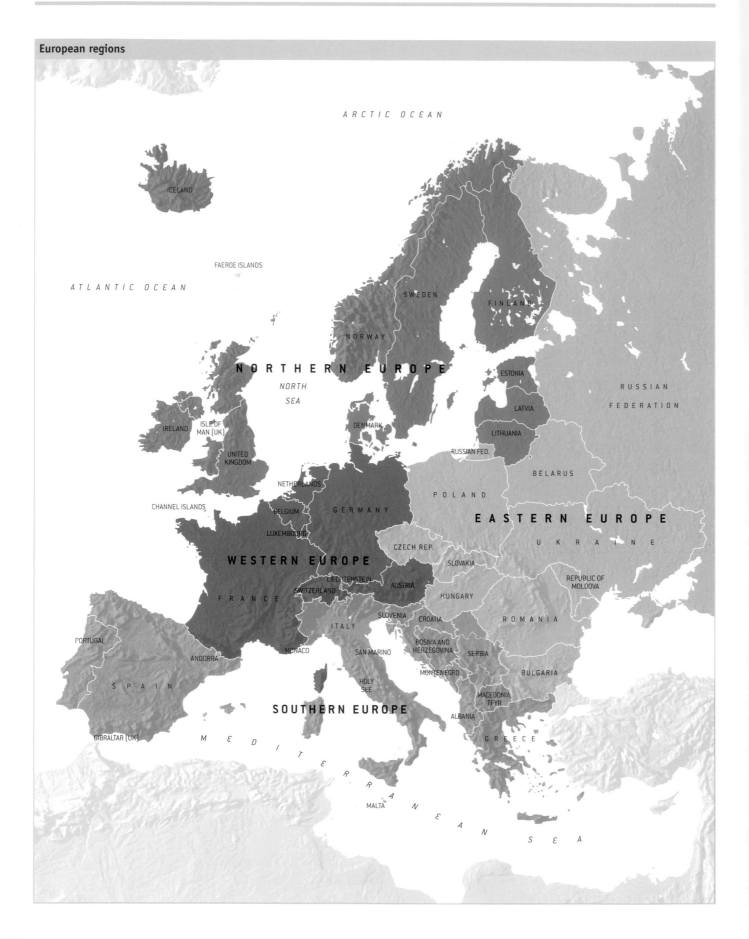

ARCTIC OCEAN

ICELAND

FAEROE ISLANDS

ATLANTIC OCEAN

NORTHERN EUROPE

NORTH SEA

SWEDEN

FINLAND

NORWAY

RUSSIAN FEDERATION

ESTONIA

LATVIA

LITHUANIA

RUSSIAN FED.

IRELAND

ISLE OF MAN (UK)

UNITED KINGDOM

DENMARK

BELARUS

CHANNEL ISLANDS

NETHERLANDS

BELGIUM

GERMANY

POLAND

EASTERN EUROPE

LUXEMBOURG

CZECH REP.

UKRAINE

WESTERN EUROPE

SLOVAKIA

LIECHTENSTEIN

SWITZERLAND

AUSTRIA

HUNGARY

REPUBLIC OF MOLDOVA

FRANCE

SLOVENIA

CROATIA

ROMANIA

PORTUGAL

ITALY

MONACO

SAN MARINO

BOSNIA AND HERZEGOVINA

SERBIA

ANDORRA

MONTENEGRO

BULGARIA

SPAIN

HOLY SEE

SOUTHERN EUROPE

MACEDONIA TFYR

ALBANIA

GIBRALTAR (UK)

GREECE

MEDITERRANEAN SEA

MALTA

Forecast Tables

Measures of Poverty, Health, Education, Infrastructure, and Governance

Multination Regional Analysis

Measures of Poverty, Health, Education, Infrastructure, and Governance

Population, Land Area, and Human Development Index

Base Case
Source: International Futures
Version 6.32, June 2010

	Population (Total in Millions)				Land Area		Population Density (Persons per Sq Km)			Population Density (Persons per Sq Mi)			Urban Population (Percent of Total Population)			
	2010	2035	2060	% Chg	Sq Km (000s)	Sq Mi (000s)	2010	2035	2060	2010	2035	2060	2010	2035	2060	% Chg
World	6815	8477	9407	38.0%	133588	51579	51	63	70	132	164	182	52.17	58.57	64.24	23.1%
Africa	1005	1696	2425	141.3%	30042	11599	33	56	81	87	146	209	41.73	46.73	52.58	26.0%
Americas	936	1134	1212	29.5%	40072	15472	23	28	30	60	73	78	80.79	83.24	84.64	4.8%
Asia with Oceania	4148	4969	5178	24.8%	40444	15615	103	123	128	266	318	332	44.52	54.28	62.84	41.2%
Europe	717.2	670	585.1	-18.4%	22970	8869	31	29	25	81	76	66	73.78	78.65	82.69	12.1%
World	6815	8477	9407	38.0%	133588	51579	51	63	70	132	164	182	52.17	58.57	64.24	23.1%
Africa-Eastern	319.6	583.3	845.9	164.7%	6358	2455	50	92	133	130	238	345	25.06	33.65	44.33	76.9%
Africa-Middle	124.4	231.7	384.4	209.0%	6613	2553	19	35	58	49	91	151	44.31	48.79	51.66	16.6%
Africa-Northern	206.5	280.3	315.9	53.0%	8259	3189	25	34	38	65	88	99	53.98	59.63	65.51	21.4%
Africa-Southern	56.03	63.46	68.15	21.6%	2675	1033	21	24	25	54	61	66	61.68	67.94	73.62	19.4%
Africa-Western	298.6	537	810.9	171.6%	6138	2370	49	87	132	126	227	342	46.28	50.82	54.8	18.4%
Africa	1005	1696	2425	141.3%	30042	11599	33	56	81	87	146	209	41.73	46.73	52.58	26.0%
America-Caribbean	39.47	47.7	51.06	29.4%	228	88	173	209	224	448	542	580	68.63	71.52	73.25	6.7%
America-Central	43.9	65.01	78.34	78.5%	522	201	84	125	150	218	323	389	55.57	60.02	64.94	16.9%
America-North	453.9	535	571	25.8%	21558	8324	21	25	26	55	64	69	81.83	85.12	87.02	6.3%
America-South	398.7	486	511.6	28.3%	17764	6859	22	27	29	58	71	75	83.57	85.44	86.14	3.1%
Americas	936	1134	1212	29.5%	40072	15472	23	28	30	60	73	78	80.79	83.24	84.64	4.8%
Asia-East	1579	1654	1516	-4.0%	11799	4556	134	140	128	347	363	333	50.72	62.6	72.44	42.8%
Asia-South Central	1717	2227	2486	44.8%	10791	4166	159	206	230	412	535	597	33.65	44.51	55.32	64.4%
Asia-South East	588.8	719.2	742.4	26.1%	4495	1735	131	160	165	339	414	428	49.31	57.23	62.44	26.6%
Asia-West	229.3	325.9	383.4	67.2%	4815	1859	48	68	80	123	175	206	66.83	69.75	72.83	9.0%
Oceania	34.3	43.71	50.04	45.9%	8543	3299	4	5	6	10	13	15	71.73	72.67	75.03	4.6%
Asia with Oceania	4148	4969	5178	24.8%	40444	15615	103	123	128	266	318	332	44.52	54.28	62.84	41.2%
Europe-East	291.5	250.9	201.3	-30.9%	18852	7279	15	13	11	40	34	28	69.77	74.37	78.82	13.0%
Europe-North	97.61	101.8	100.5	3.0%	1746	674	56	58	58	145	151	149	84.45	86.47	88.01	4.2%
Europe-South	148.5	139.2	118.3	-20.3%	1324	511	112	105	89	291	272	231	68.39	74.59	79.54	16.3%
Europe-West	188.4	186.5	172	-8.7%	1108	428	170	168	155	440	436	402	77.58	82.3	85.66	10.4%
Europe	717.2	670	585.1	-18.4%	22970	8869	31	29	25	81	76	66	73.78	78.65	82.69	12.1%

Multination Regional Analysis

Measures of Poverty, Health, Education, Infrastructure, and Governance

Population, Land Area, and Human Development Index

Base Case: Countries in Year 2060 Descending Population Sequence	Population — Total in Millions				Land Area		Population Density — Persons per Sq Km			Persons per Sq Mi			Urban Population — Percent of Total Population			
	2010	2035	2060	% Chg	Sq Km (000s)	Sq Mi (000s)	2010	2035	2060	2010	2035	2060	2010	2035	2060	% Chg
AFRICA																
Ethiopia	81.23	150.3	220.1	171.0%	1104	426	74	136	199	191	352	516	19.35	28.89	41.45	114.2%
Tanzania, United Rep	44.09	80.46	110.9	151.5%	945	355	47	85	117	121	220	304	27.23	36.67	49.71	82.6%
Uganda	33.77	69.65	105.5	212.4%	241	93	140	289	438	363	748	1134	15.47	29.85	45.7	195.4%
Kenya	38.97	68.1	92.32	136.9%	580	224	67	117	159	174	304	412	24.17	33.96	45.19	87.0%
Madagascar	21.29	39.98	62.63	194.2%	587	227	36	68	107	94	176	276	29.08	33.19	39.28	35.1%
Mozambique	22.29	38.25	51.91	132.9%	802	310	28	48	65	72	124	168	41.92	50.9	60.5	44.3%
Malawi	14.78	28.28	44.09	198.3%	119	46	125	239	372	323	618	964	20.29	27.61	36.16	78.2%
Zambia	13.15	23.97	36.01	173.8%	753	291	17	32	48	45	82	124	34.86	39.85	48.75	39.8%
Somalia	9.374	17.65	29.32	212.8%	638	246	15	28	46	38	72	119	34.59	37.51	41.95	21.3%
Rwanda	10.28	17.99	24.75	140.8%	26	10	390	683	940	1011	1769	2434	24.89	38.46	49.64	99.4%
Zimbabwe	13.99	20.05	24.15	72.6%	391	151	36	51	62	93	133	160	37.52	42.82	47.68	27.1%
Burundi	8.403	14.86	23.1	174.9%	28	11	302	534	830	782	1382	2149	10.92	16.37	23.01	110.7%
Eritrea	5.142	9.938	16.54	221.7%	118	45	44	85	141	113	219	364	20.7	24.78	30.03	45.1%
Comoros	0.694	1.259	1.968	183.6%	2.23	0.86	311	565	883	806	1462	2286	27.85	31.31	37.38	34.2%
Mauritius	1.285	1.412	1.371	6.7%	2.04	0.79	630	692	672	1631	1792	1740	45.19	57.41	67.92	50.3%
Djibouti	0.844	1.109	1.208	43.1%	23.20	8.96	36	48	52	94	124	135	94.9	98.92	96.7	1.9%
Africa-Eastern	**319.6**	**583.3**	**845.9**	**164.7%**	**6358**	**2455**	**50**	**92**	**133**	**130**	**238**	**345**	**25.06**	**33.65**	**44.33**	**76.9%**
Congo, Democratic Republic of	65.91	129.7	232.4	252.6%	2345	905	28	55	99	73	143	257	34.23	38.81	43.96	28.4%
Angola	18	32.42	46.83	160.2%	1247	481	14	26	38	37	67	97	63.79	71.88	74.41	16.6%
Cameroon	18.12	29.63	40.98	126.2%	475	184	38	62	86	99	161	223	65.15	70.51	72.27	10.9%
Chad	11.23	22.34	39.96	255.8%	1284	496	9	17	31	23	45	81	29.3	36.8	42.61	45.4%
Central African Republic	4.365	6.912	10.06	130.5%	623	241	7	11	16	18	29	42	41.7	45.75	50.51	21.1%
Congo, Republic of	4.462	7.19	9.593	115.0%	342	132	13	21	28	34	54	73	52.88	57.11	61.1	15.5%
Gabon	1.532	2.341	2.942	92.0%	268	103	6	9	11	15	23	28	89.48	95.1	94.44	5.5%
Equatorial Guinea	0.56	0.87	1.121	100.2%	28	11	20	31	40	52	80	104	54.16	70.18	77.62	43.3%
São Tomé and Príncipe	0.178	0.318	0.483	171.3%	0.96	0.37	185	331	503	480	857	1302	59.65	62.67	64.35	7.9%
Africa-Middle	**124.4**	**231.7**	**384.4**	**209.0%**	**6613**	**2553**	**19**	**35**	**58**	**49**	**91**	**151**	**44.31**	**48.79**	**51.66**	**16.6%**
Egypt	81.26	109.2	122.3	50.5%	1001	387	81	109	122	210	282	316	45.51	53.31	62.75	37.9%
Sudan	40.42	63.88	80.92	100.2%	2506	968	16	25	32	42	66	84	49.26	56.53	61.59	25.0%
Algeria	35.47	45.34	47.66	34.4%	2382	920	15	19	20	39	49	52	67.08	70.29	72.03	7.4%
Morocco	32.35	40.6	42.55	31.5%	447	172	72	91	95	188	235	247	57.22	61.07	65.91	15.2%
Tunisia	10.58	12.59	12.78	20.8%	164	63	65	77	78	167	199	202	68.42	72.55	77.1	12.7%
Libyan Arab Jamahiriya	6.452	8.674	9.724	50.7%	1760	579	4	5	6	9	13	14	78.43	80.81	84.01	7.1%
Africa-Northern	**206.5**	**280.3**	**315.9**	**53.0%**	**8259**	**3189**	**25**	**34**	**38**	**65**	**88**	**99**	**53.98**	**59.63**	**65.51**	**21.4%**

Population, Land Area, and Human Development Index

Base Case: Countries in Year 2060 Descending Population Sequence	Population Total in Millions				Land Area		Population Density Persons per Sq Km			Persons per Sq Mi			Urban Population Percent of Total Population			
	2010	2035	2060	% Chg	Sq Km (000s)	Sq Mi (000s)	2010	2035	2060	2010	2035	2060	2010	2035	2060	% Chg
AFRICA continued																
South Africa	48.79	53.55	56.71	16.2%	1221	471	40	44	46	104	114	120	64.45	70.53	75.94	17.8%
Namibia	2.249	3.427	4.21	87.2%	824	318	3	4	5	7	11	13	40.02	51.8	61.53	53.7%
Lesotho	1.89	2.42	2.641	39.7%	30	12	62	80	87	161	206	225	31.28	41.03	48.78	55.9%
Botswana	1.886	2.39	2.636	39.8%	582	225	3	4	5	8	11	12	67.99	77.78	82.02	20.6%
Swaziland	1.214	1.678	1.95	60.6%	17.36	6.70	70	97	112	181	250	291	28.17	42.75	54.6	93.8%
Africa-Southern	**56.03**	**63.46**	**68.15**	**21.6%**	**2675**	**1033**	**21**	**24**	**25**	**54**	**61**	**66**	**61.68**	**67.94**	**73.62**	**19.4%**
Nigeria	148	256.6	371.5	151.0%	924	357	160	278	402	415	719	1041	54.18	59.75	63.23	16.7%
Niger	16.49	36.83	70.11	325.2%	1267	489	13	29	55	34	75	143	17.04	23.62	31.51	84.9%
Côte d'Ivoire	20.57	36.81	55.18	168.3%	323	125	64	114	171	165	296	443	52.66	56.46	60.11	14.1%
Ghana	24.58	39.49	53.13	116.2%	239	92	103	166	223	267	429	577	51.76	55.84	59.41	14.8%
Mali	15.69	31.18	50.1	219.3%	1240	479	13	25	40	33	65	105	28.54	34.87	43.3	51.7%
Burkina Faso	15.37	30.36	49.11	219.5%	274	106	56	111	179	145	287	464	22.15	31.26	41.02	85.2%
Senegal	13.29	24.1	35.24	165.2%	197	76	68	123	179	175	317	464	41.2	44.05	50.01	21.4%
Guinea	10.38	19.67	31.87	207.0%	245	95	42	80	130	109	207	336	35.63	41.13	46.94	31.7%
Benin	9.761	18.82	30.08	208.2%	113	43	87	167	267	224	433	692	39.27	42.53	46.83	19.3%
Togo	6.98	12.57	19.32	176.8%	57	22	123	221	340	318	573	881	42.48	45.8	47.19	11.1%
Sierra Leone	6.228	10.75	15.36	146.6%	72	28	87	150	214	225	388	555	33.1	38.38	49.74	50.3%
Liberia	3.766	6.841	9.688	157.2%	111	43	34	61	87	88	159	225	64.65	73.02	79.11	22.4%
Mauritania	3.435	5.781	8.722	153.9%	1026	396	3	6	9	9	15	22	40.27	42.3	43.94	9.1%
Guinea-Bissau	1.779	3.317	5.933	233.5%	36	14	49	92	164	128	238	425	28.37	30.55	32.71	15.3%
Gambia	1.724	3.11	4.614	167.6%	11.30	4.36	153	275	408	395	713	1058	61.66	68.76	71.62	16.2%
Cape Verde	0.556	0.794	0.895	61.0%	4.03	1.56	138	197	222	357	510	575	58.58	63.99	69.94	19.4%
Africa-Western	**298.6**	**537**	**810.9**	**171.6%**	**6138**	**2370**	**49**	**87**	**132**	**126**	**227**	**342**	**46.28**	**50.82**	**54.8**	**18.4%**

Multinational Regional Analysis

Measures of Poverty, Health, Education, Infrastructure, and Governance

Population, Land Area, and Human Development Index

Base Case: Countries in Year 2060 Descending Population Sequence	Population — Total in Millions				Land Area		Population Density — Persons per Sq Km			Population Density — Persons per Sq Mi			Urban Population — Percent of Total Population			
	2010	2035	2060	% Chg	Sq Km (000s)	Sq Mi (000s)	2010	2035	2060	2010	2035	2060	2010	2035	2060	% Chg
AMERICAS																
Haiti	9.34	14.16	18.52	98.3%	28	11	337	510	667	872	1322	1729	50.94	54.84	57.05	12.0%
Dominican Republic	9.505	11.81	12.49	31.4%	49	19	195	242	256	505	628	664	75.67	80.48	83.65	10.5%
Cuba	11.45	11.48	9.956	-13.0%	111	43	103	104	90	268	268	233	76.56	78.93	82.6	7.9%
Puerto Rico	4.048	4.49	4.533	12.0%	8.95	3.46	452	502	506	1171	1299	1312	100	99.74	99.44	-0.6%
Jamaica	2.766	3.241	3.233	16.9%	10.99	4.24	252	295	294	652	764	762	54.57	59.51	64.23	17.7%
Trinidad	1.338	1.376	1.209	-9.6%	5.13	1.98	261	268	236	675	695	610	20.01	47.09	63.8	218.8%
Bahamas	0.341	0.402	0.413	21.1%	13.88	5.36	25	29	30	64	75	77	85.31	86.94	87.86	3.0%
Barbados	0.274	0.271	0.229	-16.4%	0.43	0.17	637	630	533	1651	1633	1380	40.33	55.5	67.58	67.6%
Grenada	0.114	0.149	0.164	43.9%	0.34	0.13	335	438	482	870	1137	1252	32.77	46.65	58.41	78.2%
Saint Vincent and Grenadines	0.126	0.153	0.158	25.4%	0.39	0.15	323	392	405	834	1013	1046	43.83	53.95	63.65	45.2%
Saint Lucia	0.169	0.176	0.156	-7.7%	0.62	0.24	273	284	252	707	736	653	31.91	47.67	59.76	87.3%
America-Caribbean	**39.47**	**47.7**	**51.06**	**29.4%**	**228**	**88**	**173**	**209**	**224**	**448**	**542**	**580**	**68.63**	**71.52**	**73.25**	**6.7%**
Guatemala	14.38	24.77	33.2	130.9%	109	42	132	227	305	342	589	790	49.65	55.73	62.33	25.5%
Honduras	8.015	12.09	14.41	79.8%	112	43	71	108	129	185	279	333	46.71	52.53	58.52	25.3%
El Salvador	7.345	9.276	9.953	35.5%	21.04	8.12	349	441	473	904	1142	1225	55.81	60.79	65.59	17.5%
Nicaragua	5.682	8.239	9.516	67.5%	130	50	44	63	73	113	164	190	60.48	62.55	66.18	9.4%
Costa Rica	4.677	5.841	6.148	31.5%	51	20	92	114	120	237	296	312	66.91	72.32	76.09	13.7%
Panama	3.478	4.328	4.562	31.2%	76	29	46	57	60	119	148	156	76.88	82.38	84.81	10.3%
Belize	0.323	0.473	0.546	69.0%	22.96	8.87	14	21	24	36	53	62	53.28	60.55	67.57	26.8%
America-Central	**43.9**	**65.01**	**78.34**	**78.5%**	**522**	**201**	**84**	**125**	**150**	**218**	**323**	**389**	**55.57**	**60.02**	**64.94**	**16.9%**
USA	311.1	367.3	402.8	29.5%	9629	3718	32	38	42	84	99	108	83.04	86.89	88.52	6.6%
Mexico	109.2	129.1	127.6	16.8%	1958	756	56	66	65	144	171	169	78.28	79.73	81.85	4.6%
Canada	33.57	38.54	40.64	21.1%	9971	3850	3	4	4	9	10	11	82.26	86.26	88.39	7.5%
America-North	**453.9**	**535**	**571**	**25.8%**	**21558**	**8324**	**21**	**25**	**26**	**55**	**64**	**69**	**81.83**	**85.12**	**87.02**	**6.3%**
Brazil	197	233.5	241.1	22.4%	8547	3300	23	27	28	60	71	73	87.35	89.71	89.5	2.5%
Colombia	48.99	60.81	63.66	29.9%	1139	440	43	53	56	111	138	145	71.15	73.62	76.87	8.0%
Argentina	40.72	47.33	49.61	21.8%	2780	1074	15	17	18	38	44	46	92.72	93.18	92.76	0.0%
Peru	30.28	39.04	42.7	41.0%	1285	496	24	30	33	61	79	86	71.66	75.05	80.04	11.7%
Venezuela	28.87	37.37	40.53	40.4%	912	352	32	41	44	82	106	115	95.17	96.46	95.75	0.6%
Ecuador	14.36	19.08	21.08	46.8%	284	110	51	67	74	131	174	193	64.91	66.69	67.78	4.4%
Chile	17.06	19.76	19.9	16.6%	757	292	23	26	26	58	68	68	90.25	91.98	91.54	1.4%
Bolivia	10.13	14.79	17.38	71.6%	1099	424	9	13	16	24	35	41	67.11	70.93	75	11.8%
Paraguay	6.505	9.317	10.82	66.3%	407	157	16	23	27	41	59	69	61.87	64.88	68.02	9.9%
Uruguay	3.544	3.799	3.772	6.4%	176	68	20	22	21	52	56	55	88.71	89.37	89.31	0.7%
Guyana	0.756	0.705	0.622	-17.7%	215	83	4	3	3	9	8	7	30.76	41.46	51.77	68.3%
Suriname	0.46	0.466	0.412	-10.4%	163	63	3	3	3	7	7	7	86.2	88.42	88.15	2.3%
America-South	**398.7**	**486**	**511.6**	**28.3%**	**17764**	**6859**	**22**	**27**	**29**	**58**	**71**	**75**	**83.57**	**85.44**	**86.14**	**3.1%**

Population, Land Area, and Human Development Index

Base Case: Countries in Year 2060 Descending Population Sequence	Population (Total in Millions)				Land Area		Population Density (Persons per Sq Km)			Population Density (Persons per Sq Mi)			Urban Population (Percent of Total Population)			
	2010	2035	2060	% Chg	Sq Km (000s)	Sq Mi (000s)	2010	2035	2060	2010	2035	2060	2010	2035	2060	% Chg
ASIA with OCEANIA																
China	1345	1430	1328	-1.3%	9598	3706	140	149	138	363	386	358	46.74	60.01	70.99	51.9%
Japan	127.7	113.6	92.09	-27.9%	378	146	338	301	244	875	779	631	68.86	76.95	82.07	19.2%
Korea, Repub of	49.04	47.37	36.94	-24.7%	99	38	494	477	372	1280	1236	964	83.99	86.53	87.43	4.1%
Taiwan	24.01	27.12	26.02	8.4%	36	14	667	754	723	1729	1952	1873	77.34	79.18	82.68	6.9%
Korea, Dem. People's Rep.	22.95	23.96	22.31	-2.8%	121	47	190	199	185	493	515	479	67.13	70.26	72.97	8.7%
Hong Kong SAR	7.283	8.209	7.988	9.7%	1.07	0.41	6807	7672	7465	17634	19877	19341	99.76	100	100	0.2%
Mongolia	2.672	3.234	3.31	23.9%	1566	605	2	2	2	4	5	5	57.74	62.78	70.15	21.5%
Asia-East	**1579**	**1654**	**1516**	**-4.0%**	**11799**	**4556**	**134**	**140**	**128**	**347**	**363**	**333**	**50.72**	**62.6**	**72.44**	**42.8%**
India	1169	1444	1537	31.5%	3287	1269	356	439	468	921	1138	1211	31.91	44.45	57.3	79.6%
Pakistan	173.6	281.3	380.5	119.2%	796	307	218	353	478	565	915	1238	37.59	44.57	51.21	36.2%
Bangladesh	153.6	200.2	212.5	38.3%	144	56	1067	1390	1476	2763	3601	3822	30.7	38.96	47.81	55.7%
Afghanistan	35.98	69.55	108.9	202.7%	652	252	55	107	167	143	276	432	10.3	26.52	44.29	330.0%
Iran (Islamic Republic of)	72.68	89.85	92.8	27.7%	1648	636	44	55	56	114	141	146	72.24	76.86	79.36	9.9%
Nepal	29.78	44.4	55.26	85.6%	147	57	202	302	375	524	781	972	20.4	30.38	38.06	86.6%
Uzbekistan	27.99	34.98	36.27	29.6%	447	173	63	78	81	162	203	210	37.46	45.28	54.03	44.2%
Sri Lanka	20.36	22.08	20.74	1.9%	66	25	310	337	316	804	872	819	18.48	35.61	50.12	171.2%
Kazakhstan	15.12	14.65	12.73	-15.8%	2725	1052	6	5	5	14	14	12	58.62	66.52	73.59	25.5%
Tajikistan	6.999	10.5	12.5	78.6%	143	55	49	73	87	127	190	226	27.07	35.03	43.85	62.0%
Turkmenistan	5.198	6.658	7.271	39.9%	483	189	11	14	15	28	35	39	50.67	64.14	74.07	46.2%
Kyrgyzstan	5.501	6.837	7.061	28.4%	200	77	28	34	35	71	89	91	35.45	40.54	48.16	35.9%
Bhutan	0.691	0.962	1.11	60.6%	47	18	15	20	24	38	53	61	38.11	52.7	64.28	68.7%
Maldives	0.362	0.51	0.572	58.0%	0.30	0.12	1207	1700	1907	3121	4397	4931	34.77	47.78	58.99	69.7%
Asia-South Central	**1717**	**2227**	**2486**	**44.8%**	**10791**	**4166**	**159**	**206**	**230**	**412**	**535**	**597**	**33.65**	**44.51**	**55.32**	**64.4%**
Indonesia	234.3	275.9	274.8	17.3%	1905	735	123	145	144	319	375	374	54.24	60.29	62.8	15.8%
Philippines	90.95	125.2	138.4	52.2%	300	116	303	417	461	785	1081	1195	69.39	73.36	76.17	9.8%
Viet Nam	88.6	108.7	112.1	26.5%	332	128	267	328	338	692	849	875	30.34	42.25	52.58	73.3%
Thailand	66.16	70.04	65.69	-0.7%	513	198	129	137	128	334	354	332	37.14	50.24	60.1	61.8%
Myanmar	52.96	61.81	61.38	15.9%	677	261	78	91	91	203	237	235	31.22	36.85	42.99	37.7%
Malaysia	27.47	35.77	39.15	42.5%	330	127	83	108	119	216	281	308	76.09	82.59	82.92	9.0%
Cambodia	15.47	22.94	27.61	78.5%	181	70	85	127	153	221	328	395	24.62	37.84	48.85	98.4%
LAO People's Dem Repub	6.569	10.15	12.34	87.9%	237	91	28	43	52	72	111	135	33.28	45.32	55.04	65.4%
Singapore	4.64	5.325	5.225	12.6%	0.62	0.24	7484	8589	8427	19414	22280	21862	100	99.84	100	0.0%
Timor-Leste	1.264	2.859	5.111	304.4%	14.87	5.74	85	192	344	220	498	890	25.28	33.82	43.84	73.4%
Brunei Darussalam	0.414	0.557	0.614	48.3%	5.77	2.23	72	97	106	186	250	276	77.5	83.38	85.87	10.8%
Asia-South East	**588.8**	**719.2**	**742.4**	**26.1%**	**4495**	**1735**	**131**	**160**	**165**	**339**	**414**	**428**	**49.31**	**57.23**	**62.44**	**26.6%**

Population, Land Area, and Human Development Index

Base Case: Countries in Year 2060 Descending Population Sequence	Population (Total in Millions)				Land Area		Population Density (Persons per Sq Km)			Population Density (Persons per Sq Mi)			Urban Population (Percent of Total Population)			
	2010	2035	2060	% Chg	Sq Km (000s)	Sq Mi (000s)	2010	2035	2060	2010	2035	2060	2010	2035	2060	% Chg
ASIA with OCEANIA continued																
Turkey	76.53	91.08	92.07	20.3%	775	299	99	118	119	256	304	308	69.4	72.51	76.02	9.5%
Yemen	24.44	46.8	68.6	180.7%	528	204	46	89	130	120	230	336	34	44.45	52.18	53.5%
Iraq	29.72	48.57	60.78	104.5%	438	169	68	111	139	176	287	359	65.73	70.32	75.3	14.6%
Saudi Arabia	25.86	39.2	46.65	80.4%	2150	830	12	18	22	31	47	56	82.65	83.89	85.57	3.5%
Syrian Arab Repub	21.54	34.1	42.25	96.1%	185	72	116	184	228	301	477	591	54.76	57.47	61.33	12.0%
Israel	7.639	10.2	12.03	57.5%	21.06	8.13	363	484	571	939	1254	1480	93.02	93.2	93.21	0.2%
Jordan	6.147	9.152	10.77	75.2%	89	34	69	103	121	178	266	313	81.67	84.88	86.43	5.8%
Occupied Palestinian Territory	4.185	7.64	10.35	147.3%	0.38	0.15	11013	20105	27237	28469	51973	70408	71.93	75.2	79.15	10.0%
Azerbaijan	8.822	10.28	10.27	16.4%	87	33	102	119	119	264	307	307	51.87	60.08	68.43	31.9%
United Arab Emirates	4.984	6.303	6.318	26.8%	84	32	60	75	76	154	195	196	80.4	89.13	89.08	10.8%
Oman	2.846	4.276	5.053	77.5%	310	120	9	14	16	24	36	42	76.49	81.03	83.81	9.6%
Kuwait	2.848	4.086	4.848	70.2%	17.82	6.88	160	229	272	414	594	705	100	100	100	0.0%
Lebanon	3.818	4.468	4.495	17.7%	10.40	4.02	367	430	432	951	1113	1120	100	99.49	98.54	-1.5%
Armenia	3.104	3.246	3.119	0.5%	30	12	104	109	105	270	282	271	64.35	70	77.65	20.7%
Georgia	4.354	3.594	2.99	-31.3%	70	27	62	52	43	162	134	111	53.65	58.63	65.31	21.7%
Bahrain	0.799	1.063	1.152	44.2%	0.71	0.27	1125	1497	1623	2916	3880	4204	89.75	90.21	90.18	0.5%
Qatar	0.862	1.017	0.928	7.7%	11.00	4.25	78	92	84	203	239	219	100	99.64	98.72	-1.3%
Cyprus	0.777	0.802	0.722	-7.1%	9.25	3.57	84	87	78	218	225	202	80	83.82	85.94	7.4%
Asia-West	**229.3**	**325.9**	**383.4**	**67.2%**	**4815**	**1859**	**48**	**68**	**80**	**123**	**175**	**206**	**66.83**	**69.75**	**72.83**	**9.0%**
Australia	21.37	25.66	28.46	33.2%	7741	2989	3	3	4	7	9	10	89.37	90.33	90.95	1.8%
Papua New Guinea	6.579	10.4	13.38	103.4%	463	179	14	22	29	37	58	75	15.51	29.83	42.01	170.9%
New Zealand	4.26	4.781	4.846	13.8%	271	105	16	18	18	41	46	46	87.56	88.41	89.05	1.7%
Solomon Islands	0.54	0.906	1.26	133.3%	29	11	19	31	44	48	81	113	20.48	33.36	43.24	111.1%
Fiji	0.883	0.967	0.873	-1.1%	18.27	7.05	48	53	48	125	137	124	52.7	56.69	61.28	16.3%
Vanuatu	0.237	0.378	0.471	98.7%	12.19	4.71	19	31	39	50	80	100	28.19	42.09	53.14	88.5%
Micronesia, Federated States of	0.123	0.203	0.264	114.6%	5.80	2.24	21	35	46	55	91	118	24.37	39.33	52	113.4%
Tonga	0.115	0.188	0.257	123.5%	0.75	0.29	153	251	343	397	648	886	25.88	38.84	50.01	93.2%
Samoa	0.189	0.233	0.229	21.2%	2.84	1.10	67	82	81	172	212	209	25.97	42.3	55.12	112.2%
Oceania	**34.3**	**43.71**	**50.04**	**45.9%**	**8543**	**3299**	**4**	**5**	**6**	**10**	**13**	**15**	**71.73**	**72.67**	**75.03**	**4.6%**

Population, Land Area, and Human Development Index

Base Case: Countries in Year 2060 Descending Population Sequence	Population — Total in Millions				Land Area		Population Density						Urban Population — Percent of Total Population			
	2010	2035	2060	% Chg	Sq Km (000s)	Sq Mi (000s)	Persons per Sq Km 2010	2035	2060	Persons per Sq Mi 2010	2035	2060	2010	2035	2060	% Chg
EUROPE																
Russian Federation	140.2	121.5	98.02	-30.1%	17075	6593	8	7	6	21	18	15	74.37	78.34	81.87	10.1%
Poland	38.07	34.72	28.34	-25.6%	313	121	122	111	91	315	288	235	63.03	69.74	76.33	21.1%
Ukraine	45.07	34.72	26.01	-42.3%	604	233	75	58	43	193	149	112	70.07	73.62	77.27	10.3%
Romania	21.42	19.03	15.55	-27.4%	238	92	90	80	65	233	207	169	55.5	63.03	69.96	26.1%
Czech Republic	10.23	9.334	7.779	-24.0%	128	49	80	73	61	207	189	158	74.01	77.27	81.26	9.8%
Belarus	9.594	8.492	7.007	-27.0%	208	80	46	41	34	120	106	87	74.61	79.55	83.63	12.1%
Hungary	9.886	8.473	6.825	-31.0%	93	36	106	91	73	275	236	190	68.13	73.63	78.83	15.7%
Bulgaria	7.45	5.807	4.443	-40.4%	111	43	67	52	40	174	136	104	72.02	74.66	77.93	8.2%
Slovak Republic	5.411	5.103	4.241	-21.6%	49	19	110	104	87	286	270	224	58.39	67.77	75.41	29.1%
Moldova, Repub of	4.171	3.764	3.083	-26.1%	34	13	123	111	91	319	288	236	39.29	44.41	51.21	30.3%
Europe-East	**291.5**	**250.9**	**201.3**	**-30.9%**	**18852**	**7279**	**15**	**13**	**11**	**40**	**34**	**28**	**69.77**	**74.37**	**78.82**	**13.0%**
United Kingdom	61.33	64.73	64.53	5.2%	243	94	252	266	266	654	690	688	89.48	89.57	89.85	0.4%
Sweden	9.128	9.379	9.137	0.1%	450	174	20	21	20	53	54	53	84.8	86.78	88.14	3.9%
Denmark	5.501	5.692	5.649	2.7%	43	17	128	132	131	331	342	339	85.92	87.24	88.61	3.1%
Ireland	4.381	5.165	5.499	25.5%	70	27	62	74	78	161	190	203	63.55	74.1	80.49	26.7%
Norway	4.743	5.217	5.32	12.2%	324	125	15	16	16	38	42	43	79.73	84.65	87.01	9.1%
Finland	5.314	5.337	5.061	-4.8%	338	131	16	16	15	41	41	39	64.66	74.13	80.52	24.5%
Lithuania	3.355	2.967	2.44	-27.3%	65	25	51	46	37	133	118	97	68.39	73.67	79.04	15.6%
Latvia	2.259	1.969	1.633	-27.7%	65	25	35	30	25	91	79	65	69.67	74.65	80.08	14.9%
Estonia	1.295	1.038	0.874	-32.5%	45	17	29	23	19	74	60	50	72.09	77.63	82.28	14.1%
Iceland	0.309	0.344	0.34	10.0%	103	40	3	3	3	8	9	9	92.73	92.57	92.17	-0.6%
Europe-North	**97.61**	**101.8**	**100.5**	**3.0%**	**1746**	**674**	**56**	**58**	**58**	**145**	**151**	**149**	**84.45**	**86.47**	**88.01**	**4.2%**
Italy	58.61	53.51	44.58	-23.9%	301	116	195	178	148	504	460	383	69.03	75.4	80.61	16.8%
Spain	43.98	42.11	35.83	-18.5%	506	195	87	83	71	225	216	183	77.84	81.23	84.26	8.2%
Greece	11.19	10.64	9.367	-16.3%	132	51	85	81	71	220	209	184	63.96	74.17	80.51	25.9%
Portugal	10.6	10.02	8.678	-18.1%	92	36	115	109	94	299	282	244	62.55	71.86	77.39	23.7%
Serbia	7.36	6.724	5.751	-21.9%	102	39	72	66	56	187	170	146	53.53	60.81	67.44	26.0%
Bosnia and Herzegovina	4.063	3.933	3.377	-16.9%	51	20	79	77	66	206	199	171	44.12	53.21	63.92	44.9%
Croatia	4.409	3.949	3.296	-25.2%	57	22	78	70	58	202	181	151	58.57	66.51	73.56	25.6%
Albania	3.188	3.428	3.231	1.3%	29	11	111	119	112	287	309	291	46.79	55.61	64	36.8%
Macedonia, FYR	2.06	2.021	1.76	-14.6%	26	10	80	79	68	208	204	177	67.87	70.08	72.29	6.5%
Slovenia	2.004	1.829	1.484	-25.9%	20.25	7.82	99	90	73	256	234	190	52.42	65.42	75.01	43.1%
Montenegro	0.619	0.625	0.59	-4.7%	7.76	3.00	80	81	76	207	209	197	68.97	74.62	76.41	10.8%
Malta	0.408	0.395	0.338	-17.2%	0.32	0.12	1275	1234	1056	3290	3185	2726	96.11	97.41	96.97	0.9%
Europe-South	**148.5**	**139.2**	**118.3**	**-20.3%**	**1324**	**511**	**112**	**105**	**89**	**291**	**272**	**231**	**68.39**	**74.59**	**79.54**	**16.3%**
Germany	82.59	78.05	69.01	-16.4%	357	138	231	219	193	599	566	501	74.91	80.47	84.49	12.8%
France	62.22	64.55	62.27	0.1%	552	213	113	117	113	292	303	292	77.46	81.3	84.71	9.4%
Netherlands	16.72	17.56	16.99	1.6%	42	16	403	423	409	1043	1095	1060	83.89	87.89	88.94	6.0%
Belgium	10.61	10.68	10.11	-4.7%	31	12	348	350	331	901	907	858	97.13	96.72	96.68	-0.5%
Austria	8.263	7.847	6.696	-19.0%	84	32	99	94	80	255	242	207	68.8	76.9	81.99	19.2%
Switzerland	7.504	7.237	6.17	-17.8%	41	16	182	175	149	471	454	387	75.48	81.32	84.63	12.1%
Luxembourg	0.484	0.609	0.73	50.8%	2.59	1.00	187	235	282	484	609	730	85.69	88.69	90.41	5.5%
Europe-West	**188.4**	**186.5**	**172**	**-8.7%**	**1108**	**428**	**170**	**168**	**155**	**440**	**436**	**402**	**77.58**	**82.3**	**85.66**	**10.4%**

Population, Land Area, and Human Development Index

Base Case
Source: *International Futures*
Version 6.32, June 2010

	Population Growth Rate (Annual Percent)			Total Fertility Rate (Births per Woman)				Population Below 15 Years of Age (Number in Millions)				Population 65 Years and Older (Number in Millions)			
	2010	2035	2060	2010	2035	2060	% Chg	2010	2035	2060	% Chg	2010	2035	2060	% Chg
World	1.132	0.619	0.199	2.495	2.158	1.959	-21.5%	1815	1854	1791	-1.3%	526.5	1127	1792	240.4%
Africa	2.333	1.781	1.04	4.606	3.283	2.389	-48.1%	401.7	571.7	641.6	59.7%	34.93	82.29	207.5	494.0%
Americas	1.071	0.497	0.088	2.089	1.838	1.805	-13.6%	230.4	212.7	194.2	-15.7%	86.61	191.4	292.3	237.5%
Asia with Oceania	1.07	0.389	-0.074	2.258	1.93	1.829	-19.0%	1072	981.1	879	-18.0%	285.8	679	1104	286.3%
Europe	-0.103	-0.396	-0.627	1.45	1.554	1.651	13.9%	109.3	87.82	75.59	-30.8%	118	172.2	186.6	58.1%
World	1.132	0.619	0.199	2.495	2.158	1.959	-21.5%	1815	1854	1791	-1.3%	526.5	1127	1792	240.4%
Africa-Eastern	2.693	1.988	0.968	5.135	3.351	2.078	-59.5%	138.5	208.6	213.2	53.9%	9.828	22.49	64.49	556.2%
Africa-Middle	2.611	2.274	1.745	5.595	4.238	3.374	-39.7%	55.09	91.15	129.9	135.8%	3.616	7.438	19.93	451.2%
Africa-Northern	1.715	0.774	0.112	2.835	2.01	1.811	-36.1%	64.44	63.44	56.68	-12.0%	9.745	25.84	57.38	488.8%
Africa-Southern	0.74	0.34	0.145	2.712	1.862	1.8	-33.6%	17.62	14.89	12.67	-28.1%	2.571	5.47	10.44	306.1%
Africa-Western	2.559	2.04	1.218	5.206	3.63	2.522	-51.6%	126	193.6	229.2	81.9%	9.167	21.05	55.27	502.9%
Africa	2.333	1.781	1.04	4.606	3.283	2.389	-48.1%	401.7	571.7	641.6	59.7%	34.93	82.29	207.5	494.0%
America-Caribbean	0.98	0.458	0.037	2.357	2.169	2.015	-14.5%	10.34	10.23	9.599	-7.2%	3.379	7.208	10.76	218.4%
America-Central	1.981	1.113	0.378	3.058	2.207	1.8	-41.1%	15.38	16.96	14.79	-3.8%	2.297	5.697	13.12	471.2%
America-North	0.927	0.457	0.165	1.943	1.787	1.792	-7.8%	97.62	91.82	88.12	-9.7%	52.68	107.9	146.2	177.5%
America-South	1.143	0.462	-0.038	2.121	1.812	1.8	-15.1%	107	93.7	81.7	-23.6%	28.25	70.65	122.3	332.9%
Americas	1.071	0.497	0.088	2.089	1.838	1.805	-13.6%	230.4	212.7	194.2	-15.7%	86.61	191.4	292.3	237.5%
Asia-East	0.536	-0.142	-0.551	1.67	1.707	1.743	4.4%	300.7	244.5	212.5	-29.3%	152.9	347.5	448.9	193.6%
Asia-South Central	1.421	0.677	0.162	2.694	2.062	1.883	-30.1%	531.1	502.7	460.2	-13.3%	83.11	203.3	428.7	415.8%
Asia-South East	1.189	0.411	-0.131	2.27	1.883	1.808	-20.4%	160.1	145.4	125	-21.9%	34.94	89.14	151.3	333.0%
Asia-West	1.807	1.011	0.329	3	2.245	1.856	-38.1%	72.1	79.51	72.4	0.4%	11.02	31.3	64.28	483.3%
Oceania	1.179	0.743	0.394	2.272	2.046	1.843	-18.9%	8.104	8.933	8.856	9.3%	3.836	7.792	10.65	177.6%
Asia with Oceania	1.07	0.389	-0.074	2.258	1.93	1.829	-19.0%	1072	981.1	879	-18.0%	285.8	679	1104	286.3%
Europe-East	-0.424	-0.721	-1.009	1.304	1.437	1.569	20.3%	42.53	30.72	24.34	-42.8%	40.48	56.48	66.25	63.7%
Europe-North	0.27	0.051	-0.115	1.754	1.77	1.783	1.7%	16.71	15.77	14.84	-11.2%	16.37	25.26	28.77	75.7%
Europe-South	0.007	-0.421	-0.814	1.383	1.495	1.606	16.1%	21.97	16.62	14.03	-36.1%	27.41	39.35	40.46	47.6%
Europe-West	0.127	-0.193	-0.362	1.568	1.636	1.7	8.4%	29.44	25.83	23.25	-21.0%	34.89	52.79	53.26	52.7%
Europe	-0.103	-0.396	-0.627	1.45	1.554	1.651	13.9%	109.3	87.82	75.59	-30.8%	118	172.2	186.6	58.1%

Multination Regional Analysis

Population, Land Area, and Human Development Index

Base Case: Countries in Year 2060 Descending Population Sequence	Population Growth Rate (Annual Percent)			Total Fertility Rate (Births per Woman)				Population Below 15 Years of Age (Number in Millions)				Population 65 Years and Older (Number in Millions)			
	2010	2035	2060	2010	2035	2060	% Chg	2010	2035	2060	% Chg	2010	2035	2060	% Chg
AFRICA															
Ethiopia	2.711	2.035	0.951	5.288	3.437	2.017	-61.9%	34.82	54.66	56.63	62.6%	2.643	5.722	14.97	466.4%
Tanzania, United Rep	2.837	1.875	0.83	5.166	2.941	1.8	-65.2%	19.48	27.64	24	23.2%	1.412	3.284	9.713	587.9%
Uganda	3.276	2.343	0.962	6.031	3.549	1.8	-70.2%	16.31	27.01	26.15	60.3%	0.876	1.856	7.167	718.2%
Kenya	2.616	1.77	0.736	4.649	2.979	1.8	-61.3%	16.44	22.52	19.78	20.3%	1.047	3.178	9.563	813.4%
Madagascar	2.744	2.179	1.382	4.805	3.664	2.632	-45.2%	9.026	14.6	18.29	102.6%	0.657	1.787	4.364	564.2%
Mozambique	2.436	1.741	0.696	4.973	3.044	1.8	-63.8%	9.677	13.3	12.03	24.3%	0.73	1.495	3.833	425.1%
Malawi	2.803	2.237	1.213	5.385	3.673	2.357	-56.2%	6.727	10.69	12.41	84.5%	0.459	1.05	2.829	516.3%
Zambia	2.522	2.105	1.093	5.597	3.633	2.148	-61.6%	5.986	9.037	9.537	59.3%	0.407	0.756	2.422	495.1%
Somalia	2.668	2.325	1.675	5.886	4.385	3.322	-43.6%	4.132	6.858	9.728	135.4%	0.26	0.651	1.492	473.8%
Rwanda	2.708	1.752	0.68	5.36	3.309	1.837	-65.7%	4.338	6.273	6.024	38.9%	0.257	0.628	1.886	633.9%
Zimbabwe	1.64	1.12	0.256	3.367	2.5	1.8	-46.5%	5.296	5.929	5.049	-4.7%	0.557	0.835	3.043	446.3%
Burundi	2.38	1.973	1.346	4.836	3.965	3.003	-37.9%	3.258	5.34	7.178	120.3%	0.242	0.596	1.638	576.9%
Eritrea	3.087	2.357	1.658	5.037	4.085	3.182	-36.8%	2.176	3.705	5.35	145.9%	0.133	0.282	0.935	603.0%
Comoros	2.863	2.133	1.413	4.479	3.811	2.838	-36.6%	0.27	0.436	0.584	116.3%	0.021	0.062	0.147	600.0%
Mauritius	0.59	0.063	-0.274	1.8	1.8	1.8	0.0%	0.286	0.251	0.216	-24.5%	0.098	0.248	0.344	251.0%
Djibouti	1.209	0.688	-0.147	4.006	3.074	1.828	-54.4%	0.303	0.345	0.266	-12.2%	0.028	0.063	0.138	392.9%
Africa-Eastern	**2.693**	**1.988**	**0.968**	**5.135**	**3.351**	**2.078**	**-59.5%**	**138.5**	**208.6**	**213.2**	**53.9%**	**9.828**	**22.49**	**64.49**	**556.2%**
Congo, Democratic Republic of	2.791	2.549	2.083	6.051	4.745	3.844	-36.5%	30.43	54.54	86.65	184.8%	1.755	3.321	8.683	394.8%
Angola	2.557	1.923	0.982	5.564	3.355	2.201	-60.4%	8.02	11.78	12.37	54.2%	0.454	1.222	3.553	682.6%
Cameroon	2.176	1.663	0.854	4.358	3.18	2.16	-50.4%	7.24	9.875	10.32	42.5%	0.655	1.347	3.658	458.5%
Chad	2.943	2.544	2.097	6.216	4.769	3.859	-37.9%	5.047	9.166	14.26	182.5%	0.322	0.679	1.862	478.3%
Central African Republic	1.731	1.716	1.206	4.618	3.782	2.832	-38.7%	1.738	2.426	2.978	71.3%	0.171	0.3	0.69	303.5%
Congo, Republic of	2.23	1.542	0.719	4.318	2.961	2.083	-51.8%	1.772	2.309	2.285	29.0%	0.169	0.333	0.937	454.4%
Gabon	2.058	1.286	0.508	3.382	2.529	1.83	-45.9%	0.545	0.657	0.6	10.1%	0.067	0.163	0.397	492.5%
Equatorial Guinea	2.039	1.337	0.62	5.028	3.181	2.11	-58.0%	0.226	0.286	0.265	17.3%	0.016	0.059	0.103	543.8%
São Tomé and Principe	2.657	1.986	1.304	3.969	3.37	2.781	-29.9%	0.07	0.105	0.135	92.9%	0.007	0.014	0.045	542.9%
Africa-Middle	**2.611**	**2.274**	**1.745**	**5.595**	**4.238**	**3.374**	**-39.7%**	**55.09**	**91.15**	**129.9**	**135.8%**	**3.616**	**7.438**	**19.93**	**451.2%**
Egypt	1.794	0.721	0.113	2.737	1.8	1.8	-34.2%	25.98	23.33	20.63	-20.6%	3.812	9.908	22.95	502.0%
Sudan	2.2	1.373	0.494	4.19	2.722	1.844	-56.0%	15.57	19.5	17.58	12.9%	1.499	3.548	8.804	487.3%
Algeria	1.493	0.506	-0.211	2.29	1.8	1.8	-21.4%	9.521	8.541	7.712	-19.0%	1.675	5.153	11.2	568.7%
Morocco	1.351	0.432	-0.13	2.329	1.8	1.8	-22.7%	8.979	8.148	7.161	-20.2%	1.754	4.519	8.917	408.4%
Tunisia	1.009	0.305	-0.262	1.899	1.8	1.8	-5.2%	2.452	2.242	1.975	-19.5%	0.717	1.8	3.439	379.6%
Libyan Arab Jamahiriya	1.89	0.731	0.063	2.631	1.8	1.8	-31.6%	1.941	1.684	1.626	-16.2%	0.288	0.915	2.073	619.8%
Africa-Northern	**1.715**	**0.774**	**0.112**	**2.835**	**2.01**	**1.811**	**-36.1%**	**64.44**	**63.44**	**56.68**	**-12.0%**	**9.745**	**25.84**	**57.38**	**488.8%**

Population, Land Area, and Human Development Index

Base Case: Countries in Year 2060 Descending Population Sequence	Population Growth Rate (Annual Percent)			Total Fertility Rate (Births per Woman)				Population Below 15 Years of Age (Number in Millions)				Population 65 Years and Older (Number in Millions)			
	2010	2035	2060	2010	2035	2060	% Chg	2010	2035	2060	% Chg	2010	2035	2060	% Chg
AFRICA continued															
South Africa	0.622	0.24	0.125	2.629	1.8	1.8	-31.5%	15	12.23	10.53	-29.8%	2.284	4.844	8.719	281.7%
Namibia	2.074	1.207	0.531	3.445	2.295	1.8	-47.8%	0.814	0.936	0.786	-3.4%	0.085	0.242	0.637	649.4%
Lesotho	1.116	0.664	-0.036	3.34	2.264	1.8	-46.1%	0.719	0.698	0.511	-28.9%	0.086	0.099	0.321	273.3%
Botswana	1.339	0.576	0.062	2.8	1.8	1.8	-35.7%	0.618	0.531	0.454	-26.5%	0.076	0.2	0.519	582.9%
Swaziland	1.529	0.935	0.26	3.581	2.453	1.8	-49.7%	0.466	0.499	0.383	-17.8%	0.041	0.085	0.248	504.9%
Africa-Southern	**0.74**	**0.34**	**0.145**	**2.712**	**1.862**	**1.8**	**-33.6%**	**17.62**	**14.89**	**12.67**	**-28.1%**	**2.571**	**5.47**	**10.44**	**306.1%**
Nigeria	2.435	1.867	1.077	5.151	3.354	2.409	-53.2%	62.17	89.44	99.73	60.4%	4.709	10.46	27.77	489.7%
Niger	3.393	2.993	2.076	6.791	4.913	3.338	-50.8%	7.971	15.86	24.93	212.8%	0.351	0.951	2.538	623.1%
Côte d'Ivoire	2.582	2.02	1.178	4.688	3.491	2.345	-50.0%	8.226	12.7	14.53	76.6%	0.803	1.727	4.644	478.3%
Ghana	2.111	1.57	0.761	4.19	3.257	2.143	-48.9%	9.331	12.75	13.07	40.1%	0.91	2.193	5.118	462.4%
Mali	3.005	2.436	1.288	6.217	4.164	2.556	-58.9%	7.068	12.54	15.49	119.2%	0.359	0.806	2.227	520.3%
Burkina Faso	3.03	2.395	1.357	6.029	4.319	2.595	-57.0%	6.924	11.98	15.08	117.8%	0.32	0.858	2.414	654.4%
Senegal	2.665	2.002	0.993	5.001	3.638	2.262	-54.8%	5.682	8.789	9.642	69.7%	0.325	0.717	2.171	568.0%
Guinea	2.27	2.318	1.526	5.397	3.912	2.757	-48.9%	4.457	7.371	9.535	113.9%	0.348	0.823	2.077	496.8%
Benin	2.929	2.282	1.431	5.335	3.831	2.696	-49.5%	4.172	6.888	8.78	110.5%	0.325	0.839	2.135	556.9%
Togo	2.601	1.968	1.423	4.345	3.469	2.91	-33.0%	2.757	4.281	5.516	100.1%	0.25	0.647	1.721	588.4%
Sierra Leone	2.383	1.916	0.879	5.059	3.523	2.07	-59.1%	2.686	4.032	4.273	59.1%	0.119	0.21	0.506	325.2%
Liberia	2.75	1.905	0.851	5.051	3.246	1.944	-61.5%	1.59	2.401	2.396	50.7%	0.119	0.273	0.626	426.1%
Mauritania	2.281	1.879	1.379	4.419	3.751	3.016	-31.7%	1.338	1.97	2.615	95.4%	0.093	0.244	0.602	547.3%
Guinea-Bissau	2.422	2.492	2.11	5.551	4.52	3.841	-30.8%	0.752	1.304	2.131	183.4%	0.063	0.125	0.31	392.1%
Gambia	2.565	2.02	1.122	4.968	3.53	2.336	-53.0%	0.726	1.127	1.275	75.6%	0.051	0.114	0.26	409.8%
Cape Verde	1.852	0.815	0.111	2.821	1.925	1.8	-36.2%	0.196	0.195	0.159	-18.9%	0.022	0.06	0.156	609.1%
Africa-Western	**2.559**	**2.04**	**1.218**	**5.206**	**3.63**	**2.522**	**-51.6%**	**126**	**193.6**	**229.2**	**81.9%**	**9.167**	**21.05**	**55.27**	**502.9%**

Population, Land Area, and Human Development Index

Base Case: Countries in Year 2060 Descending Population Sequence	Population Growth Rate (Annual Percent)			Total Fertility Rate (Births per Woman)				Population Below 15 Years of Age (Number in Millions)				Population 65 Years and Older (Number in Millions)			
	2010	2035	2060	2010	2035	2060	% Chg	2010	2035	2060	% Chg	2010	2035	2060	% Chg
AMERICAS															
Haiti	1.872	1.326	0.715	3.823	3.205	2.462	-35.6%	3.376	4.478	4.804	42.3%	0.404	0.779	1.816	349.5%
Dominican Republic	1.266	0.491	-0.08	2.265	1.8	1.8	-20.5%	2.848	2.365	1.97	-30.8%	0.594	1.522	2.967	399.5%
Cuba	0.255	-0.343	-0.792	1.561	1.625	1.688	8.1%	1.995	1.549	1.257	-37.0%	1.431	3.066	3.363	135.0%
Puerto Rico	0.637	0.175	-0.091	1.776	1.782	1.789	0.7%	0.811	0.745	0.684	-15.7%	0.561	0.955	1.255	123.7%
Jamaica	0.827	0.22	-0.307	2.393	1.8	1.8	-24.8%	0.794	0.679	0.541	-31.9%	0.213	0.454	0.712	234.3%
Trinidad	0.451	-0.286	-0.619	1.636	1.679	1.723	5.3%	0.274	0.217	0.172	-37.2%	0.095	0.237	0.356	274.7%
Bahamas	0.989	0.337	-0.108	1.948	1.8	1.8	-7.6%	0.085	0.074	0.065	-23.5%	0.025	0.066	0.104	316.0%
Barbados	0.257	-0.476	-0.761	1.532	.603	1.675	9.3%	0.047	0.037	0.03	-36.2%	0.029	0.069	0.073	151.7%
Grenada	1.427	0.638	0.043	2.247	1.8	1.8	-19.9%	0.031	0.03	0.027	-12.9%	0.008	0.015	0.038	375.0%
Saint Vincent and Grenadines	1.074	0.419	-0.13	2.032	1.8	1.8	-11.4%	0.033	0.029	0.025	-24.2%	0.008	0.02	0.035	337.5%
Saint Lucia	0.432	-0.308	-0.518	1.933	1.8	1.8	-6.9%	0.044	0.033	0.024	-45.5%	0.012	0.026	0.042	250.0%
America-Caribbean	**0.98**	**0.458**	**0.037**	**2.357**	**2.169**	**2.015**	**-14.5%**	**10.34**	**10.23**	**9.599**	**-7.2%**	**3.379**	**7.208**	**10.76**	**218.4%**
Guatemala	2.607	1.656	0.696	4.039	2.665	1.8	-55.4%	5.943	7.852	7.06	18.8%	0.629	1.468	4.106	552.8%
Honduras	2.104	1.093	0.359	3.069	2.08	1.8	-41.3%	2.912	3.091	2.592	-11.0%	0.345	0.923	2.437	606.4%
El Salvador	1.3	0.514	-0.019	2.338	1.8	1.8	-23.0%	2.274	1.995	1.692	-25.6%	0.518	1.037	2.113	307.9%
Nicaragua	1.973	0.937	0.231	2.734	1.984	1.8	-34.2%	1.938	2.005	1.699	-12.3%	0.252	0.666	1.682	567.5%
Costa Rica	1.415	0.505	-0.074	2.027	1.8	1.8	-11.2%	1.199	1.06	0.932	-22.3%	0.304	0.935	1.631	436.5%
Panama	1.328	0.511	-0.079	2.415	1.8	1.8	-25.5%	1.004	0.841	0.724	-27.9%	0.234	0.623	1.046	347.0%
Belize	1.971	0.947	0.211	2.964	2.067	1.8	-39.3%	0.112	0.118	0.096	-14.3%	0.013	0.045	0.105	707.7%
America-Central	**1.981**	**1.113**	**0.378**	**3.058**	**2.207**	**1.8**	**-41.1%**	**15.38**	**16.96**	**14.79**	**-3.8%**	**2.297**	**5.697**	**13.12**	**471.2%**
USA	0.903	0.534	0.336	1.935	1.8	1.8	-7.0%	61.89	61.74	62.79	1.5%	40.77	79.97	102.2	150.7%
Mexico	1.046	0.271	-0.395	2.086	1.8	1.8	-13.7%	30.35	24.54	19.53	-35.7%	7.092	18.22	32.52	358.5%
Canada	0.765	0.351	0.227	1.556	1.621	1.686	8.4%	5.38	5.545	5.794	7.7%	4.823	9.707	11.46	137.6%
America-North	**0.927**	**0.457**	**0.165**	**1.943**	**1.787**	**1.792**	**-7.8%**	**97.62**	**91.82**	**88.12**	**-9.7%**	**52.68**	**107.9**	**146.2**	**177.5%**
Brazil	0.984	0.374	-0.101	1.898	1.8	1.8	-5.2%	50.58	43.31	37.52	-25.8%	13.72	36.31	61.85	350.8%
Colombia	1.324	0.481	-0.082	2.23	1.8	1.8	-19.3%	13.9	11.86	10.38	-25.3%	2.783	8.424	14.34	415.3%
Argentina	0.899	0.398	-0.012	2.099	1.8	1.8	-14.2%	10.05	8.801	7.783	-22.6%	4.386	7.253	12.01	173.8%
Peru	1.489	0.65	0.054	2.45	1.8	1.8	-26.5%	8.938	7.699	6.837	-23.5%	1.814	4.792	9.673	433.2%
Venezuela	1.558	0.615	0.042	2.474	1.8	1.8	-27.2%	8.506	7.556	6.709	-21.1%	1.64	4.764	8.676	429.0%
Ecuador	1.568	0.672	0.105	2.521	1.821	1.8	-28.6%	4.328	4.063	3.524	-18.6%	0.928	2.366	4.512	386.2%
Chile	0.844	0.249	-0.177	1.852	1.8	1.8	-2.8%	3.781	3.44	3.019	-20.2%	1.595	3.872	5.495	244.5%
Bolivia	1.932	0.992	0.343	3.395	2.045	1.8	-47.0%	3.622	3.802	3.233	-10.7%	0.479	1.128	2.585	439.7%
Paraguay	1.905	0.917	0.306	2.997	1.988	1.8	-39.9%	2.173	2.254	1.937	-10.9%	0.335	0.866	1.914	471.3%
Uruguay	0.375	0.132	-0.2	1.885	1.8	1.8	-4.5%	0.783	0.675	0.575	-26.6%	0.493	0.696	0.992	101.2%
Guyana	-0.074	-0.599	-0.491	2.253	1.8	1.8	-20.1%	0.219	0.143	0.103	-53.0%	0.047	0.109	0.129	174.5%
Suriname	0.323	-0.377	-0.517	2.359	1.8	1.8	-23.7%	0.133	0.095	0.067	-49.6%	0.03	0.068	0.092	206.7%
America-South	**1.143**	**0.462**	**-0.038**	**2.121**	**1.812**	**1.8**	**-15.1%**	**107**	**93.7**	**81.7**	**-23.6%**	**28.25**	**70.65**	**122.3**	**332.9%**

Population, Land Area, and Human Development Index

Base Case: Countries in Year 2060 Descending Population Sequence	Population Growth Rate (Annual Percent)			Total Fertility Rate (Births per Woman)				Population Below 15 Years of Age (Number in Millions)				Population 65 Years and Older (Number in Millions)			
	2010	2035	2060	2010	2035	2060	% Chg	2010	2035	2060	% Chg	2010	2035	2060	% Chg
ASIA with OCEANIA															
China	0.603	-0.09	-0.515	1.72	1.741	1.763	2.5%	264.6	217.1	190.1	-28.2%	113	285.4	383.3	239.2%
Japan	-0.126	-0.713	-0.905	1.292	1.427	1.562	20.9%	16.92	12.21	9.705	-42.6%	29.01	36.91	36.21	24.8%
Korea, Repub of	0.21	-0.602	-1.282	1.123	1.303	1.483	32.1%	7.764	5.233	3.753	-51.7%	5.483	13.12	14.28	160.4%
Taiwan	1.041	0.164	-0.4	2.039	1.8	1.8	-11.7%	4.994	4.244	3.854	-22.8%	2.08	5.555	6.991	236.1%
Korea, Dem. People's Rep.	0.309	-0.126	-0.41	1.809	1.8	1.8	-0.5%	4.834	4.237	3.637	-24.8%	2.302	3.828	4.842	110.3%
Hong Kong SAR	0.887	0.175	-0.138	1.048	1.248	1.448	38.2%	0.883	0.856	0.921	4.3%	0.933	2.367	2.608	179.5%
Mongolia	0.933	0.275	-0.156	1.8	1.8	1.8	0.0%	0.671	0.638	0.575	-14.3%	0.112	0.333	0.717	540.2%
Asia-East	**0.536**	**-0.142**	**-0.551**	**1.67**	**1.707**	**1.743**	**4.4%**	**300.7**	**244.5**	**212.5**	**-29.3%**	**152.9**	**347.5**	**448.9**	**193.6%**
India	1.262	0.472	0.005	2.494	1.8	1.8	-27.8%	353.6	296.3	257.1	-27.3%	59.3	143.2	293.4	394.8%
Pakistan	2.215	1.534	0.796	3.964	3.117	2.184	-44.9%	62.98	86.55	91.05	44.6%	7.281	17.36	43.79	501.4%
Bangladesh	1.528	0.54	-0.081	2.421	1.818	1.8	-25.7%	47.85	43.83	37.21	-22.2%	6.169	16.33	35.35	473.0%
Afghanistan	3.281	2.31	1.216	6.675	4.224	2.254	-66.2%	16.08	27.91	31.76	97.5%	0.833	1.803	5.424	551.1%
Iran (Islamic Republic of)	1.278	0.491	-0.285	1.897	1.8	1.8	-5.1%	17.77	16.07	14.4	-19.0%	3.531	9.969	23.33	560.7%
Nepal	1.862	1.202	0.468	3.06	2.57	1.982	-35.2%	10.67	12.65	12.19	14.2%	1.247	2.789	6.556	425.7%
Uzbekistan	1.35	0.437	-0.174	2.206	1.8	1.8	-18.4%	7.973	6.918	5.987	-24.9%	1.238	3.468	7.522	507.6%
Sri Lanka	0.639	-0.042	-0.434	1.816	1.8	1.8	-0.9%	4.673	3.911	3.228	-30.9%	1.618	4.008	5.224	222.9%
Kazakhstan	-0.034	-0.343	-0.744	2.004	1.8	1.8	-10.2%	3.525	2.685	2.02	-42.7%	1.102	2.16	3.136	184.6%
Tajikistan	1.696	1.084	0.227	3.364	2.435	1.8	-46.5%	2.531	2.512	2.508	-0.9%	0.249	0.699	1.688	577.9%
Turkmenistan	1.419	0.673	0.053	2.336	1.8	1.8	-22.9%	1.506	1.319	1.176	-21.9%	0.218	0.719	1.636	650.5%
Kyrgyzstan	1.321	0.4	-0.188	2.347	1.8	1.8	-23.3%	1.568	1.405	1.214	-22.6%	0.275	0.664	1.289	368.7%
Bhutan	1.692	0.861	0.279	2.838	2.042	1.8	-36.6%	0.212	0.229	0.196	-7.5%	0.034	0.08	0.211	520.6%
Maldives	1.945	0.707	0.058	2.585	1.803	1.8	-30.4%	0.104	0.11	0.101	-2.9%	0.016	0.041	0.115	618.8%
Asia-South Central	**1.421**	**0.677**	**0.162**	**2.694**	**2.062**	**1.883**	**-30.1%**	**531.1**	**502.7**	**460.2**	**-13.3%**	**83.11**	**203.3**	**428.7**	**415.8%**
Indonesia	1.083	0.293	-0.283	2.12	1.8	1.8	-15.1%	62.44	51.98	44.38	-28.9%	14.5	35.1	58.34	302.3%
Philippines	1.732	0.742	0.083	3.006	2.032	1.8	-40.1%	30.28	30.83	24.99	-17.5%	3.963	10.96	23.01	480.6%
Viet Nam	1.198	0.42	-0.157	2.041	1.8	1.8	-11.8%	22.72	20.54	17.86	-21.4%	5.632	14.88	26.52	370.9%
Thailand	0.512	-0.088	-0.358	1.8	1.8	1.8	0.0%	14.18	12.34	10.71	-24.5%	5.186	12.63	15.27	194.4%
Myanmar	0.942	0.254	-0.292	2.04	1.8	1.8	-11.8%	13.61	11.72	10.21	-25.0%	2.969	7.358	12.48	320.3%
Malaysia	1.537	0.611	0.085	2.535	1.8	1.8	-29.0%	8.017	7.262	6.543	-18.4%	1.372	4.462	8.092	489.8%
Cambodia	1.976	1.062	0.365	3.274	2.368	1.8	-45.0%	5.126	6.199	5.495	7.2%	0.562	1.503	3.827	581.0%
LAO People's Dem Repub	2.103	1.183	0.446	3.481	2.309	1.8	-48.3%	2.401	2.807	2.378	-1.0%	0.242	0.599	1.638	576.9%
Singapore	1.097	0.137	-0.098	1.292	1.427	1.562	20.9%	0.727	0.694	0.65	-10.6%	0.464	1.479	1.698	265.9%
Timor-Leste	4.865	2.671	1.821	6.675	4.75	3.171	-52.5%	0.544	1.154	1.699	212.3%	0.039	0.099	0.276	607.7%
Brunei Darussalam	1.87	0.787	0.113	2.259	1.8	1.8	-20.3%	0.116	0.102	0.099	-14.7%	0.015	0.075	0.129	760.0%
Asia-South East	**1.189**	**0.411**	**-0.131**	**2.27**	**1.883**	**1.808**	**-20.4%**	**160.1**	**145.4**	**125**	**-21.9%**	**34.94**	**89.14**	**151.3**	**333.0%**

Population, Land Area, and Human Development Index

Base Case: Countries in Year 2060 Descending Population Sequence	Population Growth Rate (Annual Percent)			Total Fertility Rate (Births per Woman)				Population Below 15 Years of Age (Number in Millions)				Population 65 Years and Older (Number in Millions)			
	2010	2035	2060	2010	2025	2060	% Chg	2010	2035	2060	% Chg	2010	2035	2060	% Chg
ASIA with OCEANIA continued															
Turkey	1.08	0.353	-0.242	2.056	1.8	1.8	-12.5%	20.17	16.97	14.44	-28.4%	4.631	11.8	21.24	358.6%
Yemen	3.104	2.017	0.98	5.338	3.357	2.125	-60.2%	10.57	16.48	17.48	65.4%	0.597	1.696	5.528	826.0%
Iraq	2.474	1.397	0.525	3.99	2.439	1.8	-54.9%	11.87	14.24	12.01	1.2%	0.97	2.713	7.372	660.0%
Saudi Arabia	2.184	1.108	0.425	3.336	2.16	1.8	-46.0%	8.408	9.551	8.462	0.6%	0.765	3.696	7.619	895.9%
Syrian Arab Repub	2.412	1.32	0.441	3.244	2.361	1.8	-44.5%	7.629	9.018	7.997	4.8%	0.715	2.349	6.48	806.3%
Israel	1.787	0.897	0.468	2.639	1.8	1.8	-31.8%	2.09	1.944	1.935	-7.4%	0.766	1.555	2.659	247.1%
Jordan	2.219	0.972	0.332	3.293	1.973	1.8	-45.3%	2.17	2.244	1.946	-10.3%	0.235	0.677	1.841	683.4%
Occupied Palestinian Territory	2.843	1.766	0.85	4.218	2.57	1.8	-57.3%	1.801	2.397	2.071	15.0%	0.127	0.403	1.163	815.7%
Azerbaijan	0.948	0.253	-0.294	1.835	1.8	1.8	-1.9%	2.037	1.792	1.555	-23.7%	0.596	1.635	2.737	359.2%
United Arab Emirates	1.682	0.549	-0.405	2.25	1.8	1.8	-20.0%	1.016	0.906	0.893	-12.1%	0.074	1.117	1.908	2478.4%
Oman	2.096	1.039	0.372	3.194	2.232	1.8	-43.6%	0.889	1.036	0.91	2.4%	0.09	0.425	0.908	908.9%
Kuwait	2.134	1.126	0.466	2.139	1.8	1.8	-15.8%	0.665	0.684	0.774	16.4%	0.073	0.656	1.105	1413.7%
Lebanon	1.118	0.289	-0.245	2.107	1.8	1.8	-14.6%	0.978	0.834	0.713	-27.1%	0.279	0.607	1.05	276.3%
Armenia	0.555	0.006	-0.315	1.734	1.751	1.769	2.0%	0.621	0.516	0.444	-28.5%	0.34	0.593	0.915	169.1%
Georgia	-0.658	-0.612	-0.84	1.457	1.548	1.64	12.6%	0.698	0.459	0.377	-46.0%	0.61	0.816	0.955	56.6%
Bahrain	1.725	0.735	0.139	2.183	1.8	1.8	-17.5%	0.201	0.188	0.183	-9.0%	0.023	0.163	0.261	1034.8%
Qatar	1.065	0.258	-0.77	2.355	1.8	1.8	-23.6%	0.157	0.138	0.13	-17.2%	0.017	0.21	0.289	1600.0%
Cyprus	0.423	-0.224	-0.601	1.443	1.538	1.633	13.2%	0.134	0.109	0.089	-33.6%	0.106	0.196	0.25	135.8%
Asia-West	**1.807**	**1.011**	**0.329**	**3**	**2.245**	**1.856**	**-38.1%**	**72.1**	**79.51**	**72.4**	**0.4%**	**11.02**	**31.3**	**64.28**	**483.3%**
Australia	0.955	0.562	0.384	1.792	1.794	1.796	0.2%	3.97	4.172	4.38	10.3%	3.013	5.902	7.584	151.7%
Papua New Guinea	2.152	1.387	0.59	3.758	2.641	1.914	-49.1%	2.555	3.157	3.023	18.3%	0.173	0.568	1.293	647.4%
New Zealand	0.654	0.233	-0.036	1.859	1.8	1.8	-3.2%	0.849	0.794	0.732	-13.8%	0.561	1.107	1.331	137.3%
Solomon Islands	2.398	1.683	0.943	3.865	3.067	2.335	-39.6%	0.208	0.285	0.318	52.9%	0.017	0.047	0.123	623.5%
Fiji	0.695	-0.192	-0.675	2.716	1.977	1.8	-33.7%	0.274	0.227	0.153	-44.2%	0.044	0.099	0.16	263.6%
Vanuatu	2.28	1.341	0.509	3.675	2.504	1.8	-51.0%	0.089	0.109	0.092	3.4%	0.008	0.026	0.063	687.5%
Micronesia, Federated States of	2.302	1.43	0.583	3.751	2.772	1.8	-52.0%	0.044	0.061	0.055	25.0%	0.004	0.013	0.034	750.0%
Tonga	2.265	1.648	0.777	3.979	3.019	1.96	-50.7%	0.042	0.058	0.059	40.5%	0.007	0.013	0.03	328.6%
Samoa	0.473	0.293	-0.451	3.834	2.469	1.8	-53.1%	0.072	0.07	0.043	-40.3%	0.009	0.019	0.035	288.9%
Oceania	**1.179**	**0.743**	**0.394**	**2.272**	**2.046**	**1.843**	**-18.9%**	**8.104**	**8.933**	**8.856**	**9.3%**	**3.836**	**7.792**	**10.65**	**177.6%**

Population, Land Area, and Human Development Index

Base Case: Countries in Year 2060 Descending Population Sequence	Population Growth Rate (Annual Percent)			Total Fertility Rate (Births per Woman)				Population Below 15 Years of Age (Number in Millions)				Population 65 Years and Older (Number in Millions)			
	2010	2035	2060	2010	2035	2060	% Chg	2010	2035	2060	% Chg	2010	2035	2060	% Chg
EUROPE															
Russian Federation	-0.409	-0.685	-0.988	1.321	1.448	1.576	19.3%	20.74	15.39	12.32	-40.6%	18.11	26.58	31.1	71.7%
Poland	-0.091	-0.641	-0.969	1.274	1.414	1.554	22.0%	5.606	4.062	3.22	-42.6%	5.146	8.39	10.22	98.6%
Ukraine	-0.92	-1.03	-1.236	1.236	1.386	1.536	24.3%	6.122	4.935	2.965	-51.6%	7.07	8.022	8.806	24.6%
Romania	-0.267	-0.614	-0.987	1.349	1.469	1.589	17.8%	3.264	2.328	1.823	-44.1%	3.172	4.225	5.204	64.1%
Czech Republic	-0.079	-0.593	-0.858	1.313	1.442	1.572	19.7%	1.412	1.089	0.914	-35.3%	1.606	2.269	2.645	64.7%
Belarus	-0.361	-0.61	-0.905	1.245	1.393	1.54	23.7%	1.394	1.035	0.845	-39.4%	1.285	1.806	2.248	74.9%
Hungary	-0.471	-0.753	-0.959	1.339	1.462	1.584	18.3%	1.444	1.051	0.826	-42.8%	1.639	1.969	2.221	35.5%
Bulgaria	-0.878	-0.963	-1.136	1.339	1.462	1.584	18.3%	0.983	0.647	0.503	-48.8%	1.33	1.498	1.547	16.3%
Slovak Republic	0.048	-0.535	-0.934	1.283	1.421	1.558	21.4%	0.819	0.613	0.491	-40.0%	0.675	1.148	1.47	117.8%
Moldova, Repub of	-0.136	-0.696	-0.908	1.518	1.593	1.668	9.9%	0.75	0.571	0.437	-41.7%	0.447	0.575	0.793	77.4%
Europe-East	**-0.424**	**-0.721**	**-1.009**	**1.304**	**1.437**	**1.569**	**20.3%**	**42.53**	**30.72**	**24.34**	**-42.8%**	**40.48**	**56.48**	**66.25**	**63.7%**
United Kingdom	0.312	0.105	-0.086	1.781	1.786	1.791	0.6%	10.58	10.09	9.574	-9.5%	10.35	16.16	18.42	78.0%
Sweden	0.176	-0.039	-0.163	1.772	1.779	1.787	0.8%	1.466	1.428	1.335	-8.9%	1.709	2.453	2.755	61.2%
Denmark	0.223	0.025	0.011	1.8	1.8	1.8	0.0%	0.98	0.936	0.874	-10.8%	0.928	1.382	1.455	56.8%
Ireland	0.971	0.475	0.097	1.8	1.8	1.8	0.0%	0.889	0.838	0.831	-6.5%	0.523	1.047	1.468	180.7%
Norway	0.459	0.193	0.056	1.8	1.8	1.8	0.0%	0.87	0.851	0.813	-6.6%	0.735	1.267	1.43	94.6%
Finland	0.184	-0.174	-0.193	1.8	1.8	1.8	0.0%	0.873	0.827	0.762	-12.7%	0.924	1.422	1.44	55.8%
Lithuania	-0.368	-0.673	-0.923	1.302	1.434	1.567	20.4%	0.493	0.373	0.294	-40.4%	0.535	0.702	0.841	57.2%
Latvia	-0.388	-0.662	-0.878	1.339	1.462	1.584	18.3%	0.307	0.239	0.196	-36.2%	0.398	0.472	0.573	44.0%
Estonia	-0.879	-0.652	-0.736	1.518	1.593	1.668	9.9%	0.192	0.13	0.114	-40.6%	0.228	0.272	0.286	25.4%
Iceland	0.657	0.18	-0.193	1.882	1.8	1.8	-4.4%	0.063	0.057	0.05	-20.6%	0.039	0.079	0.1	156.4%
Europe-North	**0.27**	**0.051**	**-0.115**	**1.754**	**1.77**	**1.783**	**1.7%**	**16.71**	**15.77**	**14.84**	**-11.2%**	**16.37**	**25.26**	**28.77**	**75.7%**
Italy	-0.128	-0.504	-0.862	1.349	1.469	1.589	17.8%	8.143	6.116	5.12	-37.1%	12.22	16.8	15.68	28.3%
Spain	0.157	-0.341	-0.907	1.377	1.489	1.602	16.3%	6.519	4.815	4.162	-36.2%	7.759	11.87	12.62	62.6%
Greece	0.053	-0.306	-0.622	1.358	1.476	1.593	17.3%	1.583	1.253	1.11	-29.9%	2.088	2.927	3.189	52.7%
Portugal	0.002	-0.363	-0.701	1.424	1.524	1.624	14.0%	1.633	1.261	1.072	-34.4%	1.901	2.635	2.806	47.6%
Serbia	-0.245	-0.534	-0.712	1.471	1.539	1.646	11.9%	1.259	0.937	0.745	-40.8%	1.08	1.426	1.717	59.0%
Bosnia and Herzegovina	0.515	-0.426	-0.765	1.272	1.413	1.553	22.1%	0.626	0.472	0.387	-38.2%	0.554	0.923	1.144	106.5%
Croatia	-0.241	-0.61	-0.799	1.443	1.538	1.633	13.2%	0.66	0.512	0.415	-37.1%	0.772	1.014	1.062	37.6%
Albania	0.384	-0.138	-0.295	1.815	1.8	1.8	-0.8%	0.725	0.61	0.489	-32.6%	0.312	0.61	0.903	189.4%
Macedonia, FYR	0.201	-0.379	-0.726	1.499	1.579	1.659	10.7%	0.365	0.285	0.232	-36.4%	0.247	0.403	0.515	108.5%
Slovenia	-0.05	-0.626	-0.972	1.292	1.427	1.562	20.9%	0.272	0.202	0.166	-39.0%	0.335	0.531	0.547	63.3%
Montenegro	0.255	-0.147	-0.326	1.7	1.727	1.753	3.1%	0.119	0.101	0.088	-26.1%	0.08	0.12	0.157	96.3%
Malta	0.184	-0.491	-0.763	1.405	1.51	1.615	14.9%	0.064	0.05	0.04	-37.5%	0.062	0.101	0.118	90.3%
Europe-South	**0.007**	**-0.421**	**-0.814**	**1.383**	**1.495**	**1.606**	**16.1%**	**21.97**	**16.62**	**14.03**	**-36.1%**	**27.41**	**39.35**	**40.46**	**47.6%**
Germany	-0.05	-0.385	-0.518	1.368	1.483	1.598	16.8%	11.09	9.426	8.417	-24.1%	16.97	24.02	23.26	37.1%
France	0.306	0.016	-0.203	1.8	1.8	1.8	0.0%	11.28	10.13	9.19	-18.5%	10.55	16.61	17.78	68.5%
Netherlands	0.379	0.006	-0.12	1.715	1.738	1.76	2.6%	2.924	2.703	2.498	-14.6%	2.588	4.591	4.639	79.3%
Belgium	0.161	-0.103	-0.243	1.725	1.745	1.765	2.3%	1.739	1.6	1.474	-15.2%	1.879	2.821	2.903	54.5%
Austria	-0.02	-0.44	-0.767	1.433	1.531	1.628	13.6%	1.209	0.978	0.817	-32.4%	1.487	2.338	2.322	56.2%
Switzerland	0.079	-0.423	-0.771	1.443	1.538	1.633	13.2%	1.112	0.895	0.742	-33.3%	1.345	2.275	2.189	62.8%
Luxembourg	1.089	0.878	0.823	1.668	1.703	1.738	4.2%	0.085	0.097	0.115	35.3%	0.071	0.136	0.168	136.6%
Europe-West	**0.127**	**-0.193**	**-0.362**	**1.568**	**1.636**	**1.7**	**8.4%**	**29.44**	**25.83**	**23.25**	**-21.0%**	**34.89**	**52.79**	**53.26**	**52.7%**

Population, Land Area, and Human Development Index

Base Case
Source: International Futures Version 6.32, June 2010

Region	Youth Bulge (Ratio Persons 15-29 Years to Total Population)				Human Development Index (Index Range: 0-1)				HDI with Higher Ceilings (Index Range: 0-1)				Poverty below $1 per Day — Millions of People			Poverty below $1 per Day — Percent of Population		
	2010	2035	2060	% Chg	2010	2035	2060	% Chg	2010	2035	2060	% Chg	2010	2035	2060	2010	2035	2060
World	0.36	0.287	0.246	-31.7%	0.741	0.836	0.901	21.6%	0.62	0.701	0.758	22.3%	854.5	426.8	353.7	12.5%	5.0%	3.8%
Africa	0.479	0.416	0.341	-28.8%	0.554	0.706	0.803	44.9%	0.466	0.595	0.677	45.3%	304.8	292	306.2	30.3%	17.2%	12.6%
Americas	0.328	0.245	0.205	-37.5%	0.876	0.935	0.967	10.4%	0.734	0.784	0.82	11.7%	40.76	33.51	23.34	4.4%	3.0%	1.9%
Asia with Oceania	0.361	0.266	0.219	-39.3%	0.727	0.841	0.923	27.0%	0.607	0.704	0.773	27.3%	507.9	100.8	24.15	12.2%	2.0%	0.5%
Europe	0.233	0.182	0.168	-27.9%	0.904	0.957	0.978	8.2%	0.761	0.802	0.833	9.5%	1.04	0.482	0.059	0.1%	0.1%	0.0%
World	0.36	0.287	0.246	-31.7%	0.741	0.836	0.901	21.6%	0.62	0.701	0.758	22.3%	854.5	426.8	353.7	12.5%	5.0%	3.8%
Africa-Eastern	0.505	0.44	0.343	-32.1%	0.523	0.709	0.831	58.9%	0.44	0.597	0.7	59.1%	120.3	119.6	73.47	37.6%	20.5%	8.7%
Africa-Middle	0.506	0.455	0.403	-20.4%	0.473	0.613	0.691	46.1%	0.407	0.525	0.59	45.0%	45.52	71.35	110.1	36.6%	30.8%	28.6%
Africa-Northern	0.429	0.314	0.232	-45.9%	0.693	0.824	0.906	30.7%	0.573	0.689	0.759	32.5%	10.64	3.639	4.831	5.2%	1.3%	1.5%
Africa-Southern	0.429	0.345	0.242	-43.6%	0.68	0.81	0.922	35.6%	0.595	0.696	0.781	31.3%	6.287	4.125	1.375	11.2%	6.5%	2.0%
Africa-Western	0.486	0.435	0.361	-25.7%	0.5	0.668	0.776	55.2%	0.421	0.562	0.654	55.3%	122.1	93.32	116.4	40.9%	17.4%	14.4%
Africa	0.479	0.416	0.341	-28.8%	0.554	0.706	0.803	44.9%	0.466	0.595	0.677	45.3%	304.8	292	306.2	30.3%	17.2%	12.6%
America-Caribbean	0.355	0.274	0.236	-33.5%	0.771	0.835	0.89	15.4%	0.644	0.698	0.745	15.7%	6.27	8.038	8.762	15.9%	16.9%	17.2%
America-Central	0.446	0.34	0.252	-43.5%	0.757	0.847	0.918	21.3%	0.63	0.706	0.766	21.6%	7.925	11.96	8.671	18.1%	18.4%	11.1%
America-North	0.286	0.222	0.197	-31.1%	0.938	0.979	0.991	5.7%	0.787	0.822	0.856	8.8%	1.543	0.68	0.235	0.3%	0.1%	0.0%
America-South	0.361	0.254	0.203	-43.8%	0.829	0.908	0.955	15.2%	0.696	0.76	0.797	14.5%	25.03	12.83	5.67	6.3%	2.6%	1.1%
Americas	0.328	0.245	0.205	-37.5%	0.876	0.935	0.967	10.4%	0.734	0.784	0.82	11.7%	40.76	33.51	23.34	4.4%	3.0%	1.9%
Asia-East	0.292	0.203	0.178	-39.0%	0.818	0.923	0.994	21.5%	0.686	0.774	0.833	21.4%	47.84	4.296	2.451	3.0%	0.3%	0.2%
Asia-South Central	0.415	0.304	0.24	-42.2%	0.621	0.778	0.89	43.3%	0.514	0.65	0.744	44.7%	399.2	58.21	9.632	23.2%	2.6%	0.4%
Asia-South East	0.374	0.272	0.218	-41.7%	0.759	0.832	0.887	16.9%	0.639	0.699	0.743	16.3%	49.81	28.98	7.782	8.5%	4.0%	1.0%
Asia-West	0.406	0.318	0.251	-38.2%	0.779	0.864	0.924	18.6%	0.651	0.724	0.776	19.2%	9.16	7.367	2.714	4.0%	2.3%	0.7%
Oceania	0.302	0.257	0.228	-24.5%	0.874	0.916	0.938	7.3%	0.73	0.766	0.807	10.5%	1.922	1.966	1.569	5.6%	4.5%	3.1%
Asia with Oceania	0.361	0.266	0.219	-39.3%	0.727	0.841	0.923	27.0%	0.607	0.704	0.773	27.3%	507.9	100.8	24.15	12.2%	2.0%	0.5%
Europe-East	0.262	0.185	0.161	-38.5%	0.844	0.909	0.94	11.4%	0.716	0.766	0.789	10.2%	0.039	0.007	0.002	0.0%	0.0%	0.0%
Europe-North	0.234	0.199	0.186	-20.5%	0.949	0.994	0.999	5.3%	0.796	0.831	0.867	8.9%	0.003	0	0	0.0%	0.0%	0.0%
Europe-South	0.202	0.168	0.157	-22.3%	0.928	0.967	0.991	6.8%	0.776	0.806	0.832	7.2%	0.887	0.455	0.055	0.6%	0.3%	0.0%
Europe-West	0.212	0.178	0.172	-18.9%	0.956	0.991	1	4.6%	0.8	0.827	0.862	7.7%	0	0	0	0.0%	0.0%	0.0%
Europe	0.233	0.182	0.168	-27.9%	0.904	0.957	0.978	8.2%	0.761	0.802	0.833	9.5%	1.04	0.482	0.059	0.1%	0.1%	0.0%

Poverty

Multination Regional Analysis

Measures of Poverty, Health, Education, Infrastructure, and Governance

Population, Land Area, and Human Development Index

Base Case: Countries in Year 2060 Descending Population Sequence	Youth Bulge — Ratio Persons 15-29 Years to Total Population				Human Development Index — Index Range: 0-1				HDI with Higher Ceilings — Index Range: 0-1			
	2010	2035	2060	% Chg	2010	2035	2060	% Chg	2010	2035	2060	% Chg
AFRICA												
Ethiopia	0.493	0.437	0.35	-29.0%	0.424	0.643	0.807	90.3%	0.342	0.532	0.678	98.2%
Tanzania, United Rep	0.497	0.441	0.314	-36.8%	0.604	0.794	0.896	48.3%	0.515	0.672	0.754	46.4%
Uganda	0.545	0.479	0.355	-34.9%	0.577	0.77	0.897	55.5%	0.492	0.654	0.756	53.7%
Kenya	0.512	0.419	0.308	-39.8%	0.599	0.755	0.871	45.4%	0.51	0.637	0.731	43.3%
Madagascar	0.473	0.424	0.365	-22.8%	0.561	0.7	0.783	39.6%	0.471	0.592	0.661	40.3%
Mozambique	0.482	0.438	0.329	-31.7%	0.432	0.683	0.846	95.8%	0.36	0.574	0.715	98.6%
Malawi	0.506	0.455	0.369	-27.1%	0.554	0.712	0.795	43.5%	0.473	0.605	0.671	41.9%
Zambia	0.517	0.46	0.356	-31.1%	0.551	0.735	0.834	51.4%	0.482	0.601	0.704	46.1%
Somalia	0.461	0.446	0.398	-13.7%	0.476	0.625	0.722	51.7%	0.403	0.53	0.615	52.6%
Rwanda	0.536	0.447	0.336	-37.3%	0.497	0.743	0.859	72.8%	0.426	0.637	0.728	70.9%
Zimbabwe	0.566	0.396	0.292	-48.4%	0.605	0.717	0.781	29.1%	0.533	0.616	0.664	24.6%
Burundi	0.522	0.416	0.368	-29.5%	0.452	0.632	0.712	57.5%	0.384	0.537	0.603	57.0%
Eritrea	0.497	0.457	0.39	-21.5%	0.47	0.585	0.681	44.9%	0.385	0.485	0.57	48.1%
Comoros	0.465	0.419	0.366	-21.3%	0.601	0.667	0.767	27.6%	0.501	0.559	0.646	28.9%
Mauritius	0.303	0.225	0.197	-35.0%	0.815	0.904	0.966	18.5%	0.684	0.759	0.808	18.1%
Djibouti	0.47	0.374	0.304	-35.3%	0.525	0.659	0.817	55.6%	0.437	0.551	0.685	56.8%
Africa-Eastern	**0.505**	**0.44**	**0.343**	**-32.1%**	**0.523**	**0.709**	**0.831**	**58.9%**	**0.44**	**0.597**	**0.7**	**59.1%**
Congo, Democratic Republic of	0.516	0.476	0.434	-15.9%	0.418	0.545	0.636	52.2%	0.362	0.47	0.547	51.1%
Angola	0.509	0.441	0.344	-32.4%	0.591	0.817	0.862	45.9%	0.509	0.701	0.733	44.0%
Cameroon	0.491	0.407	0.329	-33.0%	0.556	0.68	0.795	43.0%	0.475	0.575	0.668	40.6%
Chad	0.5	0.463	0.413	-17.4%	0.376	0.565	0.655	74.2%	0.306	0.472	0.552	80.4%
Central African Republic	0.475	0.402	0.363	-23.6%	0.404	0.533	0.667	65.1%	0.34	0.448	0.56	64.7%
Congo, Republic of	0.486	0.403	0.313	-35.6%	0.653	0.78	0.831	27.3%	0.563	0.667	0.705	25.2%
Gabon	0.459	0.357	0.276	-39.9%	0.755	0.829	0.884	17.1%	0.644	0.704	0.749	16.3%
Equatorial Guinea	0.456	0.405	0.315	-30.9%	0.742	0.848	0.887	19.5%	0.65	0.736	0.761	17.1%
São Tomé and Príncipe	0.51	0.392	0.335	-34.3%	0.673	0.741	0.789	17.2%	0.569	0.628	0.665	16.9%
Africa-Middle	**0.506**	**0.455**	**0.403**	**-20.4%**	**0.473**	**0.613**	**0.691**	**46.1%**	**0.407**	**0.525**	**0.59**	**45.0%**
Egypt	0.433	0.314	0.218	-49.7%	0.72	0.852	0.937	30.1%	0.597	0.713	0.784	31.3%
Sudan	0.464	0.382	0.294	-36.6%	0.583	0.751	0.851	46.0%	0.488	0.631	0.72	47.5%
Algeria	0.421	0.274	0.202	-52.0%	0.748	0.846	0.903	20.7%	0.619	0.705	0.754	21.8%
Morocco	0.405	0.28	0.209	-48.4%	0.648	0.803	0.893	37.8%	0.525	0.668	0.746	42.1%
Tunisia	0.374	0.242	0.189	-49.5%	0.774	0.88	0.965	24.7%	0.641	0.732	0.804	25.4%
Libyan Arab Jamahiriya	0.4	0.299	0.21	-47.5%	0.83	0.922	0.964	16.1%	0.692	0.769	0.803	16.0%
Africa-Northern	**0.429**	**0.314**	**0.232**	**-45.9%**	**0.693**	**0.824**	**0.906**	**30.7%**	**0.573**	**0.689**	**0.759**	**32.5%**

Poverty

	Poverty below $1 per Day					
	Millions of People			Percent of Population		
	2010	2035	2060	2010	2035	2060
Ethiopia	11.51	1.623	0	14.2%	1.1%	0.0%
Tanzania, United Rep	20.62	2.631	0.009	46.8%	3.3%	0.0%
Uganda	26.06	33.71	4.297	77.2%	48.4%	4.1%
Kenya	5.04	3.822	0.285	12.9%	5.6%	0.3%
Madagascar	13.47	26.37	21.66	63.3%	66.0%	34.6%
Mozambique	6.102	0.752	0.006	27.4%	2.0%	0.0%
Malawi	2.642	4.712	0.579	17.9%	16.7%	1.3%
Zambia	9.079	9.426	4.789	69.0%	39.3%	13.3%
Somalia	4.452	9.88	15.39	47.5%	56.0%	52.5%
Rwanda	5.242	2.248	0.128	51.0%	12.5%	0.5%
Zimbabwe	9.079	13.42	12.07	64.9%	66.9%	50.0%
Burundi	3.846	5.324	5.912	45.8%	35.8%	25.6%
Eritrea	2.551	5.022	7.499	49.6%	50.5%	45.3%
Comoros	0.323	0.475	0.814	46.5%	37.7%	41.4%
Mauritius	0.039	0.007	0.001	3.0%	0.5%	0.1%
Djibouti	0.249	0.139	0.015	29.5%	12.5%	1.2%
Africa-Eastern	**120.3**	**119.6**	**73.47**	**37.6%**	**20.5%**	**8.7%**
Congo, Democratic Republic of	37.78	62.97	98.18	57.3%	48.6%	42.2%
Angola	0.254	0.009	0	1.4%	0.0%	0.0%
Cameroon	3.324	3.677	1.48	18.3%	12.4%	3.6%
Chad	1.019	0.131	5.804	9.1%	0.6%	14.5%
Central African Republic	2.896	4.301	4.392	66.3%	62.2%	43.7%
Congo, Republic of	0.169	0.041	0.011	3.8%	0.6%	0.1%
Gabon	0.016	0.054	0.016	1.0%	2.3%	0.5%
Equatorial Guinea	0	0	0	0.0%	0.0%	0.0%
São Tomé and Príncipe	0.061	0.162	0.172	34.3%	50.9%	35.6%
Africa-Middle	**45.52**	**71.35**	**110.1**	**36.6%**	**30.8%**	**28.6%**
Egypt	0.683	0.111	0.008	0.8%	0.1%	0.0%
Sudan	9.922	3.517	4.817	24.5%	5.5%	6.0%
Algeria	0.002	0	0.003	0.0%	0.0%	0.0%
Morocco	0.016	0.011	0.002	0.0%	0.0%	0.0%
Tunisia	0.002	0	0	0.0%	0.0%	0.0%
Libyan Arab Jamahiriya	0.017	0	0.001	0.3%	0.0%	0.0%
Africa-Northern	**10.64**	**3.639**	**4.831**	**5.2%**	**1.3%**	**1.5%**

Multination Regional Analysis

Measures of Poverty, Health, Education, Infrastructure, and Governance

Population, Land Area, and Human Development Index

Base Case: Countries in Year 2060 Descending Population Sequence	Youth Bulge — Ratio Persons 15-29 Years to Total Population				Human Development Index — Index Range: 0-1				HDI with Higher Ceilings — Index Range: 0-1			
	2010	2035	2060	% Chg	2010	2035	2060	% Chg	2010	2035	2060	% Chg
AFRICA continued												
South Africa	0.418	0.341	0.24	-42.6%	0.682	0.81	0.926	35.8%	0.598	0.698	0.784	31.1%
Namibia	0.474	0.358	0.255	-46.2%	0.722	0.842	0.932	29.1%	0.614	0.711	0.781	27.2%
Lesotho	0.533	0.396	0.267	-49.9%	0.565	0.728	0.824	45.8%	0.495	0.626	0.699	41.2%
Botswana	0.476	0.326	0.217	-54.4%	0.736	0.887	0.973	32.2%	0.63	0.75	0.818	29.8%
Swaziland	0.548	0.401	0.278	-49.3%	0.612	0.751	0.867	41.7%	0.534	0.643	0.735	37.6%
Africa-Southern	**0.429**	**0.345**	**0.242**	**-43.6%**	**0.68**	**0.81**	**0.922**	**35.6%**	**0.595**	**0.696**	**0.781**	**31.3%**
Nigeria	0.487	0.43	0.345	-29.2%	0.548	0.717	0.798	45.6%	0.472	0.608	0.676	43.2%
Niger	0.498	0.491	0.431	-13.5%	0.334	0.544	0.688	106.0%	0.263	0.446	0.574	118.3%
Côte d'Ivoire	0.468	0.41	0.34	-27.4%	0.513	0.673	0.8	55.9%	0.421	0.561	0.67	59.1%
Ghana	0.462	0.386	0.324	-29.9%	0.544	0.648	0.778	43.0%	0.457	0.544	0.654	43.1%
Mali	0.515	0.492	0.405	-21.4%	0.386	0.614	0.77	99.5%	0.313	0.509	0.649	107.3%
Burkina Faso	0.508	0.461	0.395	-22.2%	0.378	0.594	0.764	102.1%	0.302	0.495	0.642	112.6%
Senegal	0.51	0.437	0.362	-29.0%	0.471	0.634	0.785	66.7%	0.387	0.531	0.662	71.1%
Guinea	0.479	0.433	0.372	-22.3%	0.432	0.646	0.765	77.1%	0.345	0.537	0.639	85.2%
Benin	0.476	0.43	0.363	-23.7%	0.495	0.658	0.772	56.0%	0.398	0.543	0.643	61.6%
Togo	0.478	0.396	0.336	-29.7%	0.529	0.643	0.718	35.7%	0.433	0.532	0.598	38.1%
Sierra Leone	0.482	0.465	0.386	-19.9%	0.356	0.532	0.717	101.4%	0.294	0.444	0.606	106.1%
Liberia	0.479	0.431	0.343	-28.4%	0.446	0.654	0.807	80.9%	0.365	0.546	0.681	86.6%
Mauritania	0.468	0.396	0.36	-23.1%	0.527	0.667	0.742	40.8%	0.44	0.569	0.63	43.2%
Guinea-Bissau	0.445	0.442	0.411	-7.6%	0.477	0.647	0.687	44.0%	0.409	0.553	0.58	41.8%
Gambia	0.455	0.43	0.361	-20.7%	0.421	0.646	0.763	81.2%	0.335	0.541	0.643	91.9%
Cape Verde	0.499	0.328	0.225	-54.9%	0.739	0.85	0.925	25.2%	0.618	0.714	0.774	25.2%
Africa-Western	**0.486**	**0.435**	**0.361**	**-25.7%**	**0.5**	**0.668**	**0.776**	**55.2%**	**0.421**	**0.562**	**0.654**	**55.3%**

Poverty

	Poverty below $1 per Day					
	Millions of People			Percent of Population		
	2010	2035	2060	2010	2035	2060
South Africa	3.972	2.017	0.22	8.1%	3.8%	0.4%
Namibia	0.722	0.696	0.355	32.1%	20.3%	8.4%
Lesotho	0.68	0.678	0.384	36.0%	28.0%	14.5%
Botswana	0.304	0.129	0.092	16.1%	5.4%	3.5%
Swaziland	0.61	0.605	0.323	50.2%	36.1%	16.6%
Africa-Southern	**6.287**	**4.125**	**1.375**	**11.2%**	**6.5%**	**2.0%**
Nigeria	71.44	12.55	56.02	48.3%	4.9%	15.1%
Niger	8.914	19.72	23.72	54.1%	53.5%	33.8%
Côte d'Ivoire	3.419	4.039	2.862	16.6%	11.0%	5.2%
Ghana	9.417	16.28	9.13	38.3%	41.2%	17.2%
Mali	5.409	8.676	2.37	34.5%	27.8%	4.7%
Burkina Faso	4.395	6.971	0.912	28.6%	23.0%	1.9%
Senegal	2.319	2.33	0.659	17.4%	9.7%	1.9%
Guinea	3.87	3.749	1.88	37.3%	19.1%	5.9%
Benin	3.204	6.987	4.722	32.8%	37.1%	15.7%
Togo	3.204	4.937	8.628	45.9%	39.3%	44.7%
Sierra Leone	2.873	1.579	0.067	46.1%	14.7%	0.4%
Liberia	1.548	0.577	0.027	41.1%	8.4%	0.3%
Mauritania	0.671	2.803	2.388	19.5%	48.5%	27.4%
Guinea-Bissau	0.996	1.762	2.977	56.0%	53.1%	50.2%
Gambia	0.411	0.365	0.062	23.8%	11.7%	1.3%
Cape Verde	0.001	0.001	0	0.2%	0.1%	0.0%
Africa-Western	**122.1**	**93.32**	**116.4**	**40.9%**	**17.4%**	**14.4%**

Multination Regional Analysis

Measures of Poverty, Health, Education, Infrastructure, and Governance

Population, Land Area, and Human Development Index

Poverty

Base Case: Countries in Year 2060 Descending Population Sequence	Youth Bulge — Ratio Persons 15-29 Years to Total Population				Human Development Index — Index Range: 0-1				HDI with Higher Ceilings — Index Range: 0-1				Poverty below $1 per Day — Millions of People			Percent of Population		
	2010	2035	2060	% Chg	2010	2035	2060	% Chg	2010	2035	2060	% Chg	2010	2035	2060	2010	2035	2060
AMERICAS																		
Haiti	0.473	0.383	0.323	-31.7%	0.541	0.642	0.757	39.9%	0.447	0.537	0.636	42.3%	5.026	7.649	8.694	53.8%	54.0%	46.9%
Dominican Republic	0.396	0.269	0.202	-49.0%	0.796	0.912	0.966	21.4%	0.666	0.763	0.805	20.9%	0.119	0.018	0.004	1.3%	0.2%	0.0%
Cuba	0.247	0.174	0.159	-35.6%	0.865	0.915	0.961	11.1%	0.723	0.762	0.798	10.4%	1.085	0.316	0.029	9.5%	2.8%	0.3%
Puerto Rico	0.279	0.212	0.188	-32.6%	0.915	0.976	1	9.3%	0.764	0.814	0.854	11.8%	0	0	0	0.0%	0.0%	0.0%
Jamaica	0.375	0.286	0.21	-44.0%	0.779	0.843	0.909	16.7%	0.653	0.705	0.761	16.5%	0.009	0.033	0.032	0.3%	1.0%	1.0%
Trinidad	0.353	0.223	0.181	-48.7%	0.869	0.952	0.993	14.3%	0.737	0.801	0.832	12.9%	0.001	0	0	0.1%	0.0%	0.0%
Bahamas	0.341	0.238	0.198	-41.9%	0.878	0.945	1	13.9%	0.739	0.792	0.836	13.1%	0	0	0	0.0%	0.0%	0.0%
Barbados	0.262	0.181	0.166	-36.6%	0.899	0.939	0.991	10.2%	0.755	0.785	0.826	9.4%	0.002	0	0	0.7%	0.0%	0.0%
Grenada	0.443	0.281	0.203	-54.2%	0.827	0.89	0.942	13.9%	0.69	0.745	0.785	13.9%	0.008	0.013	0.003	7.0%	8.7%	1.8%
Saint Vincent and Grenadines	0.373	0.251	0.206	-44.8%	0.796	0.879	0.939	18.0%	0.666	0.736	0.785	18.0%	0.015	0.006	0.001	11.9%	3.9%	0.6%
Saint Lucia	0.386	0.247	0.194	-49.7%	0.829	0.893	0.941	13.5%	0.695	0.749	0.787	13.2%	0.007	0.003	0	4.1%	1.7%	0.0%
America-Caribbean	**0.355**	**0.274**	**0.236**	**-33.5%**	**0.771**	**0.835**	**0.89**	**15.4%**	**0.644**	**0.698**	**0.745**	**15.7%**	**6.27**	**8.038**	**8.762**	**15.9%**	**16.9%**	**17.2%**
Guatemala	0.484	0.399	0.293	-39.5%	0.723	0.839	0.923	27.7%	0.6	0.698	0.77	28.3%	2.244	3.635	2.684	15.6%	14.7%	8.1%
Honduras	0.473	0.335	0.236	-50.1%	0.744	0.835	0.903	21.4%	0.619	0.697	0.753	21.6%	1.178	1.827	1.529	14.7%	15.1%	10.6%
El Salvador	0.416	0.294	0.214	-48.6%	0.753	0.841	0.913	21.2%	0.627	0.704	0.765	22.0%	1.537	1.92	1.175	20.9%	20.7%	11.8%
Nicaragua	0.47	0.328	0.233	-50.4%	0.715	0.784	0.852	19.2%	0.592	0.653	0.71	19.9%	2.818	4.547	3.277	49.6%	55.2%	34.4%
Costa Rica	0.372	0.241	0.192	-48.4%	0.875	0.934	0.98	12.0%	0.731	0.779	0.815	11.5%	0.033	0.006	0.001	0.7%	0.1%	0.0%
Panama	0.355	0.268	0.205	-42.3%	0.848	0.934	0.992	17.0%	0.71	0.781	0.828	16.6%	0.09	0.012	0.002	2.6%	0.3%	0.0%
Belize	0.453	0.328	0.227	-49.9%	0.786	0.882	0.964	22.6%	0.648	0.732	0.801	23.6%	0.024	0.011	0.002	7.4%	2.3%	0.4%
America-Central	**0.446**	**0.34**	**0.252**	**-43.5%**	**0.757**	**0.847**	**0.918**	**21.3%**	**0.63**	**0.706**	**0.766**	**21.6%**	**7.925**	**11.96**	**8.671**	**18.1%**	**18.4%**	**11.1%**
USA	0.261	0.216	0.2	-23.4%	0.965	1	1	3.6%	0.809	0.841	0.872	7.8%	0	0	0	0.0%	0.0%	0.0%
Mexico	0.37	0.251	0.195	-47.3%	0.856	0.916	0.96	12.1%	0.715	0.765	0.8	11.9%	1.543	0.68	0.235	1.4%	0.5%	0.2%
Canada	0.239	0.188	0.181	-24.3%	0.964	0.998	1	3.7%	0.807	0.832	0.863	6.9%	0	0	0	0.0%	0.0%	0.0%
America-North	**0.286**	**0.222**	**0.197**	**-31.1%**	**0.938**	**0.979**	**0.991**	**5.7%**	**0.787**	**0.822**	**0.856**	**8.8%**	**1.543**	**0.68**	**0.235**	**0.3%**	**0.1%**	**0.0%**
Brazil	0.353	0.237	0.197	-44.2%	0.824	0.914	0.964	17.0%	0.692	0.766	0.805	16.3%	12.81	4.062	1.662	6.5%	1.7%	0.7%
Colombia	0.374	0.264	0.209	-44.1%	0.811	0.871	0.914	12.7%	0.682	0.732	0.765	12.2%	2.778	2.384	0.846	5.7%	3.9%	1.3%
Argentina	0.325	0.246	0.202	-37.8%	0.874	0.945	0.993	13.6%	0.735	0.791	0.828	12.7%	0.375	0.047	0.008	0.9%	0.1%	0.0%
Peru	0.392	0.276	0.206	-47.4%	0.809	0.897	0.951	18.8%	0.676	0.748	0.801	18.5%	1.902	0.813	0.353	6.3%	2.1%	0.8%
Venezuela	0.384	0.284	0.212	-44.8%	0.847	0.919	0.954	12.6%	0.711	0.771	0.798	12.2%	2.315	1.062	0.071	8.0%	2.8%	0.2%
Ecuador	0.392	0.285	0.211	-46.2%	0.826	0.877	0.898	8.7%	0.692	0.733	0.748	8.1%	1.566	2.264	1.365	10.9%	11.9%	6.5%
Chile	0.32	0.221	0.189	-40.9%	0.891	0.951	0.998	12.0%	0.745	0.794	0.83	11.4%	0.004	0	0	0.0%	0.0%	0.0%
Bolivia	0.437	0.344	0.242	-44.6%	0.742	0.847	0.894	20.5%	0.629	0.714	0.75	19.2%	2.36	1.177	0.794	23.3%	8.0%	4.6%
Paraguay	0.436	0.323	0.229	-47.5%	0.787	0.849	0.901	14.5%	0.662	0.712	0.753	13.7%	0.861	1.012	0.568	13.2%	10.9%	5.2%
Uruguay	0.288	0.222	0.192	-33.3%	0.875	0.951	1	14.3%	0.734	0.795	0.843	14.9%	0.001	0	0	0.0%	0.0%	0.0%
Guyana	0.353	0.261	0.207	-41.4%	0.767	0.825	0.885	15.4%	0.652	0.696	0.742	13.8%	0.016	0.005	0.001	2.1%	0.7%	0.2%
Suriname	0.357	0.272	0.209	-41.5%	0.788	0.881	0.948	20.3%	0.665	0.741	0.794	19.4%	0.042	0.007	0.001	9.1%	1.5%	0.2%
America-South	**0.361**	**0.254**	**0.203**	**-43.8%**	**0.829**	**0.908**	**0.955**	**15.2%**	**0.696**	**0.76**	**0.797**	**14.5%**	**25.03**	**12.83**	**5.67**	**6.3%**	**2.6%**	**1.1%**

Population, Land Area, and Human Development Index

Poverty

Base Case: Countries in Year 2060 Descending Population Sequence	Youth Bulge (Ratio Persons 15-29 Years to Total Population)				Human Development Index (Index Range: 0-1)				HDI with Higher Ceilings (Index Range: 0-1)				Poverty below $1 per Day — Millions of People			Poverty below $1 per Day — Percent of Population		
	2010	2035	2060	% Chg	2010	2035	2060	% Chg	2010	2035	2060	% Chg	2010	2035	2060	2010	2035	2060
ASIA with OCEANIA																		
China	0.303	0.209	0.181	-40.3%	0.8	0.917	0.996	24.5%	0.671	0.77	0.833	24.1%	42.56	0.578	0.011	3.2%	0.0%	0.0%
Japan	0.183	0.146	0.138	-24.6%	0.967	1	1	3.4%	0.807	0.839	0.871	7.9%	0	0	0	0.0%	0.0%	0.0%
Korea, Repub of	0.253	0.14	0.128	-49.4%	0.931	0.971	1	7.4%	0.78	0.811	0.843	8.1%	0.001	0	0	0.0%	0.0%	0.0%
Taiwan	0.301	0.228	0.196	-34.9%	0.907	0.956	1	10.3%	0.758	0.799	0.835	10.2%	0.012	0	0	0.0%	0.0%	0.0%
Korea, Dem. People's Rep.	0.303	0.222	0.201	-33.7%	0.682	0.76	0.833	22.1%	0.569	0.635	0.697	22.5%	5.228	3.716	2.441	22.8%	15.5%	10.9%
Hong Kong SAR	0.226	0.155	0.153	-32.3%	0.977	0.992	1	2.4%	0.816	0.828	0.846	3.7%	0	0	0	0.0%	0.0%	0.0%
Mongolia	0.425	0.263	0.21	-50.6%	0.757	0.831	0.906	19.7%	0.645	0.703	0.761	18.0%	0.044	0.001	0	1.6%	0.0%	0.0%
Asia-East	**0.292**	**0.203**	**0.178**	**-39.0%**	**0.818**	**0.923**	**0.994**	**21.5%**	**0.686**	**0.774**	**0.833**	**21.4%**	**47.84**	**4.296**	**2.451**	**3.0%**	**0.3%**	**0.2%**
India	0.401	0.287	0.217	-45.9%	0.625	0.8	0.918	46.9%	0.519	0.669	0.768	48.0%	321.1	20.16	0.763	27.5%	1.4%	0.0%
Pakistan	0.462	0.37	0.306	-33.8%	0.575	0.707	0.834	45.0%	0.467	0.587	0.695	48.8%	12.03	11.41	1.252	6.9%	4.1%	0.3%
Bangladesh	0.43	0.3	0.227	-47.2%	0.559	0.718	0.822	47.0%	0.454	0.597	0.687	51.3%	45.84	7.953	0.943	29.8%	4.0%	0.4%
Afghanistan	0.505	0.471	0.393	-22.2%	0.348	0.614	0.829	138.2%	0.288	0.514	0.7	143.1%	11.74	8.534	0.544	32.6%	12.3%	0.5%
Iran (Islamic Republic of)	0.445	0.268	0.204	-54.2%	0.799	0.895	0.944	18.1%	0.669	0.75	0.791	18.2%	0.001	0	0	0.0%	0.0%	0.0%
Nepal	0.455	0.348	0.288	-36.7%	0.54	0.652	0.768	42.2%	0.439	0.54	0.641	46.0%	6.847	9.282	6.043	23.0%	20.9%	10.9%
Uzbekistan	0.441	0.283	0.215	-51.2%	0.742	0.822	0.878	18.3%	0.629	0.693	0.737	17.2%	0.586	0.092	0.005	2.1%	0.3%	0.0%
Sri Lanka	0.332	0.228	0.199	-40.1%	0.786	0.859	0.917	16.7%	0.658	0.72	0.766	16.4%	0.537	0.101	0.025	2.6%	0.5%	0.1%
Kazakhstan	0.353	0.265	0.212	-39.9%	0.815	0.908	0.932	14.4%	0.697	0.768	0.785	12.6%	0	0	0	0.0%	0.0%	0.0%
Tajikistan	0.496	0.358	0.27	-45.6%	0.72	0.77	0.828	15.0%	0.613	0.651	0.696	13.5%	0.255	0.61	0.05	3.6%	5.8%	0.4%
Turkmenistan	0.431	0.283	0.212	-50.8%	0.826	0.949	0.985	19.2%	0.705	0.799	0.825	17.0%	0.067	0.001	0.001	1.3%	0.0%	0.0%
Kyrgyzstan	0.419	0.296	0.223	-46.8%	0.734	0.787	0.836	13.9%	0.623	0.665	0.703	12.8%	0.006	0.001	0	0.1%	0.0%	0.0%
Bhutan	0.457	0.314	0.226	-50.5%	0.62	0.793	0.93	50.0%	0.506	0.656	0.775	53.2%	0.107	0.02	0.005	15.5%	2.1%	0.5%
Maldives	0.485	0.313	0.212	-56.3%	0.797	0.864	0.928	16.4%	0.672	0.727	0.778	15.8%	0.058	0.04	0.005	16.0%	7.8%	0.9%
Asia-South Central	**0.415**	**0.304**	**0.24**	**-42.2%**	**0.621**	**0.778**	**0.89**	**43.3%**	**0.514**	**0.65**	**0.744**	**44.7%**	**399.2**	**58.21**	**9.632**	**23.2%**	**2.6%**	**0.4%**
Indonesia	0.36	0.258	0.211	-41.4%	0.763	0.835	0.881	15.5%	0.642	0.703	0.738	15.0%	9.233	4.311	0.694	3.9%	1.6%	0.3%
Philippines	0.426	0.326	0.236	-44.6%	0.764	0.826	0.893	16.9%	0.642	0.693	0.747	16.4%	8.752	4.813	1.728	9.6%	3.8%	1.2%
Viet Nam	0.387	0.252	0.203	-47.5%	0.768	0.845	0.904	17.7%	0.643	0.707	0.754	17.3%	0.031	0.005	0	0.0%	0.0%	0.0%
Thailand	0.299	0.231	0.209	-30.1%	0.799	0.861	0.91	13.9%	0.676	0.726	0.764	13.0%	0.056	0.02	0.006	0.1%	0.0%	0.0%
Myanmar	0.372	0.254	0.216	-41.9%	0.664	0.757	0.805	21.2%	0.566	0.639	0.676	19.4%	20.62	12.67	2.518	38.9%	20.5%	4.1%
Malaysia	0.382	0.282	0.211	-44.8%	0.848	0.919	0.968	14.2%	0.712	0.77	0.808	13.5%	0.003	0.001	0.001	0.0%	0.0%	0.0%
Cambodia	0.499	0.357	0.266	-46.7%	0.611	0.748	0.854	39.8%	0.515	0.63	0.719	39.6%	9.197	6.145	1.777	59.5%	26.8%	6.4%
LAO People's Dem Repub	0.48	0.357	0.261	-45.6%	0.639	0.774	0.878	37.4%	0.533	0.647	0.735	37.9%	1.623	0.213	0.006	24.7%	2.1%	0.0%
Singapore	0.249	0.157	0.155	-37.8%	0.958	1	1	4.4%	0.8	0.838	0.863	7.9%	0	0	0	0.0%	0.0%	0.0%
Timor-Leste	0.499	0.481	0.401	-19.6%	0.619	0.715	0.791	27.8%	0.521	0.6	0.664	27.4%	0.297	0.804	1.052	23.5%	28.1%	20.6%
Brunei Darussalam	0.346	0.265	0.215	-37.9%	0.938	0.972	0.987	5.2%	0.787	0.815	0.827	5.1%	0	0	0	0.0%	0.0%	0.0%
Asia-South East	**0.374**	**0.272**	**0.218**	**-41.7%**	**0.759**	**0.832**	**0.887**	**16.9%**	**0.639**	**0.699**	**0.743**	**16.3%**	**49.81**	**28.98**	**7.782**	**8.5%**	**4.0%**	**1.0%**

Multination Regional Analysis

Measures of Poverty, Health, Education, Infrastructure, and Governance

Population, Land Area, and Human Development Index

Base Case: Countries in Year 2060 Descending Population Sequence	Youth Bulge (Ratio Persons 15-29 Years to Total Population)				Human Development Index (Index Range: 0-1)				HDI with Higher Ceilings (Index Range: 0-1)			
	2010	2035	2060	% Chg	2010	2035	2060	% Chg	2010	2035	2050	% Chg
ASIA with OCEANIA continued												
Turkey	0.361	0.249	0.202	-44.0%	0.8	0.881	0.945	18.1%	0.671	0.738	0.791	17.9%
Yemen	0.532	0.436	0.336	-36.8%	0.585	0.741	0.837	43.1%	0.482	0.621	0.705	46.3%
Iraq	0.467	0.376	0.274	-41.3%	0.732	0.857	0.93	27.0%	0.613	0.721	0.783	27.7%
Saudi Arabia	0.393	0.319	0.241	-38.7%	0.84	0.908	0.958	14.0%	0.702	0.76	0.832	14.2%
Syrian Arab Repub	0.471	0.347	0.259	-45.0%	0.759	0.825	0.893	17.7%	0.63	0.687	0.745	18.3%
Israel	0.319	0.27	0.209	-34.5%	0.928	0.995	1	7.8%	0.774	0.829	0.873	12.8%
Jordan	0.457	0.343	0.228	-50.1%	0.791	0.872	0.957	21.0%	0.664	0.732	0.799	20.3%
Occupied Palestinian Territory	0.487	0.383	0.281	-42.3%	0.788	0.854	0.917	16.4%	0.661	0.717	0.767	16.0%
Azerbaijan	0.378	0.242	0.193	-48.9%	0.822	0.914	0.949	15.5%	0.695	0.767	0.752	14.0%
United Arab Emirates	0.263	0.206	0.187	-28.9%	0.933	1	1	7.2%	0.78	0.837	0.86	10.3%
Oman	0.412	0.309	0.236	-42.7%	0.86	0.94	0.996	15.8%	0.716	0.787	0.832	16.2%
Kuwait	0.287	0.227	0.211	-26.5%	0.945	0.997	0.994	5.2%	0.792	0.834	0.829	4.7%
Lebanon	0.356	0.256	0.203	-43.0%	0.79	0.88	0.956	21.0%	0.659	0.735	0.8	21.4%
Armenia	0.342	0.235	0.189	-44.7%	0.817	0.929	0.993	21.5%	0.688	0.778	0.823	20.3%
Georgia	0.287	0.195	0.166	-42.2%	0.729	0.851	0.922	26.5%	0.605	0.723	0.771	27.4%
Bahrain	0.329	0.232	0.208	-36.8%	0.904	0.96	1	10.6%	0.756	0.803	0.851	12.6%
Qatar	0.273	0.17	0.182	-33.3%	0.975	1	1	2.6%	0.816	0.854	0.865	6.0%
Cyprus	0.275	0.179	0.152	-44.7%	0.934	0.981	1	7.1%	0.781	0.817	0.848	8.6%
Asia-West	**0.406**	**0.318**	**0.251**	**-38.2%**	**0.779**	**0.864**	**0.924**	**18.6%**	**0.651**	**0.724**	**0.776**	**19.2%**
Australia	0.25	0.206	0.194	-22.4%	0.968	1	1	3.3%	0.809	0.837	0.871	7.7%
Papua New Guinea	0.451	0.377	0.302	-33.0%	0.569	0.715	0.804	41.3%	0.471	0.598	0.675	43.3%
New Zealand	0.267	0.208	0.19	-28.8%	0.942	0.973	1	6.2%	0.788	0.815	0.854	8.4%
Solomon Islands	0.466	0.379	0.32	-31.3%	0.627	0.702	0.782	24.7%	0.52	0.584	0.653	25.6%
Fiji	0.404	0.313	0.223	-44.8%	0.775	0.831	0.898	15.9%	0.656	0.701	0.753	14.8%
Vanuatu	0.464	0.362	0.272	-41.4%	0.718	0.814	0.901	25.5%	0.598	0.68	0.754	26.1%
Micronesia, Federated States of	0.494	0.374	0.283	-42.7%	0.749	0.806	0.888	18.6%	0.629	0.676	0.744	18.3%
Tonga	0.438	0.374	0.304	-30.6%	0.805	0.832	0.892	10.8%	0.68	0.7	0.747	9.9%
Samoa	0.468	0.35	0.255	-45.5%	0.813	0.876	0.94	15.6%	0.687	0.735	0.786	14.4%
Oceania	**0.302**	**0.257**	**0.228**	**-24.5%**	**0.874**	**0.916**	**0.938**	**7.3%**	**0.73**	**0.766**	**0.807**	**10.5%**

Poverty

	Poverty below $1 per Day					
	Millions of People			Percent of Population		
	2010	2035	2060	2010	2035	2060
Turkey	0.473	0.102	0.043	0.6%	0.1%	0.0%
Yemen	1.073	1.017	0.257	4.4%	2.2%	0.4%
Iraq	3.086	0.25	0.048	10.4%	0.5%	0.1%
Saudi Arabia	0	0	0	0.0%	0.0%	0.0%
Syrian Arab Repub	3.046	4.834	2.037	14.1%	14.2%	4.8%
Israel	0	0	0	0.0%	0.0%	0.0%
Jordan	0.001	0	0	0.0%	0.0%	0.0%
Occupied Palestinian Territory	1.233	1.059	0.316	29.5%	13.9%	3.1%
Azerbaijan	0	0	0	0.0%	0.0%	0.0%
United Arab Emirates	0	0	0	0.0%	0.0%	0.0%
Oman	0	0	0	0.0%	0.0%	0.0%
Kuwait	0	0	0	0.0%	0.0%	0.0%
Lebanon	0.117	0.082	0.011	3.1%	1.8%	0.2%
Armenia	0.009	0	0	0.3%	0.0%	0.0%
Georgia	0.123	0.023	0.003	2.8%	0.6%	0.1%
Bahrain	0	0	0	0.0%	0.0%	0.0%
Qatar	0	0	0	0.0%	0.0%	0.0%
Cyprus	0	0	0	0.0%	0.0%	0.0%
Asia-West	**9.16**	**7.367**	**2.714**	**4.0%**	**2.3%**	**0.7%**
Australia	0	0	0	0.0%	0.0%	0.0%
Papua New Guinea	1.545	1.576	1.276	23.5%	15.2%	9.5%
New Zealand	0	0	0	0.0%	0.0%	0.0%
Solomon Islands	0.107	0.148	0.205	19.8%	16.3%	16.3%
Fiji	0.165	0.081	0.011	18.7%	8.4%	1.3%
Vanuatu	0.04	0.031	0.005	16.9%	8.2%	1.1%
Micronesia, Federated States of	0.01	0.035	0.019	8.1%	17.2%	7.2%
Tonga	0.028	0.067	0.042	24.3%	35.6%	16.3%
Samoa	0.027	0.028	0.011	14.3%	12.0%	4.8%
Oceania	**1.922**	**1.966**	**1.569**	**5.6%**	**4.5%**	**3.1%**

Multination Regional Analysis

Population, Land Area, and Human Development Index

Base Case: Countries in Year 2060 Descending Population Sequence	Youth Bulge — Ratio Persons 15-29 Years to Total Population				Human Development Index — Index Range: 0-1				HDI with Higher Ceilings — Index Range: 0-1			
	2010	2035	2060	% Chg	2010	2035	2060	% Chg	2010	2035	2060	% Chg
EUROPE												
Russian Federation	0.271	0.193	0.169	-37.6%	0.837	0.912	0.932	11.4%	0.714	0.771	0.785	9.9%
Poland	0.266	0.173	0.146	-45.1%	0.889	0.943	0.979	10.1%	0.748	0.79	0.818	9.4%
Ukraine	0.257	0.178	0.156	-39.3%	0.802	0.859	0.905	12.8%	0.682	0.726	0.76	11.4%
Romania	0.247	0.178	0.155	-37.2%	0.848	0.905	0.949	11.9%	0.715	0.76	0.793	10.9%
Czech Republic	0.223	0.172	0.156	-30.0%	0.914	0.95	0.982	7.4%	0.769	0.796	0.82	6.6%
Belarus	0.27	0.184	0.161	-40.4%	0.837	0.912	0.951	13.6%	0.711	0.769	0.798	12.2%
Hungary	0.224	0.176	0.159	-29.0%	0.883	0.932	0.972	10.1%	0.746	0.783	0.814	9.1%
Bulgaria	0.219	0.167	0.152	-30.6%	0.852	0.9	0.948	11.3%	0.719	0.756	0.792	10.2%
Slovak Republic	0.266	0.176	0.15	-43.6%	0.896	0.945	0.976	8.9%	0.755	0.792	0.816	8.1%
Moldova, Repub of	0.339	0.228	0.191	-43.7%	0.746	0.785	0.841	12.7%	0.634	0.664	0.709	11.8%
Europe-East	**0.262**	**0.185**	**0.161**	**-38.5%**	**0.844**	**0.909**	**0.94**	**11.4%**	**0.716**	**0.766**	**0.789**	**10.2%**
United Kingdom	0.233	0.2	0.186	-20.2%	0.952	0.998	1	5.0%	0.797	0.832	0.869	9.0%
Sweden	0.228	0.194	0.181	-20.6%	0.962	1	1	4.0%	0.804	0.841	0.877	9.1%
Denmark	0.213	0.198	0.196	-8.0%	0.948	0.987	1	5.5%	0.796	0.826	0.863	8.4%
Ireland	0.265	0.219	0.196	-26.0%	0.964	1	1	3.7%	0.808	0.841	0.865	7.1%
Norway	0.233	0.198	0.191	-18.0%	0.983	1	1	1.7%	0.823	0.844	0.871	5.8%
Finland	0.223	0.196	0.187	-16.1%	0.952	0.996	1	5.0%	0.798	0.831	0.868	8.8%
Lithuania	0.265	0.179	0.152	-42.6%	0.872	0.927	0.975	11.8%	0.738	0.78	0.816	10.6%
Latvia	0.254	0.184	0.155	-39.0%	0.873	0.938	0.99	13.4%	0.738	0.788	0.827	12.1%
Estonia	0.246	0.196	0.171	-30.5%	0.89	0.949	1	12.4%	0.752	0.796	0.838	11.4%
Iceland	0.271	0.207	0.183	-32.5%	0.976	1	1	2.5%	0.815	0.845	0.879	7.9%
Europe-North	**0.234**	**0.199**	**0.186**	**-20.5%**	**0.949**	**0.994**	**0.999**	**5.3%**	**0.796**	**0.831**	**0.867**	**8.9%**
Italy	0.178	0.155	0.154	-13.5%	0.95	0.98	1	5.3%	0.794	0.816	0.839	5.7%
Spain	0.2	0.172	0.156	-22.0%	0.943	0.983	1	6.0%	0.788	0.82	0.843	7.0%
Greece	0.202	0.166	0.157	-22.3%	0.94	0.984	1	6.4%	0.787	0.821	0.844	7.2%
Portugal	0.209	0.174	0.163	-22.0%	0.902	0.948	0.989	9.6%	0.753	0.791	0.823	9.3%
Serbia	0.257	0.188	0.168	-34.6%	0.823	0.88	0.938	14.0%	0.688	0.737	0.784	14.0%
Bosnia and Herzegovina	0.26	0.171	0.148	-43.1%	0.833	0.906	0.957	14.9%	0.699	0.758	0.797	14.0%
Croatia	0.224	0.177	0.161	-28.1%	0.888	0.934	0.974	9.7%	0.746	0.782	0.813	9.0%
Albania	0.355	0.229	0.182	-48.7%	0.845	0.901	0.948	12.2%	0.709	0.753	0.79	11.4%
Macedonia, FYR	0.281	0.195	0.169	-39.9%	0.843	0.878	0.92	9.1%	0.71	0.737	0.769	8.3%
Slovenia	0.214	0.159	0.145	-32.2%	0.932	0.978	1	7.3%	0.782	0.817	0.847	8.3%
Montenegro	0.277	0.216	0.189	-31.8%	0.806	0.877	0.954	18.4%	0.673	0.733	0.797	18.4%
Malta	0.248	0.172	0.149	-39.9%	0.905	0.954	0.999	10.4%	0.753	0.794	0.831	10.4%
Europe-South	**0.202**	**0.168**	**0.157**	**-22.3%**	**0.928**	**0.967**	**0.991**	**6.8%**	**0.776**	**0.806**	**0.832**	**7.2%**
Germany	0.199	0.159	0.156	-21.6%	0.951	0.991	1	5.2%	0.797	0.827	0.865	8.5%
France	0.228	0.199	0.188	-17.5%	0.96	0.992	1	4.2%	0.802	0.827	0.86	7.2%
Netherlands	0.218	0.189	0.188	-13.8%	0.959	0.991	1	4.3%	0.804	0.827	0.859	6.8%
Belgium	0.216	0.192	0.184	-14.8%	0.952	0.985	1	5.0%	0.798	0.823	0.858	7.5%
Austria	0.214	0.164	0.154	-28.0%	0.959	0.994	1	4.3%	0.804	0.829	0.861	7.1%
Switzerland	0.207	0.16	0.152	-26.6%	0.973	1	1	2.8%	0.813	0.839	0.871	7.1%
Luxembourg	0.224	0.202	0.204	-8.9%	0.996	1	1	0.4%	0.836	0.853	0.864	3.3%
Europe-West	**0.212**	**0.178**	**0.172**	**-18.9%**	**0.956**	**0.991**	**1**	**4.6%**	**0.8**	**0.827**	**0.862**	**7.7%**

Poverty

	Poverty below $1 per Day					
	Millions of People			Percent of Population		
	2010	2035	2060	2010	2035	2060
Russian Federation	0.004	0	0	0.0%	0.0%	0.0%
Poland	0.001	0	0	0.0%	0.0%	0.0%
Ukraine	0.002	0	0	0.0%	0.0%	0.0%
Romania	0.01	0.002	0.001	0.0%	0.0%	0.0%
Czech Republic	0	0	0	0.0%	0.0%	0.0%
Belarus	0	0	0	0.0%	0.0%	0.0%
Hungary	0.001	0	0	0.0%	0.0%	0.0%
Bulgaria	0.009	0.001	0	0.1%	0.1%	0.0%
Slovak Republic	0.001	0	0	0.0%	0.0%	0.0%
Moldova, Repub of	0.01	0.003	0.001	0.2%	0.1%	0.0%
Europe-East	**0.039**	**0.007**	**0.002**	**0.0%**	**0.0%**	**0.0%**
United Kingdom	0	0	0	0.0%	0.0%	0.0%
Sweden	0	0	0	0.0%	0.0%	0.0%
Denmark	0	0	0	0.0%	0.0%	0.0%
Ireland	0	0	0	0.0%	0.0%	0.0%
Norway	0	0	0	0.0%	0.0%	0.0%
Finland	0	0	0	0.0%	0.0%	0.0%
Lithuania	0.002	0	0	0.0%	0.1%	0.0%
Latvia	0.001	0	0	0.0%	0.0%	0.0%
Estonia	0	0	0	0.0%	0.0%	0.0%
Iceland	0	0	0	0.0%	0.0%	0.0%
Europe-North	**0.003**	**0**	**0**	**0.0%**	**0.0%**	**0.0%**
Italy	0	0	0	0.0%	0.0%	0.0%
Spain	0	0	0	0.0%	0.0%	0.0%
Greece	0	0	0	0.0%	0.0%	0.0%
Portugal	0.001	0.003	0.004	0.0%	0.0%	0.0%
Serbia	0.277	0.061	0.007	3.8%	0.9%	0.1%
Bosnia and Herzegovina	0.553	0.36	0.04	13.6%	9.2%	1.2%
Croatia	0	0	0	0.0%	0.0%	0.0%
Albania	0.001	0.001	0	0.0%	0.0%	0.0%
Macedonia, FYR	0.001	0.001	0	0.0%	0.0%	0.0%
Slovenia	0	0	0	0.0%	0.0%	0.0%
Montenegro	0.054	0.03	0.005	8.7%	4.8%	0.8%
Malta	0	0	0	0.0%	0.0%	0.0%
Europe-South	**0.887**	**0.455**	**0.055**	**0.6%**	**0.3%**	**0.0%**
Germany	0	0	0	0.0%	0.0%	0.0%
France	0	0	0	0.0%	0.0%	0.0%
Netherlands	0	0	0	0.0%	0.0%	0.0%
Belgium	0	0	0	0.0%	0.0%	0.0%
Austria	0	0	0	0.0%	0.0%	0.0%
Switzerland	0	0	0	0.0%	0.0%	0.0%
Luxembourg	0	0	0	0.0%	0.0%	0.0%
Europe-West	**0**	**0**	**0**	**0.0%**	**0.0%**	**0.0%**

Poverty

Base Case
Source: International Futures
Version 6.32, June 2010

| | Poverty below $2 per Day | | | | | | Poverty below $5 per Day | | | | | | Poverty below $10 per Day | | | | | |
| | Millions of People | | | Percent of Population | | | Millions of People | | | Percent of Population | | | Millions of People | | | Percent of Population | | |
	2010	2035	2060	2010	2035	2060	2010	2035	2060	2010	2035	2060	2010	2035	2060	2010	2035	2060
World	2378	1397	974.3	34.9%	16.5%	10.4%	4180	3436	2415	61.3%	40.5%	25.7%	5105	5038	4110	74.9%	59.4%	43.7%
Africa	609	642.1	708.1	60.6%	37.9%	29.2%	865	1135	1241	86.1%	66.9%	51.2%	948.6	1432	1679	94.4%	84.4%	69.2%
Americas	119.5	89.94	57.73	12.8%	7.9%	4.8%	303	256.9	169.4	32.4%	22.7%	14.0%	449	434.2	319.9	48.0%	38.3%	26.4%
Asia with Oceania	1641	661.4	207.5	39.6%	13.3%	4.0%	2948	2023	996.5	71.1%	40.7%	19.2%	3526	3109	2081	85.0%	62.6%	40.2%
Europe	6.759	2.265	0.454	0.9%	0.3%	0.1%	60.54	19.19	6.494	8.4%	2.9%	1.1%	175.4	58.02	26.77	24.5%	8.7%	4.6%
World	2378	1397	974.3	34.9%	16.5%	10.4%	4180	3436	2415	61.3%	40.5%	25.7%	5105	5038	4110	74.9%	59.4%	43.7%
Africa-Eastern	233.1	240.1	147.5	72.9%	41.2%	17.4%	307.6	441.4	280.1	96.2%	75.7%	33.1%	315.9	540.5	449.6	98.8%	92.7%	53.2%
Africa-Middle	80.92	141.2	244	65.0%	60.9%	53.5%	103.3	167.8	290.5	83.0%	72.4%	75.6%	115.1	189.9	310.4	92.5%	82.0%	80.7%
Africa-Northern	55.74	25.1	17.91	27.0%	9.0%	5.7%	133.7	104.6	79.13	64.7%	37.3%	25.0%	177.3	176.4	167.6	85.9%	62.9%	53.1%
Africa-Southern	16.66	12.05	4.088	29.7%	19.0%	6.0%	33.65	28.8	12.99	60.1%	45.4%	19.1%	45.09	43.3	25.45	80.5%	68.2%	37.3%
Africa-Western	222.6	223.7	294.5	74.5%	41.7%	36.3%	286.8	392.6	578.3	96.0%	73.1%	71.3%	295.2	482.3	726.2	98.9%	89.8%	89.6%
Africa	609	642.1	708.1	60.6%	37.9%	29.2%	865	1135	1241	86.1%	66.9%	51.2%	948.6	1432	1679	94.4%	84.4%	69.2%
America-Caribbean	11.8	13.35	13.73	29.9%	28.0%	26.9%	22.72	22.88	20.27	57.6%	48.0%	39.7%	30.25	31.08	27.25	76.6%	65.2%	53.4%
America-Central	16.57	22.83	18.46	37.7%	35.1%	23.6%	29.76	39.7	36.91	67.8%	61.1%	47.1%	37.24	50.41	51.32	84.8%	77.5%	65.5%
America-North	19.91	12.75	5.822	4.4%	2.4%	1.0%	62.18	52.91	31.88	13.7%	9.9%	5.6%	96.48	94.95	69.05	21.3%	17.7%	12.1%
America-South	71.27	41.02	19.72	17.9%	8.4%	3.9%	188.4	141.4	80.3	47.3%	29.1%	15.7%	285.1	257.7	172.3	71.5%	53.0%	33.7%
Americas	119.5	89.94	57.73	12.8%	7.9%	4.8%	303	256.9	169.4	32.4%	22.7%	14.0%	449	434.2	319.9	48.0%	38.3%	26.4%
Asia-East	276.4	21.79	6.652	17.5%	1.3%	0.4%	790.6	142.5	26.25	50.1%	8.6%	1.7%	1170	420.9	88.6	74.1%	25.4%	5.8%
Asia-South Central	1071	423.6	117.6	62.4%	19.0%	4.7%	1563	1300	626.3	91.0%	58.4%	25.2%	1633	1864	1352	95.1%	83.7%	54.4%
Asia-South East	251	183.9	67.25	42.6%	25.6%	5.1%	473.3	467.5	273.5	80.4%	65.0%	36.8%	550.6	623.5	488.7	93.5%	86.7%	65.8%
Asia-West	38.09	26.96	11.61	16.6%	8.3%	3.0%	114	102.9	60.78	49.7%	31.6%	15.9%	163.3	188.3	138.1	71.2%	57.8%	36.0%
Oceania	4.378	5.176	4.475	12.8%	11.8%	8.9%	7.285	9.892	9.754	21.2%	22.6%	19.5%	8.856	12.48	13.46	25.8%	28.6%	26.9%
Asia with Oceania	1641	661.4	207.5	39.6%	13.3%	4.0%	2948	2023	996.5	71.1%	40.7%	19.2%	3526	3109	2081	85.0%	62.6%	40.2%
Europe-East	5.682	2.025	0.615	1.9%	0.8%	0.3%	48.33	11.5	4.542	16.6%	4.6%	2.3%	147.7	36.62	16.41	50.7%	14.6%	8.2%
Europe-North	0.132	0.036	0.007	0.1%	0.0%	0.0%	1.646	0.681	0.169	1.7%	0.7%	0.2%	5.424	2.92	0.934	5.6%	2.9%	0.9%
Europe-South	2.945	1.569	0.292	2.0%	1.1%	0.2%	13.28	9.455	3.403	8.9%	6.8%	2.9%	27.04	21.72	12.07	18.2%	15.6%	10.2%
Europe-West	0	0	0	0.0%	0.0%	0.0%	0.045	0.049	0.022	0.0%	0.0%	0.0%	1.813	1.284	0.446	1.0%	0.7%	0.3%
Europe	6.759	2.265	0.454	0.9%	0.3%	0.1%	60.54	19.19	6.494	8.4%	2.9%	1.1%	175.4	58.02	26.77	24.5%	8.7%	4.6%

Poverty

Base Case: Countries in Year 2060 Descending Population Sequence	Poverty below $2 per Day						Poverty below $5 per Day						Poverty below $10 per Day					
	Millions of People			Percent of Population			Millions of People			Percent of Population			Millions of People			Percent of Population		
	2010	2035	2060	2010	2035	2060	2010	2035	2060	2010	2035	2060	2010	2035	2060	2010	2035	2060
AFRICA																		
Ethiopia	50.36	23.69	0.077	62.0%	15.8%	0.0%	78.57	100.5	6.982	96.7%	66.9%	3.2%	80.41	140.8	53.5	99.0%	93.7%	24.3%
Tanzania, United Rep	34.57	11.81	0.178	78.4%	14.7%	0.2%	43.45	47.53	5.983	98.5%	59.1%	5.4%	43.65	71.16	30.62	99.0%	88.4%	27.6%
Uganda	29.51	43.84	8.893	87.4%	62.9%	8.4%	33.33	63.31	36.94	98.7%	90.9%	35.0%	33.43	68.39	67.8	99.0%	98.2%	64.3%
Kenya	23.33	25.39	5.931	59.9%	37.3%	5.4%	35.88	52.45	28.67	92.1%	77.0%	31.1%	38.54	63.93	56.39	98.9%	93.9%	61.1%
Madagascar	18.6	35.25	38.85	87.4%	88.2%	62.0%	20.97	39.37	55.39	98.5%	98.5%	88.4%	21.08	39.58	60.71	99.0%	99.0%	96.9%
Mozambique	12.57	3.495	0.095	56.4%	9.1%	0.2%	19.64	13.77	1.541	88.1%	36.0%	3.0%	21.72	24.77	6.894	97.4%	64.8%	13.3%
Malawi	10.58	20.18	8.335	71.6%	71.4%	18.9%	14.27	27.35	26.21	96.5%	96.7%	59.4%	14.63	27.99	37.99	99.0%	99.0%	86.2%
Zambia	11.59	15.64	11.77	88.1%	65.2%	32.7%	12.92	21.63	24.33	98.3%	90.2%	67.6%	13.02	23.4	31.43	99.0%	97.6%	87.3%
Somalia	8.179	15.3	23.56	87.3%	86.7%	80.4%	9.244	17.21	27.55	98.6%	97.5%	94.0%	9.281	17.48	28.77	99.0%	99.0%	98.1%
Rwanda	7.605	5.048	0.58	74.0%	28.1%	2.3%	9.777	11.46	3.66	95.1%	63.7%	14.8%	10.18	15.37	9.144	99.0%	85.4%	36.9%
Zimbabwe	13.14	18.81	20.54	93.9%	93.8%	85.1%	13.85	19.85	23.26	99.0%	99.0%	96.3%	13.85	19.85	23.91	99.0%	99.0%	99.0%
Burundi	7.135	11.61	13.66	84.9%	78.1%	59.1%	8.319	14.7	21.26	99.0%	98.9%	92.0%	8.319	14.72	22.85	99.0%	99.1%	98.9%
Eritrea	4.66	8.754	13.61	90.6%	88.1%	82.3%	5.091	9.788	15.96	99.0%	98.5%	96.5%	5.091	9.838	16.38	99.0%	99.0%	99.0%
Comoros	0.564	0.899	1.361	81.3%	71.4%	59.2%	0.678	1.187	1.786	97.7%	94.3%	90.8%	0.687	1.247	1.917	99.0%	99.0%	97.4%
Mauritius	0.206	0.058	0.016	16.0%	4.1%	1.2%	0.825	0.466	0.197	64.2%	33.0%	14.4%	1.18	0.998	0.605	91.8%	70.7%	44.1%
Djibouti	0.5	0.375	0.079	59.2%	33.8%	6.5%	0.765	0.807	0.382	90.6%	72.8%	31.6%	0.83	1.016	0.748	98.3%	91.6%	61.9%
Africa-Eastern	**233.1**	**240.1**	**147.5**	**72.9%**	**41.2%**	**17.4%**	**307.6**	**441.4**	**280.1**	**96.2%**	**75.7%**	**33.1%**	**315.9**	**540.5**	**449.6**	**98.8%**	**92.7%**	**53.2%**
Congo, Democratic Republic of	62.61	123.2	214.8	95.0%	95.0%	92.4%	65.25	128.4	230.1	99.0%	99.0%	99.0%	65.25	128.4	230.1	99.0%	99.0%	99.0%
Angola	1.206	0.098	0	6.7%	0.3%	0.0%	6.689	2.006	0.014	37.2%	6.2%	0.0%	12.81	8.6	0.304	71.2%	26.5%	0.6%
Cameroon	8.64	10.52	5.858	47.7%	35.5%	14.3%	15.4	21.92	18.51	85.0%	74.0%	45.2%	17.55	27.28	29.66	96.9%	92.1%	72.4%
Chad	3.984	1.114	16.48	35.5%	5.0%	41.2%	9.071	6.739	32.12	80.8%	30.2%	80.4%	10.84	14.08	38.07	96.5%	63.0%	95.3%
Central African Republic	3.671	5.598	6.448	84.1%	81.0%	64.1%	4.188	6.54	8.541	95.9%	94.6%	84.9%	4.319	6.806	9.438	98.9%	98.5%	93.8%
Congo, Republic of	0.625	0.21	0.064	14.0%	2.9%	0.7%	2.34	1.416	0.593	52.4%	19.7%	6.2%	3.67	3.408	1.942	82.3%	47.4%	20.2%
Gabon	0.057	0.156	0.056	3.7%	6.7%	1.9%	0.215	0.461	0.218	14.0%	19.7%	7.4%	0.449	0.841	0.486	29.3%	35.9%	16.5%
Equatorial Guinea	0	0	0	0.0%	0.0%	0.0%	0.001	0.018	0	0.2%	2.1%	0.0%	0.02	0.144	0.001	3.6%	16.6%	0.1%
São Tomé and Príncipe	0.121	0.255	0.309	68.0%	80.2%	64.0%	0.168	0.309	0.435	94.4%	97.2%	90.1%	0.176	0.315	0.471	98.9%	99.1%	97.5%
Africa-Middle	**80.92**	**141.2**	**244**	**65.0%**	**60.9%**	**63.5%**	**103.3**	**167.8**	**290.5**	**83.0%**	**72.4%**	**75.6%**	**115.1**	**189.9**	**310.4**	**92.5%**	**82.0%**	**80.7%**
Egypt	29.52	11.89	2.262	36.3%	10.9%	1.8%	69.99	57.7	23.61	86.1%	52.8%	19.3%	80.05	93.34	63.86	98.5%	85.5%	52.2%
Sudan	22.19	11.3	14.57	54.9%	17.7%	18.0%	36.97	34.55	42.84	91.5%	54.1%	52.9%	40	51.81	64.28	99.0%	81.1%	79.4%
Algeria	0.482	0.002	0.553	1.4%	0.0%	1.2%	7.469	0.308	7.817	21.1%	0.7%	16.4%	21.35	3.788	23.82	60.2%	8.4%	50.0%
Morocco	3.102	1.88	0.494	9.6%	4.6%	1.2%	15.12	11.35	4.301	46.7%	28.0%	10.1%	25.89	24.25	12.78	80.0%	59.7%	30.0%
Tunisia	0.161	0.029	0.006	1.5%	0.2%	0.0%	1.89	0.58	0.15	17.9%	4.6%	1.2%	5.377	2.622	0.916	50.8%	20.8%	7.2%
Libyan Arab Jamahiriya	0.289	0.001	0.019	4.5%	0.0%	0.2%	2.212	0.074	0.411	34.3%	0.9%	4.2%	4.624	0.635	1.943	71.7%	7.3%	20.0%
Africa-Northern	**55.74**	**25.1**	**17.91**	**27.0%**	**9.0%**	**5.7%**	**133.7**	**104.6**	**79.13**	**64.7%**	**37.3%**	**25.0%**	**177.3**	**176.4**	**167.6**	**85.9%**	**62.9%**	**53.1%**

Poverty

Base Case: Countries in Year 2060 Descending Population Sequence	Poverty below $2 per Day						Poverty below $5 per Day						Poverty below $10 per Day					
	Millions of People			Percent of Population			Millions of People			Percent of Population			Millions of People			Percent of Population		
	2010	2035	2060	2010	2035	2060	2010	2035	2060	2010	2035	2060	2010	2035	2060	2010	2035	2060
AFRICA continued																		
South Africa	13	8.383	1.649	26.6%	15.7%	2.9%	28.26	22.77	7.999	57.9%	42.5%	14.1%	38.77	35.73	18.38	79.5%	66.7%	32.4%
Namibia	1.143	1.251	0.785	50.8%	36.5%	18.6%	1.666	2.091	1.664	74.1%	61.0%	39.5%	1.953	2.654	2.45	86.8%	77.4%	58.2%
Lesotho	1.011	1.048	0.666	53.5%	43.3%	25.2%	1.493	1.672	1.276	79.0%	69.1%	48.3%	1.723	2.037	1.76	91.2%	84.2%	66.6%
Botswana	0.561	0.293	0.22	29.7%	12.3%	8.3%	1.078	0.766	0.628	57.2%	32.1%	23.8%	1.441	1.252	1.104	76.4%	52.4%	41.9%
Swaziland	0.939	1.073	0.768	77.3%	63.9%	39.4%	1.158	1.501	1.419	95.4%	89.5%	72.8%	1.202	1.633	1.75	99.0%	97.3%	89.7%
Africa-Southern	**16.66**	**12.05**	**4.088**	**29.7%**	**19.0%**	**6.0%**	**33.65**	**28.8**	**12.99**	**60.1%**	**45.4%**	**19.1%**	**45.09**	**43.3**	**25.45**	**80.5%**	**68.2%**	**37.3%**
Nigeria	113.3	44.62	136.2	76.6%	17.4%	36.7%	143.2	139.1	278	96.8%	54.2%	74.8%	146.5	209	343.3	99.0%	81.4%	92.4%
Niger	14.01	30.89	45.47	85.0%	83.9%	64.9%	16.09	35.74	61.72	97.6%	97.0%	88.0%	16.33	36.46	67.47	99.0%	93.0%	96.2%
Côte d'Ivoire	10.29	13.9	12.4	50.0%	37.8%	22.5%	17.73	28.09	32.4	86.2%	76.3%	58.7%	20	34.32	45.86	97.2%	93.2%	93.1%
Ghana	18.95	29.98	23.21	77.1%	75.9%	43.7%	23.94	37.98	41.08	97.4%	96.2%	77.3%	24.34	39.1	49.12	99.0%	99.0%	92.5%
Mali	12.76	22.5	13.58	81.3%	72.2%	27.1%	15.41	29.79	32.76	98.2%	95.5%	65.4%	15.53	30.87	43.9	99.0%	99.0%	87.6%
Burkina Faso	10.86	19.28	7.036	70.7%	63.5%	14.3%	14.78	28.5	25.74	96.2%	93.9%	52.4%	15.21	30.05	40.23	99.0%	99.0%	81.9%
Senegal	8.039	10.25	5.336	60.5%	42.5%	15.1%	12.32	19.72	17.72	92.7%	81.8%	50.3%	13.15	23.11	27.69	98.9%	95.9%	78.6%
Guinea	7.819	10.24	7.876	75.3%	52.1%	24.7%	10.14	17.6	21.52	97.7%	89.5%	67.5%	10.28	19.36	28.87	99.0%	98.4%	90.6%
Benin	7.3	14.37	13.65	74.8%	76.4%	45.4%	9.542	18.37	24.98	97.8%	97.6%	83.0%	9.663	18.63	28.92	99.0%	99.0%	96.1%
Togo	6.144	10.21	15.76	88.0%	81.2%	81.6%	6.91	12.23	18.67	99.0%	97.3%	96.6%	6.91	12.45	19.13	99.0%	99.0%	99.0%
Sierra Leone	4.182	2.939	0.227	67.1%	27.3%	1.5%	5.943	7.141	1.908	95.4%	66.4%	12.4%	6.166	9.516	5.401	99.0%	88.5%	35.2%
Liberia	3.578	4.369	1.756	95.0%	63.9%	18.1%	3.728	6.174	5.239	99.0%	90.2%	54.1%	3.728	6.688	7.823	99.0%	97.8%	80.7%
Mauritania	2.022	4.976	5.369	58.9%	86.1%	61.6%	3.262	5.723	8.101	95.0%	99.0%	92.9%	3.4	5.723	8.634	99.0%	99.0%	99.0%
Guinea-Bissau	1.69	3.151	5.636	95.0%	95.0%	95.0%	1.761	3.284	5.873	99.0%	99.0%	99.0%	1.761	3.284	5.873	99.0%	99.0%	99.0%
Gambia	1.353	1.775	0.879	78.5%	57.1%	19.1%	1.666	2.702	2.394	96.6%	86.9%	51.9%	1.707	3.006	3.563	99.0%	96.7%	77.2%
Cape Verde	0.279	0.23	0.096	50.2%	29.0%	10.7%	0.455	0.481	0.293	81.8%	60.6%	32.7%	0.525	0.646	0.502	94.4%	81.4%	56.1%
Africa-Western	**222.6**	**223.7**	**294.5**	**74.5%**	**41.7%**	**36.3%**	**286.8**	**392.6**	**578.3**	**96.0%**	**73.1%**	**71.3%**	**295.2**	**482.3**	**726.2**	**98.9%**	**89.8%**	**89.6%**

Multination Regional Analysis

Measures of Poverty, Health, Education, Infrastructure, and Governance

Poverty

Base Case: Countries in Year 2060 Descending Population Sequence	Poverty below $2 per Day						Poverty below $5 per Day						Poverty below $10 per Day					
	Millions of People			Percent of Population			Millions of People			Percent of Population			Millions of People			Percent of Population		
	2010	2035	2060	2010	2035	2060	2010	2035	2060	2010	2035	2060	2010	2035	2060	2010	2035	2060
AMERICAS																		
Haiti	7.424	11.12	13.02	79.5%	78.5%	70.3%	8.826	13.26	16.33	94.5%	93.6%	88.2%	9.205	13.9	17.65	98.6%	98.2%	95.3%
Dominican Republic	0.714	0.171	0.045	7.5%	1.4%	0.4%	3.013	1.226	0.456	31.7%	10.4%	3.7%	5.698	3.397	1.647	59.9%	28.8%	13.2%
Cuba	3.093	1.326	0.196	27.0%	11.6%	2.0%	8.358	6.035	1.988	73.0%	52.6%	20.0%	10.74	9.71	5.285	93.8%	84.6%	53.1%
Puerto Rico	0	0	0	0.0%	0.0%	0.0%	0.24	0.085	0.036	5.9%	1.9%	0.8%	0.805	0.379	0.182	19.9%	8.4%	4.0%
Jamaica	0.375	0.633	0.445	13.6%	19.5%	13.8%	1.399	1.814	1.318	50.6%	56.0%	40.8%	2.226	2.655	2.137	80.5%	81.9%	66.1%
Trinidad	0.078	0.009	0	5.8%	0.7%	0.0%	0.482	0.139	0.001	36.0%	10.1%	0.1%	0.954	0.489	0.014	71.3%	35.5%	1.2%
Bahamas	0	0	0	0.0%	0.0%	0.0%	0.002	0.001	0	0.6%	0.2%	0.0%	0.029	0.011	0.001	8.5%	2.7%	0.2%
Barbados	0.017	0.005	0.001	6.2%	1.8%	0.4%	0.114	0.055	0.012	41.6%	20.3%	5.2%	0.215	0.15	0.054	78.5%	55.4%	23.6%
Grenada	0.03	0.042	0.013	26.3%	28.2%	7.9%	0.087	0.109	0.065	76.3%	73.2%	39.6%	0.109	0.14	0.119	95.6%	94.0%	72.6%
Saint Vincent and the Grenadines	0.04	0.022	0.005	31.7%	14.4%	3.2%	0.098	0.083	0.036	77.8%	54.2%	22.8%	0.12	0.128	0.086	95.2%	83.7%	54.4%
Saint Lucia	0.03	0.015	0.004	17.8%	8.5%	2.6%	0.101	0.072	0.029	59.8%	40.9%	18.6%	0.147	0.129	0.075	87.0%	73.3%	48.1%
America-Caribbean	**11.8**	**13.35**	**13.73**	**29.9%**	**28.0%**	**26.9%**	**22.72**	**22.88**	**20.27**	**57.6%**	**48.0%**	**39.7%**	**30.25**	**31.08**	**27.25**	**76.6%**	**65.2%**	**53.4%**
Guatemala	4.933	7.551	6.111	34.3%	30.5%	18.4%	10.25	15.76	15.21	71.3%	63.6%	45.8%	12.96	20.83	22.9	90.1%	84.1%	69.0%
Honduras	3.442	4.83	4.175	42.9%	40.0%	29.0%	6.021	8.395	7.932	75.1%	69.4%	55.0%	7.274	10.41	10.66	90.8%	86.1%	74.0%
El Salvador	3.014	3.559	2.376	41.0%	38.4%	23.9%	5.517	6.456	5.08	75.1%	69.6%	51.0%	6.709	8.067	7.168	91.3%	87.0%	72.0%
Nicaragua	4.585	6.729	5.755	80.7%	81.7%	60.5%	5.555	8.006	8.289	97.8%	97.2%	87.1%	5.625	8.156	9.163	99.0%	99.0%	96.3%
Costa Rica	0.189	0.05	0.014	4.0%	0.9%	0.2%	1.084	0.481	0.178	23.2%	8.2%	2.9%	2.399	1.53	0.725	51.3%	26.2%	11.8%
Panama	0.325	0.067	0.016	9.3%	1.5%	0.4%	1.105	0.405	0.137	31.8%	9.4%	3.0%	1.967	1.064	0.47	56.6%	24.6%	10.3%
Belize	0.078	0.044	0.012	24.1%	9.3%	2.2%	0.234	0.2	0.09	72.4%	42.3%	16.5%	0.304	0.353	0.235	94.1%	74.6%	43.0%
America-Central	**16.57**	**22.83**	**18.46**	**37.7%**	**35.1%**	**23.6%**	**29.76**	**39.7**	**36.91**	**67.8%**	**61.1%**	**47.1%**	**37.24**	**50.41**	**51.32**	**84.8%**	**77.5%**	**65.5%**
USA	0	0	0	0.0%	0.0%	0.0%	0.331	0.15	0.029	0.1%	0.0%	0.0%	4.86	2.457	0.623	1.6%	0.7%	0.2%
Mexico	19.91	12.75	5.822	18.2%	9.9%	4.6%	61.84	52.76	31.85	56.6%	40.9%	25.0%	91.33	92.37	68.41	83.6%	71.5%	53.6%
Canada	0	0	0	0.0%	0.0%	0.0%	0.006	0.002	0	0.0%	0.0%	0.0%	0.286	0.128	0.015	0.9%	0.3%	0.0%
America-North	**19.91**	**12.75**	**5.822**	**4.4%**	**2.4%**	**1.0%**	**62.18**	**52.91**	**31.88**	**13.7%**	**9.9%**	**5.6%**	**96.48**	**94.95**	**69.05**	**21.3%**	**17.7%**	**12.1%**
Brazil	36.07	15.99	7.52	18.3%	6.8%	3.1%	93.64	61.91	36.1	47.5%	26.5%	15.0%	141.3	118.9	81.95	71.7%	50.9%	34.0%
Colombia	6.983	6.348	2.57	14.3%	10.4%	4.0%	19.96	20.06	10.39	40.7%	33.0%	16.3%	32.06	34.69	21.87	65.4%	57.0%	34.4%
Argentina	5.718	1.654	0.464	14.0%	3.5%	0.9%	18.14	9.101	3.689	44.5%	19.2%	7.4%	29.2	20.73	11.12	71.7%	43.8%	22.4%
Peru	6.775	3.84	1.943	22.4%	9.8%	4.6%	17	13.35	8.398	56.1%	34.2%	19.7%	24.26	23.54	17.62	80.1%	60.3%	41.3%
Venezuela	4.682	2.553	0.232	16.2%	6.8%	0.6%	14.67	11.69	2.29	50.8%	31.3%	5.7%	22.59	22.64	7.781	78.2%	60.6%	19.2%
Ecuador	4.111	5.397	3.442	28.6%	28.3%	16.3%	10.15	12.75	9.772	70.7%	66.8%	46.4%	13.16	16.88	15.17	91.6%	88.5%	72.0%
Chile	0.569	0.094	0.033	3.3%	0.5%	0.2%	2.905	0.868	0.363	17.0%	4.4%	1.8%	6.603	2.961	1.455	38.7%	15.0%	7.3%
Bolivia	4.088	2.618	1.912	40.4%	17.7%	11.0%	7.008	6.296	5.26	69.2%	42.6%	30.3%	8.676	9.541	8.828	85.6%	64.5%	50.8%
Paraguay	2.078	2.471	1.596	31.9%	26.5%	14.8%	4.058	5.069	3.932	62.4%	54.4%	36.3%	5.324	6.971	6.176	81.8%	74.8%	57.1%
Uruguay	0.024	0.001	0	0.7%	0.0%	0.0%	0.287	0.031	0.002	8.1%	0.8%	0.1%	0.986	0.22	0.026	27.8%	5.8%	0.7%
Guyana	0.042	0.016	0.004	5.6%	2.3%	0.6%	0.23	0.118	0.037	30.4%	16.7%	5.9%	0.468	0.305	0.12	61.9%	43.3%	19.3%
Suriname	0.122	0.035	0.008	26.5%	7.5%	1.9%	0.333	0.194	0.071	72.4%	41.6%	17.2%	0.43	0.355	0.194	93.5%	76.2%	47.1%
America-South	**71.27**	**41.02**	**19.72**	**17.9%**	**8.4%**	**3.9%**	**188.4**	**141.4**	**80.3**	**47.3%**	**29.1%**	**15.7%**	**285.1**	**257.7**	**172.3**	**71.5%**	**53.0%**	**33.7%**

Poverty

Base Case: Countries in Year 2060 Descending Population Sequence	Poverty below $2 per Day						Poverty below $5 per Day						Poverty below $10 per Day					
	Millions of People			Percent of Population			Millions of People			Percent of Population			Millions of People			Percent of Population		
	2010	2035	2060	2010	2035	2060	2010	2035	2050	2010	2035	2060	2010	2035	2060	2010	2035	2060
ASIA with OCEANIA																		
China	263.6	12.62	0.506	19.6%	0.9%	0.0%	758.8	119.9	20.9	56.4%	8.4%	0.8%	1109	378.9	63.25	82.5%	26.5%	4.8%
Japan	0	0	0	0.0%	0.0%	0.0%	0	0	0	0.0%	0.0%	0.0%	0.208	0.01	0	0.2%	0.0%	0.0%
Korea, Repub of	0.099	0.023	0.005	0.2%	0.0%	0.0%	4.719	1.525	0.341	9.6%	3.2%	0.9%	22.28	10.69	3.122	45.4%	22.6%	8.5%
Taiwan	0.291	0.021	0.004	1.2%	0.1%	0.0%	4.509	0.967	0.246	18.8%	3.6%	0.9%	13.42	5.988	2.094	55.9%	22.1%	8.0%
Korea, Dem. People's Rep.	11.37	8.998	6.136	49.5%	37.6%	27.5%	20.12	18.83	14.69	87.7%	78.6%	65.8%	22.48	22.73	19.61	98.0%	94.9%	87.9%
Hong Kong SAR	0	0	0	0.0%	0.0%	0.0%	0.027	0.016	0.01	0.4%	0.2%	0.1%	0.246	0.17	0.098	3.4%	2.1%	1.2%
Mongolia	1.097	0.128	0.001	41.1%	4.0%	0.0%	2.418	1.191	0.059	90.5%	36.8%	1.8%	2.645	2.488	0.44	99.0%	76.9%	13.3%
Asia-East	**276.4**	**21.79**	**6.652**	**17.5%**	**1.3%**	**0.4%**	**790.6**	**142.5**	**26.25**	**50.1%**	**8.6%**	**1.7%**	**1170**	**420.9**	**88.6**	**74.1%**	**25.4%**	**5.8%**
India	780.3	160.7	15.54	66.7%	11.1%	1.0%	1124	752.2	221.8	96.2%	52.1%	14.4%	1157	1220	702.8	99.0%	84.5%	45.7%
Pakistan	117.6	149.9	57.32	67.7%	53.3%	15.1%	170.4	266.2	245.8	98.2%	94.6%	64.6%	171.9	278.5	352	99.0%	99.0%	92.5%
Bangladesh	107.5	43.26	9.431	70.0%	21.6%	4.4%	150.2	144.2	72.53	97.8%	72.0%	34.1%	152	189.7	152	99.0%	94.8%	71.5%
Afghanistan	24.44	27.23	4.967	67.9%	39.2%	4.6%	33.89	54.74	29.28	94.2%	78.7%	26.9%	35.62	65.79	62.88	99.0%	94.6%	57.7%
Iran (Islamic Republic of)	0.054	0	0	0.1%	0.0%	0.0%	2.154	0	0.001	3.0%	0.0%	0.0%	13.23	0.023	0.047	18.2%	0.0%	0.1%
Nepal	23.49	32.78	28.54	78.9%	73.8%	51.6%	28.76	41.95	44.81	96.6%	94.5%	81.1%	29.48	43.95	51.69	99.0%	99.0%	93.5%
Uzbekistan	6.671	2.555	0.008	23.8%	7.3%	0.0%	20.95	16.69	0.51	74.8%	47.7%	1.7%	26.78	29.42	5.077	95.7%	84.1%	14.0%
Sri Lanka	6.611	2.569	0.871	32.5%	11.6%	4.2%	15.85	10.77	5.31	77.8%	48.8%	25.6%	19.43	17.71	11.65	95.4%	80.2%	56.2%
Kazakhstan	0.145	0	0	1.0%	0.0%	0.0%	3.45	0.013	0	22.8%	0.1%	0.0%	10.26	0.511	0.005	67.9%	3.5%	0.0%
Tajikistan	2.323	3.788	0.731	33.2%	36.1%	5.8%	5.909	8.668	4.235	84.4%	82.6%	33.9%	6.876	10.21	8.446	98.2%	97.2%	67.6%
Turkmenistan	0.365	0.004	0.009	7.0%	0.1%	0.1%	2.017	0.129	0.184	38.8%	1.9%	2.5%	3.799	0.809	0.937	73.1%	12.2%	12.9%
Kyrgyzstan	1.349	0.564	0.108	24.5%	8.2%	1.5%	4.456	3.689	1.477	81.0%	54.0%	20.9%	5.393	6.083	4.129	98.0%	89.0%	58.5%
Bhutan	0.255	0.073	0.02	36.9%	7.6%	1.8%	0.546	0.32	0.132	79.0%	33.3%	11.9%	0.658	0.605	0.348	95.2%	62.9%	31.4%
Maldives	0.137	0.108	0.022	37.8%	21.2%	3.8%	0.29	0.307	0.125	80.1%	50.2%	21.9%	0.347	0.436	0.28	95.9%	85.5%	49.0%
Asia-South Central	**1071**	**423.6**	**117.6**	**62.4%**	**19.0%**	**4.7%**	**1563**	**1300**	**626.3**	**91.0%**	**58.4%**	**25.2%**	**1633**	**1864**	**1352**	**95.1%**	**83.7%**	**54.4%**
Indonesia	97.97	74.09	24.3	41.8%	26.9%	8.8%	200.2	203.3	119.2	85.4%	73.7%	43.4%	229.1	260.1	210.7	97.8%	94.3%	76.7%
Philippines	34.39	25.22	11.98	37.8%	20.1%	8.7%	70.79	71.33	47.29	77.8%	57.0%	34.2%	85.78	103.5	86.25	94.3%	82.7%	62.3%
Viet Nam	42.72	20.16	3.734	48.2%	18.5%	3.3%	79.33	65.22	24.89	89.5%	60.9%	22.2%	87.48	95.42	57.97	98.7%	87.8%	51.7%
Thailand	13.71	8.87	3.173	20.7%	12.7%	4.8%	42.33	35.64	17.88	64.0%	50.9%	27.2%	59.12	57.21	37.85	89.4%	81.7%	57.6%
Myanmar	42.35	38.04	14.71	80.0%	61.5%	24.0%	51.56	56.67	37.91	97.4%	91.7%	61.8%	52.43	60.97	52.52	99.0%	98.6%	85.6%
Malaysia	1.241	0.714	0.484	4.5%	2.0%	1.2%	6.251	4.507	3.12	22.8%	12.6%	8.0%	13.4	11.57	8.605	48.8%	32.3%	22.0%
Cambodia	13.51	13.38	6.492	87.3%	58.3%	23.5%	15.3	20.63	17.11	98.9%	89.9%	62.0%	15.31	22.51	23.75	99.0%	98.1%	86.0%
LAO People's Dem Repub	4.507	1.797	0.161	68.6%	17.7%	1.3%	6.371	6.627	2.168	97.0%	65.3%	17.1%	6.503	9.317	6.235	99.0%	91.8%	50.5%
Singapore	0	0	0	0.0%	0.0%	0.0%	0.019	0.005	0.003	0.4%	0.1%	0.1%	0.19	0.081	0.045	4.1%	1.5%	0.9%
Timor-Leste	0.64	1.594	2.209	50.6%	55.8%	43.2%	1.096	2.541	4.021	86.7%	88.9%	78.7%	1.231	2.799	4.786	97.4%	97.9%	93.6%
Brunei Darussalam	0	0	0	0.0%	0.0%	0.0%	0	0	0	0.0%	0.0%	0.0%	0	0.001	0	0.0%	0.2%	0.0%
Asia-South East	**251**	**183.9**	**67.25**	**42.6%**	**25.6%**	**9.1%**	**473.3**	**467.5**	**273.5**	**80.4%**	**65.0%**	**36.8%**	**550.6**	**623.5**	**488.7**	**93.5%**	**86.7%**	**65.8%**

Multination Regional Analysis

Measures of Poverty, Health, Education, Infrastructure, and Governance

Poverty

Base Case: Countries in Year 2060 Descending Population Sequence	Poverty below $2 per Day						Poverty below $5 per Day						Poverty below $10 per Day					
	Millions of People			Percent of Population			Millions of People			Percent of Population			Millions of People			Percent of Population		
	2010	2035	2060	2010	2035	2060	2010	2035	2060	2010	2035	2060	2010	2035	2060	2010	2035	2060
ASIA with OCEANIA continued																		
Turkey	11.35	4.424	2.016	14.8%	4.9%	2.2%	43.71	28.55	16.22	57.1%	31.3%	17.6%	66.22	59.73	42.07	86.5%	65.6%	45.7%
Yemen	6.521	7.193	2.674	26.7%	15.4%	3.9%	17.87	25.63	16.15	73.1%	54.8%	23.5%	22.97	39.18	36.14	94.0%	83.7%	52.7%
Iraq	8.25	1.424	0.369	27.8%	2.9%	0.6%	21.48	11.72	5.327	72.3%	24.1%	8.8%	27.67	28.08	19.11	93.1%	57.8%	31.4%
Saudi Arabia	0	0	0	0.0%	0.0%	0.0%	0.821	1.906	0.002	3.2%	4.9%	0.0%	5.521	10.78	0.057	21.3%	27.5%	0.1%
Syrian Arab Repub	7.376	10.78	5.554	34.2%	31.6%	13.1%	16.55	23.99	17.87	76.8%	70.4%	42.3%	20.35	30.8	29.29	94.5%	90.3%	69.3%
Israel	0	0	0	0.0%	0.0%	0.0%	0.128	0.027	0.002	1.7%	0.3%	0.0%	0.952	0.325	0.042	12.5%	3.2%	0.3%
Jordan	0.28	0.102	0.001	4.6%	1.1%	0.0%	2.194	1.457	0.065	35.7%	15.9%	0.6%	4.53	4.492	0.659	73.7%	49.1%	6.1%
Occupied Palestinian Territory	2.208	2.363	0.872	52.8%	30.9%	8.4%	3.849	6.004	3.989	92.0%	78.6%	38.5%	4.143	7.346	7.265	99.0%	96.2%	70.2%
Azerbaijan	0	0	0	0.0%	0.0%	0.0%	0.012	0	0	0.1%	0.0%	0.0%	0.236	0	0	2.7%	0.0%	0.0%
United Arab Emirates	0	0	0	0.0%	0.0%	0.0%	0	0	0.003	0.0%	0.0%	0.1%	0.029	0.001	0	0.6%	0.0%	0.0%
Oman	0	0	0	0.0%	0.0%	0.0%	0.039	0.04	0	1.4%	0.9%	0.0%	0.358	0.377	0.053	12.6%	8.8%	1.0%
Kuwait	0	0	0	0.0%	0.0%	0.0%	0	0	0	0.0%	0.0%	0.0%	0.003	0	0	0.1%	0.0%	0.0%
Lebanon	0.618	0.445	0.09	16.2%	10.0%	2.0%	2.401	2.078	0.79	62.9%	46.5%	17.6%	3.464	3.543	2.096	90.7%	79.3%	46.6%
Armenia	0.721	0.016	0.001	23.2%	0.5%	0.0%	2.262	0.322	0.049	72.9%	9.9%	1.6%	2.942	1.232	0.383	94.8%	38.0%	12.3%
Georgia	0.768	0.209	0.032	17.6%	5.8%	1.1%	2.657	1.197	0.31	61.0%	33.3%	10.4%	3.848	2.395	0.948	88.4%	66.6%	31.7%
Bahrain	0	0	0	0.0%	0.0%	0.0%	0	0	0	0.0%	0.0%	0.0%	0.005	0.004	0	0.6%	0.4%	0.0%
Qatar	0	0	0	0.0%	0.0%	0.0%	0	0	0	0.0%	0.0%	0.0%	0	0	0	0.0%	0.0%	0.0%
Cyprus	0	0	0	0.0%	0.0%	0.0%	0	0	0	0.0%	0.0%	0.0%	0.013	0.009	0.003	1.7%	1.1%	0.4%
Asia-West	**38.09**	**26.96**	**11.61**	**16.6%**	**8.3%**	**3.0%**	**114**	**102.9**	**60.78**	**49.7%**	**31.6%**	**15.9%**	**163.3**	**188.3**	**138.1**	**71.2%**	**57.8%**	**36.0%**
Australia	0	0	0	0.0%	0.0%	0.0%	0.013	0.007	0.001	0.1%	0.0%	0.0%	0.334	0.199	0.029	1.6%	0.8%	0.1%
Papua New Guinea	3.495	4.236	3.766	53.1%	40.7%	28.1%	5.519	7.785	8.018	83.9%	74.9%	59.9%	6.273	9.485	10.84	95.3%	91.2%	81.0%
New Zealand	0	0	0	0.0%	0.0%	0.0%	0.018	0.01	0.001	0.4%	0.2%	0.0%	0.233	0.147	0.018	5.5%	3.1%	0.4%
Solomon Islands	0.261	0.366	0.479	48.3%	40.4%	38.0%	0.461	0.705	0.924	85.4%	77.8%	73.3%	0.524	0.849	1.143	97.0%	93.7%	90.7%
Fiji	0.38	0.237	0.05	43.0%	24.5%	5.7%	0.754	0.669	0.286	85.4%	69.2%	32.8%	0.862	0.889	0.576	97.6%	91.9%	66.0%
Vanuatu	0.091	0.087	0.023	38.4%	23.0%	4.9%	0.189	0.239	0.131	79.7%	63.2%	27.8%	0.226	0.331	0.277	95.4%	87.6%	58.8%
Micronesia, Federated States of	0.029	0.075	0.046	23.6%	36.9%	17.4%	0.085	0.158	0.13	69.1%	77.8%	49.2%	0.113	0.192	0.198	91.9%	94.6%	75.0%
Tonga	0.058	0.112	0.084	50.4%	59.6%	32.7%	0.102	0.171	0.176	88.7%	91.0%	68.5%	0.113	0.185	0.227	98.3%	98.4%	88.3%
Samoa	0.064	0.063	0.027	33.9%	27.0%	11.8%	0.145	0.149	0.088	76.7%	63.9%	38.4%	0.178	0.201	0.148	94.2%	86.3%	64.6%
Oceania	**4.378**	**5.176**	**4.475**	**12.8%**	**11.8%**	**8.9%**	**7.285**	**9.892**	**9.754**	**21.2%**	**22.6%**	**19.5%**	**8.856**	**12.48**	**13.46**	**25.8%**	**28.6%**	**26.9%**

Poverty

Base Case: Countries in Year 2060 Descending Population Sequence	$2/day Millions 2010	$2/day Millions 2035	$2/day Millions 2060	$2/day % 2010	$2/day % 2035	$2/day % 2060	$5/day Millions 2010	$5/day Millions 2035	$5/day Millions 2060	$5/day % 2010	$5/day % 2035	$5/day % 2060	$10/day Millions 2010	$10/day Millions 2035	$10/day Millions 2060	$10/day % 2010	$10/day % 2035	$10/day % 2060
EUROPE																		
Russian Federation	1.26	0	0	0.9%	0.0%	0.0%	18.21	0.058	0.029	13.0%	0.0%	0.0%	59.57	1.308	0.582	42.5%	1.1%	0.6%
Poland	0.03	0.001	0	0.1%	0.0%	0.0%	1.75	0.184	0.062	4.6%	0.5%	0.2%	10.85	2.602	0.925	28.5%	7.5%	3.3%
Ukraine	0.075	0	0	0.2%	0.0%	0.0%	5.79	0.072	0.002	12.8%	0.2%	0.0%	26.62	2.433	0.165	59.1%	7.0%	0.6%
Romania	1.413	0.423	0.117	6.6%	2.2%	0.8%	11.81	5.86	2.042	55.1%	30.8%	13.1%	19.58	14.05	6.975	91.4%	73.8%	44.9%
Czech Republic	0.007	0.002	0.001	0.1%	0.0%	0.0%	1.31	0.522	0.185	12.8%	5.6%	2.4%	6.824	4.136	1.683	66.7%	44.3%	21.6%
Belarus	0.011	0	0	0.1%	0.0%	0.0%	0.988	0.05	0.04	10.3%	0.6%	0.6%	5.104	0.737	0.424	53.2%	8.7%	6.1%
Hungary	0.017	0.003	0.003	0.2%	0.0%	0.0%	1.121	0.291	0.132	11.3%	3.4%	1.9%	5.297	2.212	0.959	53.6%	26.1%	14.1%
Bulgaria	0.108	0.021	0.001	1.4%	0.4%	0.0%	2.533	0.965	0.128	34.0%	16.6%	2.9%	6.133	3.642	0.992	82.3%	62.7%	22.3%
Slovak Republic	0.005	0.001	0.002	0.1%	0.0%	0.0%	0.752	0.193	0.148	13.9%	3.8%	3.5%	3.604	1.784	1.05	66.6%	35.0%	24.8%
Moldova, Repub of	2.755	1.573	0.489	66.1%	41.8%	15.9%	4.061	3.305	1.773	97.4%	87.8%	57.5%	4.129	3.712	2.657	99.0%	98.6%	86.2%
Europe-East	**5.682**	**2.025**	**0.615**	**1.9%**	**0.8%**	**0.3%**	**48.33**	**11.5**	**4.542**	**16.6%**	**4.6%**	**2.3%**	**147.7**	**36.62**	**16.41**	**50.7%**	**14.6%**	**8.2%**
United Kingdom	0	0	0	0.0%	0.0%	0.0%	0.052	0.022	0.002	0.1%	0.0%	0.0%	1.139	0.555	0.074	1.9%	0.9%	0.1%
Sweden	0	0	0	0.0%	0.0%	0.0%	0	0	0	0.0%	0.0%	0.0%	0.014	0.001	0	0.2%	0.0%	0.0%
Denmark	0	0	0	0.0%	0.0%	0.0%	0	0	0	0.0%	0.0%	0.0%	0.007	0.002	0	0.1%	0.0%	0.0%
Ireland	0	0	0	0.0%	0.0%	0.0%	0.002	0.001	0.001	0.0%	0.0%	0.0%	0.058	0.02	0.016	1.3%	0.4%	0.3%
Norway	0	0	0	0.0%	0.0%	0.0%	0	0	0	0.0%	0.0%	0.0%	0	0.006	0.001	0.0%	0.1%	0.0%
Finland	0	0	0	0.0%	0.0%	0.0%	0	0	0	0.0%	0.0%	0.0%	0.018	0.003	0	0.3%	0.1%	0.0%
Lithuania	0.107	0.031	0.005	3.2%	1.0%	0.2%	1.086	0.505	0.122	32.4%	17.0%	5.0%	2.433	1.571	0.572	72.5%	52.9%	23.4%
Latvia	0.007	0.001	0	0.3%	0.1%	0.0%	0.229	0.051	0.016	10.1%	2.6%	1.0%	0.966	0.355	0.128	42.8%	18.0%	7.8%
Estonia	0.018	0.004	0.001	1.4%	0.4%	0.1%	0.278	0.102	0.027	21.5%	9.8%	3.1%	0.788	0.405	0.142	60.8%	39.0%	16.2%
Iceland	0	0	0	0.0%	0.0%	0.0%	0	0	0	0.0%	0.0%	0.0%	0	0	0	0.0%	0.0%	0.0%
Europe-North	**0.132**	**0.036**	**0.007**	**0.1%**	**0.0%**	**0.0%**	**1.646**	**0.681**	**0.169**	**1.7%**	**0.7%**	**0.2%**	**5.424**	**2.92**	**0.934**	**5.6%**	**2.9%**	**0.9%**
Italy	0	0	0	0.0%	0.0%	0.0%	0.142	0.121	0.152	0.2%	0.2%	0.3%	2.425	1.848	1.499	4.1%	3.5%	3.4%
Spain	0	0	0	0.0%	0.0%	0.0%	0.088	0.068	0.047	0.2%	0.2%	0.1%	1.747	1.244	0.655	4.0%	3.0%	1.8%
Greece	0	0	0	0.0%	0.0%	0.0%	0.006	0.009	0.016	0.1%	0.1%	0.2%	0.156	0.176	0.2	1.4%	1.7%	2.1%
Portugal	0.038	0.051	0.047	0.4%	0.5%	0.5%	0.892	0.835	0.564	8.4%	8.3%	6.5%	3.712	3.138	2.014	35.0%	31.3%	23.2%
Serbia	1.207	0.401	0.054	16.4%	6.0%	0.3%	5.777	3.944	1.159	78.5%	58.7%	20.2%	7.236	6.327	3.569	98.3%	94.1%	62.1%
Bosnia and Herzegovina	1.301	0.88	0.139	32.0%	22.4%	4.1%	3.242	2.607	0.871	79.8%	66.3%	25.8%	3.923	3.561	1.921	96.6%	90.5%	56.9%
Croatia	0.008	0.001	0	0.2%	0.0%	0.0%	0.612	0.193	0.03	13.9%	4.9%	0.9%	2.734	1.434	0.346	62.0%	36.3%	10.5%
Albania	0.224	0.127	0.028	7.0%	3.7%	0.9%	1.753	1.154	0.378	55.0%	33.7%	11.7%	2.899	2.499	1.242	90.9%	72.9%	38.4%
Macedonia, FYR	0.004	0.005	0.001	0.2%	0.2%	0.1%	0.117	0.134	0.036	5.7%	6.6%	2.0%	0.569	0.598	0.211	27.6%	29.6%	12.0%
Slovenia	0.003	0	0	0.1%	0.0%	0.0%	0.203	0.022	0.004	10.1%	1.2%	0.3%	1.036	0.338	0.084	51.7%	18.5%	5.7%
Montenegro	0.162	0.103	0.022	26.2%	16.5%	3.7%	0.449	0.367	0.145	72.5%	58.7%	24.7%	0.58	0.543	0.331	93.7%	86.9%	56.1%
Malta	0	0	0	0.0%	0.0%	0.0%	0.002	0.001	0	0.5%	0.3%	0.0%	0.027	0.013	0.004	6.6%	3.3%	1.2%
Europe-South	**2.945**	**1.569**	**0.292**	**2.0%**	**1.1%**	**0.2%**	**13.28**	**9.455**	**3.403**	**8.9%**	**6.8%**	**2.9%**	**27.04**	**21.72**	**12.07**	**18.2%**	**15.6%**	**10.2%**
Germany	0	0	0	0.0%	0.0%	0.0%	0.002	0	0	0.0%	0.0%	0.0%	0.293	0.057	0.005	0.4%	0.1%	0.0%
France	0	0	0	0.0%	0.0%	0.0%	0.037	0.045	0.021	0.1%	0.1%	0.0%	1.162	1.039	0.39	1.9%	1.6%	0.6%
Netherlands	0	0	0	0.0%	0.0%	0.0%	0.003	0.002	0.001	0.0%	0.0%	0.0%	0.159	0.088	0.028	1.0%	0.5%	0.2%
Belgium	0	0	0	0.0%	0.0%	0.0%	0.004	0.002	0.001	0.0%	0.0%	0.0%	0.145	0.089	0.02	1.4%	0.8%	0.2%
Austria	0	0	0	0.0%	0.0%	0.0%	0	0	0	0.0%	0.0%	0.0%	0.033	0.006	0.002	0.2%	0.1%	0.0%
Switzerland	0	0	0	0.0%	0.0%	0.0%	0.001	0	0	0.0%	0.0%	0.0%	0.033	0.005	0.001	0.4%	0.1%	0.0%
Luxembourg	0	0	0	0.0%	0.0%	0.0%	0	0	0	0.0%	0.0%	0.0%	0	0	0	0.0%	0.0%	0.0%
Europe-West	**0**	**0**	**0**	**0.0%**	**0.0%**	**0.0%**	**0.045**	**0.049**	**0.022**	**0.0%**	**0.0%**	**0.0%**	**1.813**	**1.284**	**0.446**	**1.0%**	**0.7%**	**0.3%**

Multination Regional Analysis

Measures of Poverty, Health, Education, Infrastructure, and Governance

Poverty

Base Case
Source: International Futures
Version 6.32, June 2010

| | Poverty below $20 per Day | | | | | | GDP per Capita at PPP | | | | Gross Domestic Product | | | |
| | Millions of People | | | Percent of Population | | | Thousands in 2000 Dollars | | | | Billions in 2000 Dollars | | | |
	2010	2035	2060	2010	2035	2060	2010	2035	2060	% Chg	2010	2035	2060	% Chg
World	5729	6258	5824	84.1%	73.8%	61.9%	7.983	14.16	24.95	212.5%	39472	93138	205484	420.6%
Africa	983.3	1589	2071	97.8%	93.7%	85.4%	2.177	4.049	8.073	270.8%	904.3	3686	13675	1412.2%
Americas	571.8	604.2	498.5	61.1%	53.3%	41.1%	18.24	27.83	44.4	143.4%	14951	28690	51424	244.0%
Asia with Oceania	3830	3901	3170	92.3%	78.5%	61.2%	5.059	12.25	25.73	408.6%	13219	43858	114897	769.2%
Europe	334.9	156.2	79.66	46.7%	23.3%	13.6%	19.58	30.63	47.7	143.6%	10355	16820	25355	144.9%
World	5729	6258	5824	84.1%	73.8%	61.9%	7.983	14.16	24.95	212.5%	39472	93138	205484	420.6%
Africa-Eastern	316.4	571.8	664.3	99.0%	98.0%	78.5%	0.931	2.598	8.8	845.2%	103.4	745.4	5401	5123.4%
Africa-Middle	120.7	211.5	325.2	97.0%	91.3%	84.6%	1.566	3.079	3.679	134.9%	66.66	346.1	776.8	1065.3%
Africa-Northern	198.6	229.2	251.6	96.2%	81.8%	79.6%	4.317	8.582	15.35	255.6%	401.4	1443	3742	832.2%
Africa-Southern	52.02	54.41	40.88	92.8%	85.7%	60.0%	7.686	14.07	32.89	327.9%	204.5	580.5	1940	848.7%
Africa-Western	295.6	522.2	788.8	99.0%	97.2%	97.3%	1.251	2.492	4.476	257.8%	128.4	570.6	1815	1313.6%
Africa	983.3	1589	2071	97.8%	93.7%	85.4%	2.177	4.049	8.073	270.8%	904.3	3686	13675	1412.2%
America-Caribbean	35.03	37.72	34.76	88.8%	79.1%	68.1%	6.639	11.7	18.58	179.9%	185.9	456.9	856.3	360.6%
America-Central	41.46	57.79	62.94	94.4%	88.9%	80.3%	4.782	8.323	14.99	213.5%	101.1	330	883.2	773.6%
America-North	142.8	140.3	110	31.5%	26.2%	19.3%	29.65	43.61	68.53	131.1%	12862	22660	38631	200.3%
America-South	352.6	368.3	290.7	88.4%	75.8%	56.8%	7.89	14.64	24.55	211.2%	1802	5243	11053	513.4%
Americas	571.8	604.2	498.5	61.1%	53.3%	41.1%	18.24	27.83	44.4	143.4%	14951	28690	51424	244.0%
Asia-East	1386	860.9	276.6	87.8%	52.0%	18.2%	7.327	20.47	48.11	556.6%	9054	28019	68201	653.3%
Asia-South Central	1665	2081	2012	97.0%	93.4%	80.9%	2.543	7.276	16.4	544.9%	1426	8759	31580	2114.6%
Asia-South East	571.9	685.3	642.3	97.1%	95.3%	86.5%	3.735	6.255	10.9	191.8%	901.3	2282	5266	484.3%
Asia-West	193.9	258.1	223.3	84.6%	79.2%	58.2%	9.132	15.49	23.4	156.2%	1257	3675	7644	508.1%
Oceania	12.85	15.99	16.26	37.5%	36.6%	32.5%	22.08	29.73	48.53	119.8%	580.7	1122	2206	279.9%
Asia with Oceania	3830	3901	3170	92.3%	78.5%	61.2%	5.059	12.25	25.73	408.6%	13219	43858	114897	769.2%
Europe-East	243.8	90.84	45.42	83.6%	36.2%	22.6%	10.93	21.1	26.26	140.3%	996.9	2547	3422	243.3%
Europe-North	17.75	10.8	3.71	18.2%	10.6%	3.7%	27.65	42.58	71.77	159.6%	2612	4268	7179	174.8%
Europe-South	58.5	48.32	31.3	39.4%	34.7%	26.5%	20.72	28.08	38.41	85.4%	2156	3226	4106	90.4%
Europe-West	24.05	14.21	4.651	12.8%	7.6%	2.7%	27.57	38.33	64.26	133.1%	4633	6865	10780	132.7%
Europe	334.9	156.2	79.66	46.7%	23.3%	13.6%	19.58	30.63	47.7	143.6%	10355	16820	25355	144.9%

Poverty

Base Case: Countries in Year 2060 Descending Population Sequence	Poverty below $20 per Day						GDP per Capita at PPP				Gross Domestic Product			
	Millions of People			Percent of Population			Thousands in 2000 Dollars				Billions in 2000 Dollars			
	2010	2035	2060	2010	2035	2060	2010	2035	2060	% Chg	2010	2035	2060	% Chg
AFRICA														
Ethiopia	80.41	148.8	149.3	99.0%	99.0%	67.8%	0.642	2.103	7.374	1048.6%	15.8	136.3	1071	6678.5%
Tanzania, United Rep	43.65	79.24	73.44	99.0%	98.5%	66.2%	0.944	3.881	13.98	1380.9%	16.89	190.4	1316	7691.6%
Uganda	33.43	68.95	91.56	99.0%	99.0%	86.8%	1.202	3.793	16.18	1246.1%	11.11	114	1237	11034.1%
Kenya	38.58	67.42	78.92	99.0%	99.0%	85.5%	1.315	2.717	8.464	543.7%	18.71	81.84	520.8	2683.5%
Madagascar	21.08	39.58	62.01	99.0%	99.0%	99.0%	0.749	1.194	2.752	267.4%	4.983	15.14	69.51	1294.9%
Mozambique	22.07	33.19	19.03	99.0%	86.8%	36.7%	0.717	3.228	12.62	1660.1%	8.545	88.41	590.2	6807.0%
Malawi	14.63	27.99	42.93	99.0%	99.0%	97.4%	0.664	1.172	3.264	391.6%	2.541	9.654	60.29	2272.7%
Zambia	13.02	23.73	34.79	99.0%	99.0%	96.6%	1.168	2.963	7.548	546.2%	5.326	32.83	171.8	3125.7%
Somalia	9.281	17.48	29.02	99.0%	99.0%	99.0%	0.658	1.035	1.553	136.0%	1.173	4.079	11.8	906.0%
Rwanda	10.18	17.29	16.03	99.0%	95.1%	64.8%	0.731	3.128	12.04	1547.1%	3.258	34.91	254.6	7714.6%
Zimbabwe	13.85	19.85	23.91	99.0%	99.0%	99.0%	1.493	2.144	3.948	164.4%	5.877	13.59	38.59	556.6%
Burundi	8.319	14.72	22.87	99.0%	99.1%	99.0%	0.318	0.483	1.028	223.3%	0.942	2.061	7.174	661.6%
Eritrea	5.091	9.838	16.38	99.0%	99.0%	99.0%	0.6	0.747	1.154	92.3%	0.809	1.847	5.03	521.8%
Comoros	0.687	1.247	1.948	99.0%	99.0%	99.0%	0.948	1.159	2.239	136.2%	0.239	0.471	1.641	586.6%
Mauritius	1.272	1.323	1.068	99.0%	93.7%	77.9%	9.335	17.49	30.31	224.7%	6.331	17.56	37.26	488.5%
Djibouti	0.835	1.092	1.04	98.9%	98.5%	86.1%	1.353	3.719	9.465	384.6%	0.826	2.333	8.493	928.2%
Africa-Eastern	**316.4**	**571.8**	**664.3**	**99.0%**	**98.0%**	**78.5%**	**0.931**	**2.598**	**8.8**	**845.2%**	**103.4**	**745.4**	**5401**	**5123.4%**
Congo, Democratic Republic of	65.25	128.4	230.1	99.0%	99.0%	99.0%	0.282	0.519	0.754	167.4%	6.783	21.22	47.06	593.8%
Angola	16.66	19.85	2.887	92.6%	61.2%	6.2%	4.31	11.76	14.67	240.4%	25.32	209.9	441.8	1644.9%
Cameroon	17.94	29.19	37.08	99.0%	98.5%	90.5%	1.855	3.252	6.604	256.0%	13.99	45.44	158.2	1030.8%
Chad	11.12	19.7	39.56	99.0%	88.2%	99.0%	1.224	2.056	2.18	78.1%	2.91	12.51	24.48	741.2%
Central African Republic	4.322	6.843	9.856	99.0%	99.0%	98.0%	0.632	1.057	2.27	259.2%	1.046	2.631	9.314	790.4%
Congo, Republic of	4.297	5.499	4.315	96.3%	76.5%	45.0%	3.238	6.33	7.654	134.2%	5.202	22.42	38.95	648.8%
Gabon	0.76	1.293	0.907	49.6%	55.2%	30.8%	12.14	15.53	17.53	44.4%	6.227	15.87	28.1	351.3%
Equatorial Guinea	0.146	0.467	0.014	26.1%	53.7%	1.2%	26.85	37.85	39.89	48.5%	5.108	15.93	28.46	457.2%
São Tomé and Príncipe	0.176	0.315	0.478	98.9%	99.1%	99.0%	1.383	1.762	2.771	99.6%	0.073	0.173	0.478	554.8%
Africa-Middle	**120.7**	**211.5**	**325.2**	**97.0%**	**91.3%**	**84.6%**	**1.566**	**3.079**	**3.679**	**134.9%**	**66.66**	**346.1**	**776.8**	**1065.3%**
Egypt	80.45	107	102.2	99.0%	98.0%	83.6%	4.551	9.612	20.2	343.9%	156.8	622.5	2039	1200.4%
Sudan	40.01	60.79	76.21	99.0%	95.2%	94.2%	1.805	5.102	8.97	397.0%	24.24	164.5	449.5	1754.4%
Algeria	32.16	17.4	39.83	90.7%	38.4%	83.6%	5.606	9.068	11.75	109.6%	80.05	215.7	338.9	323.4%
Morocco	31.1	34.88	25.12	96.1%	85.9%	59.0%	3.552	6.665	12.57	253.9%	58.94	168.2	408.8	593.6%
Tunisia	8.8	6.593	3.245	83.2%	52.4%	25.4%	6.332	13.39	25.09	296.2%	30.38	110	276.9	811.5%
Libyan Arab Jamahiriya	6.062	2.618	5.016	94.0%	30.2%	51.6%	10.55	20.69	24.42	131.5%	50.97	162.2	229	349.3%
Africa-Northern	**198.6**	**229.2**	**251.6**	**96.2%**	**81.8%**	**79.6%**	**4.317**	**8.582**	**15.35**	**255.6%**	**401.4**	**1443**	**3742**	**832.2%**

Multinational Regional Analysis

Measures of Poverty, Health, Education, Infrastructure, and Governance

Poverty

Base Case: Countries in Year 2060 Descending Population Sequence	Poverty below $20 per Day						GDP per Capita at PPP				Gross Domestic Product			
	Millions of People			Percent of Population			Thousands in 2000 Dollars				Billions in 2000 Dollars			
	2010	2035	2060	2010	2035	2060	2010	2035	2060	% Chg	2010	2035	2060	% Chg
AFRICA continued														
South Africa	45.17	45.72	32.03	92.6%	85.4%	56.5%	8.021	14.52	35	336.4%	186.4	502.4	1723	824.4%
Namibia	2.123	3.05	3.165	94.4%	89.0%	75.2%	4.199	8.544	20.36	384.9%	4.959	19.55	74.74	1407.2%
Lesotho	1.835	2.26	2.157	97.1%	93.4%	81.7%	1.301	2.75	6.839	425.7%	1.166	3.495	11.95	924.9%
Botswana	1.69	1.724	1.63	89.6%	72.1%	61.8%	11.99	28.2	46.7	289.5%	10.36	49.43	110.4	965.6%
Swaziland	1.202	1.661	1.898	99.0%	99.0%	97.3%	3.935	7.195	15.17	285.5%	1.693	5.699	20.37	1103.2%
Africa-Southern	**52.02**	**54.41**	**40.88**	**92.8%**	**85.7%**	**60.0%**	**7.686**	**14.07**	**32.89**	**327.9%**	**204.5**	**580.5**	**1940**	**848.7%**
Nigeria	146.5	244.8	366.3	99.0%	95.4%	98.6%	1.467	3.29	4.719	221.7%	76.08	384	849.5	1016.6%
Niger	16.33	36.46	69.41	99.0%	99.0%	99.0%	0.564	0.92	1.91	238.7%	2.728	10.01	46.73	1613.0%
Côte d'Ivoire	20.37	36.39	52.71	99.0%	98.9%	95.5%	1.468	2.512	4.72	221.5%	11.76	39.95	132.4	1025.9%
Ghana	24.34	39.1	52.24	99.0%	99.0%	98.3%	1.16	1.687	4.297	270.4%	8.302	21	103	1140.7%
Mali	15.53	30.87	48.72	99.0%	99.0%	97.2%	0.913	1.773	5.314	482.0%	3.95	18.37	135.4	3327.8%
Burkina Faso	15.21	30.05	47.2	99.0%	99.0%	96.1%	0.959	1.817	5.474	470.8%	4.195	18.66	139.2	3218.2%
Senegal	13.15	23.86	33.21	98.9%	99.0%	94.2%	1.406	2.265	6.173	339.0%	6.827	21.67	123.1	1703.1%
Guinea	10.28	19.47	31.4	99.0%	99.0%	98.5%	1.023	2.011	4.38	328.2%	4.083	16.91	72.33	1671.5%
Benin	9.663	18.63	29.78	99.0%	99.0%	99.0%	1.132	1.726	3.496	208.8%	3.326	10.68	43.81	1217.2%
Togo	6.91	12.45	19.13	99.0%	99.0%	99.0%	0.673	0.907	1.077	60.0%	1.656	3.597	5.754	247.5%
Sierra Leone	6.166	10.49	10.02	99.0%	97.6%	65.2%	0.595	1.798	7.323	1130.8%	1.54	9.601	82.21	5238.3%
Liberia	3.728	6.773	9.194	99.0%	99.0%	94.9%	0.349	1.663	6.466	1752.7%	0.621	6.757	48.81	7759.9%
Mauritania	3.4	5.723	8.634	99.0%	99.0%	99.0%	1.552	1.411	1.898	22.3%	1.54	2.138	4.76	209.1%
Guinea-Bissau	1.761	3.284	5.873	99.0%	99.0%	99.0%	0.429	0.502	0.617	43.8%	0.239	0.422	0.803	236.0%
Gambia	1.707	3.079	4.271	99.0%	99.0%	92.6%	1.048	2.238	5.525	427.2%	0.643	2.948	14.26	2117.7%
Cape Verde	0.55	0.743	0.693	98.9%	93.6%	77.4%	2.558	6.428	16.37	540.0%	0.885	3.871	13.45	1419.8%
Africa-Western	**295.6**	**522.2**	**788.8**	**99.0%**	**97.2%**	**97.3%**	**1.251**	**2.492**	**4.476**	**257.8%**	**128.4**	**570.6**	**1815**	**1313.6%**

Poverty

Base Case: Countries in Year 2060 Descending Population Sequence	Poverty below $20 per Day						GDP per Capita at PPP				Gross Domestic Product			
	Millions of People			Percent of Population			Thousands in 2000 Dollars				Billions in 2000 Dollars			
	2010	2035	2060	2010	2035	2060	2010	2035	2060	% Chg	2010	2035	2060	% Chg
AMERICAS														
Haiti	9.246	14.02	18.24	99.0%	99.0%	98.5%	1.082	1.573	3.033	180.3%	4.106	8.641	24.69	501.3%
Dominican Republic	7.95	6.56	4.108	83.6%	55.5%	32.9%	5.16	13.25	23.51	355.6%	29.58	128.3	276.7	835.4%
Cuba	11.34	11.2	8.371	99.0%	97.6%	84.1%	6.165	10.78	18.77	204.5%	39.3	84.81	160.5	308.4%
Puerto Rico	1.814	1.12	0.625	44.8%	24.9%	13.8%	20.42	35.25	59.11	189.5%	79.38	156.6	267.1	236.5%
Jamaica	2.643	3.089	2.769	95.6%	95.3%	85.6%	5.997	7.993	13.37	122.9%	8.467	14.48	30.23	257.0%
Trinidad	1.245	0.967	0.098	93.0%	70.3%	8.1%	15.3	36.01	52.13	240.7%	15.16	45.05	61.32	304.5%
Bahamas	0.129	0.073	0.016	37.8%	18.2%	3.9%	16.94	27.08	48.1	183.9%	5.226	10.53	19.67	276.4%
Barbados	0.264	0.234	0.132	96.4%	86.3%	57.6%	13.3	19.71	36.95	177.8%	2.911	4.818	8.225	182.5%
Grenada	0.113	0.147	0.152	99.1%	98.7%	92.7%	7.953	10.33	18.05	127.0%	0.467	0.899	2.274	386.9%
Saint Vincent and Grenadines	0.124	0.148	0.131	98.4%	96.7%	82.9%	6.374	11.63	20.72	225.1%	0.452	1.25	2.884	538.1%
Saint Lucia	0.166	0.164	0.123	98.2%	93.2%	78.8%	8.404	12.82	20.6	145.1%	0.811	1.535	2.719	235.3%
America-Caribbean	**35.03**	**37.72**	**34.76**	**88.8%**	**79.1%**	**68.1%**	**6.639**	**11.7**	**18.58**	**179.9%**	**185.9**	**456.9**	**856.3**	**360.6%**
Guatemala	14.07	23.54	28.67	97.8%	95.0%	86.4%	4.406	7.655	14.31	224.8%	25.78	98.31	331.5	1185.9%
Honduras	7.821	11.5	12.63	97.6%	95.1%	87.6%	3.032	5.334	9.834	224.3%	8.482	28.59	83.52	884.7%
El Salvador	7.195	8.893	8.689	98.0%	95.9%	87.3%	4.958	7.92	14.56	193.7%	16.48	40.31	104.6	534.7%
Nicaragua	5.625	8.156	9.421	99.0%	99.0%	99.0%	2.556	3.582	6.109	159.3%	5.114	12.64	30.05	487.6%
Costa Rica	3.683	3.187	1.952	78.7%	54.6%	31.8%	8.398	15.35	26.71	218.1%	23.99	69.85	152.2	534.4%
Panama	2.746	2.068	1.179	79.0%	47.8%	25.8%	8.93	20.54	39.07	337.5%	20.05	76.44	170.6	750.9%
Belize	0.319	0.442	0.4	98.8%	93.4%	73.3%	6.568	11.56	22.3	239.5%	1.21	3.867	10.87	798.3%
America-Central	**41.46**	**57.79**	**62.94**	**94.4%**	**88.9%**	**80.3%**	**4.782**	**8.323**	**14.99**	**213.5%**	**101.1**	**330**	**883.2**	**773.6%**
USA	33.67	20.14	6.985	10.8%	5.5%	1.7%	36.37	53.69	83.05	128.3%	11315	19723	33451	195.6%
Mexico	105.2	118.1	102.6	96.3%	91.5%	80.4%	10.18	15.31	23.18	127.7%	686.8	1455	2621	281.6%
Canada	3.872	2.11	0.418	11.5%	5.5%	1.0%	30.73	42.35	67.06	118.2%	860.6	1481	2559	197.4%
America-North	**142.8**	**140.3**	**110**	**31.5%**	**26.2%**	**19.3%**	**29.55**	**43.61**	**68.53**	**131.1%**	**12862**	**22660**	**38631**	**200.3%**
Brazil	174.8	175	140.8	88.7%	74.9%	58.4%	7.977	14.97	25.78	223.2%	858.4	2535	5575	549.5%
Colombia	41.55	47.84	36.27	84.8%	78.7%	57.0%	5.541	8.675	14.54	162.4%	118.1	282.9	640.3	442.2%
Argentina	36.68	33.67	23.38	90.1%	71.1%	47.1%	11	23.14	39.54	259.5%	390	1052	1940	397.4%
Peru	28.4	32.16	28.17	93.8%	82.4%	66.0%	6.77	13.44	22.59	233.7%	91.27	331.5	799.5	776.0%
Venezuela	27.09	31.67	17.74	93.8%	84.7%	43.8%	9.53	17.42	25.95	178.1%	161.7	510.2	957.4	492.1%
Ecuador	14.17	18.61	18.87	98.7%	97.5%	89.5%	5.906	7.514	8.754	48.2%	23.01	48.96	77.37	236.2%
Chile	11.05	7.048	4.131	64.8%	35.7%	20.8%	11.57	21.1	36.58	216.2%	108.5	314.8	667.7	515.4%
Bolivia	9.606	12.19	12.36	94.8%	82.4%	71.1%	3.467	7.4	11.94	244.4%	11.82	53.45	128.4	986.3%
Paraguay	6.073	8.293	8.223	93.4%	89.0%	76.0%	3.593	5.611	10.41	189.7%	9.661	25.53	71.4	639.1%
Uruguay	2.084	0.867	0.183	58.8%	22.8%	4.9%	9.604	23.27	49.84	419.0%	27.18	82.64	184.4	578.4%
Guyana	0.656	0.517	0.268	86.8%	73.3%	43.1%	3.329	5.239	9.99	200.1%	0.895	1.629	3.695	312.8%
Suriname	0.455	0.442	0.324	98.9%	94.8%	78.6%	7.265	14.62	25.78	254.9%	1.425	4.206	8.868	522.3%
America-South	**352.6**	**368.3**	**290.7**	**88.4%**	**75.8%**	**56.8%**	**7.89**	**14.64**	**24.55**	**211.2%**	**1802**	**5243**	**11053**	**513.4%**

Poverty

Base Case: Countries in Year 2060 Descending Population Sequence	Poverty below $20 per Day						GDP per Capita at PPP				Gross Domestic Product			
	Millions of People			Percent of Population			Thousands in 2000 Dollars				Billions in 2000 Dollars			
	2010	2035	2060	2010	2035	2060	2010	2035	2060	% Chg	2010	2035	2060	% Chg
ASIA with OCEANIA														
China	1285	785.1	231.5	95.5%	54.9%	17.4%	4.862	18.55	47.47	876.3%	2998	19688	57479	1817.2%
Japan	11.24	1.559	0.108	8.8%	1.4%	0.1%	26.52	41.33	67.64	155.1%	4782	5973	7213	50.8%
Korea, Repub of	42.1	30.04	12.81	85.8%	63.4%	34.7%	19.68	31.16	50.41	156.1%	708	1331	1793	153.2%
Taiwan	21.16	16.39	8.423	88.1%	60.4%	32.4%	14.92	25.81	46.86	214.1%	307.1	664.9	1202	291.4%
Korea, Dem. People's Rep.	22.72	23.72	21.71	99.0%	99.0%	97.3%	2.795	4.207	6.318	126.0%	24.1	43.98	71.45	196.5%
Hong Kong SAR	1.203	0.947	0.565	16.5%	11.5%	7.1%	33.52	38.97	52.11	55.5%	232.7	308.7	406.9	74.9%
Mongolia	2.645	3.12	1.487	99.0%	96.5%	44.9%	2.78	6.636	15.7	464.7%	2.083	9.352	35.42	1600.4%
Asia-East	**1386**	**860.9**	**276.6**	**87.8%**	**52.0%**	**18.2%**	**7.327**	**20.47**	**48.11**	**556.6%**	**9054**	**28019**	**68201**	**653.3%**
India	1157	1409	1232	99.0%	97.6%	80.2%	2.355	8.053	20.4	766.2%	903.6	6587	25730	2747.5%
Pakistan	171.9	278.5	376.7	99.0%	99.0%	99.0%	2.122	3.228	6.627	212.3%	119.5	344.5	1297	985.4%
Bangladesh	152	198.2	199.6	99.0%	99.0%	93.9%	1.138	2.908	6.258	449.9%	81.26	326.2	861.1	959.7%
Afghanistan	35.62	68.85	91.79	99.0%	99.0%	84.3%	1.241	4.198	15.62	1158.7%	11.66	127.3	1252	10637.6%
Iran (Islamic Republic of)	38.4	0.623	0.872	52.8%	0.7%	0.9%	8.953	19.44	24.5	173.7%	168.1	763.7	1345	700.1%
Nepal	29.48	43.96	54.39	99.0%	99.0%	98.4%	0.919	1.39	2.719	195.9%	7.789	18.87	56.52	625.6%
Uzbekistan	27.71	34.28	17.61	99.0%	98.0%	48.6%	2.262	5.1	9.333	312.6%	26.41	99.13	226	755.7%
Sri Lanka	20.15	21.16	17.28	99.0%	95.8%	83.3%	3.471	6.997	13.54	290.1%	25.33	76.53	191.4	655.6%
Kazakhstan	14.4	4.475	0.225	95.2%	30.5%	1.8%	8.954	24.02	27.36	205.6%	39.49	186.6	232.5	488.8%
Tajikistan	6.929	10.4	11.34	99.0%	99.0%	90.7%	1.468	2.458	4.818	228.2%	2.002	6.663	22.58	1027.9%
Turkmenistan	4.861	2.623	2.75	93.5%	39.4%	37.8%	10.35	35.11	44.72	332.1%	36.4	206.4	313.6	761.5%
Kyrgyzstan	5.446	6.769	6.299	99.0%	99.0%	89.2%	1.678	3.007	5.35	218.8%	2.049	6.158	15.42	652.6%
Bhutan	0.684	0.829	0.646	99.0%	86.2%	58.2%	3.945	11.78	28.93	633.3%	0.952	6.76	27.02	2738.2%
Maldives	0.358	0.494	0.438	98.9%	96.9%	76.6%	3.965	8.488	18.92	377.2%	1.011	3.535	10.19	907.9%
Asia-South Central	**1665**	**2081**	**2012**	**97.0%**	**93.4%**	**80.9%**	**2.543**	**7.276**	**16.4**	**544.9%**	**1426**	**8759**	**31580**	**2114.6%**
Indonesia	232	273.1	260.5	99.0%	99.0%	94.8%	3.205	5.341	8.821	175.2%	262.7	652.6	1355	415.8%
Philippines	90.04	119.7	117.6	99.0%	95.6%	85.0%	2.944	5.285	10.02	240.4%	120	358	934.7	678.9%
Viet Nam	87.71	106.5	89.99	98.4%	98.0%	80.3%	2.2	4.814	10.25	365.9%	59.81	226.4	701.2	1072.4%
Thailand	65.07	67.44	55.12	98.4%	96.3%	83.9%	6.367	9.528	16.06	152.2%	170.4	336.4	718.6	321.7%
Myanrar	52.43	61.19	59.28	99.0%	99.0%	96.6%	0.911	1.818	3.113	241.7%	14	39.95	77.46	453.3%
Malaysia	20.69	21.14	17.42	75.3%	59.1%	44.5%	10.7	17.89	28.98	170.8%	131.5	389.7	931.7	608.5%
Cambodia	15.31	22.71	26.74	99.0%	99.0%	96.8%	1.417	3.881	8.187	477.8%	7.347	42.19	139.6	1800.1%
LAO People's Dem Repub	6.503	10.05	10.31	99.0%	99.0%	83.5%	1.767	5	12.38	600.6%	3.081	21.44	99.4	3126.2%
Singapore	0.938	0.579	0.339	20.2%	10.9%	6.5%	36.65	46.21	61.98	69.1%	125	198.4	280.9	124.7%
Timor-Leste	1.251	2.831	5.049	99.0%	99.0%	98.8%	2	3.21	4.806	140.3%	0.464	2.286	8.245	1676.9%
Brunei Darussalam	0.024	0.029	0	5.8%	5.2%	0.0%	38.56	46.1	45.41	17.8%	6.918	14.7	19.57	182.9%
Asia-South East	**571.9**	**685.3**	**642.3**	**97.1%**	**95.3%**	**86.5%**	**3.735**	**6.255**	**10.9**	**191.8%**	**901.3**	**2282**	**5266**	**484.3%**

Poverty

Base Case: Countries in Year 2060 Descending Population Sequence	Poverty below $20 per Day						GDP per Capita at PPP				Gross Domestic Product			
	Millions of People			Percent of Population			Thousands in 2000 Dollars				Billions in 2000 Dollars			
	2010	2035	2060	2010	2035	2060	2010	2035	2060	% Chg	2010	2035	2060	% Chg
ASIA with OCEANIA continued														
Turkey	74.91	82.08	70.18	97.9%	90.1%	76.2%	7.068	13.48	22.39	216.8%	275.1	834.9	1790	550.7%
Yemen	24.19	45.28	55.14	99.0%	96.8%	80.4%	2.049	4.267	7.619	271.8%	14.4	80.83	275.3	1811.8%
Iraq	29.42	41.94	39.57	99.0%	86.3%	65.1%	5.894	13.68	25.51	332.8%	93.69	504.6	1425	1421.0%
Saudi Arabia	15.65	26.58	0.906	60.5%	67.8%	1.9%	18.74	27.21	32.48	73.3%	259.4	748.8	1280	393.4%
Syrian Arab Repub	21.33	33.44	37.43	99.0%	98.1%	88.6%	3.727	5.406	9.529	155.7%	29.01	79.59	228.8	688.7%
Israel	3.278	1.813	0.409	42.9%	17.8%	3.4%	19.95	38.57	80.48	303.4%	147.6	389.5	965.3	554.0%
Jordan	5.834	7.59	3.03	94.9%	82.9%	28.1%	4.259	8.591	24.67	479.2%	14.64	54.89	237	1518.9%
Occupied Palestinian Territory	4.143	7.564	9.435	99.0%	99.0%	91.2%	3.291	6.169	13.82	319.9%	4.667	21.39	96.24	1962.1%
Azerbaijan	1.722	0	0.001	19.5%	0.0%	0.0%	5.889	16.08	20.86	254.2%	17.92	101	157.6	779.5%
United Arab Emirates	0.54	0.043	0.002	10.8%	0.7%	0.0%	32.38	50.13	63.32	95.6%	131.5	281.4	371	182.1%
Oman	1.321	1.553	0.415	46.4%	36.3%	8.2%	19.71	29	45.48	130.7%	32.19	93.23	204.3	534.7%
Kuwait	0.188	0.047	0	6.6%	1.2%	0.0%	38.22	51.82	41.08	7.5%	60.37	146.1	154.8	156.4%
Lebanon	3.779	4.278	3.494	99.0%	95.7%	77.7%	9.33	16.47	28.05	200.6%	25.15	63.68	120.8	380.3%
Armenia	3.073	2.432	1.351	99.0%	74.9%	43.3%	4.401	19.01	38.65	778.2%	4.727	38.8	103.6	2091.7%
Georgia	4.278	3.241	1.858	98.3%	90.2%	62.1%	3.705	8.667	15.15	308.9%	5.546	16.15	31.7	471.6%
Bahrain	0.091	0.087	0.001	11.4%	8.2%	0.1%	32.32	44.05	68.59	112.2%	13.92	33.29	62.74	350.7%
Qatar	0	0	0	0.0%	0.0%	0.0%	96.54	129.1	101.6	5.2%	114.9	164.6	108.3	-5.7%
Cyprus	0.125	0.085	0.035	16.1%	10.6%	4.8%	22.41	32.35	46.66	108.2%	12.13	22.3	31.18	157.0%
Asia-West	**193.9**	**258.1**	**223.3**	**84.6%**	**79.2%**	**58.2%**	**9.132**	**15.49**	**23.4**	**156.2%**	**1257**	**3675**	**7644**	**508.1%**
Australia	3.064	2.073	0.469	14.3%	8.1%	1.6%	30.29	42.99	72.23	138.5%	507.9	971.8	1893	272.7%
Papua New Guinea	6.513	10.18	12.5	99.0%	97.9%	93.4%	1.734	3.606	5.647	225.7%	4.657	18.88	41.36	788.1%
New Zealand	1.203	0.904	0.188	28.2%	18.9%	3.9%	21.47	30.15	54.47	153.7%	64.72	123.6	248.4	283.8%
Solomon Islands	0.534	0.896	1.233	98.9%	98.9%	97.9%	1.719	2.783	4.642	170.0%	0.422	1.194	3.022	616.1%
Fiji	0.874	0.957	0.784	99.0%	99.0%	89.8%	3.734	5.81	12.52	235.3%	1.88	3.454	8.612	358.1%
Vanuatu	0.235	0.369	0.399	99.2%	97.6%	84.7%	3.38	6.076	12.2	260.9%	0.328	1.177	3.953	1105.2%
Micronesia, Federated States of	0.122	0.201	0.241	99.2%	99.0%	91.3%	5.233	7.107	13.31	154.3%	0.27	0.702	2.325	761.1%
Tonga	0.113	0.186	0.249	98.3%	98.9%	96.9%	4.313	5.2	10.01	132.1%	0.172	0.382	1.418	724.4%
Samoa	0.187	0.225	0.195	98.9%	96.6%	85.2%	4.799	9.302	19.2	300.1%	0.343	1.14	3.362	880.2%
Oceania	**12.85**	**15.99**	**16.26**	**37.5%**	**36.6%**	**32.5%**	**22.08**	**29.73**	**48.53**	**119.8%**	**580.7**	**1122**	**2206**	**279.9%**

Poverty

Base Case: Countries in Year 2060 Descending Population Sequence	Poverty below $20 per Day						GDP per Capita at PPP				Gross Domestic Product			
	Millions of People			Percent of Population			Thousands in 2000 Dollars				Billions in 2000 Dollars			
	2010	2035	2060	2010	2035	2060	2010	2035	2060	% Chg	2010	2035	2060	% Chg
EUROPE														
Russian Federation	108.4	11.91	5.413	77.3%	9.8%	5.5%	11.77	24.66	26.63	126.3%	432.7	1322	1491	244.6%
Poland	26.98	12.94	5.697	70.9%	37.3%	20.1%	13.23	23.39	33.21	151.0%	237.8	542	807.3	239.5%
Ukraine	42.56	16.17	2.761	94.4%	46.6%	10.6%	5.495	10.05	15.14	175.5%	53.18	115.9	191	259.2%
Romania	21.21	18.32	12.53	99.0%	96.3%	80.6%	9.113	15.06	22.76	149.8%	58.33	123.8	219.1	275.6%
Czech Republic	9.998	8.437	5.135	97.7%	90.4%	66.0%	18.91	26.12	34.97	84.9%	77.1	131	200.1	159.5%
Belarus	8.855	3.557	1.983	92.3%	41.9%	28.3%	9.009	21.1	30.19	235.1%	24.57	87.62	146.8	497.5%
Hungary	9.07	5.981	3.171	91.7%	70.6%	46.5%	14.88	23.94	35.57	139.0%	59.76	116.2	193.5	223.8%
Bulgaria	7.363	5.5	2.872	98.8%	94.7%	64.6%	9.066	13.96	22.24	145.3%	18.95	32.15	58.4	208.2%
Slovak Republic	5.27	4.296	2.854	97.4%	84.2%	67.3%	15.94	25.82	33.72	111.5%	32.48	72.09	106.4	227.6%
Moldova, Repub of	4.129	3.726	3.011	99.0%	99.0%	97.7%	2.078	3.175	6.499	212.8%	2.046	3.553	8.77	328.6%
Europe-East	**243.8**	**90.84**	**45.42**	**83.6%**	**36.2%**	**22.6%**	**10.93**	**21.1**	**26.26**	**140.3%**	**996.9**	**2547**	**3422**	**243.3%**
United Kingdom	9.274	5.487	1.134	15.1%	8.5%	1.8%	27.26	41.87	72.03	164.2%	1635	2691	4639	183.7%
Sweden	0.719	0.114	0.006	7.9%	1.2%	0.1%	28.86	46.9	80.67	179.5%	279.7	459.5	757.8	170.9%
Denmark	0.397	0.134	0.01	7.2%	2.4%	0.2%	29.17	42.79	74.33	154.8%	169.2	253.2	430.3	154.3%
Ireland	0.584	0.273	0.188	13.3%	5.3%	3.4%	32.96	51.66	69.81	111.8%	130.6	246.9	365.1	179.6%
Norway	0.049	0.198	0.043	1.0%	3.8%	0.8%	43.53	54.07	77.75	78.6%	199.2	274.7	406.7	104.2%
Finland	0.488	0.139	0.021	9.2%	2.6%	0.4%	27.55	42.69	74.55	170.6%	143.4	226.6	376.7	162.7%
Lithuania	3.191	2.565	1.407	95.1%	86.5%	57.7%	13.54	23.39	37.5	177.0%	19.41	42.3	76.65	294.9%
Latvia	1.849	1.079	0.499	81.9%	54.8%	30.6%	13	25.43	42.15	224.2%	14	34.78	60.88	334.9%
Estonia	1.178	0.798	0.402	91.0%	76.9%	46.0%	16.24	29	50.3	209.7%	9.899	20.52	37.34	277.2%
Iceland	0.016	0.01	0	5.2%	2.9%	0.0%	33.63	49.05	80.91	140.6%	11.76	18.45	29.11	147.5%
Europe-North	**17.75**	**10.8**	**3.71**	**18.2%**	**10.6%**	**3.7%**	**27.65**	**42.58**	**71.77**	**159.6%**	**2612**	**4268**	**7179**	**174.8%**
Italy	15.04	11.4	7.576	25.7%	21.3%	17.0%	23.2	29.69	39.62	70.8%	1076	1431	1695	57.5%
Spain	11.64	8.565	4.3	26.5%	20.3%	12.0%	23.22	32.51	44.4	91.2%	686.4	1127	1440	109.8%
Greece	1.488	1.399	1.237	13.3%	13.1%	13.2%	26.4	35.88	46.69	76.9%	193.3	308.7	384.5	98.9%
Portugal	7.722	6.601	4.512	72.8%	65.9%	52.0%	16.67	23.09	33.1	98.6%	111.8	175.6	260.5	133.0%
Serbia	7.286	6.657	5.328	99.0%	99.0%	92.6%	8.243	11.65	18.81	128.2%	12.85	23.57	51.36	299.7%
Bosnia and Herzegovina	4.022	3.879	2.838	99.0%	98.6%	84.0%	5.73	12.51	21.39	273.3%	8.304	26.5	53.73	547.0%
Croatia	4.211	3.278	1.45	95.5%	83.0%	44.0%	12.27	19.41	29.3	138.8%	25.53	48.21	80.37	214.8%
Albania	3.156	3.255	2.348	99.0%	95.0%	72.7%	5.383	10.52	17.64	227.7%	5.866	17.85	38.62	558.4%
Macedonia, FYR	1.345	1.349	0.671	65.3%	66.7%	38.1%	6.935	9.213	14.38	107.4%	4.376	7.291	14	219.9%
Slovenia	1.83	1.234	0.509	91.3%	67.5%	34.3%	21.36	33.63	51.79	142.5%	26.18	50	68.7	162.4%
Montenegro	0.613	0.612	0.494	99.0%	97.9%	83.7%	6.957	11.54	22.7	226.3%	1.245	2.916	8.635	593.6%
Malta	0.141	0.084	0.035	34.6%	21.3%	10.4%	18.36	25.17	35.43	93.0%	4.297	7.094	10.68	148.5%
Europe-South	**58.5**	**48.32**	**31.3**	**39.4%**	**34.7%**	**26.5%**	**20.72**	**28.08**	**38.41**	**85.4%**	**2156**	**3226**	**4106**	**90.4%**
Germany	7.804	2.429	0.312	9.4%	3.1%	0.5%	26.58	38.76	67.9	155.5%	1974	2927	4599	133.0%
France	11.13	8.943	3.497	17.9%	13.9%	5.6%	26.97	36.21	59.7	121.4%	1475	2244	3629	146.0%
Netherlands	2.352	1.399	0.464	14.1%	8.0%	2.7%	30.31	40.19	64.22	111.9%	423.6	641.1	1025	142.0%
Belgium	1.639	1.069	0.294	15.4%	10.0%	2.9%	27.47	36.85	62.35	127.0%	250.5	370.8	606.5	142.1%
Austria	0.573	0.224	0.061	6.9%	2.9%	0.9%	30.32	40.91	63.95	110.9%	215.6	295.9	406.2	88.4%
Switzerland	0.55	0.15	0.023	7.3%	2.1%	0.4%	32.29	44.68	71.83	122.5%	269	348.8	464.8	72.8%
Luxembourg	0.001	0	0	0.2%	0.0%	0.0%	61.23	70.08	74.36	21.4%	24.93	37.52	49.91	100.2%
Europe-West	**24.05**	**14.21**	**4.651**	**12.8%**	**7.6%**	**2.7%**	**27.57**	**38.33**	**64.26**	**133.1%**	**4633**	**6865**	**10780**	**132.7%**

Health

Base Case
Source: International Futures
Version 6.32, June 2010

	Life Expectancy at Birth (Years)				Infant Mortality Rate (Deaths per 1,000 Infants before 1 Year of Age)				Child Mortality Probability (Deaths per 1,000 Children before Age 5)				Adult Mortality Probability (Deaths per 1,000 Adults before Age 60)			
	2010	2035	2060	% Chg	2010	2035	2060	% Chg	2010	2035	2060	% Chg	2010	2035	2060	% Chg
World	70.15	74.92	78.53	11.9%	31.52	14.47	7.039	-77.7%	61.38	30.75	15.68	-74.5%	164.2	128.8	103.2	-37.1%
Africa	57.97	67.05	71.99	24.2%	67.84	31.14	15.55	-77.1%	116.3	56.66	31.58	-72.8%	303.9	193.7	141.7	-53.4%
Americas	76.55	80.64	83.7	9.3%	13.46	5.51	2.649	-80.3%	19.12	7.989	3.742	-80.4%	119.5	95.18	78.55	-34.3%
Asia with Oceania	70.55	75.52	79.78	13.1%	31.12	12.3	4.611	-85.2%	49.46	20.72	6.968	-85.9%	151.1	120.2	93.09	-38.4%
Europe	76.53	80.74	83.94	9.7%	6.925	3.703	2.404	-65.3%	8.658	4.441	2.84	-67.2%	136.4	99.26	78.04	-42.8%
World	70.15	74.92	78.53	11.9%	31.52	14.47	7.039	-77.7%	61.38	30.75	15.68	-74.5%	164.2	128.8	103.2	-37.1%
Africa-Eastern	57.37	68.08	73.67	28.4%	64.11	24.79	8.801	-86.3%	103.4	41.12	15.44	-85.1%	325.9	187	122.7	-62.4%
Africa-Middle	50.31	58.79	64.21	27.6%	102	59.4	36.86	-63.9%	169.5	104.2	68.34	-59.7%	369	283.5	229.1	-37.9%
Africa-Northern	70.09	75.14	78.74	12.3%	33.18	13.85	7.334	-77.9%	45.95	18.9	9.621	-79.1%	143.4	106.3	87.43	-39.0%
Africa-Southern	51.05	62.89	73.48	43.9%	59.96	36.83	13.32	-77.8%	83.69	51.62	19.2	-77.1%	546.7	328.9	178.9	-67.3%
Africa-Western	54.73	65.77	71.18	30.1%	83.05	34.19	15.87	-80.9%	139.4	59.07	27.7	-80.1%	311.6	199.3	144.9	-53.5%
Africa	57.97	67.05	71.99	24.2%	67.84	31.14	15.55	-77.1%	116.3	56.66	31.58	-72.8%	303.9	193.7	141.7	-53.4%
America-Caribbean	73.18	76.63	79.81	9.1%	25.96	18.27	10.39	-60.0%	44.36	34.9	18.8	-57.6%	143.5	118.3	92.29	-35.7%
America-Central	73.59	78.23	81.55	10.8%	21.62	8.321	3.521	-83.7%	28.68	10.79	4.493	-84.3%	151.2	119.3	100.5	-33.5%
America-North	79.04	82.63	85.51	8.2%	7.842	3.742	1.935	-75.3%	10.39	4.702	2.363	-77.3%	90.75	70.57	56.42	-37.8%
America-South	74.36	79.17	82.4	10.8%	17.72	5.828	2.541	-85.7%	22.86	7.597	3.295	-85.6%	149.2	114.7	97.02	-35.0%
Americas	76.55	80.64	83.7	9.3%	13.46	5.51	2.649	-80.3%	19.12	7.989	3.742	-80.4%	119.5	95.18	78.55	-34.3%
Asia-East	74.84	79.01	82.94	10.8%	17.6	6.442	2.836	-83.9%	22.73	8.377	3.684	-83.8%	112.5	89.07	65.95	-41.4%
Asia-South Central	65.93	72.69	78.04	18.4%	47.06	16.91	4.914	-89.6%	70.84	28.71	7.867	-88.9%	201	150.5	111.5	-44.5%
Asia-South East	71.47	75.61	79.06	10.6%	24.04	11.79	5.971	-75.2%	31.88	15.65	7.913	-75.2%	149.7	111.9	87.44	-41.6%
Asia-West	72.2	76.24	79.43	10.0%	25.71	12.34	7.112	-72.3%	33.32	16.25	9.078	-72.8%	123.4	96.62	81.68	-33.8%
Oceania	77.41	80.48	83.19	7.5%	13.02	7.004	3.968	-69.5%	25.94	12.75	6.326	-75.6%	98.53	86.8	78.23	-20.6%
Asia with Oceania	70.55	75.52	79.78	13.1%	31.12	12.3	4.611	-85.2%	49.46	20.72	6.968	-85.9%	151.1	120.2	93.09	-38.4%
Europe-East	70.7	75.62	78.81	11.5%	10.99	6.557	4.969	-54.8%	13.8	8.262	6.242	-54.8%	218.1	160.7	141.3	-35.2%
Europe-North	79.74	83.72	86.75	8.8%	4.149	1.933	1	-75.9%	5.14	2.374	1.225	-76.2%	76.84	54.21	41.22	-46.4%
Europe-South	80.26	83.22	85.81	6.9%	4.563	2.422	1.454	-68.1%	5.668	2.99	1.781	-68.6%	71.58	55.1	43.93	-38.6%
Europe-West	80.84	83.98	86.83	7.4%	3.532	1.755	0.889	-74.8%	4.332	2.16	1.1	-74.6%	69.08	53.58	42.97	-37.8%
Europe	76.53	80.74	83.94	9.7%	6.925	3.703	2.404	-65.3%	8.658	4.441	2.84	-67.2%	136.4	99.26	78.04	-42.8%

Health

Base Case: Countries in Year 2060 Descending Population Sequence	Life Expectancy at Birth (Years)				Infant Mortality Rate (Deaths per 1,000 Infants before 1 Year of Age)				Child Mortality Probability (Deaths per 1,000 Children before Age 5)				Adult Mortality Probability (Deaths per 1,000 Adults before Age 60)			
	2010	2035	2060	% Chg	2010	2035	2060	% Chg	2010	2035	2060	% Chg	2010	2035	2060	% Chg
AFRICA																
Ethiopia	58.17	68.26	72.76	25.1%	67.12	19.39	5.079	-92.4%	109.8	32.99	8.696	-92.1%	283	183.9	131.7	-53.5%
Tanzania, United Rep	60.64	71.22	76.87	26.8%	49.76	15.68	5.095	-89.8%	81.25	25.46	8.195	-89.9%	297	150.7	88.16	-70.3%
Uganda	57.28	68.49	75.58	31.9%	58.97	22.71	5.54	-90.6%	96.36	38.02	9.135	-90.5%	348.1	183.9	113.5	-67.4%
Kenya	58.94	70.58	77.26	31.1%	56.92	26.25	8.51	-85.0%	89.85	42.68	14.1	-84.3%	316.8	141.1	73.12	-76.9%
Madagascar	61.45	68.48	72.81	18.5%	62.09	32.68	13.76	-77.8%	93.5	50.54	21.69	-76.8%	236.6	173.3	137.8	-41.8%
Mozambique	53.21	65.44	71.71	34.8%	76.47	25.29	8.131	-89.4%	127.9	42.36	13.38	-89.5%	373.7	223.3	145.5	-61.1%
Malawi	57.97	68.54	73.24	26.3%	67.57	29.45	14.05	-79.2%	97.26	43.83	21.25	-78.2%	336.2	176.2	108.3	-67.8%
Zambia	49.99	63.43	72.74	45.5%	81.06	40.06	14.94	-81.6%	134.6	68.34	25.96	-80.7%	454.1	224.5	103.9	-77.1%
Somalia	53.8	63.07	67.53	25.5%	89.72	42.81	24.23	-73.0%	143.1	71.23	41.1	-71.3%	315.6	236.7	196.5	-37.7%
Rwanda	52.34	64.23	71.7	37.0%	89.56	31.35	6.017	-93.3%	135.2	49.74	9.713	-92.8%	361.8	245.1	168.8	-53.3%
Zimbabwe	50.05	63.36	68.8	37.5%	49.35	29.91	18.33	-62.9%	79.94	49.69	31.12	-61.1%	576.1	301.7	225	-60.9%
Burundi	54.2	65.41	69.87	28.9%	84.19	35.61	13.7	-83.7%	139.2	61.67	24.33	-82.5%	320.5	199	159.4	-50.3%
Eritrea	60.52	66.69	70.43	16.4%	50.93	29.68	16.59	-67.4%	69.31	41.13	23.25	-66.5%	324.9	238.5	192.3	-40.8%
Comoros	65.47	68.91	73.06	11.6%	51.55	38.39	19.31	-62.5%	65.76	49.48	25.31	-61.5%	198.9	164.8	128.9	-35.2%
Mauritius	72.81	77.54	81.73	12.3%	13.81	7.478	4.449	-67.8%	16.36	8.91	5.315	-67.5%	166	121.2	89.23	-46.2%
Djibouti	57.23	64.9	73.05	27.6%	79.07	40.68	10.29	-87.0%	112.7	59.76	15.49	-86.3%	300.7	218.7	144.5	-51.9%
Africa-Eastern	**57.37**	**68.08**	**73.67**	**28.4%**	**64.11**	**24.79**	**8.801**	**-86.3%**	**103.4**	**41.12**	**15.44**	**-85.1%**	**325.9**	**187**	**122.7**	**-62.4%**
Congo, Democratic Republic of	48.45	55.85	61.2	26.3%	109.9	66.94	41.56	-62.2%	181.3	114.7	73.37	-59.5%	391.3	330.2	276.3	-29.4%
Angola	51.39	64.25	70.21	36.6%	90.39	33.55	18.79	-79.2%	153.9	59.92	34.32	-77.7%	356.2	235	180.1	-49.4%
Cameroon	54.02	64.02	71.61	32.6%	79.96	42.96	17.48	-78.1%	129.1	71.53	29.9	-76.8%	347.5	219.6	143.9	-58.6%
Chad	49.79	58.24	64.27	29.1%	129	80.4	56.18	-56.4%	198.6	129.2	92.49	-53.4%	324.4	241.7	180.8	-44.3%
Central African Republic	49.28	57.8	66.01	33.9%	102.2	66.07	29.12	-71.5%	168.1	112.5	51.71	-69.2%	392.5	281.8	203.3	-48.2%
Congo, Republic of	56.14	64.98	71.22	26.9%	71.17	40.32	21.75	-69.4%	111.8	65.04	35.84	-67.9%	332.3	216.7	154.9	-53.4%
Gabon	61.83	67.62	72.41	17.1%	52.11	40.88	29.08	-44.2%	79.26	62.84	45.41	-42.7%	267.5	191.3	150.2	-43.9%
Equatorial Guinea	50.14	58.33	64.61	28.9%	101.5	75.5	57.34	-43.5%	164.3	125	97.2	-40.8%	382.7	273.8	201	-47.5%
São Tomé and Príncipe	66.18	69.64	73.84	11.6%	70.13	54.69	31.72	-54.8%	89.05	70.23	41.51	-53.4%	141.3	113.1	88.26	-37.5%
Africa-Middle	**50.31**	**58.79**	**64.21**	**27.6%**	**102**	**59.4**	**36.86**	**-63.9%**	**169.5**	**104.2**	**68.34**	**-59.7%**	**369**	**283.5**	**229.1**	**-37.9%**
Egypt	71.34	76.25	80.55	12.9%	29.8	12.56	6.459	-78.3%	34.27	14.66	7.581	-77.9%	128	90.73	64.76	-49.4%
Sudan	60.91	69.24	73.23	20.2%	54.34	16.63	7.632	-86.0%	86.49	27.31	12.67	-85.4%	259.9	185.9	148.2	-43.0%
Algeria	73.41	77.63	80.32	9.4%	28.88	16.45	11.66	-59.6%	30.5	17.57	12.48	-59.1%	105.6	77.96	65.97	-37.5%
Morocco	72.07	76.08	79.67	10.5%	28.67	13.61	6.153	-78.5%	33.82	16.28	7.413	-78.1%	118.4	91.86	71.01	-40.0%
Tunisia	75.15	79.93	83.75	11.4%	17.59	7.718	4.089	-76.8%	19.6	8.678	4.609	-76.5%	87.74	54.34	38.28	-56.4%
Libyan Arab Jamahiriya	75.37	80.36	83.38	10.6%	15.08	6.131	4.087	-72.9%	16.3	6.68	4.459	-72.6%	113.8	76.93	61	-46.4%
Africa-Northern	**70.09**	**75.14**	**78.74**	**12.3%**	**33.18**	**13.85**	**7.334**	**-77.9%**	**45.95**	**18.9**	**9.621**	**-79.1%**	**143.4**	**106.3**	**87.43**	**-39.0%**

Health

Base Case: Countries in Year 2060 Descending Population Sequence	Life Expectancy at Birth (Years)				Infant Mortality Rate (Deaths per 1,000 Infants before 1 Year of Age)				Child Mortality Probability (Deaths per 1,000 Children before Age 5)				Adult Mortality Probability (Deaths per 1,000 Adults before Age 60)			
	2010	2035	2060	% Chg	2010	2035	2060	% Chg	2010	2035	2060	% Chg	2010	2035	2060	% Chg
AFRICA continued																
South Africa	50.18	61.85	72.98	45.4%	61.74	39.09	13.97	-77.4%	85.75	54.58	19.92	-76.8%	560.2	347.8	189.4	-66.2%
Namibia	64.43	73.33	79.51	23.4%	35.57	16.06	6.758	-81.0%	51.39	23.63	10.04	-80.5%	266.4	141.2	82.64	-69.0%
Lesotho	49.84	62.9	71.05	42.6%	64.03	34.41	13.08	-79.6%	92.43	50.26	19.54	-78.9%	540.4	274.4	160.4	-70.3%
Botswana	59.65	71.72	78.52	31.6%	34.74	17.88	8.164	-76.5%	52.36	26.7	12.54	-76.1%	382	187	110.1	-71.2%
Swaziland	49.5	62.45	71.42	44.3%	66.54	37.68	16.05	-75.9%	101.4	57.85	25.28	-75.1%	524.6	285	169.9	-67.6%
Africa-Southern	**51.05**	**62.89**	**73.48**	**43.9%**	**59.96**	**36.83**	**13.32**	**-77.8%**	**83.69**	**51.62**	**19.2**	**-77.1%**	**546.7**	**328.9**	**178.9**	**-67.3%**
Nigeria	52.18	65.52	70.73	35.6%	89.04	30.84	17.35	-80.5%	150.1	54.6	31.39	-79.1%	347.6	215.2	157	-54.8%
Niger	53.64	64.9	70.06	30.6%	82.23	32.91	11.55	-86.0%	155.5	65.68	23.65	-84.8%	304	196.4	150.2	-50.6%
Côte d'Ivoire	60	68.26	74.86	24.8%	83.66	48.13	19.43	-76.8%	115.3	68.15	28.24	-75.5%	239.3	132	79.95	-66.6%
Ghana	58.81	65.8	72.21	22.8%	66.46	43.23	18.53	-72.0%	103.3	68.59	30.3	-70.7%	279.1	198.8	143.3	-48.7%
Mali	52.5	65.83	70.03	33.4%	87.54	23.22	7.404	-91.5%	155.5	44	14.27	-90.8%	331.3	202.9	159.7	-51.8%
Burkina Faso	53.97	63.03	70.19	30.1%	80.39	39.46	11.37	-85.9%	153.1	78.74	23.45	-84.7%	287.5	205.2	146.3	-49.1%
Senegal	56.4	64.25	70.48	25.0%	56.99	28.49	9.125	-84.0%	114.7	59.27	19.44	-83.1%	292.6	211.3	151	-48.4%
Guinea	59.2	67.7	72.96	23.2%	92.27	43.09	19.13	-79.3%	136.5	66.44	30.22	-77.9%	211.8	149.6	112.1	-47.1%
Benin	63.64	70.93	75.06	17.9%	74.12	36.16	17.02	-77.0%	103.4	52.05	24.95	-75.9%	171.9	112	82.64	-51.9%
Togo	65.15	71.3	74.92	15.0%	64.62	39.91	27.56	-57.4%	86.92	54.71	38.19	-56.1%	178.5	107.8	74.01	-58.5%
Sierra Leone	48.76	57.58	63.93	31.1%	92.73	38.27	10.05	-89.2%	133.9	57.63	15.46	-88.5%	479.5	383.8	289	-39.7%
Liberia	60.05	67.59	71.74	19.5%	79.39	23.09	7.409	-90.7%	116.2	35.3	11.46	-90.1%	229.8	175.5	126.7	-44.9%
Mauritania	57.51	63.12	69.1	20.2%	68.79	51.51	25.97	-62.2%	110.4	84.02	43.53	-60.6%	274.1	202.1	148.6	-45.8%
Guinea-Bissau	52.86	65.35	70.35	33.1%	94.16	40.6	21.35	-77.3%	158.6	72.02	38.78	-75.5%	321.8	198.9	153.7	-52.2%
Gambia	58.23	65.11	69.53	19.4%	68.78	34.75	13.94	-79.7%	101.2	52.71	21.58	-78.7%	272.7	199.3	158.6	-41.8%
Cape Verde	72.18	76.31	80.38	11.4%	23.23	9.834	2.812	-87.9%	27.48	11.79	3.397	-87.6%	129.4	91.67	67.01	-48.2%
Africa-Western	**54.73**	**65.77**	**71.18**	**30.1%**	**83.05**	**34.19**	**15.87**	**-80.9%**	**139.4**	**59.07**	**27.7**	**-80.1%**	**311.6**	**199.3**	**144.9**	**-53.5%**

Health

Base Case: Countries in Year 2060 Descending Population Sequence	Life Expectancy at Birth (Years)				Infant Mortality Rate (Deaths per 1,000 Infants before 1 Year of Age)				Child Mortality Probability (Deaths per 1,000 Children before Age 5)				Adult Mortality Probability (Deaths per 1,000 Adults before Age 60)			
	2010	2035	2060	% Chg	2010	2035	2060	% Chg	2010	2035	2060	% Chg	2010	2035	2060	% Chg
AMERICAS																
Haiti	61.98	66.38	72.08	16.3%	64.26	49.23	24.76	-61.5%	84.16	65.17	33.46	-60.2%	241	180.9	124.7	-48.3%
Dominican Republic	74.28	80.14	84.28	13.5%	25.72	7.651	2.764	-89.3%	28.34	8.649	3.123	-89.0%	150.7	106	79.32	-47.4%
Cuba	79.43	82.85	85.53	7.7%	4.601	2.098	1.132	-75.4%	6.293	2.879	1.556	-75.3%	86.93	68.81	57.1	-34.3%
Puerto Rico	79.6	83.15	85.61	7.6%	6.248	2.593	1.336	-78.6%	7.455	3.101	1.599	-78.6%	90.82	69.89	59.74	-34.2%
Jamaica	72.06	76.29	79.6	10.5%	22.55	10.46	4.419	-80.4%	26.84	12.68	5.337	-80.1%	178.7	144.5	126.3	-29.3%
Trinidad	71.26	77.41	81.08	13.8%	21.12	6.698	3.028	-85.7%	26.15	8.431	3.812	-85.4%	171.4	114.5	86.1	-49.8%
Bahamas	74.52	79.41	83.39	11.9%	9.157	4.166	2.032	-77.8%	13.67	6.267	3.078	-77.5%	158.3	107.3	76.97	-51.4%
Barbados	77.87	81.09	84.12	8.0%	9.053	3.606	1.297	-85.7%	10.17	4.075	1.468	-85.6%	79.28	59.13	42.46	-46.4%
Grenada	75.88	79.14	82.48	8.7%	12.25	5.396	2.189	-82.1%	13.81	6.121	2.491	-82.0%	89.18	69.48	51.51	-42.2%
Saint Vincent and Grenadines	73.62	77.6	80.63	9.5%	19.73	6.682	2.976	-84.9%	23.1	7.925	3.543	-84.7%	102.1	76.98	60.26	-41.0%
Saint Lucia	74.52	78.03	80.95	8.6%	11.16	4.531	2.172	-80.5%	14.3	5.833	2.798	-80.4%	132.7	107.2	90.3	-32.0%
America-Caribbean	**73.18**	**76.63**	**79.81**	**9.1%**	**25.96**	**18.27**	**10.39**	**-60.0%**	**44.36**	**34.9**	**18.8**	**-57.6%**	**143.5**	**118.3**	**92.29**	**-35.7%**
Guatemala	71.68	77.92	81.67	13.9%	27.34	8.273	3.018	-89.0%	34.39	10.67	3.903	-88.7%	174.5	127.7	104.5	-40.1%
Honduras	73.7	78.4	81.53	10.6%	23.53	8.414	3.651	-84.5%	32.39	11.75	5.124	-84.2%	134.2	98.35	80.98	-39.7%
El Salvador	72.09	76.34	79.52	10.3%	19.95	8.046	3.298	-83.5%	23.15	9.495	3.883	-83.2%	196.9	162.6	143.8	-27.0%
Nicaragua	73.45	76.44	79.49	8.2%	21.71	13.75	7.108	-67.3%	25.78	16.46	8.545	-66.9%	160.9	133.7	113.5	-29.5%
Costa Rica	79.54	82.76	85.48	7.5%	8.376	3.458	1.744	-79.2%	9.627	3.992	2.016	-79.1%	85.49	67.16	54.14	-36.7%
Panama	76.28	80.6	83.8	9.9%	15.41	5.35	2.236	-85.5%	19.95	7.017	2.932	-85.3%	107	79.15	61.39	-42.6%
Belize	77.35	81.36	84.95	9.8%	15.14	6.429	2.955	-80.5%	19.01	8.139	3.754	-80.3%	100	75.78	58.29	-41.7%
America-Central	**73.59**	**78.23**	**81.55**	**10.8%**	**21.62**	**8.321**	**3.521**	**-83.7%**	**28.68**	**10.79**	**4.493**	**-84.3%**	**151.2**	**119.3**	**100.5**	**-33.5%**
USA	79.6	83.26	86.15	8.2%	5.444	2.765	1.517	-72.1%	6.754	3.441	1.89	-72.0%	88.49	66.43	52.52	-40.6%
Mexico	76.82	80.42	83.19	8.3%	15.76	6.992	3.509	-77.7%	18.83	8.426	4.236	-77.5%	107.9	86.46	72.2	-33.1%
Canada	81.11	84.02	86.48	6.6%	4.294	2.162	1.128	-73.7%	5.226	2.638	1.378	-73.6%	65.8	52.46	43.67	-33.6%
America-North	**79.04**	**82.63**	**85.51**	**8.2%**	**7.842**	**3.742**	**1.935**	**-75.3%**	**10.39**	**4.702**	**2.363**	**-77.3%**	**90.75**	**70.57**	**56.42**	**-37.8%**
Brazil	73.86	79.38	83	12.4%	19.29	5.488	2.166	-88.8%	23.76	6.855	2.714	-88.6%	166.2	124.8	103.4	-37.8%
Colombia	73.74	77.17	79.63	8.0%	15.88	6.302	2.773	-82.5%	21.63	8.672	3.828	-82.3%	148	129.7	123.8	-16.4%
Argentina	76.25	80.54	83.82	9.9%	11.34	4.314	2.113	-81.4%	13.01	4.984	2.444	-81.2%	118.3	86.17	66.63	-43.7%
Peru	74.69	80.03	83.71	12.1%	19.25	6.827	3.072	-84.0%	26.89	9.651	4.361	-83.8%	123.2	86.46	64.87	-47.3%
Venezuela	74.78	78.68	81.07	8.4%	14.12	4.863	2.311	-83.6%	17.95	6.237	2.972	-83.4%	131.2	109.4	101.9	-22.3%
Ecuador	75.92	79.59	81.78	7.7%	19.26	8.515	4.711	-75.5%	22.98	10.28	5.696	-75.2%	125.1	104.9	99.09	-20.8%
Chile	79.19	82.55	85.48	7.9%	6.436	2.783	1.43	-77.8%	7.785	3.379	1.738	-77.7%	92.68	72.31	57.88	-37.5%
Bolivia	67.48	74.28	77.95	15.5%	39.45	11.6	4.946	-87.5%	50.61	15.27	6.548	-87.1%	190.3	135.5	107.3	-43.6%
Paraguay	72.94	77.43	80.69	10.6%	26.87	10.3	4.206	-84.3%	31.63	12.37	5.067	-84.0%	145.8	114.9	96.29	-34.0%
Uruguay	77.17	81.52	84.95	10.1%	10.8	3.769	1.673	-84.5%	13.18	4.63	2.059	-84.4%	102.9	71.88	52.45	-49.0%
Guyana	68.82	73.78	78.25	13.7%	35.85	17.95	7.891	-78.0%	47.56	24.2	10.74	-77.4%	188.8	141.8	108.2	-42.7%
Suriname	69.67	75.21	80.02	14.9%	19.18	7.112	2.955	-84.6%	26.42	9.912	4.137	-84.3%	204.9	152.5	112.5	-45.1%
America-South	**74.36**	**79.17**	**82.4**	**10.8%**	**17.72**	**5.828**	**2.541**	**-85.7%**	**22.86**	**7.597**	**3.295**	**-85.6%**	**149.2**	**114.7**	**97.02**	**-35.0%**

Health

Base Case: Countries in Year 2060 Descending Population Sequence	Life Expectancy at Birth (Years)				Infant Mortality Rate (Deaths per 1,000 Infants before 1 Year of Age)				Child Mortality Probability (Deaths per 1,000 Children before Age 5)				Adult Mortality Probability (Deaths per 1,000 Adults before Age 60)			
	2010	2035	2060	% Chg	2010	2035	2060	% Chg	2010	2035	2060	% Chg	2010	2035	2060	% Chg
ASIA with OCEANIA																
China	73.89	78.38	82.6	11.8%	19.35	6.786	2.906	-85.0%	24.04	8.546	3.674	-84.7%	119	92.93	67.54	-43.2%
Japan	83.14	86.16	88.64	6.6%	2.765	1.463	0.839	-69.7%	3.782	2.004	1.15	-69.6%	58.23	47.13	40.68	-30.1%
Korea, Repub of	79.63	82.26	84.57	6.2%	3.901	1.897	0.994	-74.5%	5.091	2.481	1.302	-74.4%	76.89	63.76	54.13	-29.6%
Taiwan	79.3	81.46	83.35	5.1%	4.02	2.061	1.171	-70.9%	5.245	2.695	1.533	-70.8%	78.48	64.75	53.53	-31.8%
Korea, Dem. People's Rep.	68.24	72.71	76.61	12.3%	43.27	24.13	12.4	-71.3%	54.9	31.12	16.16	-70.6%	145	114.3	91.28	-37.0%
Hong Kong SAR	82.66	83.88	85.15	3.0%	3.314	2.183	1.342	-59.5%	4.198	2.768	1.702	-59.5%	53.7	49.39	44.21	-17.7%
Mongolia	68	72.66	77.47	13.9%	33.01	11.89	3.238	-90.2%	33.84	12.42	3.41	-89.9%	231.2	182.3	142.8	-38.2%
Asia-East	**74.84**	**79.01**	**82.94**	**10.8%**	**17.6**	**6.442**	**2.836**	**-83.9%**	**22.73**	**8.377**	**3.684**	**-83.8%**	**112.5**	**89.07**	**65.95**	**-41.4%**
India	65.57	73.32	78.97	20.4%	45.09	11.31	1.977	-95.6%	65.19	16.89	2.991	-95.4%	209.1	154.3	112	-46.4%
Pakistan	66.62	71.21	77.86	16.9%	64.1	41.76	13.69	-78.6%	87.31	57.93	19.5	-77.7%	152.6	124.5	89.1	-41.6%
Bangladesh	67.53	72.3	75.87	12.4%	37.62	13.37	5.872	-84.4%	48.37	17.58	7.781	-83.9%	184.1	145.4	113.2	-38.5%
Afghanistan	45.25	60.19	69.85	54.4%	151.9	45	5.27	-96.5%	214.4	69.53	8.439	-96.1%	426.6	314.4	214.5	-49.7%
Iran (Islamic Republic of)	72.42	76.96	79.81	10.2%	24.53	10.27	6.939	-71.7%	28.02	11.89	8.047	-71.3%	118.2	89.8	73.63	-37.7%
Nepal	66.47	70.23	75.01	12.8%	44.57	29.11	11.6	-74.0%	56.62	37.44	15.15	-73.2%	191.9	157.2	115.5	-39.8%
Uzbekistan	68.89	73.55	77.58	12.6%	41.35	18.13	7.489	-81.9%	48.43	21.66	9.026	-81.4%	183.2	146.3	119	-35.0%
Sri Lanka	74.74	77.9	80.91	8.3%	14.72	9.178	5.456	-62.9%	18.23	11.42	6.812	-62.6%	133.8	110.6	90.63	-32.3%
Kazakhstan	66.76	73.58	76.61	14.8%	24.09	9.918	8.12	-66.3%	28.14	11.74	9.621	-65.8%	260.2	178.4	157.5	-39.5%
Tajikistan	67.75	71.48	75.18	11.0%	52.49	33.46	18.42	-64.9%	66.38	42.96	23.97	-63.9%	175.1	148.9	126.1	-28.0%
Turkmenistan	67.18	77.14	81.11	20.7%	39.38	12.42	9.116	-76.9%	48.97	15.83	11.65	-76.2%	210.6	121.5	97.28	-53.8%
Kyrgyzstan	69.02	72.59	75.69	9.7%	31.99	17.08	9.229	-71.2%	37.95	20.54	11.17	-70.6%	185	147.8	121.8	-34.2%
Bhutan	67.18	74.48	80.63	20.0%	40.8	17.21	6.386	-84.3%	58.4	25.19	9.451	-83.8%	183.5	123.4	81.99	-55.3%
Maldives	72.65	76.11	79.6	9.6%	23.76	11.15	4.981	-79.0%	28.12	13.35	5.996	-78.7%	118.2	94.82	70.59	-40.3%
Asia-South Central	**65.93**	**72.69**	**78.04**	**18.4%**	**47.06**	**16.91**	**4.914**	**-89.6%**	**70.84**	**28.71**	**7.867**	**-88.9%**	**201**	**150.5**	**111.5**	**-44.5%**
Indonesia	71.72	75.52	78.78	9.8%	24.48	13.2	7.189	-70.6%	29.19	15.92	8.707	-70.2%	136.3	104.2	82.19	-39.7%
Philippines	72.47	75.94	79.67	9.9%	21.71	12.13	5.294	-75.6%	25.44	14.34	6.303	-75.2%	127.3	100.4	78.52	-38.3%
Viet Nam	75.12	78.29	81.35	8.3%	16.48	6.668	2.671	-83.8%	19.68	8.079	3.234	-83.6%	110.6	84.16	64.72	-41.5%
Thailand	70.09	74.35	78	11.3%	7.681	4.559	2.551	-66.8%	11.32	6.752	3.803	-66.4%	217.7	166.8	130	-40.3%
Myanmar	65.01	72.14	75.48	16.1%	55.7	20.92	12.43	-77.7%	80.66	31.29	18.77	-76.7%	202.5	148.8	119.7	-40.9%
Malaysia	74.98	79.12	82.42	9.9%	8.616	4.888	2.877	-66.6%	10.98	6.251	3.669	-66.6%	117.5	83.49	63.84	-45.7%
Cambodia	62.47	69.82	75.36	20.6%	58.43	24.56	8.757	-85.0%	81.28	35.17	12.72	-84.4%	240	171.2	125	-47.9%
LAO People's Dem Repub	66.4	72.86	77.5	16.7%	43.93	13.75	3.231	-92.6%	57.02	18.34	4.357	-92.4%	193.8	137.9	101.9	-47.4%
Singapore	80.96	84.54	87.65	8.3%	2.599	1.463	0.812	-68.8%	3.537	1.989	1.104	-68.8%	60.84	45.8	36.14	-40.6%
Timor-Leste	62.16	68.84	73.14	17.7%	65.05	32.84	18.48	-71.6%	87.37	45.3	25.84	-70.4%	234.2	175.3	140.2	-40.1%
Brunei Darussalam	77.45	79.92	81.47	5.2%	5.332	2.996	2.006	-62.4%	6.49	3.662	2.458	-62.1%	77.19	60.98	54.26	-29.7%
Asia-South East	**71.47**	**75.61**	**79.06**	**10.6%**	**24.04**	**11.79**	**5.971**	**-75.2%**	**31.88**	**15.65**	**7.913**	**-75.2%**	**149.7**	**111.9**	**87.44**	**-41.6%**

Health

Base Case: Countries in Year 2060 Descending Population Sequence	Life Expectancy at Birth (Years)				Infant Mortality Rate (Deaths per 1,000 Infants before 1 Year of Age)				Child Mortality Probability (Deaths per 1,000 Children before Age 5)				Adult Mortality Probability (Deaths per 1,000 Adults before Age 60)			
	2010	2035	2060	% Chg	2010	2035	2060	% Chg	2010	2035	2060	% Chg	2010	2035	2060	% Chg
ASIA with OCEANIA continued																
Turkey	72.62	77.17	80.94	11.5%	26.42	13.17	7.766	-70.6%	29.86	15.06	8.92	-70.1%	113.3	79.09	57.3	-49.4%
Yemen	64.43	70.14	74.21	15.2%	50.65	21.44	10.33	-79.6%	67.18	29.16	14.2	-78.9%	217.5	172.3	137.9	-36.6%
Iraq	68.82	73.55	76.92	11.8%	31.33	11.18	5.648	-82.0%	37.7	13.7	6.957	-81.5%	158.2	127.1	109	-31.1%
Saudi Arabia	73.36	77.22	80.14	9.2%	19.41	13.04	10.23	-47.3%	22.35	15.1	11.87	-46.9%	116.6	85.89	69.21	-40.6%
Syrian Arab Repub	74.84	77.8	80.72	7.9%	14.95	9.223	5.161	-65.5%	17.01	10.55	5.921	-65.2%	99.55	76.79	59.67	-40.1%
Israel	81.13	84.4	86.93	7.1%	4.18	1.784	0.856	-79.5%	5.004	2.141	1.028	-79.5%	58.46	42.66	34.61	-40.8%
Jordan	73.55	77.33	82.1	11.6%	17.61	8.507	3.738	-78.8%	19.58	9.546	4.205	-78.5%	134.1	104.2	73.72	-45.0%
Occupied Palestinian Territory	74.36	77.53	80.71	8.5%	15.53	5.706	2.447	-84.2%	17.84	6.616	2.846	-84.0%	104.5	82.38	64.39	-38.4%
Azerbaijan	72.14	78.65	82.3	14.1%	32.1	10.98	7.224	-77.5%	38.53	13.44	8.859	-77.0%	137.8	93.7	72.53	-47.4%
United Arab Emirates	78.55	83.02	86.29	9.9%	7.466	2.725	1.499	-79.9%	8.29	3.042	1.674	-79.8%	67.64	43.7	31.33	-53.7%
Oman	76.32	79.66	82.92	8.6%	11.79	7.244	4.345	-63.1%	13.24	8.172	4.914	-62.9%	85.58	61.92	44.48	-48.0%
Kuwait	78.17	81.81	83.59	6.9%	8.428	4.5	3.196	-62.1%	9.328	5.001	3.54	-62.0%	70.02	50.2	43.81	-37.4%
Lebanon	72.92	77.26	81.2	11.4%	20.36	10.64	5.909	-71.0%	23.72	12.51	6.977	-70.6%	121.8	88.26	64.99	-46.6%
Armenia	74.43	79.66	84.14	13.0%	22.14	7.118	3.644	-83.5%	23.99	7.84	4.009	-83.3%	117.8	85.39	61.36	-47.9%
Georgia	72.47	76.67	80.74	11.4%	30.82	14.08	7.881	-74.4%	31.73	14.78	8.238	-74.0%	132.3	102.7	78.07	-41.0%
Bahrain	76.53	79.66	82.74	8.1%	8.832	4.758	2.548	-71.2%	11.25	6.085	3.265	-71.0%	84.13	60.66	41.3	-50.9%
Qatar	77.88	81.41	82.88	6.4%	6.18	3.643	3.018	-51.2%	7.411	4.38	3.628	-51.0%	91.03	65.19	59.97	-34.1%
Cyprus	80.36	84.07	87.31	8.6%	4.768	2.313	1.243	-73.9%	5.662	2.754	1.48	-73.9%	54.8	37.8	27.5	-49.8%
Asia-West	**72.2**	**76.24**	**79.43**	**10.0%**	**25.71**	**12.34**	**7.112**	**-72.3%**	**33.32**	**16.25**	**9.078**	**-72.8%**	**123.4**	**96.62**	**81.68**	**-33.8%**
Australia	82.01	85.15	87.8	7.1%	4.249	2.124	1.098	-74.2%	4.923	2.466	1.276	-74.1%	56.97	43.8	35.85	-37.1%
Papua New Guinea	62.79	69.36	73.62	17.2%	42.88	18.08	9.204	-78.5%	57.64	24.84	12.75	-77.9%	286.7	212.7	166.1	-42.1%
New Zealand	80.71	83.87	86.62	7.3%	4.165	2.119	1.034	-75.2%	5.345	2.727	1.333	-75.1%	67.64	52.29	42.51	-37.2%
Solomon Islands	67.07	70.63	74.24	10.7%	41.27	27.88	17.42	-57.8%	52.61	35.93	22.66	-56.9%	187.4	156.1	126.2	-32.7%
Fiji	69.83	73.92	78.2	12.0%	18.77	11.76	6.422	-65.8%	23.07	14.54	7.972	-65.4%	178.7	134.4	96.27	-46.1%
Vanuatu	71.12	75.53	79.6	11.9%	27.05	15.57	8.37	-69.1%	32.25	18.76	10.15	-68.5%	142	105.2	76.87	-45.9%
Micronesia, Federated States of	69.49	73.41	77.81	12.0%	32.25	22.78	12.92	-59.9%	39.23	27.93	15.98	-59.3%	159.3	122	89.01	-44.1%
Tonga	72.16	75.21	79.44	10.1%	23.66	20.32	11.37	-51.9%	27.73	23.88	13.47	-51.4%	147.7	118.7	89.07	-39.7%
Samoa	72.54	77.22	81.59	12.5%	20.57	10.79	5.892	-71.4%	24.33	12.88	7.065	-71.0%	148.7	107.7	75.34	-49.3%
Oceania	**77.41**	**80.48**	**83.19**	**7.5%**	**13.02**	**7.004**	**3.968**	**-69.5%**	**25.94**	**12.75**	**6.326**	**-75.6%**	**98.53**	**86.8**	**78.23**	**-20.6%**

Health

Base Case: Countries in Year 2060 Descending Population Sequence	Life Expectancy at Birth (Years)				Infant Mortality Rate (Deaths per 1,000 Infants before 1 Year of Age)				Child Mortality Probability (Deaths per 1,000 Children before Age 5)				Adult Mortality Probability (Deaths per 1,000 Adults before Age 60)			
	2010	2035	2060	% Chg	2010	2035	2060	% Chg	2010	2035	2060	% Chg	2010	2035	2060	% Chg
EUROPE																
Russian Federation	68.18	74.01	76.8	12.6%	12.63	7.157	5.828	-53.9%	16.01	9.093	7.357	-54.0%	266	193.6	177.4	-33.3%
Poland	76.3	80.07	83.16	9.0%	5.992	3.673	2.728	-54.5%	7.002	4.302	3.198	-54.3%	120.4	90.92	75.07	-37.6%
Ukraine	69.33	73.48	77.6	11.9%	12.23	8.076	5.451	-55.4%	15.19	10.07	6.726	-55.7%	234.4	185.5	150.3	-35.9%
Romania	73.54	77.6	81.4	10.7%	13.76	8.703	6.046	-56.1%	16.41	10.43	7.263	-55.7%	136.1	102.1	80.89	-40.6%
Czech Republic	77.08	80.24	83.08	7.8%	3.415	2.304	1.698	-50.3%	4.279	2.89	2.131	-50.2%	95.35	74.52	62.88	-34.1%
Belarus	70.59	75.48	79.03	12.0%	8.218	4.641	3.517	-57.2%	10.22	5.788	4.384	-57.1%	213.3	157.5	131.7	-38.3%
Hungary	73.99	77.85	81.18	9.7%	6.448	3.909	2.724	-57.8%	7.841	4.764	3.324	-57.6%	157	119.5	97.97	-37.6%
Bulgaria	74.04	77.6	81.51	10.1%	11.11	7.739	5.527	-50.3%	13.57	9.485	6.788	-50.0%	128.5	99.4	76.45	-40.5%
Slovak Republic	75.56	79.41	82.45	9.1%	6.132	3.779	2.915	-52.5%	7.283	4.5	3.474	-52.3%	122.1	93.03	78.12	-36.0%
Moldova, Repub of	69.12	71.66	74.61	7.9%	15.39	11.72	7.258	-52.8%	19.09	14.59	9.071	-52.5%	210.8	178.9	150.1	-28.8%
Europe-East	**70.7**	**75.62**	**78.81**	**11.5%**	**10.99**	**6.557**	**4.969**	**-54.8%**	**13.8**	**8.262**	**6.242**	**-54.8%**	**218.1**	**160.7**	**141.3**	**-35.2%**
United Kingdom	80.11	84.18	87.17	8.8%	4.228	1.868	0.916	-78.3%	5.183	2.295	1.126	-78.3%	68.62	47.3	36.42	-46.9%
Sweden	81.37	85.12	87.91	8.0%	2.65	1.236	0.637	-76.0%	3.585	1.674	0.863	-75.9%	56.61	40.3	32.62	-42.4%
Denmark	78.77	82.05	85.14	8.1%	3.862	1.833	0.911	-76.4%	5.002	2.377	1.182	-76.4%	85.65	66.29	51.66	-39.7%
Ireland	80.42	83.88	86.38	7.4%	3.986	1.954	1.151	-71.1%	5.006	2.459	1.449	-71.1%	61.71	45.41	38.25	-38.0%
Norway	81.1	83.99	86.56	6.7%	3.039	1.747	1.015	-66.6%	4.058	2.335	1.359	-66.5%	59.62	47.17	38.57	-35.3%
Finland	80.12	83.58	86.3	7.7%	2.744	1.317	0.65	-76.3%	3.303	1.587	0.784	-76.3%	77.17	58.14	47.24	-38.8%
Lithuania	72.89	77.26	81.18	11.4%	7.867	4.884	3.389	-56.9%	10.03	6.249	4.343	-56.7%	186.6	143.8	119.9	-35.7%
Latvia	73.44	78.29	82.68	12.6%	8.138	4.489	2.947	-63.8%	9.99	5.531	3.636	-63.6%	171.5	122.3	93.14	-45.7%
Estonia	74.27	78.96	83.32	12.2%	6.411	3.719	2.348	-63.4%	8.291	4.824	3.048	-63.2%	166.8	120.6	90.9	-45.5%
Iceland	82.4	85.66	88.41	7.3%	2.513	1.274	0.827	-67.1%	3.314	1.679	1.08	-67.4%	46.54	34.02	26.69	-42.7%
Europe-North	**79.74**	**83.72**	**86.75**	**8.8%**	**4.149**	**1.933**	**1**	**-75.9%**	**5.14**	**2.374**	**1.225**	**-76.2%**	**76.84**	**54.21**	**41.22**	**-46.4%**
Italy	81.51	84.37	86.84	6.5%	3.447	1.598	0.859	-75.1%	4.063	1.887	1.014	-75.0%	61.37	47.03	37.71	-38.6%
Spain	81.27	84.02	86.3	6.2%	3.408	1.637	0.911	-73.3%	4.231	2.036	1.134	-73.2%	66.52	51.81	42	-36.9%
Greece	79.77	83.16	86.12	8.0%	3.401	1.74	1.016	-70.1%	3.852	1.975	1.154	-70.0%	66.12	48.81	38.3	-42.1%
Portugal	79.08	82.16	84.9	7.4%	3.7	1.848	1.012	-72.6%	4.803	2.403	1.317	-72.6%	81.91	62.13	48.6	-40.7%
Serbia	74.79	77.98	81.45	8.9%	11.14	7.655	5.107	-54.2%	13.04	8.99	6.012	-53.9%	115.4	90.97	72.29	-37.4%
Bosnia and Herzegovina	75.71	79.66	83.44	10.2%	12.29	6.613	4.05	-67.0%	14.34	7.761	4.765	-66.8%	101.8	75.12	56.77	-44.2%
Croatia	76.87	80.4	83.46	8.6%	5.804	3.715	2.554	-56.0%	6.888	4.418	3.041	-55.9%	100.8	75.51	61.73	-38.8%
Albania	77.25	80.64	83.89	8.6%	14.83	7.789	5.009	-66.2%	16.14	8.527	5.497	-65.9%	74.22	57.19	45.26	-39.0%
Macedonia, FYR	74.86	77.74	80.79	7.9%	14.12	9.352	6.181	-56.2%	15.93	10.59	7.022	-55.9%	103.6	82.93	68.59	-33.8%
Slovenia	79.09	82.75	85.58	8.2%	3.047	1.349	0.712	-76.6%	3.628	1.609	0.85	-76.6%	85.81	63.29	52.42	-38.9%
Montenegro	74.75	78.34	82.48	10.3%	9.679	5.713	3.335	-65.5%	10.76	6.377	3.732	-65.3%	133.1	103.3	79.32	-40.4%
Malta	80.23	83.3	85.99	7.2%	6.063	4.604	3.517	-42.0%	7.026	5.341	4.081	-41.9%	54.39	39.19	29.38	-46.0%
Europe-South	**80.26**	**83.22**	**85.81**	**6.9%**	**4.563**	**2.422**	**1.454**	**-68.1%**	**5.668**	**2.99**	**1.781**	**-68.6%**	**71.58**	**55.1**	**43.93**	**-38.6%**
Germany	80.27	83.64	86.89	8.2%	3.588	1.771	0.879	-75.5%	4.44	2.196	1.091	-75.4%	69.07	52.19	40.52	-41.3%
France	81.72	84.63	87.13	6.6%	3.305	1.617	0.823	-75.1%	4.061	1.989	1.013	-75.1%	71.71	56.59	46.58	-35.0%
Netherlands	80.44	83.29	85.93	6.8%	3.997	2.125	1.115	-72.1%	4.868	2.594	1.362	-72.0%	63.21	49.11	38.7	-38.8%
Belgium	80.14	83.17	85.97	7.3%	3.585	1.839	0.947	-73.6%	4.482	2.304	1.187	-73.5%	72.91	57.24	46.99	-35.6%
Austria	80.44	83.61	86.45	7.5%	3.644	1.693	0.845	-76.8%	4.316	2.009	1.004	-76.7%	69.7	54.33	44.65	-35.9%
Switzerland	82.26	85.15	87.73	6.6%	3.54	1.826	0.957	-73.0%	4.404	2.276	1.193	-72.9%	57.57	45.44	36.95	-35.8%
Luxembourg	80.05	83.03	85.22	6.5%	3.781	2.085	1.274	-66.3%	5.486	3.031	1.855	-66.2%	66.37	50.02	41.4	-37.6%
Europe-West	**80.84**	**83.98**	**86.83**	**7.4%**	**3.532**	**1.755**	**0.889**	**-74.8%**	**4.332**	**2.16**	**1.1**	**-74.6%**	**69.08**	**53.58**	**42.97**	**-37.8%**

Multination Regional Analysis

Measures of Poverty, Health, Education, Infrastructure, and Governance

Health

Base Case
Source: International Futures
Version 6.32, June 2010

	Calories per Capita				Undernourished Children				Adult Obesity Rate				Adult Smoking Rate			
	Available per Person per Day				Percent of All Children				Percent of Adults 30 Years and Older				Percentage of Adults Who Smoke Tobacco			
	2010	2035	2060	% Chg	2010	2035	2060	% Chg	2010	2035	2060	% Chg	2010	2035	2060	% Chg
World	2856	3082	3247	13.7%	15.63	8.663	5.608	-64.1%	11.33	12.88	14.23	25.6%	28.87	26.39	25.25	-12.5%
Africa	2464	2675	2885	17.1%	21.83	12.62	8.012	-63.3%	9.159	9.225	9.996	9.1%	17.67	18.82	20.88	18.2%
Americas	3216	3344	3456	7.5%	4.262	3.504	2.942	-31.0%	32.89	35.47	37.97	15.4%	20.3	20.53	21.31	5.0%
Asia with Oceania	2779	3108	3334	20.0%	19.05	9.476	5.616	-70.5%	4.978	7.41	9.436	89.6%	33.6	30.27	28.26	-15.9%
Europe	3378	3480	3533	4.6%	2.041	1.386	1.1	-46.1%	22.78	24.24	24.91	9.4%	28.49	26.74	25	-12.2%
World	2856	3082	3247	13.7%	15.63	8.663	5.608	-64.1%	11.33	12.88	14.23	25.6%	28.87	26.39	25.25	-12.5%
Africa-Eastern	2085	2481	2928	40.4%	25.4	13.57	6.889	-72.9%	1.963	3.47	6.372	224.6%	12.82	15.54	19.06	48.7%
Africa-Middle	1908	2227	2400	25.8%	26.51	18.51	14.02	-47.1%	3.688	4.885	5.731	55.4%	22.94	22.4	22.57	-1.6%
Africa-Northern	3076	3227	3321	8.0%	12.61	6.69	4.619	-63.4%	24.33	25.84	26.88	10.5%	23.37	22.96	23.93	2.4%
Africa-Southern	2925	3161	3505	19.8%	13.56	8.058	4.492	-66.9%	26.9	30.47	37.13	38.0%	15	18.74	21.62	44.1%
Africa-Western	2591	2733	2849	10.0%	24	12.68	7.956	-66.9%	5.316	6.169	6.939	30.5%	17.24	18.67	20.72	20.2%
Africa	2464	2675	2885	17.1%	21.83	12.62	8.012	-63.3%	9.159	9.225	9.996	9.1%	17.67	18.82	20.88	18.2%
America-Caribbean	2731	2898	3088	13.1%	10.53	8.973	6.563	-37.7%	22.75	25.71	28.94	27.2%	19.18	19.9	20.92	9.1%
America-Central	2441	2736	3089	26.5%	12.17	8.228	5.153	-57.7%	24.08	30.28	38.74	60.9%	23.75	22.63	23.45	-1.3%
America-North	3587	3626	3633	1.3%	2.439	2.252	2.167	-11.2%	41.95	42.8	42.85	2.1%	15.57	16.27	17.27	10.9%
America-South	2927	3160	3352	14.5%	4.848	3.713	3.108	-35.9%	24.54	29.06	33.31	35.7%	25.42	24.99	25.53	0.4%
Americas	3216	3344	3456	7.5%	4.262	3.504	2.942	-31.0%	32.89	35.47	37.97	15.4%	20.3	20.53	21.31	5.0%
Asia-East	3026	3446	3658	20.9%	4.61	3.186	2.612	-43.3%	3.698	7.148	9.274	150.8%	36.45	33.24	29.45	-19.2%
Asia-South Central	2527	2904	3209	27.0%	32.73	13.62	7.045	-78.5%	3.495	5.225	7.153	104.7%	32.71	29.6	28.45	-13.0%
Asia-South East	2761	2941	3117	12.9%	21.9	12.53	7.576	-65.4%	3.62	4.533	5.755	59.0%	30.74	26.76	26	-15.4%
Asia-West	2982	3136	3283	10.1%	10.75	7.046	4.744	-55.9%	25.32	27.37	29.34	15.9%	29.85	28.73	27.76	-7.0%
Oceania	2998	3167	3349	11.7%	5.843	4.2	3.304	-43.5%	25.5	27.2	29.9	17.3%	20.62	20.87	20.02	-2.9%
Asia with Oceania	2779	3108	3334	20.0%	19.05	9.476	5.616	-70.5%	4.978	7.41	9.436	89.6%	33.6	30.27	28.26	-15.9%
Europe-East	3210	3386	3397	5.8%	4.852	3.514	2.985	-38.5%	23.74	26.64	26.91	13.4%	33.25	31.26	29.13	-12.4%
Europe-North	3413	3529	3633	6.4%	0.073	0.092	0.106	45.2%	25.48	27.32	29.12	14.3%	17	15.98	15.66	-7.9%
Europe-South	3443	3467	3495	1.5%	0.698	0.597	0.525	-24.8%	22.11	22.77	23.54	6.5%	28.6	28.11	26.54	-7.2%
Europe-West	3543	3569	3645	2.9%	0	0	0		20.45	20.52	21.25	3.9%	26.73	25.42	24.55	-8.2%
Europe	3378	3480	3533	4.6%	2.041	1.386	1.1	-46.1%	22.78	24.24	24.91	9.4%	28.49	26.74	25	-12.2%

Health

Base Case: Countries in Year 2060 Descending Population Sequence	Calories per Capita (Available per Person per Day)				Undernourished Children (Percent of All Children)				Adult Obesity Rate (Percent of Adults 30 Years and Older)				Adult Smoking Rate (Percentage of Adults Who Smoke Tobacco)			
	2010	2035	2060	% Chg	2010	2035	2060	% Chg	2010	2035	2060	% Chg	2010	2035	2060	% Chg
AFRICA																
Ethiopia	1958	2427	2939	50.1%	34.68	16.55	6.883	-80.2%	0.252	1.556	4.066	1513.5%	3.888	9.446	15	285.8%
Tanzania, United Rep	2031	2595	3145	54.8%	17.14	5.558	3.242	-81.1%	2.993	6.986	13.13	338.7%	13.2	16.34	20.07	52.0%
Uganda	2412	2807	3297	36.7%	20.82	9.922	3.56	-82.9%	1.126	2.263	4.976	341.9%	17.93	18.47	21.73	21.2%
Kenya	2205	2514	2992	35.7%	18.44	10.93	5.636	-69.4%	1.497	2.47	5.191	246.8%	11.56	15.09	18.72	61.9%
Madagascar	2078	2275	2606	25.4%	35.27	26.41	12.32	-55.1%	2.119	2.876	4.756	124.4%	24.84	22.27	22.72	-8.5%
Mozambique	2159	2704	3190	47.8%	21.33	7.436	3.856	-81.7%	2.551	5.425	9.71	280.6%	22.54	22.63	24.07	6.8%
Malawi	2187	2371	2714	24.1%	17.53	11.2	6.315	-64.0%	2.056	2.966	5.296	157.6%	14.28	16.06	18.74	31.2%
Zambia	2046	2458	2905	42.0%	22.83	11.36	5.495	-75.9%	1.075	2.445	5.2	383.7%	9.214	13.42	17.49	89.8%
Somalia	2042	2229	2404	17.7%	35.87	25.68	17.23	-52.0%	2.216	2.798	3.569	61.1%	23.59	22.18	22.42	-5.0%
Rwanda	2146	2673	3154	47.0%	17.73	7.061	3.509	-80.2%	0.853	2.441	5.398	532.8%	7.026	11.74	16.96	141.4%
Zimbabwe	2038	2285	2640	29.5%	14.15	11.77	7.777	-45.0%	11.58	13.48	17.54	51.5%	11.1	14.84	17.92	61.4%
Burundi	1709	1906	2231	30.5%	44.11	28.5	16.07	-63.6%	1.372	2.033	3.769	174.7%	16.44	17.61	19.43	18.2%
Eritrea	1500	1500	1642	9.5%	38.43	31.99	24.94	-35.1%	0.08	0.079	0	-100.0%	22.69	22.25	22.39	-1.3%
Comoros	1790	1992	2410	34.6%	31.04	24.76	15.25	-50.9%	5.399	6.691	10.4	92.6%	23.54	22.31	22.6	-4.0%
Mauritius	3006	3237	3442	14.5%	13.8	9.044	5.903	-57.2%	15.53	18.19	20.82	34.1%	16.68	19.64	22.47	34.7%
Djibouti	2325	2606	3015	29.7%	22.27	12.6	6.155	-72.4%	5.623	7.543	11.37	102.2%	47.43	39.09	34.1	-28.1%
Africa-Eastern	**2085**	**2481**	**2928**	**40.4%**	**25.4**	**13.57**	**6.889**	**-72.9%**	**1.963**	**3.47**	**6.372**	**224.6%**	**12.82**	**15.54**	**19.06**	**48.7%**
Congo, Democratic Republic of	1604	1951	2135	33.1%	28.42	22	17.17	-39.5%	0.601	1.211	1.875	212.0%	23.79	22.34	22.38	-5.9%
Angola	2223	2730	3015	35.6%	31.07	14.19	7.749	-75.1%	7.128	11.69	15.1	111.8%	23.07	23.78	24.06	4.3%
Cameroon	2326	2573	2889	24.2%	18.92	11.34	6.444	-65.9%	12.69	15.41	19.61	54.5%	21.09	22.88	23.31	10.5%
Chad	2150	2395	2490	15.8%	30.36	18.37	14.04	-53.8%	1.458	2.094	2.448	67.9%	19.85	19.7	20.82	4.9%
Central African Republic	1983	2212	2530	27.6%	24.87	20.94	12.32	-50.5%	1.049	1.643	3.053	191.0%	23.47	22.11	22.4	-4.6%
Congo, Republic of	2267	2629	2859	26.1%	9.812	7.508	5.921	-39.7%	2.671	4.582	6.269	134.7%	23.39	23.2	23.34	-0.2%
Gabon	2713	2926	3109	14.6%	11.21	8.014	5.562	-50.4%	12.25	14.16	16.13	31.7%	24.59	24.36	24.56	-0.1%
Equatorial Guinea	3400	3487	3475	2.2%	16.74	10.23	6.47	-61.4%	14.96	15.87	15.74	5.2%	27.49	24.68	24.63	-10.4%
São Tomé and Príncipe	2513	2555	2677	6.5%	11.5	12.55	8.96	-22.1%	4.048	4.203	4.805	18.7%	21.99	22.51	22.71	3.3%
Africa-Middle	**1908**	**2227**	**2400**	**25.8%**	**26.51**	**18.51**	**14.02**	**-47.1%**	**3.688**	**4.885**	**5.731**	**55.4%**	**22.94**	**22.4**	**22.57**	**-1.6%**
Egypt	3374	3474	3537	4.8%	6.26	4.455	3.489	-44.3%	42.12	44.39	45.93	9.0%	33.82	29.66	28.8	-14.8%
Sudan	2343	2761	3023	29.0%	37.25	13.15	7.195	-80.7%	4.841	7.621	9.989	106.3%	14.25	16.89	19.61	37.6%
Algeria	3067	3173	3201	4.4%	8.45	6.223	5.011	-40.7%	12.65	13.66	13.99	10.6%	16.93	19.21	21.08	24.5%
Morocco	3128	3235	3322	6.2%	8.596	6.095	4.425	-48.5%	16.51	17.58	18.49	12.0%	14.46	17.27	20.29	40.3%
Tunisia	3277	3433	3517	7.3%	1.189	1.482	1.811	52.3%	26.68	29.11	30.5	14.3%	26.08	26.08	26.57	1.9%
Libyan Arab Jamahiriya	3362	3493	3427	1.9%	0	0	0		22.02	23.97	23.15	5.1%	24.47	25.04	25.24	3.1%
Africa-Northern	**3076**	**3227**	**3321**	**8.0%**	**12.61**	**6.69**	**4.619**	**-63.4%**	**24.33**	**25.84**	**26.88**	**10.5%**	**23.37**	**22.96**	**23.93**	**2.4%**

Multination Regional Analysis

Measures of Poverty, Health, Education, Infrastructure, and Governance

Health

Base Case: Countries in Year 2060 Descending Population Sequence	Calories per Capita (Available per Person per Day)				Undernourished Children (Percent of All Children)				Adult Obesity Rate (Percent of Adults 30 Years and Older)				Adult Smoking Rate (Percentage of Adults Who Smoke Tobacco)			
	2010	2035	2060	% Chg	2010	2035	2060	% Chg	2010	2035	2060	% Chg	2010	2035	2060	% Chg
AFRICA continued																
South Africa	2999	3230	3568	19.0%	13.46	7.999	4.477	-66.7%	28.9	33.03	40.25	39.3%	14.53	18.48	21.55	48.3%
Namibia	2345	2736	3213	37.0%	20.84	10.62	5.174	-75.2%	4.076	6.293	10.45	156.4%	17.91	19.21	22.23	24.1%
Lesotho	2661	2851	3084	15.9%	16.1	9.725	5.275	-67.2%	23.18	24.71	27.89	20.3%	19.44	21.28	22.67	16.6%
Botswana	2307	2846	3307	43.3%	6.411	4.414	3.212	-49.9%	14.95	23.04	31.92	113.5%	24.41	25.62	24.32	-0.4%
Swaziland	2382	2716	3136	31.7%	11.54	7.469	4.133	-64.2%	12.97	16.98	23.55	81.6%	6.982	12.36	17.41	149.4%
Africa-Southern	**2925**	**3161**	**3505**	**19.8%**	**13.56**	**8.058**	**4.492**	**-66.9%**	**26.9**	**30.47**	**37.13**	**38.0%**	**15**	**18.74**	**21.62**	**44.1%**
Nigeria	2735	2925	2919	6.7%	22.8	7.949	6.643	-70.9%	5.653	6.849	6.815	20.6%	11.02	14.34	17.63	60.0%
Niger	2193	2334	2553	16.4%	38.84	27.56	14.16	-63.5%	2.103	2.544	3.496	66.2%	32.1	28.3	26.46	-17.6%
Côte d'Ivoire	2645	2759	2899	9.6%	20.6	13.14	7.66	-62.8%	3.733	4.243	4.968	33.1%	23.19	22.66	22.98	-0.9%
Ghana	2713	2715	2912	7.3%	20.73	16.77	8.184	-60.5%	5.187	5.199	6.543	26.1%	5.095	10.09	15.02	194.8%
Mali	2256	2495	2892	28.2%	29.06	14.72	5.939	-79.6%	4.544	5.669	8.481	86.6%	23.74	22.51	23.21	-2.2%
Burkina Faso	2514	2673	2991	19.0%	36.62	21.97	8.377	-77.1%	0.996	1.27	2.264	127.3%	10.7	14.18	17.8	66.4%
Senegal	2395	2564	2931	22.4%	17.34	11.26	5.685	-67.2%	7.641	8.688	11.75	53.8%	23.35	22.49	23.2	-0.6%
Guinea	2461	2651	2865	16.4%	24.08	13.81	7.695	-68.0%	4.115	4.996	6.275	52.5%	63.86	48.48	39.59	-38.0%
Benin	2584	2641	2794	8.1%	19.29	14.16	7.852	-59.3%	6.893	7.153	8.116	17.7%	24.29	22.59	22.96	-5.5%
Togo	2305	1968	1921	-16.7%	20.74	19.42	18.15	-12.5%	4.051	3.09	3.038	-25.0%	22.56	22.31	22.44	-0.5%
Sierra Leone	2010	2433	2971	47.8%	24.66	12.08	4.941	-80.0%	10.91	15.15	22.77	108.7%	32.99	27.29	26.53	-19.6%
Liberia	2026	2587	3021	49.1%	25.26	9.077	4.446	-82.4%	11.06	17.81	24.88	125.0%	23.99	22.42	23.29	-2.9%
Mauritania	2785	2617	2605	-6.5%	20.72	22.43	14.01	-32.4%	17.91	16.18	16.11	-10.1%	24.96	22.35	22.48	-9.9%
Guinea-Bissau	2001	1662	1734	-13.3%	27.33	26.06	21.98	-19.6%	2.285	1.861	1.865	-18.4%	24.34	22.08	22.31	-8.3%
Gambia	2330	2593	2906	24.7%	5.898	4.595	3.541	-40.0%	1.94	2.693	4.159	114.4%	23.9	23.14	23.53	-1.5%
Cape Verde	3240	3415	3547	9.5%	12.15	6.935	4.391	-63.9%	12.1	13.56	14.88	23.0%	23.88	22.9	24.42	2.3%
Africa-Western	**2591**	**2733**	**2849**	**10.0%**	**24**	**12.68**	**7.956**	**-66.9%**	**5.316**	**6.169**	**6.939**	**30.5%**	**17.24**	**18.67**	**20.72**	**20.2%**

Health

Base Case: Countries in Year 2060 Descending Population Sequence	Calories per Capita (Available per Person per Day)				Undernourished Children (Percent of All Children)				Adult Obesity Rate (Percent of Adults 30 Years and Older)				Adult Smoking Rate (Percentage of Adults Who Smoke Tobacco)			
	2010	2035	2060	% Chg	2010	2035	2060	% Chg	2010	2035	2060	% Chg	2010	2035	2060	% Chg
AMERICAS																
Haiti	2144	2323	2615	22.0%	16.27	17	11.22	-38.6%	10.34	11.77	14.77	42.8%	7.076	11.21	15.55	119.8%
Dominican Republic	2366	2859	3246	37.2%	2.773	2.557	2.406	-13.2%	26.71	36.5	45.78	71.4%	12.95	17.42	20.91	61.5%
Cuba	3289	3363	3425	4.1%	17.05	11.8	8.029	-52.9%	25.44	26.63	27.66	8.7%	33.78	31.84	29.83	-11.7%
Puerto Rico	3301	3471	3633	10.1%	0	0	0		25.39	28.12	30.88	21.6%	13.44	17.44	19.09	42.0%
Jamaica	2697	2869	3131	16.1%	3.63	3.523	3.133	-3.7%	26.67	29.52	34.42	29.1%	26.55	25.18	25.14	-5.3%
Trinidad	2864	3261	3482	21.6%	5.189	3.58	2.858	-44.9%	37.41	46.61	52.41	40.1%	27.1	27.05	25.21	-7.0%
Bahamas	2751	3069	3439	25.0%	10.59	7.111	4.48	-57.7%	27.49	33.38	41.32	50.3%	13.23	17.46	19.07	44.1%
Barbados	3142	3295	3534	12.5%	0.138	0.875	1.346	616.0%	40.75	44.12	50.02	22.7%	12.14	16.17	19.56	61.1%
Grenada	2993	3098	3319	10.9%	3.459	3.345	2.783	-19.8%	20.38	21.8	25.26	23.9%	23.55	23.78	24.68	4.8%
Saint Vincent and Grenadines	2676	2968	3260	21.8%	12.21	7.429	4.745	-61.1%	18.92	23.33	28.44	50.3%	16.42	18.89	21.68	32.0%
Saint Lucia	2994	3154	3353	12.0%	3.748	3.203	2.798	-25.3%	26.23	28.61	32.09	22.3%	25.64	24.78	25.4	-0.9%
America-Caribbean	**2731**	**2898**	**3088**	**13.1%**	**10.53**	**8.973**	**6.563**	**-37.7%**	**22.75**	**25.71**	**28.94**	**27.2%**	**19.18**	**19.9**	**20.92**	**9.1%**
Guatemala	2282	2642	3067	34.4%	18.39	10.72	6.004	-67.4%	30.78	38.42	49.19	59.8%	17.8	17.62	20.65	16.0%
Honduras	2416	2700	3023	25.1%	11.98	7.755	5.027	-58.0%	13.9	17.58	22.61	62.7%	20.6	21.99	22.97	11.5%
El Salvador	2596	2843	3169	22.1%	8.975	6.495	4.21	-53.1%	17.67	21.14	26.46	49.7%	26.28	26.07	25.84	-1.7%
Nicaragua	2324	2554	2844	22.4%	9.904	8.558	5.781	-41.6%	30.39	35.02	41.66	37.1%	47.31	37.11	32.23	-31.9%
Costa Rica	2867	3143	3406	18.8%	4.824	3.629	2.893	-40.0%	26.38	31.38	36.73	39.2%	21.8	22.4	24.22	11.1%
Panama	2403	2904	3343	39.1%	7.302	4.686	3.237	-55.7%	20.52	29.33	38.83	89.2%	14.34	18.29	20.65	44.0%
Belize	2894	3109	3341	15.4%	10.86	6.993	4.489	-58.7%	17.81	20.72	24.31	36.5%	24.7	23.94	25.15	1.8%
America-Central	**2441**	**2736**	**3089**	**26.5%**	**12.17**	**8.228**	**5.153**	**-57.7%**	**24.08**	**30.28**	**38.74**	**60.9%**	**23.75**	**22.63**	**23.45**	**-1.3%**
USA	3730	3744	3701	-0.8%	1.733	1.821	1.992	14.9%	44.95	45.27	44.31	-1.4%	17.53	16.99	16.98	-3.1%
Mexico	3178	3291	3402	7.0%	5.2	4.15	3.409	-34.4%	37.47	39.81	42.27	12.8%	9.512	14.2	18.69	96.5%
Canada	3594	3621	3682	2.4%	0	0	0		28.77	29.22	30.19	4.9%	17.07	16.32	15.75	-7.7%
America-North	**3587**	**3626**	**3633**	**1.3%**	**2.439**	**2.252**	**2.167**	**-11.2%**	**41.95**	**42.8**	**42.85**	**2.1%**	**15.57**	**16.27**	**17.27**	**10.9%**
Brazil	3169	3353	3471	9.5%	5.375	3.817	3.118	-42.0%	18.48	21	22.76	23.2%	18.46	20.63	23.06	24.9%
Colombia	2621	2869	3157	20.5%	4.742	3.837	3.148	-33.6%	24.62	28.99	34.71	41.0%	22.89	22.1	23.27	1.7%
Argentina	3028	3318	3507	15.8%	2.595	2.303	2.227	-14.6%	42.27	49.43	54.48	28.9%	31.1	28.91	27.31	-12.2%
Peru	2670	3008	3284	23.0%	4.316	3.569	3.065	-29.0%	31.42	38.42	44.95	43.1%	41.24	34.94	32.05	-22.3%
Venezuela	2359	2804	3194	35.4%	4.074	3.43	2.945	-27.7%	31.87	41.93	52.28	64.0%	31.58	29.98	28.82	-8.7%
Ecuador	2668	2839	2982	11.8%	10.39	7.718	5.893	-43.3%	16.07	18.34	20.45	27.3%	34.3	30.72	28.06	-18.2%
Chile	2922	3194	3431	17.4%	0.569	1.247	1.678	194.9%	32.2	37.65	42.95	33.4%	49.59	39.47	34.51	-30.4%
Bolivia	2281	2689	3026	32.7%	6.917	4.865	3.899	-43.6%	32.25	41.34	50.18	55.6%	37.37	31.11	28.97	-22.5%
Paraguay	2568	2768	3040	18.4%	5.09	4.271	3.479	-31.7%	16.63	19.42	23.73	42.7%	15.66	17.9	20.39	30.2%
Uruguay	2960	3295	3550	19.9%	4.23	3.234	2.598	-38.6%	30.62	37.24	42.94	40.2%	28.6	29.04	26.62	-6.9%
Guyana	2820	2957	3160	12.1%	7.948	6.118	4.446	-44.1%	16.6	18.47	21.46	29.3%	24.81	22.91	23.57	-5.0%
Suriname	2766	3074	3334	20.5%	9.847	6.28	4.305	-56.3%	17.1	21.47	25.75	50.6%	23.84	24.18	25.3	6.1%
America-South	**2927**	**3160**	**3352**	**14.5%**	**4.848**	**3.713**	**3.108**	**-35.9%**	**24.54**	**29.06**	**33.31**	**35.7%**	**25.42**	**24.99**	**25.53**	**0.4%**

Health

Base Case: Countries in Year 2060 Descending Population Sequence	Calories per Capita (Available per Person per Day)				Undernourished Children (Percent of All Children)				Adult Obesity Rate (Percent of Adults 30 Years and Older)				Adult Smoking Rate (Percentage of Adults Who Smoke Tobacco)			
	2010	2035	2060	% Chg	2010	2035	2060	% Chg	2010	2035	2060	% Chg	2010	2035	2060	% Chg
ASIA with OCEANIA																
China	3054	3496	3695	21.0%	4.134	2.892	2.479	-40.0%	2.924	6.521	8.501	190.7%	37.74	34.24	30.15	-20.1%
Japan	2818	3122	3447	22.3%	8.941	6.196	4.141	-53.7%	2.674	4.694	7.472	179.4%	29.71	26.86	24.43	-17.8%
Korea, Repub of	3075	3278	3485	13.3%	2.259	2.243	2.192	-3.0%	10.3	12.56	15.13	46.9%	33.81	31.86	27.81	-17.7%
Taiwan	3188	3377	3573	12.1%	0.207	0.897	1.386	569.6%	23.4	26.44	29.81	27.4%	24.67	25.53	24.33	-1.4%
Korea, Dem. People's Rep.	2249	2510	2796	24.3%	18.76	11.64	7.097	-62.2%	10.24	13.44	17.63	72.2%	23.33	22.58	22.84	-2.1%
Hong Kong SAR	3480	3487	3542	1.8%	0	0	0		27.89	28.11	29	4.0%	12.26	11.56	10.88	-11.3%
Mongolia	2346	2760	3182	35.6%	10.94	6.251	3.989	-63.5%	21.88	29.5	38.89	77.7%	42.35	37.97	33.59	-20.7%
Asia-East	**3026**	**3446**	**3658**	**20.9%**	**4.61**	**3.186**	**2.612**	**-43.3%**	**3.698**	**7.148**	**9.274**	**150.8%**	**36.45**	**33.24**	**29.45**	**-19.2%**
India	2552	2999	3336	30.7%	34.97	12.7	6.512	-81.4%	2.122	4.115	6.368	200.1%	33.87	30.33	29.24	-13.7%
Pakistan	2372	2572	2900	22.3%	30.35	19.48	9.422	-69.0%	3.302	4.221	6.304	90.9%	27.22	25.1	24.85	-8.7%
Bangladesh	2264	2627	2923	29.1%	38.29	14.87	7.91	-79.3%	0.072	0.199	0.638	786.1%	42.45	35.72	31.5	-25.8%
Afghanistan	2276	2736	3254	43.0%	33.99	13.76	4.792	-85.9%	1.379	2.989	6.338	359.6%	52.94	42.92	36.95	-30.2%
Iran (Islamic Republic of)	3131	3364	3388	8.2%	9.814	6.236	4.815	-50.9%	25.29	29.03	29.56	16.9%	12.19	17.04	20.21	65.8%
Nepal	2505	2569	2719	8.5%	39.47	27.83	13.6	-65.5%	0.183	0.15	0.294	60.7%	31.92	31.03	28.17	-11.7%
Uzbekistan	2419	2762	3042	25.8%	2.422	2.584	2.716	12.1%	19.42	25.01	30.35	56.3%	12.93	16.15	19.08	47.6%
Sri Lanka	2491	2805	3137	25.9%	24.56	13.99	7.864	-68.0%	0.258	0.935	2.043	691.9%	13.31	16.1	19.52	46.7%
Kazakhstan	2932	3303	3356	14.5%	10.55	6.099	4.6	-56.4%	14.9	19.96	20.74	39.2%	35.64	34.06	30.97	-13.1%
Tajikistan	1986	2297	2693	35.6%	34.57	20.6	10.41	-69.9%	10.16	13.94	20.03	97.1%	22.45	22.51	22.9	2.0%
Turkmenistan	2965	3417	3497	17.9%	7.138	4.08	3.344	-53.2%	19.47	26.67	28.12	44.4%	14.08	18.89	20.26	43.9%
Kyrgyzstan	3172	3168	3114	-1.8%	5.642	4.656	4.281	-24.1%	14.31	14.28	13.76	-3.8%	27.77	26.24	25.12	-9.5%
Bhutan	2702	3111	3466	28.3%	7.444	4.29	2.92	-60.8%	14.16	19.28	24.7	74.4%	24.75	24.1	25.68	3.8%
Maldives	2620	2942	3295	25.8%	26.54	12.89	6.476	-75.6%	21.09	25.66	31.67	50.2%	27.92	26.57	26.73	-4.3%
Asia-South Central	**2527**	**2904**	**3209**	**27.0%**	**32.73**	**13.62**	**7.045**	**-78.5%**	**3.495**	**5.225**	**7.153**	**104.7%**	**32.71**	**29.6**	**28.45**	**-13.0%**
Indonesia	2931	3036	3136	7.0%	20.66	12.13	7.555	-63.4%	2.034	2.298	2.611	28.4%	37.57	30.79	28.5	-24.1%
Philippines	2542	2794	3074	20.9%	24.64	14.23	8.112	-67.1%	3.434	4.919	7.052	105.4%	24.88	24.28	24.49	-1.6%
Viet Nam	2676	2928	3156	17.9%	25.06	13.14	7.451	-70.3%	0.287	0.642	1.256	337.6%	25.69	21.66	23.05	-10.3%
Thailand	2478	2771	3116	25.7%	16.31	10.75	5.656	-59.2%	8.454	11.21	15.22	80.0%	29.54	26.23	26.06	-11.8%
Myanmar	2970	3018	2931	-1.3%	28.79	14.99	10.27	-64.3%	8.575	9.024	8.181	-4.6%	25.18	23.84	23.52	-6.6%
Malaysia	2906	3157	3391	16.7%	8.459	5.889	4.165	-50.8%	7.131	9.02	11.13	56.1%	22.74	23.82	25.05	10.2%
Cambodia	2140	2577	2946	37.7%	29.25	13.99	6.515	-77.7%	0.38	2.341	4.983	1211.3%	33.61	31.96	29.23	-13.0%
LAO People's Dem Repub	2389	2789	3150	31.9%	34.27	13.77	6.797	-80.2%	9.692	14.58	20.13	107.7%	36.19	32.37	29.99	-17.1%
Singapore	3511	3534	3593	2.3%	3.354	3.091	2.773	-17.3%	2.049	2.146	2.377	16.0%	11.28	10.84	10.79	-4.3%
Timor-Leste	2738	2886	2933	7.1%	50.94	28.92	15.51	-69.6%	13.75	15.24	15.76	14.6%	20.31	20.94	21.9	7.8%
Brunei Darussalam	2880	3131	3332	15.7%	7.006	5.234	3.995	-43.0%	27.38	32.03	36.13	32.0%	24.03	23.82	23.77	-1.1%
Asia-South East	**2761**	**2941**	**3117**	**12.9%**	**21.9**	**12.53**	**7.576**	**-65.4%**	**3.62**	**4.533**	**5.755**	**59.0%**	**30.74**	**26.76**	**26**	**-15.4%**

Health

Base Case: Countries in Year 2060 Descending Population Sequence	Calories per Capita (Available per Person per Day)				Undernourished Children (Percent of All Children)				Adult Obesity Rate (Percent of Adults 30 Years and Older)				Adult Smoking Rate (Percentage of Adults Who Smoke Tobacco)			
	2010	2035	2060	% Chg	2010	2035	2060	% Chg	2010	2035	2060	% Chg	2010	2035	2060	% Chg
ASIA with OCEANIA continued																
Turkey	3319	3424	3456	4.1%	2.558	2.596	2.559	-13.5%	29.68	31.54	32.23	8.6%	33	31.03	29.44	-10.8%
Yemen	2082	2473	2850	36.9%	43.3	20.05	9.68	-77.6%	5.367	8.526	12.66	135.9%	57.97	46.41	38.36	-33.8%
Iraq	2850	3163	3419	20.0%	19.17	9.671	5.731	-70.1%	16.64	20.75	24.66	48.2%	24.43	24.9	25.72	5.3%
Saudi Arabia	2879	3111	3293	14.4%	13.26	8.911	5.966	-55.0%	37.44	42.95	47.62	27.2%	14.68	18.19	20.67	40.8%
Syrian Arab Repub	3062	3085	3190	4.2%	3.134	3.275	2.906	-7.3%	21.59	21.89	23.41	8.4%	28.95	27.84	26.63	-8.0%
Israel	3538	3659	3688	4.2%	0	0	0		28.73	30.75	31.27	8.8%	21.58	23.99	23.43	8.6%
Jordan	2732	2991	3380	23.7%	3.82	3.203	2.53	-33.8%	39.23	45.41	55.88	42.4%	34.05	29.63	29.18	-14.3%
Occupied Palestinian Territory	2296	2643	3090	34.6%	5.376	3.932	2.957	-45.0%	10.88	14.13	19.67	80.8%	22.32	22.97	24.01	7.6%
Azerbaijan	2878	3233	3311	15.0%	9.387	5.355	4.19	-55.4%	31.67	39.02	40.75	28.7%	15.39	19.31	21.7	41.0%
United Arab Emirates	3286	3433	3516	7.0%	0	0	0		37.17	41.53	44.88	20.7%	11.69	8.891	7.967	-31.8%
Oman	3289	3404	3531	7.4%	11.51	7.996	5.302	-53.9%	14.89	16.45	18.21	22.3%	11.64	15.76	17.94	54.1%
Kuwait	3096	3290	3326	7.4%	0.206	0.92	1.622	687.4%	49.5	56.33	58.57	18.3%	27.31	20.59	18.28	-33.1%
Lebanon	3202	3339	3448	7.7%	3.824	3.255	2.864	-25.1%	29.12	31.41	33.33	14.5%	34.84	32.99	31.02	-11.0%
Armenia	2453	3060	3409	39.0%	3.727	2.538	2.257	-39.4%	24.67	36.43	44.71	81.2%	29.97	30.49	28.75	-4.1%
Georgia	2722	3023	3216	18.1%	0.328	1.203	1.831	458.2%	14.76	18.66	21.49	45.6%	29.08	27.83	27.21	-6.4%
Bahrain	3466	3539	3678	6.1%	8.111	6.279	4.443	-45.2%	35.08	36.94	40.26	14.8%	11.43	8.94	8.323	-27.2%
Qatar	3793	3681	3605	-5.0%	4.999	4.548	3.941	-21.2%	27.89	26.71	26.67	-4.4%	27.12	22.75	18.22	-32.8%
Cyprus	3269	3383	3492	6.8%	0	0	0		21.87	23.53	25.18	15.1%	17.22	21.29	21.59	25.4%
Asia-West	**2982**	**3136**	**3283**	**10.1%**	**10.75**	**7.046**	**4.744**	**-55.9%**	**25.32**	**27.37**	**29.34**	**15.9%**	**29.85**	**28.73**	**27.76**	**-7.0%**
Australia	3165	3357	3568	12.7%	0.185	0.84	1.327	617.3%	30.15	33.83	38.18	26.6%	14.86	14.4	14.04	-5.5%
Papua New Guinea	2401	2702	2879	19.9%	25.89	12.75	7.553	-70.8%	2.037	3.668	4.891	140.1%	37.71	33.93	30.11	-20.2%
New Zealand	3211	3350	3567	11.1%	0.198	0.904	1.385	599.5%	35.2	38.01	42.75	21.4%	19.54	23.84	22.85	16.9%
Solomon Islands	2324	2541	2780	19.6%	18.46	12.4	8.088	-56.2%	14.27	17.16	20.81	45.8%	39.56	31.64	28.82	-27.1%
Fiji	2960	3051	3259	10.1%	9.948	6.829	4.388	-55.9%	27.47	28.9	32.62	18.7%	17.39	18.46	21.12	21.4%
Vanuatu	2651	2885	3174	19.7%	9.402	6.122	4	-57.5%	26.04	30.27	36.14	38.8%	28.02	26.63	26.17	-6.6%
Micronesia, Federated States of	2807	2936	3194	13.8%	8.944	7.122	4.561	-49.0%	75.32	81.37	94.13	25.0%	25.63	25.52	25.54	-0.4%
Tonga	2735	2814	3079	12.6%	10.84	10.1	5.952	-45.1%	72.11	75.73	88.48	22.7%	33.13	29.74	27.96	-15.6%
Samoa	2959	3167	3401	14.9%	10.17	6.996	4.623	-54.5%	59.81	67.06	75.86	26.8%	43.11	37.82	33.84	-21.5%
Oceania	**2998**	**3167**	**3349**	**11.7%**	**5.843**	**4.2**	**3.304**	**-43.5%**	**25.5**	**27.2**	**29.9**	**17.3%**	**20.62**	**20.87**	**20.02**	**-2.9%**

Health

Base Case: Countries in Year 2060 Descending Population Sequence	Calories per Capita (Available per Person per Day)				Undernourished Children (Percent of All Children)				Adult Obesity Rate (Percent of Adults 30 Years and Older)				Adult Smoking Rate (Percentage of Adults Who Smoke Tobacco)			
	2010	2035	2060	% Chg	2010	2035	2060	% Chg	2010	2035	2060	% Chg	2010	2035	2060	% Chg
EUROPE																
Russian Federation	3168	3404	3383	6.8%	5.954	4.272	3.746	-37.1%	25.94	29.97	29.66	14.3%	37.79	34.58	31.19	-17.5%
Poland	3396	3506	3516	3.5%	0	0	0		23.43	25.13	25.32	8.1%	31.56	30.73	28.91	-8.4%
Ukraine	3089	3227	3281	6.2%	8.375	6.172	4.826	-42.4%	20.86	22.84	23.67	13.5%	30.98	28.77	27.37	-11.7%
Romania	3590	3570	3494	-2.7%	2.043	2.243	2.501	22.4%	13.12	12.95	12.24	-6.7%	20.66	22.36	23.8	15.2%
Czech Republic	3330	3403	3467	4.1%	0	0	0		29.28	30.56	31.73	8.4%	25.52	25.99	25.57	0.2%
Belarus	2966	3273	3388	14.2%	5.749	4.079	3.376	-41.3%	28.65	34.5	36.9	28.8%	28.86	28.55	27.91	-3.3%
Hungary	3527	3555	3545	0.5%	0	0	0		22.62	23.02	22.87	1.1%	33.29	31.76	29.34	-11.9%
Bulgaria	2938	3109	3298	12.3%	5.858	4.655	3.668	-37.4%	26.18	29.16	32.72	25.0%	35.47	31.55	29.79	-16.0%
Slovak Republic	2858	3124	3330	16.5%	8.416	5.949	4.353	-48.3%	23.43	27.91	31.8	35.7%	28.77	28.21	27.08	-5.9%
Moldova, Repub of	2749	2817	2991	8.8%	3.359	3.699	3.512	4.6%	11.79	12.45	14.47	22.7%	15.83	18.51	20.32	28.4%
Europe-East	3210	3386	3397	5.8%	4.852	3.514	2.985	-38.5%	23.74	26.64	26.91	13.4%	33.25	31.26	29.13	-12.4%
United Kingdom	3444	3542	3643	5.8%	0	0	0		30.51	32.28	34.17	12.0%	13.7	12.89	12.9	-5.8%
Sweden	3235	3431	3581	10.7%	0	0	0		16.19	18.9	21.16	30.7%	13.93	13.58	13.58	-2.5%
Denmark	3465	3552	3660	5.6%	0	0	0		12.25	13.24	14.54	18.7%	28.39	26.24	25.17	-11.3%
Ireland	3694	3733	3700	0.2%	0	0	0		13.34	13.78	13.4	0.4%	26.78	24.8	24.11	-10.0%
Norway	3529	3584	3661	3.7%	0	0	0		14.16	14.82	15.77	11.4%	22.24	21.49	21.25	-4.5%
Finland	3175	3368	3556	12.0%	0.184	0.833	1.335	625.5%	25.61	28.96	32.5	26.9%	17.58	17.03	17.02	-3.2%
Lithuania	3395	3498	3551	4.6%	0	0	0		21.47	22.95	23.74	10.6%	27.82	27.61	26.56	-4.5%
Latvia	3069	3320	3492	13.8%	2.739	2.477	2.362	-13.8%	18.79	22.3	24.98	32.9%	35.3	32.97	29.55	-16.3%
Estonia	3268	3438	3578	9.5%	0	0	0		12.44	14.33	16.04	28.9%	31.25	30.4	27.22	-12.9%
Iceland	3316	3464	3597	8.5%	0	0	0		27.12	29.69	32.14	18.5%	18.2	17.55	17.55	-3.6%
Europe-North	3413	3529	3633	6.4%	0.073	0.092	0.106	45.2%	25.48	27.32	29.12	14.3%	17	15.98	15.66	-7.9%
Italy	3632	3576	3539	-2.6%	0	0	0		18.22	17.52	17.09	-6.2%	23.79	24.72	24.17	1.6%
Spain	3408	3475	3528	3.5%	0	0	0		22.61	23.62	24.43	8.0%	31.92	29.82	27.21	-14.8%
Greece	3655	3618	3567	-2.4%	0	0	0		31.36	30.71	29.81	-4.9%	34.76	32.33	28.89	-16.9%
Portugal	3691	3623	3566	-3.4%	0	0	0		20.19	19.3	18.59	-7.9%	18.28	21.31	22.92	25.4%
Serbia	2760	2962	3203	16.1%	2.329	2.51	2.518	8.1%	28.41	32.24	37.3	31.3%	47.48	42.43	36.65	-22.8%
Bosnia and Herzegovina	2721	3038	3272	20.2%	3.565	2.87	2.568	-28.0%	26.53	32.36	37.18	40.1%	44.79	33.74	31.17	-10.4%
Croatia	2844	3072	3296	15.9%	0.775	1.36	1.769	128.3%	25.44	29.54	33.98	33.6%	26.81	27.72	27.52	2.6%
Albania	2921	3137	3292	12.7%	17.54	11.08	7.275	-58.5%	31.67	36.04	39.39	24.4%	37.51	34.15	31.26	-16.7%
Macedonia, FYR	2889	3000	3177	10.0%	0.301	1.32	1.984	559.1%	22.08	23.77	26.69	20.9%	35.81	32.34	29.77	-16.9%
Slovenia	3010	3243	3456	14.8%	4.153	3.301	2.751	-33.8%	25.58	29.66	33.81	32.2%	20.4	23.41	22.78	11.7%
Montenegro	2911	3103	3364	15.6%	6.074	4.577	3.357	-44.7%	19.78	22.33	26.23	32.6%	22.96	23.69	25.04	9.1%
Malta	3513	3538	3590	2.2%	0	0	0		41.2	41.7	42.89	4.1%	21.87	24.01	24.31	11.2%
Europe-South	3443	3467	3495	1.5%	0.698	0.597	0.525	-24.8%	22.11	22.77	23.54	6.5%	28.6	28.11	26.54	-7.2%
Germany	3476	3541	3645	4.9%	0	0	0		28.62	29.74	31.58	10.3%	29.45	27.87	26.6	-9.7%
France	3608	3598	3651	1.2%	0	0	0		10.28	10.19	10.7	4.1%	23.44	22.75	22.58	-3.7%
Netherlands	3491	3514	3600	3.1%	0	0	0		15.8	16.08	17.17	8.7%	30.26	28.51	26.62	-12.0%
Belgium	3611	3591	3645	0.9%	0	0	0		16.17	15.92	16.58	2.5%	24.86	23.91	23.33	-6.2%
Austria	3714	3680	3686	-0.8%	0	0	0		29.63	29.06	29.17	-1.6%	23.14	23.72	21.26	-8.1%
Switzerland	3554	3589	3661	3.0%	0	0	0		21.23	21.71	22.76	7.2%	22.58	21.37	21.11	-6.5%
Luxembourg	3697	3688	3664	-0.9%	0	0	0		18.59	18.49	18.2	-2.1%	28.53	26.66	26.03	-8.8%
Europe-West	3543	3569	3645	2.9%	0	0	0		20.45	20.52	21.25	3.9%	26.73	25.42	24.55	-8.2%

Multination Regional Analysis

Measures of Poverty, Health, Education, Infrastructure, and Governance

Health

Base Case
Source: International Futures
Version 6.32, June 2010

	HIV Prevalence Rate (Percent of Population Infected)				Government Spending on Health (Percent of GDP)				Disability-Adjusted Life Years (Millions of Life Years Lost plus Life Years Lived with Disability)									
									Communicable Diseases			Noncommunicable Diseases			Injuries		
	2010	2035	2060	% Chg	2010	2035	2060	% Chg	2010	2035	2060	2010	2035	2060	2010	2035	2060
World	0.759	0.549	0.217	-71.4%	5.549	5.329	5.204	-6.2%	522	256.2	113.6	758.2	906	955.8	173.2	201.4	215.4
Africa	4.145	2.191	0.648	-84.4%	2.468	2.784	3.502	41.9%	259.5	153.9	80.84	103.2	150.1	218.5	39.6	58.98	79.9
Americas	0.558	0.363	0.129	-76.9%	6.087	6.807	7.212	18.5%	20.59	9.462	4.162	105.5	126.2	130.5	18.84	21.66	22.44
Asia with Oceania	0.178	0.108	0.038	-78.7%	4.03	3.694	3.919	-2.8%	234.8	89.9	27.36	453.9	547.3	542.8	101	110.5	104.6
Europe	0.406	0.266	0.091	-77.6%	6.975	7.617	7.851	12.6%	7.129	2.895	1.225	94.24	81.15	63.07	13.62	10.11	8.335
World	0.759	0.549	0.217	-71.4%	5.549	5.329	5.204	-6.2%	522	256.2	113.6	758.2	906	955.8	173.2	201.4	215.4
Africa-Eastern	5.853	3.043	0.87	-85.1%	2.582	2.578	2.989	15.8%	84.27	43.33	13.56	29.04	44.15	65.27	12.65	19.26	27.23
Africa-Middle	3.286	1.814	0.538	-83.6%	1.598	1.901	2.284	42.9%	52.77	46.84	38.67	14.6	24.26	40.08	7.233	13.1	20.79
Africa-Northern	0.287	0.189	0.072	-74.9%	2.396	2.97	4.048	68.9%	11.38	3.94	1.501	19.27	25.61	31.01	5.347	6.671	7.241
Africa-Southern	18.64	10.86	3.62	-80.6%	3.375	4.34	5.82	72.4%	16.09	7.907	2.182	6.727	6.878	6.901	2.5	2.914	2.821
Africa-Western	2.647	1.441	0.423	-84.0%	1.611	1.536	1.947	20.9%	94.96	51.9	24.93	33.59	49.22	75.19	11.87	17.03	21.81
Africa	4.145	2.191	0.648	-84.4%	2.468	2.784	3.502	41.9%	259.5	153.9	80.84	103.2	150.1	218.5	39.6	58.98	79.9
America-Caribbean	0.916	0.648	0.245	-73.3%	4.966	6.216	6.838	37.7%	2.458	1.86	0.904	4.39	5.324	5.655	0.853	1.053	1.045
America-Central	0.641	0.364	0.121	-81.1%	3.733	4.237	4.421	18.4%	2.114	0.944	0.341	4.531	6.297	7.975	1.16	1.709	2.035
America-North	0.603	0.416	0.146	-75.8%	6.445	7.382	7.866	22.0%	4.869	2.732	1.295	51.88	60.5	59.87	5.353	5.836	6.097
America-South	0.463	0.282	0.1	-78.4%	3.775	4.534	5.181	37.2%	11.15	3.925	1.621	44.74	54.09	57.01	11.47	13.06	13.26
Americas	0.558	0.363	0.129	-76.9%	6.087	6.807	7.212	18.5%	20.59	9.462	4.162	105.5	126.2	130.5	18.84	21.66	22.44
Asia-East	0.068	0.048	0.018	-73.5%	4.634	4.16	4.254	-8.2%	29.29	10.09	4.237	171.4	183.5	153.3	30.77	29.7	22.34
Asia-South Central	0.247	0.133	0.045	-81.8%	1.502	2.071	2.833	88.6%	167.9	61.99	15.16	192.7	241.4	254	52.81	60.83	61.7
Asia-South East	0.351	0.2	0.067	-80.9%	1.589	2.08	2.628	65.4%	28.21	13.42	5.902	63.23	85.49	91.05	12.37	12.93	12.38
Asia-West	0.024	0.013	0.004	-83.3%	3.333	4.082	5.442	63.3%	8.229	3.783	1.755	22.77	32.12	39.23	4.627	6.5	7.664
Oceania	0.244	0.181	0.064	-73.8%	6.128	6.756	6.907	12.7%	1.101	0.605	0.308	3.73	4.725	5.165	0.415	0.501	0.571
Asia with Oceania	0.178	0.108	0.038	-78.7%	4.03	3.694	3.919	-2.8%	234.8	89.9	27.36	453.9	547.3	542.8	101	110.5	104.6
Europe-East	0.623	0.413	0.157	-74.8%	4.566	5.053	5.934	30.0%	4.782	1.743	0.66	46.47	35.55	25.84	10.41	7.138	5.614
Europe-North	0.17	0.114	0.038	-77.6%	7.036	7.942	8.019	14.0%	0.606	0.313	0.172	10.93	10.21	8.747	0.836	0.772	0.727
Europe-South	0.342	0.236	0.084	-75.4%	6.196	6.854	7.125	15.0%	0.841	0.376	0.16	17.06	16.24	13.26	1.14	0.97	0.81
Europe-West	0.197	0.142	0.049	-75.1%	7.82	8.727	8.632	10.4%	0.918	0.493	0.244	21.07	20.32	16.18	1.42	1.391	1.307
Europe	0.406	0.266	0.091	-77.6%	6.975	7.617	7.851	12.6%	7.129	2.895	1.225	94.24	81.15	63.07	13.62	10.11	8.335

Health

Base Case: Countries in Year 2060 Descending Population Sequence	HIV Prevalence Rate (Percent of Population Infected)				Government Spending on Health (Percent of GDP)				Disability-Adjusted Life Years (Millions of Life Years Lost plus Life Years Lived with Disability)								
									Communicable Diseases			Noncommunicable Diseases			Injuries		
	2010	2035	2060	% Chg	2010	2035	2060	% Chg	2010	2035	2060	2010	2035	2060	2010	2035	2060
AFRICA																	
Ethiopia	2.298	1.28	0.368	-84.0%	2.313	2.387	3.018	30.5%	21.39	8.557	1.781	7.437	11.75	17.66	2.488	3.909	5.8
Tanzania, United Rep	6.804	3.597	1.032	-84.8%	2.838	3.153	3.554	25.2%	9.619	4.025	0.975	3.377	4.903	7.134	1.278	1.951	2.909
Uganda	6.298	3.111	0.864	-86.3%	1.815	1.396	1.833	1.0%	8.964	4.953	0.849	2.604	4.242	6.321	1.739	2.971	4.665
Kenya	5.685	2.881	0.853	-85.0%	2.035	2.3	3.38	66.1%	9.579	5.466	1.542	3.063	4.404	6.088	1.394	1.927	2.372
Madagascar	0.117	0.067	0.02	-82.9%	1.978	1.375	1.39	-29.7%	4.083	3.055	1.407	2.22	3.645	5.661	0.676	1.055	1.407
Mozambique	12.08	6.493	1.861	-84.6%	2.364	2.175	2.51	6.2%	7.249	2.856	0.615	2.464	3.208	4.181	1.119	1.627	2.423
Malawi	13.33	7.242	2.1	-84.2%	6.885	6.831	7.125	3.5%	3.813	2.585	1.223	1.019	1.752	3.027	0.381	0.698	1.058
Zambia	16.35	8.787	2.524	-84.6%	3.485	3.342	3.364	-3.5%	5.269	3.641	1.302	1.233	1.763	2.578	0.604	0.893	1.132
Somalia	0.52	0.298	0.09	-82.7%	1.134	0.845	1.032	-9.0%	2.952	1.978	1.289	1.271	1.958	3.166	0.856	1.296	1.8
Rwanda	2.787	1.432	0.421	-84.9%	4.258	4.571	5.184	21.7%	3.704	1.506	0.228	1.11	1.701	2.238	0.554	0.829	1.111
Zimbabwe	15.23	7.058	2.282	-85.0%	3.739	2.575	2.809	-24.9%	3.825	2.183	1.07	1.66	2.282	3.083	0.943	1.186	1.26
Burundi	2.277	1.234	0.389	-82.9%	0.61	0.503	0.691	13.3%	2.678	1.575	0.693	0.806	1.275	2.156	0.373	0.537	0.738
Eritrea	1.652	0.941	0.295	-82.1%	1.817	0.983	1.091	-40.0%	0.859	0.743	0.506	0.457	0.855	1.516	0.177	0.303	0.47
Comoros	0.057	0.034	0.011	-80.7%	1.58	1.157	1.261	-20.2%	0.087	0.096	0.056	0.064	0.119	0.182	0.014	0.023	0.031
Mauritius	1.066	0.715	0.254	-76.2%	2.244	2.886	3.533	57.4%	0.017	0.008	0.003	0.153	0.166	0.142	0.019	0.018	0.015
Djibouti	3.051	1.814	0.559	-81.7%	5.078	3.356	4.293	-15.5%	0.18	0.1	0.019	0.104	0.132	0.13	0.038	0.042	0.042
Africa-Eastern	**5.853**	**3.043**	**0.87**	**-85.1%**	**2.582**	**2.578**	**2.989**	**15.8%**	**84.27**	**43.33**	**13.56**	**29.04**	**44.15**	**65.27**	**12.65**	**19.26**	**27.23**
Congo, Democratic Republic of	2.547	1.456	0.443	-82.6%	1.202	0.991	0.97	-19.3%	31.79	31.8	28.64	7.911	14.35	25.5	4.203	8.049	14.01
Angola	1.975	1.08	0.318	-83.9%	1.716	2.272	2.874	67.5%	6.742	3.181	1.62	2.05	2.885	4.265	1.16	2.218	2.953
Cameroon	5.746	3.229	0.988	-82.8%	1.005	1.098	1.356	34.9%	5.28	3.513	1.324	2.111	2.96	3.975	0.813	1.125	1.426
Chad	3.66	2.113	0.643	-82.4%	1.862	0.997	1.026	-44.9%	5.56	5.693	5.752	1.321	2.314	3.897	0.466	0.842	1.338
Central African Republic	6.47	3.719	1.15	-82.2%	1.777	1.763	2.014	13.3%	1.716	1.433	0.681	0.533	0.783	1.095	0.273	0.389	0.48
Congo, Republic of	3.472	1.918	0.593	-82.9%	1.546	1.553	1.932	25.0%	1.21	0.824	0.419	0.441	0.625	0.889	0.211	0.315	0.382
Gabon	5.424	3.104	0.989	-81.8%	2.818	2.36	2.727	-3.2%	0.24	0.194	0.108	0.147	0.224	0.295	0.07	0.106	0.131
Equatorial Guinea	3.635	2.109	0.616	-83.1%	1.504	1.249	1.636	8.8%	0.206	0.173	0.105	0.071	0.101	0.127	0.032	0.049	0.065
São Tomé and Príncipe	0.017	0.01	0.003	-82.4%	4.489	4.134	4.111	-8.4%	0.027	0.029	0.021	0.013	0.023	0.038	0.004	0.006	0.008
Africa-Middle	**3.286**	**1.814**	**0.538**	**-83.6%**	**1.598**	**1.901**	**2.284**	**42.9%**	**52.77**	**46.84**	**38.67**	**14.6**	**24.26**	**40.08**	**7.233**	**13.1**	**20.79**
Egypt	0.017	0.01	0.003	-82.4%	2.566	3.475	4.722	84.0%	2.661	0.829	0.354	8.273	10.31	12.12	0.934	1.067	1.004
Sudan	1.405	0.785	0.242	-82.8%	1.624	2.148	2.825	74.0%	6.059	1.96	0.543	4.094	5.684	7.605	3.239	4.233	4.842
Algeria	0.084	0.051	0.019	-77.4%	2.869	2.465	2.602	-9.3%	1.094	0.53	0.336	2.613	3.779	4.648	0.5	0.589	0.628
Morocco	0.088	0.053	0.019	-78.4%	1.521	2.342	3.299	116.9%	1.098	0.438	0.171	2.888	3.94	4.4	0.478	0.548	0.534
Tunisia	0.045	0.029	0.011	-75.6%	2.65	3.946	4.951	86.8%	0.314	0.127	0.063	0.86	1.118	1.267	0.121	0.141	0.129
Libyan Arab Jamahiriya	0.015	0.009	0.003	-80.0%	2.355	2.53	2.83	20.2%	0.153	0.056	0.035	0.546	0.781	0.977	0.075	0.094	0.104
Africa-Northern	**0.287**	**0.189**	**0.072**	**-74.9%**	**2.396**	**2.97**	**4.048**	**68.9%**	**11.38**	**3.94**	**1.501**	**19.27**	**25.61**	**31.01**	**5.347**	**6.671**	**7.241**

Multination Regional Analysis

Measures of Poverty, Health, Education, Infrastructure, and Governance

Health

Base Case: Countries in Year 2060 Descending Population Sequence	HIV Prevalence Rate (Percent of Population Infected)				Government Spending on Health (Percent of GDP)				Disability-Adjusted Life Years (Millions of Life Years Lost plus Life Years Lived with Disability)								
									Communicable Diseases			Noncommunicable Diseases			Injuries		
	2010	2035	2060	% Chg	2010	2035	2060	% Chg	2010	2035	2060	2010	2035	2060	2010	2035	2060
AFRICA continued																	
South Africa	18.13	10.63	3.557	-80.4%	3.174	3.861	5.383	69.6%	14.54	7.124	1.937	6.005	6.065	5.923	2.154	2.497	2.4
Namibia	14.47	8.19	2.633	-81.8%	4.078	5.464	7.359	80.5%	0.316	0.167	0.057	0.167	0.231	0.29	0.064	0.099	0.115
Lesotho	25.68	13.6	4.322	-83.2%	3.192	4.779	7.86	146.2%	0.561	0.278	0.079	0.219	0.225	0.285	0.115	0.124	0.115
Botswana	25.48	14.35	5.124	-79.9%	6.435	8.62	11.02	71.3%	0.318	0.146	0.049	0.174	0.179	0.21	0.083	0.083	0.079
Swaziland	26.79	14.81	4.627	-82.7%	4.792	5.273	7.753	61.8%	0.354	0.192	0.06	0.162	0.178	0.193	0.084	0.112	0.112
Africa-Southern	**18.64**	**10.86**	**3.62**	**-80.6%**	**3.375**	**4.34**	**5.82**	**72.4%**	**16.09**	**7.907**	**2.182**	**6.727**	**6.878**	**6.901**	**2.5**	**2.914**	**2.821**
Nigeria	3.399	1.887	0.569	-83.3%	1.379	1.385	1.534	11.2%	53.04	23.54	13.15	18.81	25.22	37.58	7.182	9.721	11.67
Niger	0.787	0.444	0.129	-83.6%	2.703	2.375	2.545	-5.8%	6.498	4.602	2.22	1.522	2.777	5.42	0.465	0.873	1.432
Côte d'Ivoire	4.203	2.141	0.648	-84.6%	0.994	1.066	1.501	51.0%	4.936	3.871	1.622	1.598	2.575	3.902	0.568	0.85	1.048
Ghana	1.975	1.147	0.352	-82.2%	1.887	1.452	1.507	-20.1%	5.143	4.064	1.618	2.754	4.008	5.23	0.832	1.131	1.309
Mali	1.336	0.761	0.218	-83.7%	2.494	2.197	2.49	-0.2%	6.114	2.267	0.676	1.772	2.62	4.332	0.588	0.916	1.43
Burkina Faso	1.591	0.825	0.24	-84.9%	3.406	3.368	3.766	10.6%	5.462	4.14	1.255	1.489	2.705	4.239	0.529	0.888	1.315
Senegal	0.759	0.425	0.126	-83.4%	2.671	2.582	2.967	11.1%	3.189	2.209	0.665	1.46	2.368	3.523	0.483	0.721	0.9
Guinea	1.514	0.862	0.257	-83.0%	0.947	0.735	0.862	-9.0%	2.77	1.942	0.989	0.984	1.602	2.537	0.317	0.5	0.7
Benin	1.314	0.744	0.223	-83.0%	2.124	2.141	2.403	13.1%	1.909	1.367	0.722	0.805	1.342	2.189	0.183	0.294	0.41
Togo	3.363	1.947	0.614	-81.7%	1.26	1.136	1.185	-6.0%	1.124	0.961	0.785	0.498	0.855	1.444	0.111	0.164	0.223
Sierra Leone	2.336	1.312	0.374	-84.0%	1.805	1.317	1.625	-10.0%	2.129	1.182	0.283	0.791	1.338	2.007	0.265	0.432	0.636
Liberia	1.584	0.879	0.253	-84.0%	1.729	2.067	2.629	52.1%	0.92	0.369	0.097	0.281	0.529	0.814	0.089	0.162	0.204
Mauritania	0.718	0.42	0.133	-81.5%	1.573	1.085	1.059	-32.7%	0.728	0.733	0.445	0.367	0.605	0.909	0.114	0.165	0.214
Guinea-Bissau	1.824	1.075	0.337	-81.5%	1.495	1.063	1.104	-26.2%	0.643	0.412	0.31	0.223	0.309	0.52	0.078	0.117	0.179
Gambia	0.893	0.505	0.148	-83.4%	3.113	2.423	2.452	-21.2%	0.336	0.226	0.089	0.204	0.312	0.474	0.055	0.085	0.123
Cape Verde	0.016	0.009	0.003	-81.3%	3.525	3.295	4.111	16.6%	0.022	0.008	0.002	0.037	0.058	0.076	0.009	0.012	0.015
Africa-Western	**2.647**	**1.441**	**0.423**	**-84.0%**	**1.611**	**1.536**	**1.947**	**20.9%**	**94.96**	**51.5**	**24.93**	**33.59**	**49.22**	**75.19**	**11.87**	**17.03**	**21.81**

Multination Regional Analysis

Measures of Poverty, Health, Education, Infrastructure, and Governance

Health

Base Case: Countries in Year 2060 Descending Population Sequence	HIV Prevalence Rate (Percent of Population Infected)				Government Spending on Health (Percent of GDP)				Disability-Adjusted Life Years (Millions of Life Years Lost plus Life Years Lived with Disability)									
									Communicable Diseases			Noncommunicable Diseases			Injuries		
	2010	2035	2060	% Chg	2010	2035	2060	% Chg	2010	2035	2060	2010	2035	2060	2010	2035	2060
AMERICAS																	
Haiti	2.124	1.244	0.395	-81.4%	3.006	3.058	3.119	3.8%	1.691	1.56	0.796	1.028	1.559	2.125	0.32	0.435	0.466
Dominican Republic	1.057	0.61	0.219	-79.3%	1.757	2.273	2.668	51.8%	0.452	0.154	0.049	0.938	1.152	1.253	0.235	0.277	0.24
Cuba	0.063	0.045	0.016	-74.6%	9.004	12.89	14.56	61.7%	0.072	0.039	0.022	1.241	1.295	1.009	0.118	0.125	0.119
Puerto Rico	0.015	0.01	0.003	-80.0%	5.026	7.352	7.945	58.1%	0.032	0.015	0.009	0.54	0.571	0.545	0.047	0.049	0.051
Jamaica	1.524	0.921	0.317	-79.2%	2.215	2.767	3.621	63.5%	0.136	0.064	0.019	0.308	0.364	0.371	0.101	0.137	0.142
Trinidad	1.347	0.901	0.348	-74.2%	3.347	3.364	4.62	38.0%	0.051	0.017	0.005	0.216	0.231	0.206	0.019	0.017	0.015
Bahamas	2.683	1.73	0.617	-77.0%	3.335	3.98	4.466	33.9%	0.013	0.006	0.002	0.041	0.049	0.048	0.007	0.007	0.007
Barbados	1.114	0.816	0.293	-73.7%	4.486	5.722	6.948	54.9%	0.004	0.002	0.001	0.031	0.039	0.031	0.001	0.001	0.001
Grenada	0.015	0.009	0.003	-80.0%	3.766	4.044	4.838	28.5%	0.002	0.001	0	0.011	0.015	0.02	0.001	0.001	0.001
Saint Vincent and Grenadines	0.015	0.009	0.003	-80.0%	3.659	5.118	6.617	80.8%	0.003	0.001	0	0.015	0.021	0.023	0.002	0.002	0.001
Saint Lucia	0.015	0.009	0.003	-80.0%	3.153	3.911	4.878	54.7%	0.003	0.001	0	0.022	0.026	0.025	0.003	0.003	0.003
America-Caribbean	**0.916**	**0.648**	**0.245**	**-73.3%**	**4.966**	**6.216**	**6.838**	**37.7%**	**2.458**	**1.86**	**0.904**	**4.39**	**5.324**	**5.655**	**0.853**	**1.053**	**1.045**
Guatemala	0.839	0.452	0.138	-83.6%	1.769	1.911	2.298	29.9%	0.973	0.428	0.151	1.416	2.029	2.822	0.396	0.714	0.986
Honduras	0.602	0.317	0.106	-82.4%	3.071	3.084	3.288	7.1%	0.46	0.174	0.058	0.828	1.211	1.624	0.171	0.205	0.229
El Salvador	0.765	0.436	0.154	-79.9%	3.554	3.651	3.993	12.4%	0.324	0.147	0.05	0.887	1.068	1.166	0.317	0.458	0.478
Nicaragua	0.206	0.116	0.039	-81.1%	4.04	4.015	4.001	-1.0%	0.209	0.13	0.058	0.613	0.966	1.24	0.137	0.168	0.175
Costa Rica	0.29	0.185	0.068	-76.6%	5.072	6.424	7.198	41.9%	0.038	0.016	0.007	0.426	0.562	0.611	0.066	0.079	0.081
Panama	0.855	0.515	0.181	-78.8%	5.067	6.06	6.951	37.2%	0.102	0.045	0.016	0.332	0.418	0.463	0.067	0.078	0.077
Belize	1.815	1.047	0.352	-80.6%	2.71	3.183	4.545	67.7%	0.009	0.004	0.002	0.029	0.042	0.05	0.006	0.008	0.009
America-Central	**0.641**	**0.364**	**0.121**	**-81.1%**	**3.733**	**4.237**	**4.421**	**18.4%**	**2.114**	**0.944**	**0.341**	**4.531**	**6.297**	**7.975**	**1.16**	**1.709**	**2.035**
USA	0.746	0.53	0.179	-76.0%	6.6	7.614	8.158	23.6%	2.688	1.778	0.905	35.81	40.36	39.09	3.361	3.653	4.03
Mexico	0.292	0.177	0.065	-77.7%	3.04	3.946	4.47	47.0%	2.039	0.86	0.334	12.52	15.91	16.84	1.72	1.884	1.737
Canada	0.282	0.201	0.068	-75.9%	7.128	7.677	7.52	5.5%	0.143	0.094	0.056	3.558	4.224	3.938	0.272	0.299	0.331
America-North	**0.603**	**0.416**	**0.146**	**-75.8%**	**6.445**	**7.382**	**7.866**	**22.0%**	**4.869**	**2.732**	**1.295**	**51.88**	**60.5**	**59.87**	**5.353**	**5.836**	**6.097**
Brazil	0.554	0.35	0.127	-77.1%	3.526	4.49	5.194	47.3%	5.357	1.611	0.62	23.55	27.64	27.53	5.958	6.317	6.156
Colombia	0.526	0.322	0.114	-78.3%	6.568	7.581	8.582	30.7%	1.495	0.623	0.215	4.737	6.468	7.155	2.218	2.85	3.077
Argentina	0.475	0.287	0.102	-78.5%	4.611	5.487	6.055	31.3%	0.733	0.345	0.176	4.832	5.211	5.481	0.602	0.615	0.622
Peru	0.384	0.225	0.081	-78.9%	2.718	3.185	3.613	32.9%	1.1	0.445	0.225	2.872	3.661	4.215	0.55	0.593	0.546
Venezuela	0.015	0.009	0.003	-80.0%	2.415	2.795	3.378	39.9%	0.592	0.193	0.089	3.103	4.006	4.586	0.948	1.229	1.332
Ecuador	0.283	0.167	0.058	-79.5%	2.251	2.212	2.42	7.5%	0.448	0.212	0.105	1.378	1.908	2.297	0.335	0.464	0.54
Chile	0.257	0.173	0.062	-75.9%	2.931	3.742	4.347	48.3%	0.136	0.071	0.034	1.692	2.021	1.944	0.241	0.258	0.254
Bolivia	0.136	0.075	0.024	-82.4%	5.039	4.642	5.128	1.8%	0.85	0.251	0.096	1.279	1.629	2.046	0.324	0.388	0.381
Paraguay	0.491	0.281	0.094	-80.9%	3.245	3.548	4.262	31.3%	0.315	0.126	0.045	0.705	0.984	1.244	0.217	0.278	0.286
Uruguay	0.406	0.252	0.089	-78.1%	3.49	4.167	4.578	31.2%	0.049	0.02	0.007	0.414	0.385	0.357	0.047	0.043	0.04
Guyana	2.414	1.509	0.501	-79.2%	3.966	2.669	3.021	-23.8%	0.054	0.021	0.006	0.107	0.108	0.091	0.02	0.017	0.015
Suriname	1.978	1.212	0.417	-78.9%	2.999	3.68	4.324	44.2%	0.021	0.008	0.002	0.067	0.068	0.057	0.012	0.013	0.01
America-South	**0.463**	**0.282**	**0.1**	**-78.4%**	**3.775**	**4.534**	**5.181**	**37.2%**	**11.15**	**3.925**	**1.621**	**44.74**	**54.09**	**57.01**	**11.47**	**13.06**	**13.26**

Multination Regional Analysis

Health

Base Case: Countries in Year 2060 Descending Population Sequence	HIV Prevalence Rate (Percent of Population Infected)				Government Spending on Health (Percent of GDP)				Disability-Adjusted Life Years (Millions of Life Years Lost plus Life Years Lived with Disability)								
									Communicable Diseases			Noncommunicable Diseases			Injuries		
	2010	2035	2060	% Chg	2010	2035	2060	% Chg	2010	2035	2060	2010	2035	2060	2010	2035	2060
ASIA with OCEANIA																	
China	0.077	0.053	0.02	-74.0%	2.073	3.137	3.823	84.4%	26.82	8.674	3.52	146.1	155.8	130	28.63	27.68	20.64
Japan	0.011	0.008	0.003	-72.7%	6.59	7.351	7.177	8.9%	0.878	0.542	0.297	12.17	11.09	8.544	1.108	0.986	0.83
Korea, Repub of	0.031	0.023	0.009	-71.0%	3.216	4.381	4.928	53.2%	0.196	0.13	0.077	4.759	5.865	4.583	0.536	0.549	0.43
Taiwan	0.014	0.01	0.003	-78.6%	4.69	6.103	6.765	44.2%	0.046	0.016	0.007	3.838	5.243	5.085	0.097	0.079	0.063
Korea, Dem. People's Rep.	0.014	0.009	0.003	-78.6%	1.915	2.822	4.26	122.5%	1.248	0.699	0.33	3.095	3.522	3.214	0.312	0.306	0.279
Hong Kong SAR	0.013	0.01	0.004	-69.2%	1.975	2.793	3.077	55.8%	0.006	0.004	0.002	1.095	1.605	1.529	0.01	0.01	0.01
Mongolia	0.027	0.017	0.006	-77.8%	1.305	1.216	2.449	87.7%	0.095	0.028	0.005	0.345	0.423	0.386	0.074	0.085	0.08
Asia-East	**0.068**	**0.048**	**0.018**	**-73.5%**	**4.634**	**4.16**	**4.254**	**-8.2%**	**29.29**	**10.09**	**4.237**	**171.4**	**183.5**	**153.3**	**30.77**	**29.7**	**22.34**
India	0.322	0.177	0.062	-80.7%	1.084	1.887	2.837	161.7%	104.5	25.76	4.96	135.5	160.6	157.9	39.21	43.61	42.01
Pakistan	0.086	0.05	0.016	-81.4%	0.994	1.198	1.825	83.6%	23.76	19.99	6.431	15.49	24	30.19	3.451	5.063	6.094
Bangladesh	0.013	0.007	0.003	-76.9%	1.032	1.036	1.249	21.0%	11.47	3.991	1.501	14.77	21.96	25.28	3.585	4.035	4.108
Afghanistan	0.019	0.011	0.003	-84.2%	2.903	3.167	3.273	12.7%	19.38	7.575	0.281	7.427	10.16	12.03	1.813	2.927	4.562
Iran (Islamic Republic of)	0.156	0.096	0.037	-76.3%	2.943	2.851	3.147	6.9%	2.299	0.748	0.39	6.479	8.359	10.4	1.718	2.05	1.96
Nepal	0.401	0.228	0.073	-81.8%	1.351	1.429	1.682	24.5%	2.982	2.388	0.917	2.803	4.45	5.908	0.62	0.89	0.964
Uzbekistan	0.056	0.033	0.012	-78.6%	2.885	3.657	4.444	54.0%	1.468	0.532	0.167	3.482	4.536	4.816	0.6	0.639	0.583
Sri Lanka	0.026	0.018	0.006	-76.9%	1.841	2.266	2.94	59.7%	0.232	0.111	0.053	2.006	2.486	2.317	0.784	0.713	0.568
Kazakhstan	0.014	0.009	0.003	-78.6%	3.407	3.243	4.068	19.4%	0.493	0.138	0.074	2.453	1.993	1.701	0.591	0.446	0.39
Tajikistan	0.184	0.105	0.034	-81.5%	1.154	1.009	1.367	18.5%	0.745	0.544	0.279	0.813	1.205	1.552	0.128	0.167	0.176
Turkmenistan	0.015	0.009	0.003	-80.0%	3.978	5.561	5.888	48.0%	0.289	0.08	0.049	0.681	0.7	0.785	0.135	0.1	0.098
Kyrgyzstan	0.098	0.058	0.02	-79.6%	2.387	2.23	2.675	12.1%	0.233	0.103	0.045	0.689	0.868	0.959	0.139	0.158	0.147
Bhutan	0.048	0.028	0.01	-79.2%	2.634	2.415	3.336	26.7%	0.065	0.025	0.009	0.068	0.084	0.09	0.022	0.026	0.025
Maldives	0.015	0.009	0.003	-80.0%	7.543	8.553	9.672	28.2%	0.01	0.004	0.002	0.029	0.046	0.059	0.009	0.011	0.011
Asia-South Central	**0.247**	**0.133**	**0.045**	**-81.8%**	**1.502**	**2.071**	**2.833**	**88.6%**	**167.9**	**61.99**	**15.16**	**192.7**	**241.4**	**254**	**52.81**	**60.83**	**61.7**
Indonesia	0.134	0.081	0.029	-78.4%	1.175	1.58	2.044	74.0%	8.447	4.185	1.933	21.92	30.73	32.71	6.191	6.224	5.596
Philippines	0.013	0.008	0.003	-76.9%	1.369	1.72	2.173	58.7%	4.113	2.761	1.403	9.811	14.26	17.09	0.834	1.076	1.266
Viet Nam	0.455	0.283	0.103	-77.4%	1.675	1.713	2.171	29.6%	3.109	1.329	0.437	7.727	10.82	11.7	1.106	1.257	1.377
Thailand	1.316	0.895	0.309	-76.5%	2.268	2.824	3.295	45.3%	3.069	1.351	0.485	10.17	12.12	10.21	2.163	2.109	1.878
Myanmar	0.349	0.196	0.07	-79.9%	1.201	1.772	2.264	88.5%	5.145	1.665	0.76	6.97	8.33	8.449	1.277	1.231	1.124
Malaysia	0.409	0.248	0.086	-79.0%	2.084	3.085	4.171	100.1%	0.617	0.381	0.213	2.769	3.958	4.521	0.276	0.341	0.352
Cambodia	0.686	0.323	0.105	-84.7%	1.533	1.614	1.725	12.5%	2.586	1.166	0.388	2.601	3.402	4.035	0.298	0.376	0.394
LAO People's Dem Repub	0.098	0.054	0.017	-82.7%	1.019	0.756	0.974	-4.4%	0.81	0.303	0.073	0.643	0.921	1.209	0.159	0.203	0.233
Singapore	0.12	0.093	0.032	-73.3%	1.161	1.767	2.221	91.3%	0.042	0.04	0.023	0.407	0.588	0.541	0.024	0.027	0.027
Timor-Leste	0.018	0.011	0.003	-83.3%	10.49	9.163	8.735	-16.7%	0.268	0.238	0.185	0.159	0.283	0.465	0.039	0.077	0.128
Brunei Darussalam	0.014	0.009	0.003	-78.6%	2.482	2.304	2.683	8.1%	0.004	0.003	0.002	0.042	0.086	0.113	0.004	0.004	0.004
Asia-South East	**0.351**	**0.2**	**0.067**	**-80.9%**	**1.589**	**2.08**	**2.628**	**65.4%**	**28.21**	**13.42**	**5.902**	**63.23**	**85.49**	**91.05**	**12.37**	**12.93**	**12.38**

Health

Base Case: Countries in Year 2060 Descending Population Sequence	HIV Prevalence Rate (Percent of Population Infected)				Government Spending on Health (Percent of GDP)				Communicable Diseases			Disability-Adjusted Life Years Noncommunicable Diseases (Millions of Life Years Lost plus Life Years Lived with Disability)			Injuries		
	2010	2035	2060	% Chg	2010	2035	2060	% Chg	2010	2035	2060	2010	2035	2060	2010	2035	2060
ASIA with OCEANIA continued																	
Turkey	0.004	0.002	0.001	-75.0%	4.04	5.252	6.114	51.3%	1.974	0.847	0.43	8.076	9.939	10.29	0.783	0.806	0.738
Yemen	0.018	0.01	0.003	-83.3%	1.767	1.879	3.038	71.9%	2.715	1.334	0.481	2.78	4.457	6.614	1.023	1.622	2.057
Iraq	0.017	0.009	0.003	-82.4%	3.366	4.471	6.291	86.9%	1.455	0.499	0.203	2.304	3.31	4.455	1.412	2.363	3.053
Saudi Arabia	0.015	0.009	0.003	-80.0%	3.295	3.539	5.585	69.5%	0.591	0.4	0.295	2.412	4.224	5.486	0.602	0.697	0.73
Syrian Arab Repub	0.016	0.009	0.003	-81.3%	2.361	2.933	3.98	68.6%	0.506	0.325	0.161	2.036	3.416	4.798	0.22	0.33	0.402
Israel	0.105	0.062	0.021	-80.0%	4.658	6.362	6.882	47.7%	0.049	0.026	0.018	0.769	0.958	1.134	0.054	0.071	0.084
Jordan	0.03	0.016	0.006	-80.0%	4.738	4.736	5.707	20.5%	0.168	0.07	0.029	0.593	0.847	1.022	0.103	0.14	0.134
Occupied Palestinian Territory	0.018	0.01	0.003	-83.3%	2.466	2.285	2.704	9.7%	0.106	0.04	0.013	0.343	0.548	0.836	0.081	0.132	0.167
Azerbaija¬	0.091	0.059	0.022	-75.8%	1.021	1.587	2.093	105.0%	0.284	0.083	0.044	1.087	1.178	1.166	0.088	0.073	0.061
United Arab Emirates	0.013	0.009	0.004	-69.2%	2.272	2.381	2.751	21.1%	0.041	0.022	0.012	0.288	0.638	0.705	0.044	0.05	0.039
Oman	0.015	0.009	0.003	-80.0%	2.432	2.678	3.506	44.2%	0.039	0.024	0.012	0.231	0.42	0.537	0.026	0.029	0.03
Kuwait	0.053	0.036	0.013	-75.5%	2.518	2.779	4.727	87.7%	0.018	0.015	0.012	0.2	0.426	0.549	0.027	0.03	0.035
Lebanon	0.115	0.071	0.026	-77.4%	3.675	4.173	4.762	29.6%	0.097	0.043	0.02	0.429	0.503	0.515	0.076	0.081	0.074
Armenia	0.114	0.074	0.028	-75.4%	1.725	1.82	2.184	26.6%	0.069	0.019	0.007	0.415	0.387	0.355	0.03	0.028	0.023
Georgia	0.047	0.032	0.012	-74.5%	1.626	1.877	2.386	46.7%	0.097	0.027	0.011	0.603	0.506	0.372	0.034	0.027	0.02
Bahrain	0.189	0.126	0.044	-76.7%	2.907	3.35	3.647	25.5%	0.008	0.006	0.004	0.071	0.142	0.162	0.008	0.008	0.006
Qatar	0.012	0.009	0.004	-66.7%	2.737	2.938	4.411	61.2%	0.005	0.006	0.004	0.066	0.143	0.158	0.011	0.009	0.008
Cyprus	0.094	0.065	0.025	-73.4%	2.756	4.052	4.85	76.0%	0.007	0.003	0.002	0.07	0.077	0.071	0.005	0.004	0.003
Asia-West	**0.024**	**0.013**	**0.004**	**-83.3%**	**3.333**	**4.082**	**5.442**	**63.3%**	**8.229**	**3.788**	**1.755**	**22.77**	**32.12**	**39.23**	**4.627**	**6.5**	**7.664**
Australia	0.123	0.084	0.029	-76.4%	6.071	6.656	6.76	11.3%	0.111	0.066	0.038	1.963	2.365	2.326	0.171	0.187	0.206
Papua New Guinea	0.918	0.518	0.159	-82.7%	3.964	3.808	4.263	7.5%	0.864	0.454	0.224	0.967	1.388	1.849	0.179	0.244	0.296
New Zealand	0.047	0.032	0.011	-76.6%	6.855	8.178	8.636	26.0%	0.021	0.011	0.005	0.436	0.496	0.441	0.041	0.041	0.041
Solomon Islands	0.017	0.01	0.003	-82.4%	4.229	3.222	3.481	-17.7%	0.046	0.039	0.025	0.105	0.163	0.216	0.01	0.013	0.015
Fiji	0.015	0.009	0.003	-80.0%	2.86	3.432	4.808	68.1%	0.029	0.014	0.006	0.158	0.175	0.163	0.008	0.008	0.005
Vanuatu	0.017	0.009	0.003	-82.4%	2.502	3.104	5.107	104.1%	0.011	0.007	0.003	0.036	0.051	0.064	0.002	0.003	0.003
Micronesia, Federated States of	0.016	0.01	0.003	-81.3%	11.07	9.177	10.26	-7.3%	0.008	0.006	0.003	0.021	0.031	0.039	0.002	0.002	0.002
Tonga	0.017	0.01	0.003	-82.4%	3.38	3.251	3.733	10.4%	0.005	0.005	0.003	0.018	0.027	0.035	0.001	0.001	0.002
Samoa	0.017	0.01	0.003	-82.4%	3.843	3.803	4.3	11.9%	0.007	0.003	0.001	0.025	0.029	0.031	0.001	0.002	0.001
Oceania	**0.244**	**0.181**	**0.064**	**-73.8%**	**6.128**	**6.756**	**6.907**	**12.7%**	**1.101**	**0.605**	**0.308**	**3.73**	**4.725**	**5.165**	**0.415**	**0.501**	**0.571**

Health

Base Case: Countries in Year 2060 Descending Population Sequence	HIV Prevalence Rate (Percent of Population Infected)				Government Spending on Health (Percent of GDP)				Disability-Adjusted Life Years (Millions of Life Years Lost plus Life Years Lived with Disability)								
									Communicable Diseases			Noncommunicable Diseases			Injuries		
	2010	2035	2060	% Chg	2010	2035	2060	% Chg	2010	2035	2060	2010	2035	2060	2010	2035	2060
EUROPE																	
Russian Federation	0.862	0.589	0.225	-73.9%	4.269	4.417	5.448	27.6%	3.02	1.066	0.423	24.15	17.7	12.82	7.099	4.682	3.877
Poland	0.065	0.045	0.018	-72.3%	4.547	5.669	6.301	38.6%	0.177	0.079	0.04	4.535	4.117	3.226	0.579	0.462	0.352
Ukraine	1.158	0.773	0.3	-74.1%	4.334	5.795	7.226	66.7%	1.044	0.373	0.099	8.06	5.62	3.666	1.501	1.038	0.674
Romania	0.098	0.065	0.025	-74.5%	3.891	4.283	4.675	20.1%	0.223	0.089	0.041	2.929	2.471	1.891	0.354	0.272	0.189
Czech Republic	0.019	0.013	0.005	-73.7%	6.366	6.868	7.213	13.3%	0.041	0.02	0.01	1.215	1.124	0.885	0.128	0.114	0.098
Belarus	0.182	0.122	0.047	-74.2%	5.336	6.953	7.357	37.9%	0.083	0.029	0.011	1.528	1.199	0.895	0.35	0.246	0.18
Hungary	0.046	0.03	0.011	-76.1%	4.531	5.314	5.576	23.1%	0.052	0.02	0.01	1.536	1.194	0.861	0.136	0.115	0.094
Bulgaria	0.014	0.01	0.004	-71.4%	4.848	5.519	6.499	34.1%	0.045	0.017	0.008	1.148	0.858	0.576	0.088	0.059	0.039
Slovak Republic	0.013	0.009	0.003	-76.9%	5.311	6.01	6.244	17.6%	0.025	0.012	0.006	0.65	0.628	0.508	0.074	0.061	0.047
Moldova, Repub of	0.188	0.119	0.045	-76.1%	4.328	4.898	5.495	27.0%	0.071	0.038	0.012	0.718	0.642	0.516	0.099	0.089	0.063
Europe-East	**0.623**	**0.413**	**0.157**	**-74.8%**	**4.566**	**5.053**	**5.934**	**30.0%**	**4.782**	**1.743**	**0.66**	**46.47**	**35.55**	**25.84**	**10.41**	**7.138**	**5.614**
United Kingdom	0.167	0.115	0.039	-76.6%	6.834	7.818	7.873	15.2%	0.396	0.206	0.117	6.865	6.455	5.588	0.366	0.358	0.361
Sweden	0.099	0.068	0.023	-76.8%	7.393	8.523	8.634	16.8%	0.041	0.023	0.013	0.927	0.848	0.715	0.065	0.064	0.065
Denmark	0.12	0.082	0.027	-77.5%	8.922	10.51	10.65	19.4%	0.027	0.014	0.007	0.728	0.686	0.551	0.051	0.05	0.049
Ireland	0.182	0.12	0.043	-76.4%	6.298	6.645	6.374	1.2%	0.025	0.016	0.01	0.415	0.484	0.509	0.026	0.029	0.034
Norway	0.091	0.062	0.021	-76.9%	8.409	8.773	9.165	9.0%	0.02	0.014	0.009	0.455	0.494	0.447	0.045	0.047	0.047
Finland	0.066	0.046	0.015	-77.3%	6.111	7.098	7.073	15.7%	0.023	0.013	0.006	0.531	0.469	0.364	0.079	0.071	0.065
Lithuania	0.088	0.059	0.023	-73.9%	3.974	4.895	5.611	41.2%	0.028	0.011	0.004	0.476	0.377	0.276	0.115	0.088	0.064
Latvia	0.619	0.412	0.161	-74.0%	3.5	4.483	5.236	49.6%	0.027	0.01	0.003	0.322	0.244	0.179	0.057	0.041	0.028
Estonia	1.055	0.72	0.264	-75.0%	3.982	4.812	5.214	30.9%	0.017	0.006	0.002	0.182	0.131	0.093	0.032	0.02	0.014
Iceland	0.249	0.17	0.06	-75.9%	7.63	8.687	9.13	19.7%	0.001	0.001	0	0.024	0.027	0.024	0.002	0.002	0.002
Europe-North	**0.17**	**0.114**	**0.038**	**-77.6%**	**7.036**	**7.942**	**8.019**	**14.0%**	**0.606**	**0.313**	**0.172**	**10.93**	**10.21**	**8.747**	**0.836**	**0.772**	**0.727**
Italy	0.388	0.274	0.095	-75.5%	6.579	7.221	7.503	14.0%	0.26	0.109	0.04	6.641	6.175	4.777	0.39	0.339	0.296
Spain	0.472	0.327	0.12	-74.6%	5.707	6.412	6.544	14.7%	0.272	0.128	0.057	4.755	4.772	4.11	0.324	0.269	0.222
Greece	0.133	0.091	0.033	-75.2%	5.602	6.483	6.84	22.1%	0.043	0.022	0.012	1.206	1.128	0.957	0.093	0.07	0.053
Portugal	0.45	0.304	0.109	-75.8%	7.01	7.931	8.753	24.9%	0.092	0.041	0.016	1.39	1.322	1.107	0.095	0.081	0.065
Serbia	0.117	0.076	0.028	-76.1%	4.975	5.803	6.852	37.7%	0.054	0.026	0.012	1.044	0.92	0.729	0.063	0.057	0.047
Bosnia and Herzegovina	0.018	0.012	0.005	-72.2%	4.992	5.703	6.411	28.4%	0.028	0.01	0.005	0.505	0.488	0.392	0.039	0.031	0.023
Croatia	0.016	0.011	0.004	-75.0%	6.004	7.06	7.807	30.0%	0.026	0.011	0.005	0.587	0.492	0.373	0.052	0.044	0.036
Albania	0.015	0.009	0.003	-80.0%	2.495	2.625	3.157	26.5%	0.031	0.012	0.006	0.301	0.318	0.3	0.035	0.032	0.026
Macedonia, FYR	0.035	0.023	0.008	-77.1%	5.264	5.192	5.631	7.0%	0.018	0.009	0.004	0.266	0.275	0.234	0.02	0.02	0.018
Slovenia	0.035	0.026	0.01	-71.4%	6.263	7.442	7.737	23.5%	0.01	0.005	0.002	0.232	0.22	0.17	0.022	0.02	0.016
Montenegro	0.015	0.009	0.003	-80.0%	6.46	6.909	7.578	17.3%	0.004	0.002	0.001	0.086	0.08	0.066	0.006	0.006	0.005
Malta	0.071	0.049	0.019	-73.2%	6.389	7.141	7.661	19.9%	0.003	0.002	0.001	0.045	0.048	0.041	0.002	0.002	0.002
Europe-South	**0.342**	**0.236**	**0.084**	**-75.4%**	**6.196**	**6.854**	**7.125**	**15.0%**	**0.841**	**0.376**	**0.16**	**17.06**	**16.24**	**13.26**	**1.14**	**0.97**	**0.81**
Germany	0.091	0.065	0.022	-75.8%	7.974	8.766	8.453	6.0%	0.387	0.207	0.101	9.926	9.156	7.01	0.53	0.481	0.428
France	0.325	0.223	0.075	-76.9%	8.701	9.766	9.861	13.3%	0.311	0.161	0.083	6.385	6.282	5.248	0.57	0.594	0.58
Netherlands	0.154	0.109	0.036	-76.6%	5.763	6.35	6.256	8.6%	0.088	0.057	0.029	1.847	1.996	1.637	0.088	0.094	0.096
Belgium	0.201	0.139	0.047	-76.6%	7.137	7.997	7.973	11.7%	0.051	0.026	0.013	1.167	1.128	0.916	0.104	0.099	0.094
Austria	0.148	0.107	0.038	-74.3%	7.728	8.713	8.57	10.9%	0.032	0.014	0.006	0.997	0.987	0.767	0.071	0.065	0.055
Switzerland	0.475	0.351	0.122	-74.3%	5.912	7.079	7.171	21.3%	0.043	0.023	0.009	0.708	0.715	0.541	0.055	0.054	0.048
Luxembourg	0.16	0.109	0.035	-78.1%	6.773	5.71	6.557	-3.2%	0.006	0.004	0.002	0.045	0.056	0.061	0.004	0.005	0.006
Europe-West	**0.197**	**0.142**	**0.049**	**-75.1%**	**7.82**	**8.727**	**8.632**	**10.4%**	**0.918**	**0.493**	**0.244**	**21.07**	**20.32**	**16.18**	**1.42**	**1.391**	**1.307**

Multination Regional Analysis

Health

Base Case
Source: International Futures Version 6.32, June 2010

	Years Living with Disabilities — Millions of Life Years Lived with Disability									Total Deaths — Annual Deaths in Millions				Deaths and Death Rates from Communicable Diseases — AIDS					
	Communicable Diseases			Noncommunicable Diseases			Injuries							Annual Deaths (in thousands)			Age Standardized Death Rates per 100,000		
	2010	2035	2060	2010	2035	2060	2010	2035	2060	2010	2035	2060	% Chg	2010	2035	2060	2010	2035	2060
World	111	63.08	31.3	450.1	509.8	532.7	54.17	60.98	63.1	56.74	75.4	98.79	74.1%	1744	1157	359.7	30.19	14.51	3.951
Africa	42.02	31.38	19.69	58.38	80.25	111.2	12.12	17.5	22.61	11.68	12.71	18.29	56.6%	1341	938.7	306.4	165.4	59.05	12.74
Americas	6.77	3.36	1.669	69.32	82.07	85.94	6.288	6.966	6.925	6.185	9.25	12.76	106.3%	106.1	68.49	17.75	11.36	6.005	1.612
Asia with Oceania	59.52	27.14	9.392	272.4	303.1	299.2	32.55	34.05	31.6	30.42	44.45	58.57	92.5%	245	127.6	31.29	5.705	2.7	0.722
Europe	2.722	1.181	0.54	49.37	43.74	35.88	3.165	2.426	1.939	8.362	8.869	9.044	8.2%	52.63	22.18	4.255	7.264	4.006	0.961
World	111	63.08	31.3	450.1	509.8	532.7	54.17	60.98	63.1	56.74	75.4	98.79	74.1%	1744	1157	359.7	30.19	14.51	3.951
Africa-Eastern	14.4	9.527	3.631	17.04	23.91	32.87	3.665	5.452	7.033	3.553	3.688	5.424	52.7%	541.7	391.6	132	237.5	74.55	15.51
Africa-Middle	8.55	9.23	8.995	8.209	12.92	20.35	2.055	3.557	5.527	2.021	2.428	3.41	68.7%	134.3	136.5	53.47	131.3	63.39	14.18
Africa-Northern	2.343	1.036	0.449	10.9	13.83	16.56	1.975	2.317	2.407	1.283	1.9	3.068	139.1%	22.42	15.16	4.425	12.27	5.497	1.457
Africa-Southern	2.049	1.081	0.381	3.645	3.648	3.618	0.592	0.646	0.59	0.882	0.758	0.722	-18.1%	410.4	222.7	56.07	777.3	349.2	86.28
Africa-Western	14.68	10.51	6.237	18.59	25.95	37.76	3.831	5.526	7.055	3.937	3.938	5.662	43.8%	231.9	172.7	60.43	93.48	34	7.401
Africa	42.02	31.38	19.69	58.38	80.25	111.2	12.12	17.5	22.61	11.68	12.71	18.29	56.6%	1341	938.7	306.4	165.4	59.05	12.74
America-Caribbean	0.675	0.533	0.303	2.918	3.448	3.607	0.286	0.343	0.344	0.288	0.413	0.552	91.7%	12.28	7.19	1.982	34.4	15.59	4.245
America-Central	0.611	0.301	0.123	3.106	4.192	5.184	0.391	0.552	0.629	0.23	0.355	0.597	159.6%	11.91	8.784	2.576	30.53	13.53	3.567
America-North	1.758	1.06	0.577	34.62	40.47	40.76	1.518	1.592	1.537	3.242	4.718	6.172	90.4%	43.33	29.73	7.494	8.961	5.393	1.389
America-South	3.726	1.465	0.665	28.68	33.96	36.39	4.093	4.479	4.415	2.425	3.764	5.442	124.4%	38.59	22.79	5.697	9.708	4.732	1.3
Americas	6.77	3.36	1.669	69.32	82.07	85.94	6.288	6.966	6.925	6.185	9.25	12.76	106.3%	106.1	68.49	17.75	11.36	6.005	1.612
Asia-East	10.61	4.025	1.772	101.8	100.2	86.08	8.036	6.672	4.84	11.56	17.93	21.47	85.7%	44.32	24.4	5.33	2.626	1.645	0.442
Asia-South Central	37.91	17.07	4.667	113.2	128.9	132.1	18.8	20.85	20.11	13.6	18.02	24.57	80.7%	107.9	56.15	14.64	6.211	2.56	0.694
Asia-South East	8.324	4.504	2.116	41.03	51.88	54.42	3.838	4.049	3.826	3.769	6.071	8.555	127.0%	88.47	44.18	10.52	14.34	6.548	1.692
Asia-West	2.263	1.291	0.692	13.9	19.04	23.25	1.765	2.345	2.68	1.246	2.066	3.49	180.1%	2.541	1.526	0.405	1.013	0.495	0.129
Oceania	0.412	0.257	0.145	2.452	3.054	3.333	0.115	0.135	0.145	0.243	0.368	0.492	102.5%	1.776	1.309	0.388	5.163	2.887	0.797
Asia with Oceania	59.52	27.14	9.392	272.4	303.1	299.2	32.55	34.05	31.6	30.42	44.45	58.57	92.5%	245	127.6	31.29	5.705	2.7	0.722
Europe-East	1.685	0.649	0.27	20.84	16.04	12.32	2.246	1.564	1.171	4.112	3.821	3.597	-12.5%	41.99	17.16	3.199	14.63	8.489	2.183
Europe-North	0.259	0.136	0.075	6.419	6.172	5.51	0.232	0.215	0.192	0.973	1.112	1.227	26.1%	2.033	1.003	0.227	1.937	1.034	0.248
Europe-South	0.354	0.166	0.075	10.14	9.702	8.222	0.338	0.295	0.251	1.517	1.778	1.96	29.2%	5.545	2.562	0.514	3.288	2.177	0.545
Europe-West	0.432	0.241	0.123	12.62	12.41	10.3	0.397	0.395	0.358	1.86	2.275	2.378	27.8%	3.102	1.468	0.318	1.421	0.781	0.195
Europe	2.722	1.181	0.54	49.37	43.74	35.88	3.165	2.426	1.939	8.362	8.869	9.044	8.2%	52.63	22.18	4.255	7.264	4.006	0.961

Health

Base Case: Countries in Year 2060 Descending Population Sequence	Years Living with Disabilities									Total Deaths				Deaths and Death Rates from Communicable Diseases					
	Communicable Diseases			Noncommunicable Diseases			Injuries			Annual Deaths in Millions				AIDS Annual Deaths (in thousands)			Age Standardized Death Rates per 100,000		
				Millions of Life Years Lived with Disability															
	2010	2035	2060	2010	2035	2060	2010	2035	2060	2010	2035	2060	% Chg	2010	2035	2060	2010	2035	2060
AFRICA																			
Ethiopia	3.809	2.135	0.558	4.257	5.973	8.186	0.683	1.048	1.414	0.892	0.916	1.417	58.9%	62.64	50.31	17.43	100.3	36.98	7.83
Tanzania, United Rep	1.633	0.802	0.204	2.083	2.785	3.802	0.358	0.508	0.65	0.412	0.421	0.642	55.8%	94.81	75.08	24.49	279.6	100.7	21.87
Uganda	1.471	1.06	0.197	1.623	2.511	3.531	0.468	0.764	1.015	0.364	0.372	0.543	49.2%	68.64	54.65	19.6	305.7	90.1	18.52
Kenya	1.673	1.217	0.445	1.951	2.673	3.406	0.393	0.538	0.602	0.389	0.398	0.579	48.8%	87.27	54.99	17.64	343.9	92.77	18.11
Madagascar	0.62	0.587	0.344	1.246	1.947	2.837	0.22	0.351	0.462	0.197	0.263	0.406	106.1%	1.435	1.333	0.494	7.167	3.322	0.774
Mozambique	1.251	0.601	0.137	1.377	1.568	1.956	0.308	0.418	0.533	0.304	0.28	0.372	22.4%	60.34	44.93	14.43	310.6	119.6	28.06
Malawi	0.646	0.568	0.342	0.637	1.04	1.611	0.11	0.201	0.293	0.154	0.17	0.255	65.6%	27.54	22.87	8.439	299.8	105.7	19.8
Zambia	0.795	0.685	0.32	0.742	1.028	1.404	0.171	0.248	0.297	0.2	0.151	0.218	9.0%	58.06	45.92	16.33	624.5	217.6	45.17
Somalia	0.565	0.484	0.375	0.682	0.995	1.564	0.373	0.573	0.798	0.128	0.15	0.22	71.9%	2	1.864	0.732	24.2	11.24	2.509
Rwanda	0.611	0.353	0.07	0.628	0.831	1.026	0.149	0.211	0.258	0.145	0.136	0.182	25.5%	10.24	6.462	2.103	134.3	39.24	8.337
Zimbabwe	0.684	0.495	0.29	0.918	1.191	1.51	0.259	0.331	0.346	0.191	0.181	0.252	31.9%	54.7	23.18	6.609	614.1	115.8	27.75
Burundi	0.438	0.343	0.198	0.462	0.681	1.021	0.098	0.145	0.199	0.108	0.114	0.183	69.4%	9.102	5.444	2.002	144.8	40.34	9.108
Eritrea	0.148	0.154	0.131	0.263	0.467	0.734	0.05	0.087	0.136	0.044	0.064	0.112	154.5%	3.891	4.006	1.578	92.07	43.8	9.662
Comoros	0.015	0.017	0.012	0.038	0.067	0.098	0.005	0.008	0.01	0.005	0.009	0.014	180.0%	0.071	0.056	0.021	10.34	4.831	1.08
Mauritius	0.003	0.001	0.001	0.075	0.08	0.072	0.006	0.005	0.005	0.009	0.014	0.017	88.9%	0.259	0.141	0.032	17.55	9.378	2.46
Djibouti	0.035	0.024	0.006	0.058	0.069	0.064	0.015	0.016	0.015	0.009	0.01	0.011	22.2%	0.731	0.417	0.107	95.17	38.19	9.237
Africa-Eastern	**14.4**	**9.527**	**3.631**	**17.04**	**23.91**	**32.87**	**3.665**	**5.452**	**7.033**	**3.553**	**3.688**	**5.424**	**52.7%**	**541.7**	**391.6**	**132**	**237.5**	**74.55**	**15.51**
Congo, Democratic Republic of	5.42	6.445	6.838	4.501	7.57	12.74	1.129	2.099	3.57	1.162	1.505	2.169	86.7%	60.91	80.77	34.25	116.1	69.37	15.21
Angola	0.952	0.609	0.369	1.123	1.535	2.203	0.352	0.598	0.803	0.269	0.254	0.356	32.3%	13.96	12.38	4.232	91.34	39.16	8.933
Cameroon	0.728	0.603	0.29	1.146	1.561	2.01	0.261	0.357	0.43	0.24	0.252	0.321	33.8%	32.79	23.26	7.615	217.1	80.12	18.72
Chad	0.838	1.019	1.161	0.752	1.29	2.134	0.151	0.272	0.442	0.199	0.247	0.349	75.4%	9.496	8.196	3.47	92.91	37.26	8.393
Central African Republic	0.305	0.297	0.179	0.296	0.414	0.534	0.071	0.101	0.124	0.072	0.08	0.094	30.6%	8.911	6.123	2.109	238	89.3	21.12
Congo, Republic of	0.234	0.189	0.114	0.26	0.355	0.479	0.057	0.081	0.096	0.054	0.058	0.081	50.0%	5.595	3.912	1.235	161.1	56.87	12.82
Gabon	0.039	0.035	0.022	0.086	0.127	0.161	0.022	0.033	0.04	0.015	0.019	0.027	80.0%	1.597	1.059	0.315	116.6	44.83	11.23
Equatorial Guinea	0.028	0.027	0.018	0.037	0.053	0.066	0.01	0.015	0.019	0.009	0.01	0.011	22.2%	0.993	0.787	0.24	204.9	97.09	21.21
São Tomé and Príncipe	0.005	0.006	0.005	0.008	0.014	0.022	0.001	0.002	0.003	0.001	0.002	0.003	200.0%	0.001	0.001	0	0.806	0.316	0.075
Africa-Middle	**8.55**	**9.23**	**8.995**	**8.209**	**12.92**	**20.35**	**2.055**	**3.557**	**5.527**	**2.021**	**2.428**	**3.41**	**68.7%**	**134.3**	**136.5**	**53.47**	**131.3**	**63.39**	**14.18**
Egypt	0.575	0.227	0.11	4.537	5.49	6.488	0.387	0.4	0.351	0.457	0.704	1.121	145.3%	1.019	0.677	0.18	1.297	0.607	0.168
Sudan	1.154	0.515	0.177	2.301	3.026	3.945	1.164	1.443	1.58	0.381	0.445	0.685	79.8%	18.39	12.61	3.781	53	19.99	4.727
Algeria	0.19	0.099	0.064	1.541	2.069	2.457	0.158	0.182	0.194	0.17	0.301	0.553	225.3%	1.354	0.856	0.213	3.53	2.043	0.575
Morocco	0.232	0.11	0.05	1.606	2.068	2.274	0.191	0.208	0.196	0.188	0.308	0.469	149.5%	1.344	0.835	0.207	4.085	2.099	0.571
Tunisia	0.123	0.056	0.03	0.564	0.698	0.792	0.045	0.049	0.045	0.061	0.093	0.147	141.0%	0.265	0.156	0.037	2.346	1.335	0.363
Libyan Arab Jamahiriya	0.068	0.028	0.018	0.351	0.479	0.603	0.029	0.036	0.041	0.026	0.049	0.092	253.8%	0.044	0.026	0.007	0.637	0.308	0.088
Africa-Northern	**2.343**	**1.036**	**0.449**	**10.9**	**13.83**	**16.56**	**1.975**	**2.317**	**2.407**	**1.283**	**1.9**	**3.068**	**139.1%**	**22.42**	**15.16**	**4.425**	**12.27**	**5.497**	**1.457**

Health

Base Case: Countries in Year 2060 Descending Population Sequence	Years Living with Disabilities — Millions of Life Years Lived with Disability									Total Deaths — Annual Deaths in Millions				Deaths and Death Rates from Communicable Diseases					
	Communicable Diseases			Noncommunicable Diseases			Injuries							AIDS — Annual Deaths (in thousands)			AIDS — Age Standardized Death Rates per 100,000		
	2010	2035	2060	2010	2035	2060	2010	2035	2060	2010	2035	2060	% Chg	2010	2035	2060	2010	2035	2060
AFRICA continued																			
South Africa	1.768	0.92	0.319	3.228	3.192	3.1	0.496	0.536	0.485	0.802	0.682	0.621	-22.6%	386.1	208.5	52.27	827.3	387.6	96.74
Namibia	0.063	0.037	0.015	0.106	0.14	0.167	0.017	0.024	0.026	0.017	0.021	0.032	88.2%	4.039	2.671	0.777	233.7	79.6	17.76
Lesotho	0.112	0.063	0.022	0.123	0.121	0.139	0.033	0.035	0.031	0.028	0.022	0.026	-7.1%	8.196	4.552	1.176	616.9	184.7	45.48
Botswana	0.046	0.023	0.01	0.099	0.1	0.115	0.023	0.021	0.019	0.018	0.018	0.025	38.9%	7.017	3.859	1.007	436.5	157.1	42.26
Swaziland	0.06	0.038	0.015	0.089	0.095	0.098	0.024	0.03	0.028	0.017	0.016	0.018	5.9%	5.097	3.058	0.841	552.3	182.9	44.77
Africa-Southern	**2.049**	**1.081**	**0.381**	**3.645**	**3.648**	**3.618**	**0.592**	**0.646**	**0.59**	**0.882**	**0.758**	**0.722**	**-18.1%**	**410.4**	**222.7**	**56.07**	**777.3**	**349.2**	**86.28**
Nigeria	8.554	5.131	3.357	10.21	12.93	18.58	2.346	3.177	3.892	2.166	1.934	2.818	30.1%	139.1	104.6	35.86	112.2	42.63	9.523
Niger	0.86	0.861	0.555	0.877	1.561	2.845	0.15	0.291	0.479	0.235	0.251	0.364	54.9%	5.038	5.567	2.508	37.22	17.03	3.6
Côte d'Ivoire	0.821	0.79	0.423	1.001	1.581	2.251	0.155	0.231	0.284	0.215	0.255	0.349	62.3%	33.94	20.05	7.114	206.3	58.89	12.99
Ghana	0.825	0.752	0.376	1.465	2.032	2.463	0.271	0.377	0.429	0.26	0.329	0.436	67.7%	16.8	11.71	3.729	82.94	31.16	7.074
Mali	0.925	0.523	0.207	0.98	1.37	2.104	0.191	0.3	0.428	0.233	0.188	0.298	27.9%	4.384	3.781	1.438	33.66	13.53	2.846
Burkina Faso	0.691	0.694	0.303	0.853	1.469	2.153	0.17	0.287	0.394	0.206	0.238	0.306	48.5%	7.101	4.922	1.885	60.89	18.84	3.908
Senegal	0.453	0.407	0.167	0.804	1.25	1.734	0.156	0.238	0.293	0.148	0.174	0.251	69.6%	1.572	1.411	0.488	12.39	5.543	1.353
Guinea	0.399	0.367	0.235	0.573	0.898	1.363	0.101	0.161	0.222	0.116	0.135	0.191	64.7%	3.109	2.556	0.98	34.18	13.44	3.037
Benin	0.272	0.251	0.165	0.492	0.794	1.227	0.06	0.098	0.133	0.085	0.106	0.169	98.8%	2.94	2.459	0.93	35.41	13.87	3.108
Togo	0.165	0.17	0.159	0.312	0.518	0.632	0.036	0.056	0.078	0.053	0.075	0.128	141.5%	6.71	5.244	1.908	115.5	43.81	10.04
Sierra Leone	0.3	0.22	0.068	0.399	0.604	0.831	0.083	0.135	0.184	0.097	0.103	0.134	38.1%	5.487	5.54	1.874	99.58	54.26	11.78
Liberia	0.146	0.08	0.026	0.171	0.265	0.367	0.028	0.05	0.062	0.038	0.044	0.067	76.3%	3.009	2.69	0.902	96.37	41.62	9.11
Mauritania	0.115	0.131	0.097	0.205	0.329	0.479	0.037	0.055	0.073	0.036	0.051	0.072	100.0%	1.403	1.169	0.417	42.14	19.88	4.772
Guinea-Bissau	0.099	0.085	0.077	0.118	0.161	0.269	0.025	0.04	0.063	0.027	0.027	0.039	44.4%	0.847	0.686	0.29	53.98	22.35	5.095
Gambia	0.053	0.046	0.022	0.109	0.157	0.226	0.018	0.027	0.037	0.018	0.023	0.034	88.9%	0.39	0.306	0.107	25.61	10.26	2.27
Cape Verde	0.004	0.002	0	0.023	0.033	0.041	0.003	0.004	0.004	0.003	0.004	0.007	133.3%	0.004	0.002	0.001	0.789	0.29	0.079
Africa-Western	**14.68**	**10.51**	**6.237**	**18.59**	**25.95**	**37.76**	**3.831**	**5.526**	**7.055**	**3.937**	**3.938**	**5.662**	**43.8%**	**231.9**	**172.7**	**60.43**	**93.48**	**34**	**7.401**

Multination Regional Analysis

Health

Base Case: Countries in Year 2060 Descending Population Sequence	Years Living with Disabilities (Millions of Life Years Lived with Disability)									Total Deaths (Annual Deaths in Millions)				Deaths and Death Rates from Communicable Diseases					
	Communicable Diseases			Noncommunicable Diseases			Injuries							AIDS (Annual Deaths in thousands)			Age Standardized Death Rates per 100,000		
	2010	2035	2060	2010	2035	2060	2010	2035	2060	2010	2035	2060	% Chg	2010	2035	2060	2010	2035	2060
AMERICAS																			
Haiti	0.425	0.43	0.261	0.691	1.023	1.314	0.118	0.16	0.173	0.087	0.115	0.157	80.5%	5.567	3.662	1.133	71.51	26.94	6.22
Dominican Republic	0.149	0.055	0.02	0.64	0.753	0.81	0.081	0.086	0.076	0.052	0.078	0.118	126.9%	3.68	1.895	0.474	40.21	16.12	4.586
Cuba	0.027	0.014	0.007	0.786	0.79	0.624	0.028	0.03	0.03	0.08	0.126	0.158	97.5%	0.144	0.071	0.015	1.288	0.779	0.198
Puerto Rico	0.012	0.007	0.004	0.378	0.403	0.389	0.011	0.01	0.009	0.031	0.043	0.052	67.7%	0.028	0.014	0.003	0.673	0.293	0.077
Jamaica	0.038	0.019	0.007	0.202	0.235	0.241	0.036	0.046	0.046	0.021	0.027	0.035	66.7%	1.96	1.136	0.268	74.64	36.34	9.742
Trinidad	0.016	0.005	0.002	0.142	0.149	0.135	0.007	0.006	0.005	0.01	0.014	0.018	80.0%	0.704	0.314	0.065	48.36	24.66	6.541
Bahamas	0.004	0.002	0.001	0.027	0.032	0.031	0.003	0.003	0.003	0.002	0.003	0.005	150.0%	0.145	0.074	0.018	40.92	17.69	4.758
Barbados	0.001	0.001	0	0.02	0.025	0.02	0.001	0	0	0.002	0.003	0.004	100.0%	0.049	0.021	0.004	16.15	8.63	2.194
Grenada	0.001	0	0	0.007	0.01	0.013	0	0	0	0.001	0.001	0.002	100.0%	0.001	0	0	0.761	0.267	0.053
Saint Vincent and Grenadines	0.001	0	0	0.01	0.014	0.015	0.001	0.001	0.001	0.001	0.001	0.002	100.0%	0.004	0.002	0.001	3.117	1.278	0.339
Saint Lucia	0.001	0	0	0.015	0.017	0.016	0.001	0.001	0.001	0.001	0.001	0.002	100.0%	0.001	0.001	0.001	0.684	0.325	0.086
America-Caribbean	**0.675**	**0.533**	**0.303**	**2.918**	**3.448**	**3.607**	**0.286**	**0.343**	**0.344**	**0.288**	**0.413**	**0.552**	**91.7%**	**12.28**	**7.19**	**1.982**	**34.4**	**15.59**	**4.245**
Guatemala	0.236	0.118	0.047	0.96	1.366	1.849	0.125	0.216	0.284	0.077	0.109	0.19	146.8%	5.867	5.001	1.586	47.53	20.24	5.008
Honduras	0.171	0.075	0.029	0.576	0.815	1.059	0.066	0.078	0.084	0.038	0.059	0.11	189.5%	1.399	0.828	0.234	20.31	6.736	1.749
El Salvador	0.104	0.051	0.02	0.608	0.71	0.76	0.105	0.145	0.147	0.049	0.069	0.099	102.0%	2.275	1.422	0.361	34.13	15.41	4.265
Nicaragua	0.054	0.037	0.019	0.409	0.616	0.766	0.045	0.056	0.057	0.027	0.048	0.084	211.1%	0.692	0.496	0.136	12.87	5.975	1.617
Costa Rica	0.013	0.006	0.003	0.298	0.373	0.404	0.024	0.028	0.029	0.019	0.039	0.064	236.8%	0.271	0.167	0.042	5.791	2.728	0.755
Panama	0.029	0.013	0.006	0.233	0.283	0.311	0.025	0.026	0.025	0.018	0.03	0.046	155.6%	1.35	0.831	0.207	38.95	19.6	5.353
Belize	0.003	0.001	0.001	0.022	0.03	0.035	0.002	0.003	0.003	0.001	0.002	0.004	300.0%	0.061	0.039	0.011	23.61	8.222	1.965
America-Central	**0.611**	**0.301**	**0.123**	**3.106**	**4.192**	**5.184**	**0.391**	**0.552**	**0.629**	**0.23**	**0.355**	**0.597**	**159.6%**	**11.91**	**8.784**	**2.576**	**30.53**	**13.53**	**3.567**
USA	1.021	0.713	0.414	23.47	26.84	26.71	0.823	0.856	0.858	2.46	3.411	4.245	72.6%	28.29	20.94	5.435	8.228	5.443	1.357
Mexico	0.678	0.304	0.135	8.854	10.89	11.42	0.631	0.666	0.606	0.525	0.905	1.441	174.5%	14.62	8.548	1.999	13.47	6.685	1.884
Canada	0.059	0.043	0.028	2.3	2.734	2.633	0.064	0.07	0.072	0.258	0.403	0.486	88.4%	0.421	0.239	0.06	1.071	0.587	0.147
America-North	**1.758**	**1.06**	**0.577**	**34.62**	**40.47**	**40.76**	**1.518**	**1.592**	**1.537**	**3.242**	**4.718**	**6.172**	**90.4%**	**43.33**	**29.73**	**7.494**	**8.961**	**5.393**	**1.389**
Brazil	1.957	0.689	0.289	14.62	16.95	17.45	2.093	2.141	2.044	1.223	1.882	2.656	117.2%	6.968	3.584	0.876	3.45	1.525	0.421
Colombia	0.488	0.212	0.088	3.264	4.209	4.645	0.774	0.954	0.987	0.272	0.486	0.721	165.1%	12.93	7.942	1.968	26.19	13.4	3.699
Argentina	0.238	0.118	0.069	3.082	3.311	3.541	0.239	0.232	0.226	0.312	0.394	0.521	67.0%	6.72	3.865	0.959	16.91	8.09	2.19
Peru	0.28	0.125	0.066	1.903	2.342	2.683	0.214	0.227	0.209	0.155	0.249	0.406	161.9%	4.072	2.598	0.672	13.55	6.691	1.886
Venezuela	0.228	0.085	0.042	2.121	2.629	2.994	0.327	0.399	0.422	0.147	0.264	0.411	179.6%	0.891	0.503	0.129	3.169	1.325	0.355
Ecuador	0.116	0.063	0.036	0.932	1.261	1.498	0.111	0.147	0.162	0.073	0.124	0.203	178.1%	1.769	1.163	0.304	12.78	6.229	1.69
Chile	0.042	0.023	0.012	1.114	1.275	1.245	0.088	0.092	0.088	0.094	0.166	0.228	142.6%	1.575	0.903	0.215	8.868	4.659	1.235
Bolivia	0.227	0.085	0.037	0.793	0.978	1.205	0.126	0.149	0.146	0.072	0.093	0.15	108.3%	0.692	0.5	0.139	7.412	3.327	0.857
Paraguay	0.114	0.05	0.02	0.489	0.66	0.816	0.09	0.111	0.109	0.035	0.056	0.091	160.0%	1.383	0.98	0.269	22.35	10.57	2.824
Uruguay	0.015	0.006	0.003	0.251	0.233	0.218	0.019	0.016	0.015	0.033	0.035	0.043	30.3%	0.642	0.34	0.08	18.34	8.912	2.351
Guyana	0.016	0.007	0.002	0.071	0.068	0.058	0.007	0.006	0.005	0.006	0.007	0.008	33.3%	0.691	0.28	0.058	93.5	42.08	10.92
Suriname	0.006	0.002	0.001	0.042	0.042	0.036	0.004	0.004	0.003	0.004	0.004	0.005	25.0%	0.257	0.129	0.027	56.98	28.28	7.494
America-South	**3.726**	**1.465**	**0.665**	**28.68**	**33.96**	**36.39**	**4.093**	**4.479**	**4.415**	**2.425**	**3.764**	**5.442**	**124.4%**	**38.59**	**22.79**	**5.697**	**9.708**	**4.732**	**1.3**

Health

| Base Case: Countries in Year 2060 Descending Population Sequence | Years Living with Disabilities — Millions of Life Years Lived with Disability | | | | | | | | | Total Deaths — Annual Deaths in Millions | | | | Deaths and Death Rates from Communicable Diseases | | | | | |
| | Communicable Diseases | | | Noncommunicable Diseases | | | Injuries | | | | | | | AIDS — Annual Deaths (in thousands) | | | Age Standardized Death Rates per 100,000 | | |
	2010	2035	2060	2010	2035	2060	2010	2035	2060	2010	2035	2060	% Chg	2010	2035	2060	2010	2035	2060
ASIA with OCEANIA																			
China	9.878	3.603	1.557	85.57	82.34	70.68	7.511	6.177	4.431	9.618	15.07	18.43	91.6%	41.85	23.28	5.114	2.928	1.826	0.487
Japan	0.35	0.197	0.101	7.428	6.969	5.638	0.27	0.242	0.197	1.231	1.622	1.487	20.8%	1.601	0.705	0.135	1.025	0.548	0.145
Korea, Repub of	0.067	0.044	0.027	3.064	3.592	2.796	0.114	0.118	0.093	0.294	0.572	0.706	140.1%	0.637	0.304	0.056	1.09	0.679	0.196
Taiwan	0.016	0.006	0.003	2.927	3.946	3.835	0.023	0.018	0.013	0.124	0.254	0.352	183.9%	0	0	0	0	0	0
Korea, Dem. People's Rep.	0.26	0.161	0.082	1.787	1.961	1.806	0.099	0.097	0.089	0.231	0.29	0.321	39.0%	0.158	0.072	0.016	0.754	0.388	0.099
Hong Kong SAR	0.002	0.001	0.001	0.829	1.205	1.154	0.002	0.002	0.002	0.002	0.093	0.125	166.0%	0	0	0	0	0	0
Mongolia	0.034	0.012	0.003	0.193	0.194	0.174	0.017	0.019	0.016	0.017	0.03	0.04	135.3%	0.072	0.038	0.009	2.417	1.383	0.362
Asia-East	**10.61**	**4.025**	**1.772**	**101.8**	**100.2**	**86.08**	**8.036**	**6.672**	**4.84**	**11.56**	**17.93**	**21.47**	**85.7%**	**44.32**	**24.4**	**5.33**	**2.626**	**1.645**	**0.442**
India	24.01	7.567	1.346	79.68	85.6	82.67	13.75	14.54	13.18	9.392	12.17	16.01	70.5%	88.77	42.53	10.72	7.435	2.985	0.843
Pakistan	5.156	4.838	1.948	9.32	13.86	16.54	1.514	2.209	2.596	1.276	1.849	2.595	103.4%	5.45	4.369	1.399	3.371	1.564	0.381
Bangladesh	2.717	1.191	0.497	8.934	11.28	12.21	1.242	1.403	1.423	0.985	1.587	2.464	150.2%	1.926	1.242	0.312	1.092	0.681	0.195
Afghanistan	3.335	1.985	0.127	3.569	4.317	5.083	0.748	1.097	1.388	0.732	0.608	0.704	-3.8%	0.248	0.209	0.077	0.436	0.214	0.065
Iran (Islamic Republic of)	1.021	0.377	0.214	3.959	4.728	5.772	0.615	0.645	0.64	0.404	0.64	1.164	188.1%	4.006	2.45	0.599	5.053	2.873	0.8
Nepal	0.625	0.568	0.268	1.796	2.671	3.282	0.19	0.265	0.294	0.205	0.313	0.479	133.7%	6.192	4.569	1.346	23.92	10.28	2.487
Uzbekistan	0.42	0.192	0.071	2.077	2.418	2.483	0.226	0.219	0.183	0.18	0.28	0.419	132.8%	0.351	0.217	0.053	1.157	0.693	0.2
Sri Lanka	0.071	0.037	0.02	1.259	1.5	1.41	0.225	0.21	0.169	0.135	0.229	0.266	97.0%	0.26	0.14	0.031	1.267	0.702	0.185
Kazakhstan	0.19	0.061	0.034	1.218	0.941	0.832	0.118	0.09	0.075	0.162	0.165	0.186	14.8%	0.206	0.087	0.018	1.315	0.642	0.175
Tajikistan	0.206	0.175	0.103	0.54	0.728	0.861	0.054	0.066	0.065	0.045	0.068	0.11	144.4%	0.27	0.2	0.056	3.462	1.822	0.526
Turkmenistan	0.077	0.029	0.018	0.372	0.368	0.424	0.053	0.031	0.028	0.037	0.044	0.072	94.6%	0.074	0.041	0.011	1.42	0.617	0.179
Kyrgyzstan	0.07	0.037	0.018	0.404	0.456	0.485	0.054	0.062	0.058	0.04	0.06	0.085	112.5%	0.134	0.082	0.02	2.27	1.294	0.363
Bhutan	0.014	0.007	0.003	0.041	0.048	0.05	0.007	0.008	0.008	0.005	0.006	0.01	100.0%	0.005	0.003	0.001	0.562	0.321	0.09
Maldives	0.002	0.001	0.001	0.02	0.028	0.033	0.004	0.004	0.004	0.002	0.003	0.006	200.0%	0.011	0.007	0.002	2.911	1.415	0.379
Asia-South Central	**37.91**	**17.07**	**4.667**	**113.2**	**128.9**	**132.1**	**18.8**	**20.85**	**20.11**	**13.6**	**18.02**	**24.57**	**80.7%**	**107.9**	**56.15**	**14.64**	**6.211**	**2.56**	**0.694**
Indonesia	2.567	1.388	0.667	13.75	17.94	18.84	2.006	2.109	1.942	1.469	2.435	3.442	134.3%	5.195	3.026	0.714	2.102	1.334	0.374
Philippines	1.443	1.02	0.509	6.912	9.628	11.32	0.192	0.235	0.252	0.44	0.792	1.233	180.2%	1.14	0.777	0.203	1.226	0.631	0.172
Viet Nam	1.002	0.464	0.177	5.206	6.483	6.773	0.296	0.327	0.339	0.479	0.826	1.287	168.7%	22.72	13.8	3.366	24.49	13.5	3.741
Thailand	0.772	0.376	0.163	6.443	7.517	6.393	0.732	0.728	0.655	0.582	0.849	0.918	57.7%	31.13	14.3	3.174	43.63	22.26	5.595
Myanmar	1.109	0.448	0.235	4.18	4.346	4.243	0.413	0.403	0.371	0.462	0.619	0.843	82.5%	18.02	7.381	1.735	32.13	11.97	3.195
Malaysia	0.197	0.132	0.082	1.917	2.645	2.998	0.064	0.073	0.072	0.126	0.247	0.379	200.8%	3.533	2.276	0.59	12.61	6.525	1.766
Cambodia	0.857	0.462	0.179	1.789	2.135	2.431	0.071	0.084	0.085	0.13	0.169	0.249	91.5%	6.31	2.35	0.67	45.13	10.18	2.491
LAO People's Dem Repub	0.294	0.134	0.037	0.426	0.543	0.664	0.045	0.056	0.061	0.044	0.059	0.1	127.3%	0.139	0.106	0.031	1.902	1.018	0.287
Singapore	0.015	0.012	0.006	0.269	0.393	0.38	0.006	0.006	0.006	0.025	0.055	0.07	180.0%	0.268	0.152	0.035	5.49	3.335	0.856
Timor-Leste	0.065	0.068	0.06	0.104	0.184	0.294	0.013	0.026	0.042	0.012	0.017	0.027	125.0%	0.009	0.009	0.004	0.704	0.306	0.068
Brunei Darussalam	0.003	0.002	0.001	0.032	0.064	0.085	0.001	0.001	0.001	0.001	0.004	0.007	600.0%	0.003	0.002	0	0.646	0.301	0.08
Asia-South East	**8.324**	**4.504**	**2.116**	**41.03**	**51.88**	**54.42**	**3.838**	**4.049**	**3.826**	**3.769**	**6.071**	**8.555**	**127.0%**	**88.47**	**44.18**	**10.52**	**14.34**	**6.548**	**1.692**

Health

Base Case: Countries in Year 2060 Descending Population Sequence	Years Living with Disabilities (Millions of Life Years Lived with Disability)									Total Deaths (Annual Deaths in Millions)				Deaths and Death Rates from Communicable Diseases					
	Communicable Diseases			Noncommunicable Diseases			Injuries							AIDS (Annual Deaths in thousands)			Age Standardized Death Rates per 100,000		
	2010	2035	2060	2010	2035	2060	2010	2035	2060	2010	2035	2060	% Chg	2010	2035	2060	2010	2035	2060
ASIA with OCEANIA continued																			
Turkey	0.604	0.304	0.168	4.69	5.547	5.77	0.288	0.28	0.252	0.459	0.728	1.096	138.8%	0.527	0.274	0.066	0.649	0.332	0.09
Yemen	0.528	0.341	0.144	1.514	2.313	3.332	0.412	0.626	0.763	0.171	0.247	0.441	157.9%	0.168	0.141	0.049	0.63	0.266	0.072
Iraq	0.301	0.142	0.067	1.383	1.956	2.557	0.505	0.781	0.979	0.167	0.255	0.472	182.6%	0.205	0.146	0.043	0.397	0.265	0.092
Saudi Arabia	0.239	0.179	0.14	1.629	2.741	3.623	0.247	0.281	0.29	0.098	0.224	0.414	322.4%	0.178	0.118	0.033	0.618	0.312	0.079
Syrian Arab Repub	0.209	0.149	0.081	1.44	2.33	3.196	0.095	0.14	0.165	0.073	0.155	0.328	349.3%	0.148	0.103	0.03	0.434	0.289	0.099
Israel	0.026	0.015	0.011	0.56	0.7	0.833	0.014	0.016	0.017	0.042	0.066	0.099	135.7%	0.138	0.091	0.026	1.869	0.827	0.202
Jordan	0.073	0.035	0.015	0.384	0.503	0.608	0.04	0.05	0.045	0.025	0.046	0.083	232.0%	0.077	0.05	0.014	1.05	0.575	0.155
Occupied Palestinian Territory	0.05	0.022	0.008	0.241	0.367	0.535	0.034	0.054	0.063	0.014	0.028	0.059	321.4%	0.029	0.023	0.007	0.868	0.29	0.068
Azerbaijan	0.086	0.032	0.019	0.621	0.631	0.636	0.037	0.027	0.022	0.058	0.085	0.123	112.1%	0.132	0.076	0.018	1.473	0.957	0.264
United Arab Emirates	0.019	0.01	0.006	0.212	0.412	0.47	0.014	0.016	0.012	0.009	0.04	0.094	944.4%	0.076	0.042	0.01	1.349	0.801	0.195
Oman	0.016	0.011	0.006	0.158	0.276	0.361	0.01	0.012	0.011	0.008	0.022	0.042	425.0%	0.02	0.013	0.004	0.637	0.315	0.078
Kuwait	0.008	0.006	0.005	0.142	0.274	0.361	0.01	0.011	0.013	0.006	0.026	0.058	866.7%	0.077	0.048	0.014	2.119	1.371	0.337
Lebanon	0.041	0.02	0.01	0.259	0.299	0.313	0.029	0.03	0.027	0.026	0.037	0.052	100.0%	0.268	0.155	0.037	6.872	3.506	0.95
Armenia	0.024	0.008	0.003	0.247	0.223	0.211	0.012	0.008	0.006	0.027	0.031	0.038	40.7%	0.258	0.134	0.03	8.334	4.495	1.251
Georgia	0.03	0.01	0.005	0.282	0.234	0.18	0.011	0.008	0.005	0.053	0.051	0.049	-7.5%	0.122	0.05	0.01	3.63	2.397	0.588
Bahrain	0.004	0.003	0.002	0.051	0.096	0.114	0.003	0.003	0.003	0.002	0.008	0.014	600.0%	0.076	0.044	0.011	7.918	4.472	1.162
Qatar	0.003	0.003	0.002	0.045	0.095	0.109	0.003	0.003	0.003	0.002	0.008	0.017	750.0%	0.006	0.003	0.001	0.548	0.403	0.096
Cyprus	0.004	0.002	0.001	0.044	0.048	0.046	0.001	0.001	0.001	0.006	0.008	0.01	66.7%	0.035	0.016	0.003	4.459	2.317	0.634
Asia-West	**2.263**	**1.291**	**0.692**	**13.9**	**19.04**	**23.25**	**1.765**	**2.345**	**2.68**	**1.246**	**2.066**	**3.49**	**180.1%**	**2.541**	**1.526**	**0.405**	**1.013**	**0.495**	**0.129**
Australia	0.062	0.037	0.021	1.271	1.553	1.569	0.048	0.05	0.049	0.15	0.232	0.297	98.0%	0.268	0.159	0.042	1.087	0.574	0.142
Papua New Guinea	0.301	0.184	0.102	0.642	0.849	1.098	0.048	0.065	0.079	0.049	0.072	0.112	128.6%	1.401	1.096	0.334	21.76	10.19	2.571
New Zealand	0.012	0.006	0.003	0.284	0.324	0.291	0.011	0.011	0.009	0.031	0.045	0.055	77.4%	0.072	0.035	0.008	1.615	0.744	0.196
Solomon Islands	0.016	0.015	0.011	0.076	0.113	0.147	0.003	0.004	0.005	0.003	0.006	0.01	233.3%	0.004	0.003	0.001	0.791	0.314	0.073
Fiji	0.01	0.006	0.003	0.108	0.118	0.111	0.003	0.002	0.002	0.006	0.008	0.01	66.7%	0.027	0.013	0.003	3.153	1.385	0.369
Vanuatu	0.004	0.003	0.001	0.026	0.036	0.044	0.001	0.001	0.002	0.002	0.002	0.003	200.0%	0.002	0.001	0	0.854	0.306	0.068
Micronesia, Federated States of	0.003	0.003	0.001	0.015	0.022	0.027	0	0.001	0.001	0.001	0.001	0.002	100.0%	0.001	0.001	0	0.793	0.314	0.071
Tonga	0.002	0.002	0.001	0.012	0.019	0.025	0	0	0	0.001	0.001	0.002	100.0%	0.001	0.001	0	0.779	0.316	0.072
Samoa	0.002	0.001	0.001	0.018	0.02	0.022	0	0	0	0.001	0.001	0.002	100.0%	0.001	0.001	0	0.879	0.313	0.073
Oceania	**0.412**	**0.257**	**0.145**	**2.452**	**3.054**	**3.333**	**0.115**	**0.135**	**0.145**	**0.243**	**0.368**	**0.492**	**102.5%**	**1.776**	**1.309**	**0.388**	**5.163**	**2.887**	**0.797**

Multination Regional Analysis

Measures of Poverty, Health, Education, Infrastructure, and Governance

Health

Base Case: Countries in Year 2060 Descending Population Sequence	Years Living with Disabilities — Millions of Life Years Lived with Disability									Total Deaths — Annual Deaths in Millions				Deaths and Death Rates from Communicable Diseases					
	Communicable Diseases			Noncommunicable Diseases			Injuries							AIDS — Annual Deaths (in thousands)			AIDS — Age Standardized Death Rates per 100,000		
	2010	2035	2060	2010	2035	2060	2010	2035	2060	2010	2035	2060	% Chg	2010	2035	2060	2010	2035	2060
EUROPE																			
Russian Federation	1.067	0.397	0.176	10.49	7.814	5.966	1.407	0.939	0.734	2.11	1.87	1.775	-15.9%	24.48	10.44	1.993	18.04	10.87	2.844
Poland	0.053	0.023	0.012	2.261	2.029	1.683	0.191	0.149	0.111	0.392	0.47	0.47	19.9%	0.477	0.215	0.042	1.188	0.744	0.196
Ukraine	0.388	0.15	0.047	3.55	2.397	1.645	0.298	0.207	0.132	0.736	0.608	0.506	-31.3%	15.61	5.948	1.055	34.24	20.62	5.401
Romania	0.062	0.028	0.013	1.356	1.143	0.924	0.137	0.101	0.067	0.267	0.264	0.268	0.4%	0.341	0.132	0.026	2.078	1.09	0.283
Czech Republic	0.017	0.008	0.004	0.612	0.57	0.474	0.042	0.038	0.033	0.114	0.134	0.132	15.8%	0.071	0.028	0.006	0.635	0.376	0.094
Belarus	0.032	0.012	0.005	0.67	0.522	0.414	0.069	0.05	0.035	0.139	0.125	0.123	-11.5%	0.676	0.261	0.051	6.574	3.339	0.905
Hungary	0.022	0.009	0.005	0.715	0.569	0.438	0.026	0.023	0.018	0.137	0.129	0.117	-14.6%	0.124	0.053	0.01	1.035	0.52	0.129
Bulgaria	0.013	0.005	0.003	0.512	0.392	0.285	0.03	0.02	0.012	0.11	0.098	0.082	-25.5%	0.051	0.017	0.003	0.693	0.384	0.097
Slovak Republic	0.006	0.003	0.002	0.32	0.303	0.257	0.025	0.02	0.015	0.054	0.067	0.071	31.5%	0.037	0.015	0.003	0.632	0.417	0.106
Moldova, Repub of	0.024	0.013	0.005	0.355	0.301	0.235	0.02	0.018	0.013	0.053	0.056	0.054	1.9%	0.124	0.056	0.011	3.168	1.815	0.461
Europe-East	1.685	0.649	0.27	20.84	16.04	12.32	2.246	1.564	1.171	4.112	3.821	3.597	-12.5%	41.99	17.16	3.199	14.63	8.489	2.183
United Kingdom	0.172	0.09	0.051	4.099	3.977	3.572	0.108	0.104	0.098	0.605	0.685	0.778	28.6%	0.769	0.402	0.095	1.159	0.631	0.157
Sweden	0.018	0.011	0.006	0.555	0.525	0.459	0.019	0.018	0.017	0.093	0.105	0.111	19.4%	0.127	0.064	0.015	1.198	0.647	0.162
Denmark	0.013	0.007	0.004	0.437	0.417	0.346	0.016	0.015	0.014	0.057	0.069	0.068	19.3%	0.127	0.065	0.015	2.011	1.057	0.26
Ireland	0.01	0.006	0.003	0.267	0.307	0.334	0.007	0.007	0.008	0.029	0.045	0.062	113.8%	0.132	0.077	0.019	2.727	1.62	0.399
Norway	0.009	0.007	0.004	0.28	0.306	0.287	0.016	0.017	0.016	0.042	0.055	0.062	47.6%	0.129	0.07	0.017	2.2	1.199	0.298
Finland	0.009	0.005	0.002	0.3	0.262	0.211	0.027	0.023	0.019	0.052	0.066	0.062	19.2%	0.127	0.063	0.014	2.398	1.29	0.304
Lithuania	0.01	0.004	0.002	0.227	0.181	0.142	0.022	0.017	0.012	0.045	0.042	0.04	-11.1%	0.123	0.054	0.01	3.468	1.841	0.496
Latvia	0.01	0.004	0.002	0.15	0.116	0.093	0.012	0.008	0.006	0.031	0.028	0.026	-16.1%	0.246	0.106	0.021	11	6.936	1.762
Estonia	0.006	0.002	0.001	0.09	0.065	0.051	0.006	0.004	0.003	0.017	0.016	0.013	-23.5%	0.241	0.096	0.019	17.98	10.73	2.66
Iceland	0.001	0	0	0.015	0.017	0.015	0.001	0.001	0.001	0.002	0.003	0.004	100.0%	0.011	0.006	0.001	3.625	1.729	0.449
Europe-North	0.259	0.136	0.075	6.419	6.172	5.51	0.232	0.215	0.192	0.973	1.112	1.227	26.1%	2.033	1.003	0.227	1.937	1.034	0.248
Italy	0.113	0.05	0.019	4.017	3.769	3.031	0.114	0.107	0.099	0.628	0.726	0.764	21.7%	2.006	0.906	0.179	3.133	2.017	0.515
Spain	0.122	0.06	0.029	2.972	2.952	2.621	0.093	0.079	0.065	0.411	0.501	0.614	49.4%	2.414	1.144	0.23	4.563	3.284	0.802
Greece	0.015	0.008	0.004	0.665	0.637	0.572	0.029	0.022	0.017	0.117	0.134	0.147	25.6%	0.14	0.066	0.014	1.118	0.672	0.173
Portugal	0.038	0.017	0.007	0.868	0.839	0.726	0.026	0.023	0.019	0.113	0.128	0.138	22.1%	0.63	0.295	0.06	5.394	3.265	0.844
Serbia	0.02	0.011	0.005	0.526	0.469	0.388	0.019	0.016	0.012	0.087	0.09	0.088	1.1%	0.124	0.056	0.011	1.671	0.909	0.249
Bosnia and Herzegovina	0.01	0.004	0.002	0.256	0.246	0.228	0.015	0.011	0.008	0.04	0.05	0.054	35.0%	0.028	0.012	0.002	0.631	0.308	0.084
Croatia	0.011	0.005	0.002	0.307	0.264	0.211	0.014	0.013	0.011	0.053	0.056	0.052	-1.9%	0.034	0.013	0.003	0.674	0.303	0.072
Albania	0.01	0.004	0.002	0.18	0.179	0.167	0.013	0.011	0.009	0.02	0.031	0.038	90.0%	0.022	0.01	0.002	0.716	0.322	0.088
Macedonia, FYR	0.007	0.004	0.002	0.146	0.148	0.13	0.005	0.005	0.004	0.019	0.025	0.027	42.1%	0.035	0.015	0.003	1.59	0.789	0.211
Slovenia	0.004	0.002	0.001	0.133	0.128	0.105	0.006	0.006	0.005	0.02	0.025	0.025	25.0%	0.069	0.027	0.005	3.403	2.07	0.514
Montenegro	0.002	0.001	0	0.043	0.041	0.035	0.002	0.002	0.002	0.006	0.007	0.007	16.7%	0.004	0.002	0	0.694	0.321	0.086
Malta	0.001	0.001	0	0.029	0.031	0.027	0.001	0.001	0.001	0.003	0.005	0.005	66.7%	0.038	0.016	0.003	8.835	4.511	1.203
Europe-South	0.354	0.166	0.075	10.14	9.702	8.222	0.338	0.295	0.251	1.517	1.778	1.96	29.2%	5.545	2.562	0.514	3.288	2.177	0.545
Germany	0.18	0.099	0.05	5.746	5.456	4.443	0.145	0.133	0.115	0.898	1.052	1.049	16.8%	1.036	0.484	0.101	1.052	0.593	0.151
France	0.155	0.086	0.047	3.954	3.931	3.35	0.166	0.176	0.167	0.558	0.696	0.767	37.5%	0.845	0.383	0.087	1.255	0.612	0.15
Netherlands	0.039	0.025	0.013	1.145	1.247	1.054	0.024	0.026	0.025	0.145	0.205	0.217	49.7%	0.257	0.134	0.031	1.294	0.747	0.181
Belgium	0.022	0.012	0.006	0.587	0.677	0.575	0.027	0.025	0.022	0.109	0.127	0.133	22.0%	0.133	0.066	0.015	1.154	0.623	0.152
Austria	0.015	0.007	0.003	0.628	0.632	0.509	0.019	0.018	0.015	0.081	0.099	0.107	32.1%	0.126	0.059	0.012	1.305	0.766	0.199
Switzerland	0.018	0.01	0.004	0.436	0.434	0.334	0.015	0.015	0.013	0.065	0.089	0.098	50.8%	0.633	0.302	0.061	6.806	4.138	1.075
Luxembourg	0.003	0.002	0.001	0.026	0.034	0.038	0.001	0.002	0.002	0.004	0.006	0.008	100.0%	0.073	0.04	0.011	14.33	6.81	1.634
Europe-West	0.432	0.241	0.123	12.62	12.41	10.3	0.397	0.395	0.358	1.86	2.275	2.378	27.8%	3.102	1.468	0.318	1.421	0.781	0.195

Health

Base Case
Source: International Futures
Version 6.32, June 2010

	Diarrheal Diseases						Deaths and Death Rates from Communicable Diseases											
	Annual Deaths (in thousands)			Age Standardized Death Rates per 100,000			Malaria						Respiratory Infections					
							Annual Deaths (in thousands)			Age Standardized Death Rates per 100,000			Annual Deaths (in thousands)			Age Standardized Death Rates per 100,000		
	2010	2035	2060	2010	2035	2060	2010	2035	2060	2010	2035	2060	2010	2035	2060	2010	2035	2060
World	1726	693.5	438	21.07	7.807	3.41	798.7	304.4	128.2	5.987	2.23	0.994	3669	2619	2355	54.36	24.14	11.19
Africa	892.3	405.2	247.2	66.52	22.42	9.265	764.8	294.1	124.5	37.53	10.58	3.73	1316	683.7	490.7	120	45.11	19.92
Americas	49.63	25.33	23.02	4.865	1.453	0.589	1.652	0.559	0.209	0.167	0.047	0.015	221.7	221.7	253	20.22	8.578	4.283
Asia with Oceania	778.3	258.7	163.9	17.34	5.315	1.707	32.17	9.68	3.52	0.705	0.183	0.055	1955	1569	1485	53.78	23.13	9.669
Europe	5.547	4.239	3.889	0.445	0.181	0.102	0.055	0.021	0.008	0.006	0.002	0.001	172.7	141.5	124.1	10.72	5.067	2.848
World	1726	693.5	438	21.07	7.807	3.41	798.7	304.4	128.2	5.987	2.23	0.994	3669	2619	2355	54.36	24.14	11.19
Africa-Eastern	281.3	93.75	36.72	63.14	16.05	4.569	195.8	47.93	7.105	32.52	5.773	0.823	404.4	153.9	79.52	112.7	31.8	9.921
Africa-Middle	205.1	140.9	106.4	106.5	47.69	23.79	179.1	118.4	77.98	66.06	27.46	12.68	301.5	222.4	189.3	194.4	95.87	50.73
Africa-Northern	39.32	15.27	14.8	18.75	5.437	2.091	28.11	4.167	0.696	8.421	1.265	0.24	69.56	43.12	45.48	41.5	13.86	5.722
Africa-Southern	16.6	7.534	5.889	32.76	11.75	4.582	0.973	0.339	0.146	1.447	0.509	0.159	25.85	16.84	15.63	62.75	25.69	11.34
Africa-Western	350	147.8	83.43	92.83	28.55	10.47	360.9	123.3	38.59	57.91	14.57	4.179	514.5	247.4	160.8	162	56.27	22
Africa	892.3	405.2	247.2	66.52	22.42	9.265	764.8	294.1	124.5	37.53	10.58	3.73	1316	683.7	490.7	120	45.11	19.92
America-Caribbean	6.646	5.128	2.488	12.86	8.998	3.992	0.341	0.259	0.097	0.688	0.48	0.186	17.69	17.51	15.19	37.79	23.82	11.62
America-Central	6.241	2.476	2.157	12.83	3.759	1.398	0.017	0.004	0.001	0.029	0.006	0.002	13.52	9.819	10.93	37.33	13.72	6.011
America-North	8.568	8.881	10.09	1.377	0.597	0.301	0.006	0.003	0.001	0.0012	0.0005	0.0002	81.93	97.37	112.9	10.41	5.36	2.971
America-South	28.18	8.847	8.281	7.168	1.346	0.446	1.288	0.292	0.109	0.319	0.062	0.017	108.5	97.01	113.9	27.77	9.936	4.751
Americas	49.63	25.33	23.02	4.865	1.453	0.589	1.652	0.559	0.209	0.167	0.047	0.015	221.7	221.7	253	20.22	8.578	4.283
Asia-East	53.91	15.31	10.22	4.258	0.939	0.284	0.64	0.401	0.315	0.04	0.011	0.005	374.4	420.2	444.9	18.56	7.735	3.708
Asia-South Central	609.5	188.6	108.5	30.88	8.572	2.315	17.7	4.716	1.18	0.949	0.207	0.036	1250	817.4	670.2	86.75	34.04	12.22
Asia-South East	78.21	38.84	30.8	13.85	5.015	2.037	10.89	3.476	1.586	1.694	0.455	0.195	269.6	290.5	324.9	64.58	31.48	16.33
Asia-West	34.45	14.91	13.51	16.58	6.282	2.807	0.816	0.324	0.123	0.283	0.096	0.032	53.15	32.98	35.75	25.99	9.852	4.296
Oceania	2.24	1.051	0.828	6.423	2.73	1.266	2.137	0.764	0.316	4.936	1.648	0.643	7.78	8.149	9.158	24.71	11.84	6.065
Asia with Oceania	778.3	258.7	163.9	17.34	5.315	1.707	32.17	9.68	3.52	0.705	0.183	0.055	1955	1569	1485	53.78	23.13	9.669
Europe-East	0.875	0.312	0.188	0.38	0.143	0.091	0.007	0.002	0.001	0.0022	0.0007	0.0003	50.97	31.99	22.02	12.3	5.609	3.278
Europe-North	1.724	1.608	1.629	0.602	0.298	0.17	0.008	0.003	0.001	0.008	0.003	0.001	46.21	42.69	42.73	16.37	8.014	4.449
Europe-South	0.635	0.447	0.417	0.224	0.093	0.046	0.014	0.006	0.002	0.007	0.003	0.001	30.65	23.52	19.86	7.419	3.35	1.71
Europe-West	2.054	1.838	1.645	0.388	0.18	0.094	0.026	0.011	0.004	0.011	0.004	0.002	48.19	45.88	41.35	8.429	4.286	2.307
Europe	5.547	4.239	3.889	0.445	0.181	0.102	0.055	0.021	0.008	0.006	0.002	0.001	172.7	141.5	124.1	10.72	5.067	2.848

Health

Deaths and Death Rates from Communicable Diseases

Base Case: Countries in Year 2060 Descending Population Sequence	Diarrheal Diseases — Annual Deaths (in thousands)			Diarrheal Diseases — Age Standardized Death Rates per 100,000			Malaria — Annual Deaths (in thousands)			Malaria — Age Standardized Death Rates per 100,000			Respiratory Infections — Annual Deaths (in thousands)			Respiratory Infections — Age Standardized Death Rates per 100,000		
	2010	2035	2060	2010	2035	2060	2010	2035	2060	2010	2035	2060	2010	2035	2060	2010	2035	2060
AFRICA																		
Ethiopia	86.74	18.66	3.763	76.34	12.81	2.103	35.19	6.368	0.537	25.52	3.183	0.254	128.1	34.89	10.06	140.1	29.95	5.462
Tanzania, United Rep	23.07	3.717	1.693	42.4	5.791	1.497	29.04	3.233	0.156	33.2	2.943	0.152	34.28	8.396	4.899	82.98	15.51	4.29
Uganda	26.29	8.983	1.958	49.28	14.06	2.416	33.41	8.219	0.18	43.63	7.347	0.186	36.08	12.74	5.758	89.49	25.79	7.048
Kenya	24.95	10.5	5.074	43.83	15.49	4.773	27.38	9.618	1.462	40.24	11.01	1.764	33.24	16.22	11.38	78.44	29.32	10.26
Madagascar	22.03	13.37	5.743	77.91	29.72	9.333	2.352	1.167	0.331	6.304	1.988	0.462	30.69	20.76	11.83	138.6	56.3	20.44
Mozambique	17.12	2.501	0.695	54.79	7.581	1.69	24.61	2.705	0.109	59.57	5.105	0.231	24.49	4.478	1.706	102.7	17.57	4.058
Malawi	13.09	5.533	2.386	59.38	17.2	6.118	10.1	3.883	1.19	34.48	8.811	2.503	18.7	8.797	5.285	107.3	34.61	14.48
Zambia	14.5	7.167	2.726	69.16	27.92	8.933	15.8	6.687	1.456	57.03	17.38	3.873	20.95	11.03	6.366	125	53.99	21.93
Somalia	12.51	6.477	4.101	114.9	38.24	15.95	2.58	1.023	0.46	16.51	4.009	1.279	18.77	8.836	4.868	124.6	37.92	14.81
Rwanda	16.56	3.971	0.775	101.4	21.88	3.577	7.188	1.575	0.106	41.71	6.818	0.449	23.98	6.844	2.019	176.9	46.54	9.363
Zimbabwe	7.642	4.773	4.179	52.13	25.74	15.43	1.509	0.746	0.381	8.607	3.439	1.666	11.28	7.669	8.188	94.47	45.77	28.52
Burundi	12.01	4.944	1.659	99.29	28.15	6.868	6.052	2.303	0.577	42.41	10.7	2.044	17.44	8.431	3.568	172	56.81	16.26
Eritrea	3.891	2.463	1.552	55.91	22.01	9.076	0.195	0.113	0.057	2.181	0.783	0.279	4.948	3.499	2.657	97.13	40.63	17.89
Comoros	0.314	0.375	0.279	52.18	33.21	14.63	0.272	0.251	0.099	23.5	14.17	4.384	0.501	0.72	0.624	110.7	74.69	34.04
Mauritius	0.014	0.008	0.007	1.233	0.417	0.162	0	0	0	0.026	0.005	0.001	0.213	0.228	0.23	17.43	7.332	3.246
Djibouti	0.619	0.307	0.134	72.24	34.04	8.634	0.08	0.037	0.005	7.756	3.074	0.443	0.797	0.341	0.074	71.92	29.89	5.415
Africa-Eastern	**281.3**	**93.75**	**36.72**	**63.14**	**16.05**	**4.569**	**195.8**	**47.93**	**7.105**	**32.52**	**5.773**	**0.823**	**404.4**	**153.9**	**79.52**	**112.7**	**31.8**	**9.921**
Congo, Democratic Republic of	125.6	96.4	75.47	115.5	53.76	27.18	103.8	76.34	55.04	67.03	29.03	13.82	182.1	145.9	127.7	205.2	103.8	57.03
Angola	32.32	10.88	5.895	121.8	34.34	12.72	14.34	3.879	1.502	39.99	8.26	3.03	48.51	20.55	13.64	225.3	78.03	30.05
Cameroon	18.97	10.41	5.13	82.17	34.66	12.17	22.73	10.62	2.602	68.83	25.4	6.314	28.61	18.77	12.29	155.2	74.05	29.1
Chad	19.64	16.68	16.04	110.9	58.99	34.41	23.34	18.85	15.53	87.43	42.71	23.44	29.2	26.22	27.28	214.4	123.9	71.8
Central African Republic	5.006	3.738	1.642	87.8	47.29	16.33	5.547	3.679	1.132	71.39	34.19	9.072	7.512	5.859	3.123	161	89.5	33.81
Congo, Republic of	2.267	1.488	1.207	45.36	24.22	11.48	7.186	3.473	1.345	90.92	36.58	14.73	3.368	2.747	2.939	94.61	54.78	27.18
Gabon	0.529	0.55	0.524	39.2	24.75	12.8	1.231	0.882	0.427	55.23	33.29	17.92	0.939	1.149	1.316	86.71	55.12	28.09
Equatorial Guinea	0.759	0.646	0.426	106.9	65.37	37.43	0.893	0.661	0.381	80.74	51.85	34.9	1.144	1.097	0.825	196.1	125.5	70.92
São Tomé and Príncipe	0.07	0.07	0.041	25.04	17.47	7.584	0.017	0.016	0.009	6.057	3.846	1.688	0.103	0.116	0.121	67.25	44.41	23.44
Africa-Middle	**205.1**	**140.9**	**106.4**	**106.5**	**47.69**	**23.79**	**179.1**	**118.4**	**77.98**	**66.06**	**27.46**	**12.68**	**301.5**	**222.4**	**189.3**	**194.4**	**95.87**	**50.73**
Egypt	10.45	3.054	2.807	12.11	3.068	1.131	0.407	0.082	0.03	0.441	0.081	0.022	18.51	9.929	10.48	28.45	8.843	3.849
Sudan	15.98	3.365	1.694	31.83	6.163	1.722	27.43	4.002	0.638	41.49	5.268	0.871	22.89	7.083	4.123	56.44	13.8	4.183
Algeria	7.5	6.487	8.274	29.27	12.17	6.133	0.01	0.003	0.001	0.024	0.009	0.005	15.21	16.49	21.75	68	28.67	14.25
Morocco	4.267	1.947	1.595	13.78	5.07	1.748	0.246	0.076	0.024	0.733	0.207	0.053	6.755	5.11	4.651	25.82	10.9	4.312
Tunisia	0.704	0.29	0.281	7.48	1.918	0.678	0.016	0.004	0.002	0.166	0.031	0.009	5.315	3.721	3.481	57.27	18.52	7.918
Libyan Arab Jamahiriya	0.408	0.131	0.147	5.832	1.542	0.776	0	0	0	0	0	0	0.879	0.786	0.998	19.46	7.13	3.556
Africa-Northern	**39.32**	**15.27**	**14.8**	**18.75**	**5.437**	**2.091**	**28.11**	**4.167**	**0.696**	**8.421**	**1.265**	**0.24**	**69.56**	**43.12**	**45.48**	**41.5**	**13.86**	**5.722**

Health

Deaths and Death Rates from Communicable Diseases

Base Case: Countries in Year 2060 Descending Population Sequence	Diarrheal Diseases						Malaria						Respiratory Infections					
	Annual Deaths (in thousands)			Age Standardized Death Rates per 100,000			Annual Deaths (in thousands)			Age Standardized Death Rates per 100,000			Annual Deaths (in thousands)			Age Standardized Death Rates per 100,000		
	2010	2035	2060	2010	2035	2060	2010	2035	2060	2010	2035	2060	2010	2035	2060	2010	2035	2060
AFRICA continued																		
South Africa	14.54	6.371	4.682	32.45	11.35	4.367	0.237	0.119	0.088	0.612	0.206	0.08	22.42	14.2	12.43	60.74	24.36	10.76
Namibia	0.296	0.291	0.418	21.86	9.928	4.409	0.681	0.206	0.054	20.66	5.786	1.395	0.613	0.768	1.157	56.34	26.61	12
Lesotho	0.594	0.255	0.206	37.54	16.05	6.359	0.009	0.003	0.001	0.386	0.11	0.025	0.975	0.5	0.515	81.13	35.33	15.61
Botswana	0.502	0.306	0.411	33.8	11.99	5.689	0.025	0.005	0.002	1.167	0.221	0.069	0.852	0.777	1.089	74.73	29.25	13.77
Swaziland	0.677	0.31	0.172	56.16	21.78	7.294	0.021	0.007	0.002	1.478	0.39	0.087	0.994	0.595	0.438	108.5	46.99	17.79
Africa-Southern	**16.6**	**7.534**	**5.889**	**32.76**	**11.75**	**4.582**	**0.973**	**0.339**	**0.146**	**1.447**	**0.509**	**0.159**	**25.85**	**16.84**	**15.63**	**62.75**	**25.69**	**11.34**
Nigeria	165.7	44.55	32.63	84.61	18.29	8.998	196.9	47.43	19.32	63.66	12.14	4.666	262.2	104.2	85.69	166.3	51.08	24.28
Niger	33.45	15.37	5.225	126.7	33.08	7.905	21.34	8.884	2.294	50.25	11.53	2.111	49.81	24.94	11.37	234.1	70.33	20.44
Côte d'Ivoire	16.96	12.25	5.838	65.36	16.05	10.77	13.67	8.333	2.089	34.61	15.03	3.619	24.37	20.06	12.65	125.2	67.02	23.8
Ghana	23.05	24.74	20.51	144.8	82.4	33.78	28.24	16.86	4.084	69.61	31.76	7.889	16.63	13.74	8.141	68.41	36.76	13.99
Mali	25.71	5.056	1.193	106.5	15.42	3.104	20.07	3.317	0.449	51.56	5.817	0.724	37.63	8.869	3.189	199.5	35.42	8.797
Burkina Faso	27.06	15.87	4.07	117.9	46.94	10.51	26.12	13.54	1.995	71.09	23.88	3.215	38.37	24.99	9.062	216.6	96.07	25.85
Senegal	15.89	8.385	2.59	97.34	36.29	8.946	10.89	5.037	0.754	40.15	13.01	1.934	22.16	13.56	6.102	187.5	77.3	21.99
Guinea	11.08	5.835	2.973	77.05	27.56	10.08	14.37	6.54	2.062	66.07	19.71	5.204	16.05	9.666	6.284	145	58.25	23.3
Benin	7.962	4.522	2.421	63.37	22.81	8.329	10.18	4.608	1.553	50.06	15.09	4.362	11.63	7.533	5.364	119.7	46.53	19.52
Togo	3.437	2.553	2.491	41.85	19.45	11.54	5.312	3.34	2.364	41.99	18.47	10.25	5.098	4.31	4.895	82.25	39.47	23.47
Sierra Leone	10.13	3.726	0.866	146.3	44.31	10.4	4.752	1.498	0.149	36.61	8.723	0.951	15.92	7.15	2.478	293.3	108.2	28.55
Liberia	3.118	0.58	0.173	65	9.992	2.386	2.62	0.434	0.045	34.11	4.32	0.497	4.912	1.445	0.576	128.6	30.38	7.633
Mauritania	2.693	2.754	1.498	75.92	45.54	16.93	2.329	1.823	0.8	44.71	23.03	7.739	4.021	4.133	2.899	155.9	84.95	35.96
Guinea-Bissau	2.527	1.027	0.61	98.43	23.84	8.812	2.24	0.87	0.457	59	13.88	4.703	3.789	1.728	1.237	178.8	50.26	21.61
Gambia	1.106	0.53	0.26	65.16	20.24	7.566	1.913	0.786	0.177	57.89	16.31	3.521	1.719	1.003	0.683	140.3	50.28	20.4
Cape Verde	0.104	0.062	0.076	26.28	9.717	3.733	0.011	0.002	0	1.364	0.26	0.008	0.197	0.146	0.191	60.48	23.08	9.556
Africa-Western	**350**	**147.8**	**83.43**	**92.83**	**28.55**	**10.47**	**360.9**	**123.3**	**38.59**	**57.91**	**14.57**	**4.179**	**514.5**	**247.4**	**160.8**	**162**	**56.27**	**22**

Health

Deaths and Death Rates from Communicable Diseases

Base Case: Countries in Year 2060 Descending Population Sequence	Diarrheal Diseases — Annual Deaths (in thousands) 2010	2035	2060	Diarrheal Diseases — Age Standardized Death Rates per 100,000 2010	2035	2060	Malaria — Annual Deaths (in thousands) 2010	2035	2060	Malaria — Age Standardized Death Rates per 100,000 2010	2035	2060	Respiratory Infections — Annual Deaths (in thousands) 2010	2035	2060	Respiratory Infections — Age Standardized Death Rates per 100,000 2010	2035	2060
AMERICAS																		
Haiti	5.29	4.53	1.987	40.76	27.83	10.37	0.32	0.256	0.096	2.703	1.59	0.508	8.287	7.757	4.808	88.67	59.39	24.73
Dominican Republic	0.868	0.261	0.197	9.168	1.753	0.51	0.02	0.003	0.001	0.193	0.03	0.007	1.775	1.261	1.27	20.22	6.49	2.613
Cuba	0.202	0.207	0.19	1.176	0.487	0.235	0	0	0	0	0	0	5.446	6.452	7.101	27.53	12.32	6.539
Puerto Rico	0.009	0.01	0.01	0.093	0.045	0.025	0	0	0	0	0	0	1.064	1.089	0.991	13.16	5.997	3.18
Jamaica	0.24	0.087	0.068	7.898	2.186	0.706	0	0	0	0	0	0	0.71	0.49	0.489	22.75	9.299	4.265
Trinidad	0.022	0.019	0.019	1.88	0.655	0.325	0	0	0	0	0	0	0.19	0.223	0.252	15.03	6.827	3.344
Bahamas	0.004	0.006	0.009	1.293	0.608	0.32	0	0	0	0.114	0.033	0.009	0.054	0.078	0.103	17.34	8.348	4.265
Barbados	0.003	0.003	0.004	0.52	0.253	0.139	0.001	0	0	0.16	0.06	0.019	0.077	0.083	0.083	16.84	8.471	4.455
Grenada	0.004	0.002	0.003	2.654	1.312	0.632	0	0	0	0	0	0	0.037	0.032	0.042	33.71	16.56	7.901
Saint Vincent and Grenadines	0.004	0.002	0.002	3.299	0.808	0.332	0	0	0	0	0	0	0.025	0.023	0.023	21.99	8.966	4.223
Saint Lucia	0.001	0.001	0.001	0.635	0.196	0.079	0	0	0	0	0	0	0.03	0.023	0.029	15.79	6.741	3.417
America-Caribbean	**6.646**	**5.128**	**2.488**	**12.86**	**8.998**	**3.992**	**0.341**	**0.259**	**0.097**	**0.688**	**0.48**	**0.186**	**17.69**	**17.51**	**15.19**	**37.79**	**23.82**	**11.62**
Guatemala	3.479	1.292	1.211	22.55	5.609	2.031	0.01	0.002	0.001	0.054	0.009	0.002	7.344	4.952	5.769	69.75	22.05	9.127
Honduras	1.076	0.29	0.232	10.52	2.381	0.741	0.004	0.001	0	0.035	0.007	0.001	1.461	0.624	0.61	17.6	5.201	2.055
El Salvador	0.656	0.238	0.164	8.268	2.119	0.588	0	0	0	0	0	0	2.666	2.167	1.941	37.28	15.43	6.382
Nicaragua	0.705	0.425	0.269	10.72	5.41	2.063	0.002	0.001	0	0.026	0.01	0.004	0.961	0.796	0.843	18.22	9.3	4.312
Costa Rica	0.104	0.123	0.162	2.323	0.914	0.436	0.001	0	0	0.017	0.005	0.002	0.445	0.563	0.744	9.706	4.045	1.931
Panama	0.212	0.101	0.11	5.984	1.517	0.652	0	0	0	0	0	0	0.585	0.645	0.879	18.29	7.795	4.063
Belize	0.009	0.007	0.008	3.231	1.19	0.514	0	0	0	0	0	0	0.058	0.073	0.143	25.23	12.13	5.994
America-Central	**6.241**	**2.476**	**2.157**	**12.83**	**3.759**	**1.398**	**0.017**	**0.004**	**0.001**	**0.029**	**0.006**	**0.002**	**13.52**	**9.819**	**10.93**	**37.33**	**13.72**	**6.011**
USA	4.207	5.171	5.659	0.65	0.367	0.217	0.006	0.003	0.001	0.002	0.001	0	59.82	72.63	82.33	8.758	4.973	2.917
Mexico	3.74	2.897	3.592	3.619	1.292	0.578	0	0	0	0	0	0	16.54	17.51	22.74	16.24	6.94	3.391
Canada	0.621	0.813	0.84	0.813	0.452	0.266	0	0	0	0	0	0	5.571	7.23	7.871	6.793	3.752	2.182
America-North	**8.568**	**8.881**	**10.09**	**1.377**	**0.597**	**0.301**	**0.006**	**0.003**	**0.001**	**0.0012**	**0.0005**	**0.0002**	**81.93**	**97.37**	**112.9**	**10.41**	**5.36**	**2.971**
Brazil	16.48	4.193	3.503	9.007	1.341	0.357	0.755	0.144	0.047	0.388	0.064	0.016	51.81	39.72	42.2	27.28	7.977	3.324
Colombia	2.278	0.987	1.001	4.726	1.161	0.414	0.303	0.073	0.026	0.593	0.127	0.035	6.479	6.067	6.921	15.81	5.819	2.715
Argentina	0.319	0.241	0.263	0.614	0.218	0.107	0	0	0	0	0	0	15.64	15.34	17.2	25.36	12.23	6.661
Peru	2.436	0.646	0.607	7.315	1.414	0.461	0.054	0.012	0.005	0.165	0.033	0.01	15.83	19.12	27.46	65.9	28.35	14.76
Venezuela	1.704	1.166	1.419	6.471	1.913	0.868	0.029	0.009	0.004	0.102	0.023	0.008	3.481	3.845	5.078	15.17	5.752	2.903
Ecuador	1.04	0.376	0.318	6.45	1.767	0.654	0.071	0.025	0.012	0.458	0.142	0.059	3.335	3.462	4.455	23.63	10.26	5.433
Chile	0.21	0.277	0.337	0.945	0.419	0.222	0	0	0	0	0	0	3.546	4.823	6.048	15.14	6.824	3.584
Bolivia	2.775	0.601	0.52	22.51	4.326	1.556	0.028	0.006	0.002	0.23	0.039	0.011	5.689	2.479	2.256	60.75	17.71	7.557
Paraguay	0.689	0.203	0.172	9.002	2.011	0.665	0	0	0	0	0	0	1.244	0.918	1.113	22.65	7.773	3.605
Uruguay	0.076	0.051	0.05	1.269	0.429	0.205	0	0	0	0	0	0	1.122	0.847	0.854	15.57	6.588	3.401
Guyana	0.112	0.059	0.045	15.63	6.002	2.231	0.024	0.013	0.007	3.281	1.55	0.563	0.238	0.247	0.213	36.78	19.98	9.669
Suriname	0.062	0.048	0.045	15.26	6.046	2.544	0.023	0.009	0.005	5.169	1.584	0.516	0.13	0.137	0.143	33.43	16.14	7.22
America-South	**28.18**	**8.847**	**8.281**	**7.168**	**1.346**	**0.446**	**1.288**	**0.292**	**0.109**	**0.319**	**0.062**	**0.017**	**108.5**	**97.01**	**113.9**	**27.77**	**9.936**	**4.751**

Health

Deaths and Death Rates from Communicable Diseases

Base Case: Countries in Year 2060 Descending Population Sequence	Diarrheal Diseases						Malaria						Respiratory Infections					
	Annual Deaths (in thousands)			Age Standardized Death Rates per 100,000			Annual Deaths (in thousands)			Age Standardized Death Rates per 100,000			Annual Deaths (in thousands)			Age Standardized Death Rates per 100,000		
	2010	2035	2060	2010	2035	2060	2010	2035	2060	2010	2035	2060	2010	2035	2060	2010	2035	2060
ASIA with OCEANIA																		
China	46.56	10.82	7.254	4.43	0.858	3.238	0.303	0.058	0.023	0.025	0.004	0.001	216	231.1	290.7	16.8	6.48	2.987
Japan	1.709	1.874	1.442	0.422	0.199	3.109	0.001	0	0	0	0	0	122.1	148	114.1	24.09	12.85	7.415
Korea, Repub of	0.111	0.196	0.246	0.186	0.098	0.056	0.003	0.001	0	0.006	0.002	0.001	5.904	11.79	14.66	8.978	5.425	3.228
Taiwan	0.248	0.231	0.205	0.999	0.369	0.169	0.248	0.227	0.2	1	0.361	0.164	0.48	0.555	0.516	1.906	0.792	0.394
Korea, Dem. People's Rep.	4.889	2.007	0.933	27.72	11.51	4.264	0.085	0.115	0.092	0.694	0.371	0.174	29.28	28.3	24.63	133.5	73.6	37.55
Hong Kong SAR	0.085	0.117	0.095	0.698	0.378	0.179	0	0	0	0	0	0	0.214	0.303	0.246	1.522	0.859	0.422
Mongolia	0.31	0.073	0.047	13.28	2.629	0.405	0	0	0	0	0	0	0.503	0.147	0.068	21.01	4.689	0.962
Asia-East	**53.91**	**15.31**	**10.22**	**4.258**	**0.939**	**0.284**	**0.64**	**0.401**	**0.315**	**0.04**	**0.011**	**0.005**	**374.4**	**420.2**	**444.9**	**18.56**	**7.735**	**3.708**
India	357.5	72.62	59.26	28.45	4.908	1.152	12.35	2.705	0.682	1.01	0.185	0.026	801.1	522	473.7	88.37	30.75	11.49
Pakistan	79.34	65.63	30.28	37.61	22.04	5.95	1.585	1.144	0.261	0.678	0.355	0.069	145.9	157.5	107.3	99.71	62.77	20.12
Bangladesh	38.71	11.44	9.459	26.51	7.075	2.579	3.525	0.802	0.228	2.035	0.436	0.106	80.04	56.04	52.8	84.47	31.25	12.75
Afghanistan	102.3	24.16	2.636	175.9	39.95	5.048	0.165	0.04	0.002	0.315	0.051	0.002	165.1	37.93	1.736	227.6	38.91	1.892
Iran (Islamic Republic of)	5.496	1.265	1.172	7.438	1.668	0.768	0.007	0.002	0.001	0.01	0.002	0.001	8.742	4.666	5.887	15.08	4.624	2.173
Nepal	13.14	9.524	4.33	40.49	22.82	6.765	0.019	0.013	0.003	0.052	0.027	0.006	22.77	25.02	18.58	116.2	71.82	25.14
Uzbekistan	5.779	1.257	0.251	17.98	4.853	1.125	0.001	0	0	0.003	0.001	0	9.132	3.081	1.72	32.71	9.483	3.056
Sri Lanka	0.281	0.157	0.117	1.578	0.504	0.195	0.001	0	0	0.003	0.001	0	4.384	4.632	3.567	21.16	8.908	4.203
Kazakhstan	1.182	0.188	0.095	8.04	1.796	1.245	0.012	0.002	0.001	0.085	0.017	0.008	3.959	1.471	0.901	26.08	8.143	4.995
Tajikistan	3.329	1.787	0.641	30.56	15.9	6.819	0.001	0.001	0	0.016	0.008	0.003	4.791	3.128	2.283	55.84	30.74	15.55
Turkmenistan	1.286	0.204	0.131	21.49	3.576	2.013	0	0	0	0	0	0	2.483	0.903	0.855	49.44	12.37	6.527
Kyrgyzstan	0.841	0.239	0.075	12.95	4.58	1.673	0	0	0	0	0	0	1.423	0.619	0.423	26.8	9.688	4.347
Bhutan	0.279	0.102	0.073	34.96	11.25	3.071	0.022	0.006	0.001	2.702	0.608	0.115	0.459	0.364	0.373	84.91	38.38	12.9
Maldives	0.041	0.01	0.005	9.072	2.589	0.706	0.004	0.001	0	0.78	0.213	0.049	0.056	0.046	0.065	25.51	11.24	4.347
Asia-South Central	**609.5**	**188.6**	**108.5**	**30.88**	**8.572**	**2.315**	**17.7**	**4.716**	**1.18**	**0.949**	**0.207**	**0.036**	**1250**	**817.4**	**670.2**	**86.75**	**34.04**	**12.22**
Indonesia	19.45	8.829	7.582	9.146	3.221	1.27	1.48	0.578	0.252	0.641	0.212	0.076	111.3	123.8	130.1	66.51	31.55	16.14
Philippines	12.83	9.89	8.912	15.54	7.958	3.567	0.17	0.087	0.036	0.166	0.072	0.024	51.01	84.09	115.4	106.3	65.66	36.21
Viet Nam	4.705	1.324	0.863	5.52	1.267	0.325	0.131	0.03	0.009	0.15	0.03	0.006	21.37	15.4	15.88	28.06	9.43	4.032
Thailand	11.57	9.735	7.77	18.45	7.786	3.422	0.684	0.247	0.087	1.043	0.351	0.118	16.15	16.54	13.99	25.69	11.59	5.44
Myanmar	17.13	3.812	2.24	32.26	6.851	2.722	6.289	1.309	0.519	11.74	2.314	0.859	39.38	21.54	19.32	89.88	27.06	13.21
Malaysia	0.891	0.347	0.226	2.965	1.136	0.505	0.013	0.005	0.002	0.045	0.014	0.005	7.164	10.87	13.54	42.36	19.37	9.752
Cambodia	8.946	3.856	2.424	55.12	20.03	6.106	0.397	0.128	0.033	2.127	0.554	0.117	15.44	8.375	5.861	117.5	44.3	14.86
LAO People's Dem Repub	2.19	0.71	0.568	33.25	9.215	2.994	0.054	0.014	0.003	0.69	0.141	0.023	4.122	2.009	1.744	79.33	26.26	9.241
Singapore	0.021	0.03	0.033	0.374	0.168	0.075	0	0	0	0	0	0	3.496	7.531	8.551	57.85	30.36	15.52
Timor-Leste	0.476	0.311	0.179	18.33	7.309	3.116	1.667	1.08	0.644	70.72	25.97	10.89	0.133	0.258	0.409	42.38	22.82	12.82
Brunei Darussalam	0.001	0	0	0.162	0.045	0.016	0	0	0	0	0	0	0.025	0.041	0.043	9.454	5.38	3.055
Asia-South East	**78.21**	**38.84**	**30.8**	**13.85**	**5.015**	**2.037**	**10.89**	**3.476**	**1.586**	**1.694**	**0.455**	**0.195**	**269.6**	**290.5**	**324.9**	**64.58**	**31.48**	**16.33**

Health

Deaths and Death Rates from Communicable Diseases

Base Case: Countries in Year 2060 Descending Population Sequence	Diarrheal Diseases — Annual Deaths (in thousands) 2010	2035	2060	Diarrheal Diseases — Age Standardized Death Rates per 100,000 2010	2035	2060	Malaria — Annual Deaths (in thousands) 2010	2035	2060	Malaria — Age Standardized Death Rates per 100,000 2010	2035	2060	Respiratory Infections — Annual Deaths (in thousands) 2010	2035	2060	Respiratory Infections — Age Standardized Death Rates per 100,000 2010	2035	2060
ASIA with OCEANIA continued																		
Turkey	7.071	2.531	1.666	9.865	3.361	1.45	0	0	0	0	0	0	14.05	9.737	10.52	23.26	8.633	3.982
Yemen	11.93	5.034	3.521	45.37	15.21	5.709	0.8	0.315	0.118	2.59	0.648	0.174	19.03	8.535	4.728	63.92	20.35	7.164
Iraq	8.931	4.297	5.618	43.82	14.13	5.976	0	0	0	0	0	0	7.352	1.844	1.229	20.05	4.608	1.556
Saudi Arabia	1.993	1.133	1.079	7.032	3.254	1.874	0.012	0.006	0.003	0.045	0.016	0.008	4.001	5.314	9.764	32.37	15.85	7.736
Syrian Arab Repub	2.021	1.182	0.981	8.444	3.863	1.509	0	0	0	0	0	0	2.49	2.252	2.601	16.47	7.598	3.498
Israel	0.1	0.115	0.144	0.817	0.391	0.217	0.001	0.001	0.001	0.008	0.004	0.003	0.667	0.761	0.929	5.384	2.611	1.432
Jordan	0.42	0.129	0.119	5.349	1.606	0.496	0	0	0	0	0	0	0.86	0.651	1.052	20.83	7.985	3.767
Occupied Palestinian Territory	0.055	0.024	0.026	1.659	0.456	0.191	0	0	0	0	0	0	0.382	0.202	0.272	13.85	4.175	1.786
Azerbaijan	1.041	0.167	0.08	12.61	2.329	1.142	0	0	0	0	0	0	2.021	0.88	0.749	24.96	6.249	3.05
United Arab Emirates	0.051	0.011	0.018	1.385	0.188	0.047	0	0	0	0.006	0.001	0	0.327	0.849	1.177	24.91	7.533	2.744
Oman	0.187	0.116	0.11	6.535	2.93	1.231	0.001	0.001	0	0.047	0.018	0.006	0.126	0.088	0.098	4.584	2.197	0.95
Kuwait	0.004	0.004	0.011	0.248	0.082	0.032	0.001	0.001	0	0.031	0.011	0.006	0.168	0.713	1.36	22.03	11.29	5.156
Lebanon	0.182	0.065	0.046	4.939	1.611	0.593	0	0	0	0.017	0.002	0.001	0.54	0.429	0.467	16	6.566	3.111
Armenia	0.15	0.018	0.005	5.582	0.844	0.259	0	0	0	0	0	0	0.283	0.103	0.101	8.785	1.859	0.793
Georgia	0.297	0.054	0.02	10.64	2.959	1.195	0	0	0	0	0	0	0.544	0.164	0.088	14.88	4.441	1.861
Bahrain	0.008	0.026	0.055	3.188	1.776	1.029	0	0	0	0	0	0	0.029	0.082	0.22	11.63	6.33	3.267
Qatar	0.003	0.005	0.009	0.684	0.293	0.157	0	0	0	0	0	0	0.015	0.062	0.091	5.562	2.912	1.598
Cyprus	0.009	0.002	0	1.962	0.405	0.089	0	0	0	0	0	0	0.271	0.31	0.311	19.51	9.679	5.202
Asia-West	**34.45**	**14.91**	**13.51**	**16.58**	**6.282**	**2.807**	**0.816**	**0.324**	**0.123**	**0.283**	**0.096**	**0.032**	**53.15**	**32.98**	**35.75**	**25.99**	**9.852**	**4.296**
Australia	0.041	0.05	0.057	0.084	0.043	0.025	0.001	0	0	0.009	0.003	0.001	3.948	4.727	5.491	7.504	3.704	2.091
Papua New Guinea	1.988	0.826	0.611	29.52	9.566	3.825	1.944	0.638	0.251	23.35	5.808	1.932	2.875	2.439	2.584	90.45	34.92	15.75
New Zealand	0.009	0.008	0.01	0.113	0.044	0.021	0	0	0	0	0	0	0.455	0.529	0.658	4.467	2.199	1.25
Solomon Islands	0.087	0.08	0.096	20.39	11.86	6.359	0.164	0.113	0.059	24.76	11.44	4.61	0.121	0.122	0.142	32.74	18.66	9.639
Fiji	0.053	0.042	0.034	8.564	3.701	1.65	0	0	0	0	0	0	0.242	0.2	0.151	39.65	17.52	7.706
Vanuatu	0.016	0.008	0.005	6.233	2.245	0.767	0.025	0.011	0.004	7.877	2.754	0.857	0.035	0.038	0.042	28.98	12.52	5.257
Micronesia, Federated States of	0.018	0.014	0.008	13.08	7.062	2.783	0	0	0	0.281	0.142	0.055	0.035	0.035	0.034	29.84	20.38	9.394
Tonga	0.018	0.018	0.006	10.6	8.151	2.634	0.001	0.001	0	0.863	0.584	0.203	0.03	0.032	0.031	31.13	18.15	8.268
Samoa	0.011	0.004	0.002	4.942	1.669	0.612	0.001	0	0	0.564	0.182	0.064	0.038	0.026	0.024	26.79	11.15	5.223
Oceania	**2.24**	**1.051**	**0.828**	**6.423**	**2.73**	**1.266**	**2.137**	**0.764**	**0.316**	**4.936**	**1.648**	**0.643**	**7.78**	**8.149**	**9.158**	**24.71**	**11.84**	**6.065**

Health

Deaths and Death Rates from Communicable Diseases

Base Case: Countries in Year 2060 Descending Population Sequence	Diarrheal Diseases — Annual Deaths (in thousands) 2010	2035	2060	Diarrheal Diseases — Age Standardized Death Rates per 100,000 2010	2035	2060	Malaria — Annual Deaths (in thousands) 2010	2035	2060	Malaria — Age Standardized Death Rates per 100,000 2010	2035	2060	Respiratory Infections — Annual Deaths (in thousands) 2010	2035	2060	Respiratory Infections — Age Standardized Death Rates per 100,000 2010	2035	2060
EUROPE																		
Russian Federation	0.634	0.22	0.139	0.548	0.193	0.137	0.003	0.001	0	0.002	0.001	0	27.7	14.13	8.087	14.83	6.432	4.016
Poland	0.017	0.016	0.015	0.031	0.013	0.007	0.001	0	0	0.003	0.001	0	8.933	8.65	7.357	12.81	6.135	3.303
Ukraine	0.066	0.018	0.007	0.223	0.087	0.043	0.001	0	0	0.002	0.001	0	1.309	0.619	0.313	2.252	1.024	0.546
Romania	0.082	0.027	0.013	0.616	0.27	0.138	0	0	0	0	0	0	5.167	2.98	2.173	19.74	8.791	4.507
Czech Republic	0.008	0.005	0.003	0.092	0.043	0.023	0	0	0	0	0	0	2.41	1.91	1.42	11.87	5.407	2.763
Belarus	0.014	0.005	0.002	0.159	0.05	0.025	0	0	0	0	0	0	0.442	0.246	0.165	3.353	1.444	0.827
Hungary	0.003	0.001	0	0.042	0.016	0.008	0.001	0	0	0.005	0.001	0	0.934	0.559	0.393	5.231	2.233	1.138
Bulgaria	0.014	0.005	0.002	0.302	0.138	0.068	0.001	0	0	0.008	0.003	0.001	1.414	0.824	0.574	12.54	6.031	3.115
Slovak Republic	0.007	0.005	0.004	0.106	0.043	0.023	0	0	0	0	0	0	1.691	1.428	1.233	19.81	8.536	4.453
Moldova, Repub of	0.028	0.011	0.003	0.903	0.502	0.19	0	0	0	0	0	0.001	0.962	0.642	0.309	21.39	13.28	6.616
Europe-East	**0.875**	**0.312**	**0.188**	**0.38**	**0.143**	**0.091**	**0.007**	**0.002**	**0.001**	**0.0022**	**0.0007**	**0.0003**	**50.97**	**31.99**	**22.02**	**12.3**	**5.609**	**3.278**
United Kingdom	1.444	1.321	1.347	0.785	0.384	0.216	0.007	0.003	0.001	0.011	0.004	0.001	35.6	31.73	31.99	19.22	9.17	5.011
Sweden	0.087	0.089	0.084	0.298	0.162	0.096	0.005	0.002	0	0.01	0.003	0	2.958	2.994	2.907	9.463	5.103	2.993
Denmark	0.056	0.05	0.044	0.469	0.2	0.106	0	0	0	0	0	0	1.23	1.211	1.116	7.796	3.857	2.177
Ireland	0.012	0.011	0.013	0.17	0.069	0.035	0.007	0.003	0.002	0.048	0.018	0.007	1.92	2.397	2.89	23.6	11.98	6.679
Norway	0.098	0.106	0.115	0.652	0.363	0.217	0.001	0	0	0.013	0.005	0.002	1.512	1.609	1.675	10.01	5.544	3.25
Finland	0.021	0.027	0.023	0.129	0.071	0.042	0	0	0	0	0	0	1.847	2.098	1.683	12.38	6.53	3.699
Lithuania	0.004	0.001	0	0.211	0.074	0.034	0	0	0	0	0	0	0.522	0.284	0.188	10.52	4.486	2.286
Latvia	0.001	0	0	0.019	0.006	0.002	0	0	0	0	0	0	0.355	0.191	0.131	9.902	4.053	1.987
Estonia	0	0	0	0	0	0	0	0	0	0	0	0	0.211	0.112	0.069	10.27	4.449	2.124
Iceland	0.001	0.002	0.002	0.132	0.075	0.045	0	0	0	0	0	0	0.056	0.066	0.083	7.589	3.585	1.967
Europe-North	**1.724**	**1.608**	**1.629**	**0.602**	**0.298**	**0.17**	**0.008**	**0.003**	**0.001**	**0.008**	**0.003**	**0.001**	**46.21**	**42.69**	**42.73**	**16.37**	**8.014**	**4.449**
Italy	0.048	0.036	0.03	0.022	0.01	0.005	0.002	0.001	0	0.003	0.001	0	10.18	7.107	5.488	4.989	2.108	1.044
Spain	0.4	0.333	0.342	0.293	0.137	0.074	0.005	0.002	0.001	0.01	0.003	0.001	8.635	6.936	6.661	6.56	3.107	1.666
Greece	0	0	0	0	0	0	0	0	3.001	0	0.002	3.001	3.783	3.309	3.027	13.6	6.641	3.604
Portugal	0.039	0.028	0.021	0.174	0.069	0.03	0.007	0.003	3.002	0.048	0.018	3.002	4.184	3.143	2.367	15.18	6.886	3.207
Serbia	0.002	0.001	0.001	0.032	0.016	0.008	0	0	0	0	0	0	0.461	0.309	0.233	3.731	1.778	0.895
Bosnia and Herzegovina	0.005	0.001	0	0.191	0.057	0.02	0	0	0	0	0	0	0.213	0.179	0.147	3.868	1.577	0.692
Croatia	0.012	0.006	0.003	0.147	0.047	0.02	0	0	0	0	0	0	1.52	1.015	0.682	15.16	6.177	2.939
Albania	0.108	0.033	0.015	4.076	1.257	0.522	0	0	0	0	0	0	0.455	0.393	0.358	13.04	5.127	2.452
Macedonia, FYR	0.018	0.008	0.003	1.145	0.524	0.239	0	0	0	0	0	0	0.108	0.076	0.06	4.484	1.928	0.929
Slovenia	0.003	0.001	0.001	0.117	0.029	0.011	0	0	0	0	0	0	0.864	0.765	0.609	17.6	7.307	3.535
Montenegro	0	0	0	0.027	0.01	0.004	0	0	0	0	0	0	0.031	0.022	0.017	3.492	1.464	0.661
Malta	0	0.001	0.001	0.038	0.018	0.009	0	0	0	0	0	0	0.207	0.265	0.207	22.87	11.94	6.283
Europe-South	**0.635**	**0.447**	**0.417**	**0.224**	**0.093**	**0.046**	**0.014**	**0.006**	**0.002**	**0.007**	**0.003**	**0.001**	**30.65**	**23.52**	**19.86**	**7.419**	**3.35**	**1.71**
Germany	0.911	0.871	0.783	0.388	0.195	0.104	0.006	0.003	0.001	0.006	0.002	0.001	21.04	20.78	18.89	8.432	4.488	2.418
France	0.893	0.728	0.644	0.505	0.21	0.106	0.015	0.006	0.002	0.019	0.007	0.003	14.13	11.81	10.48	6.708	3.053	1.616
Netherlands	0.104	0.114	0.1	0.268	0.138	0.074	0	0	0	0	0	0	5.928	6.867	6.016	14.33	7.804	4.242
Belgium	0.084	0.067	0.063	0.263	0.117	0.064	0.003	0.002	0.001	0.019	0.008	0.003	3.823	3.074	2.727	12.04	5.675	3.053
Austria	0.018	0.012	0.01	0.103	0.041	0.019	0.001	0	0	0.011	0.003	0.001	1.45	1.295	1.247	5.946	2.835	1.509
Switzerland	0.039	0.042	0.042	0.18	0.088	0.046	0.001	0	0	0.008	0.004	0.002	1.647	1.852	1.775	6.741	3.71	2.041
Luxembourg	0.004	0.004	0.004	0.566	0.247	0.121	0	0	0	0	0	0.002	0.167	0.201	0.212	15	8.855	5.015
Europe-West	**2.054**	**1.838**	**1.645**	**0.388**	**0.18**	**0.094**	**0.026**	**0.011**	**0.004**	**0.011**	**0.004**	**0.002**	**48.19**	**45.88**	**41.35**	**8.429**	**4.286**	**2.307**

Multination Regional Analysis

Measures of Poverty, Health, Education, Infrastructure, and Governance

Health

Base Case
Source: International Futures
Version 6.32, June 2010

	Other Communicable Diseases — Annual Deaths (in thousands)			Other Communicable Diseases — Age Standardized Death Rates per 100,000			Cardiovascular Diseases — Annual Deaths (in thousands)			Cardiovascular Diseases — Age Standardized Death Rates per 100,000			Diabetes — Annual Deaths (in thousands)			Diabetes — Age Standardized Death Rates per 100,000		
	2010	2035	2060	2010	2035	2060	2010	2035	2060	2010	2035	2060	2010	2035	2060	2010	2035	2060
World	7427	4061	2062	97.17	40.27	16.49	17177	26682	34177	283.9	235.9	179.8	1141	2139	3392	21.11	19.83	18.48
Africa	2872	1933	1150	214	87.62	39.29	1511	3168	6203	356	352.5	300.6	172.1	341.4	699.5	39.92	35.31	31.46
Americas	347.2	203.6	145.5	35.44	13.52	5.563	1932	2778	3387	163.7	107.8	68.09	253.8	493.4	771.4	26.55	23.51	20.69
Asia with Oceania	4086	1869	734.5	97.22	34.95	9.919	9422	16425	20558	292.1	233.5	157.5	578.1	1114	1686	17.57	15.39	13.23
Europe	122.2	54.53	31.96	14.83	5.609	2.948	4267	4255	3972	292	174.9	107	135.5	188.5	233.2	8.274	7.481	6.69
World	7427	4061	2062	97.17	40.27	16.49	17177	26682	34177	283.9	235.9	179.8	1141	2139	3392	21.11	19.83	18.48
Africa-Eastern	900.9	506.4	162.8	213.5	69.34	18.34	380.8	961.3	2090	315.2	364.9	308.2	46.59	91.76	193.7	36.83	30.98	25.33
Africa-Middle	577.3	596.7	558.9	325.8	179.2	106.4	175.2	351.8	737.1	391.8	407.2	372.8	23.2	46.07	105.3	49.23	45.81	43.34
Africa-Northern	170.1	66.78	31.28	73.9	24.94	9.663	438.6	844.2	1401	375.5	291.3	199	24.64	53.22	102.2	20.34	17.46	15.28
Africa-Southern	95.38	36.8	14.28	165.4	59.07	20.4	98.94	137.7	153.5	306.7	205.3	114.8	21.7	36.43	55.17	63.72	54.16	45.11
Africa-Western	1128	726.6	383.2	274	104.1	42.48	417.7	872.7	1821	380.5	364.8	313.7	56	113.9	243.2	48.43	42.57	37.38
Africa	2872	1933	1150	214	87.62	39.29	1511	3168	6203	356	352.5	300.6	172.1	341.4	699.5	39.92	35.31	31.46
America-Caribbean	37.42	32.93	20.62	96.53	67.73	35.06	82.97	129.7	182.9	213.1	167	142.1	11.98	21.57	33.25	34.24	32.59	30.82
America-Central	28.46	12.86	6.823	58.41	18.96	6.3	47.72	94.2	171.7	155.9	120.1	84.69	9.857	21.62	43.06	34.89	31.28	27.89
America-North	95.95	70.13	56.2	17.71	7.31	3.119	1097	1364	1434	137.3	81.98	46.46	131.9	245.2	358.6	23.46	20.94	18.09
America-South	185.3	87.71	61.82	47.06	14.31	5.235	704.1	1191	1599	189.8	128.8	82.3	100	205	336.5	28.39	24.42	21.48
Americas	347.2	203.6	145.5	35.44	13.52	5.563	1932	2778	3387	163.7	107.8	68.09	253.8	493.4	771.4	26.55	23.51	20.69
Asia-East	589.5	267.2	143.6	40.34	13.31	5.259	3956	5914	5374	222.2	140.3	70.29	213.5	375	478.1	11.62	9.454	7.901
Asia-South Central	2853	1234	389.5	158.2	52.5	11.6	3779	7268	10313	357.2	303.4	206.7	210.4	408.5	670.5	19.37	16.64	13.69
Asia-South East	507.9	295.2	158.3	94.43	38.18	14.34	1076	2163	3162	258	214.9	156.7	116.8	240.8	358	26.02	22.74	19.79
Asia-West	118.2	62.12	36.12	46.37	19.21	8.77	527.7	949.7	1557	388	279.7	190.7	31.08	77.42	159.4	23.55	20.84	18.47
Oceania	17.24	10.94	6.943	52.81	23.17	10.67	83.62	129.4	152.1	196	161.1	118.2	6.267	12.41	19.59	15.99	15.29	14.18
Asia with Oceania	4086	1869	734.5	97.22	34.95	9.919	9422	16425	20558	292.1	233.5	157.5	578.1	1114	1686	17.57	15.39	13.23
Europe-East	62.59	19.27	8.952	22.64	9.059	5.793	2497	2323	2219	493.3	305.8	205.9	27.98	31.55	32.55	5.983	5.406	4.919
Europe-North	10.65	5.854	4.131	8.522	2.887	1.082	399.1	401.4	340.5	166.9	95.87	51.29	13.44	19.88	26.24	6.13	5.469	4.851
Europe-South	19.07	9.662	5.632	9.761	3.876	1.745	671.9	755.5	768.9	174.7	118.6	77.23	43.63	60.11	76.6	11.33	10.12	9.101
Europe-West	30.2	20.15	13.35	9.33	3.632	1.448	744.7	831.1	700.2	139.7	86.68	47.05	51.81	78.96	100.2	10.55	9.433	8.225
Europe	122.2	54.53	31.96	14.83	5.609	2.948	4267	4255	3972	292	174.9	107	135.5	188.5	233.2	8.274	7.481	6.69

Column group notes: Columns 1–6 fall under **Deaths and Death Rates from Communicable Diseases** (Other Communicable Diseases); columns 7–18 fall under **Deaths and Death Rates from Noncommunicable Diseases** (Cardiovascular Diseases and Diabetes).

Health

Base Case: Countries in Year 2060 Descending Population Sequence	Deaths and Death Rates from Communicable Diseases						Deaths and Death Rates from Noncommunicable Diseases											
	Other Communicable Diseases						Cardiovascular Diseases						Diabetes					
	Annual Deaths (in thousands)			Age Standardized Death Rates per 103,000			Annual Deaths (in thousands)			Age Standardized Death Rates per 100,000			Annual Deaths (in thousands)			Age Standardized Death Rates per 100,000		
	2010	2035	2060	2010	2035	2060	2010	2035	2060	2010	2035	2060	2010	2035	2060	2010	2035	2060
AFRICA																		
Ethiopia	259.3	113	18.48	232.9	57.43	8.606	108.4	305.6	550.5	347.2	473.3	429.3	13.15	23.61	44	39.35	32.08	24.73
Tanzania, United Rep	89.85	28.96	3.695	144.2	28.72	3.633	46.14	130.5	268.6	280.7	336.2	236	5.722	10.95	24.3	32.8	25.79	20.76
Uganda	81.81	50.45	4.684	187.8	58.12	5.104	30.88	72.29	169.3	287	304.1	200.7	3.864	7.677	19.46	35.46	29.4	22
Kenya	101.2	67.04	20.41	209.3	87.36	23.17	31.96	83.24	202	233.2	221.7	174.6	3.823	9.75	23.33	27.66	24.48	20.44
Madagascar	56.13	47.71	23.41	201.1	91.35	33.27	26.42	62.83	146.2	301.7	293.7	287.4	3.603	8.318	16.87	40.08	36.22	31.81
Mozambique	70.72	24.25	2.473	227.9	48.76	5.345	26.74	81.82	151.5	367.8	484.5	357.2	4.061	6.706	12.59	43.2	33.91	26.47
Malawi	38.97	30.64	16.46	219.2	84.09	35.71	15.46	38.33	96.2	318.1	341.5	348.4	1.784	3.701	8.25	33.41	29.33	25.64
Zambia	40.91	32.47	13.1	221.7	105.3	36.12	14.31	27.83	72.78	296.8	293.6	232.9	1.832	3.266	7.997	36.62	32.22	27.35
Somalia	38.01	28.95	19.81	254	105.2	50.35	17.52	38.41	78.23	492.3	485.7	438.1	1.386	2.888	5.837	35.47	31.68	28.92
Rwanda	40.4	20.58	2.849	302.3	96.01	12.51	12.89	35.63	71.02	352.6	442.3	332.4	1.66	3.383	6.506	44.61	37.38	28.3
Zimbabwe	40.26	27.72	17.31	277.6	132.5	73.57	20.33	33.15	57.91	294.9	254	212.4	2.623	4.823	10.98	38.43	36.14	34.22
Burundi	27.73	20.25	9.912	250	103.3	35.01	10.93	26.29	73.8	352.4	371.5	447.4	1.409	3.028	6.266	43.08	38.15	33.61
Eritrea	11.38	10.95	8.718	213.5	100.9	48.62	5.805	13.33	35.25	340.9	312.5	296.8	0.89	2.107	4.893	49.8	44.91	40.95
Comoros	1.368	1.566	0.94	143.7	97.92	42.27	0.764	1.695	4.052	277.5	232.4	224.4	0.175	0.46	0.943	60.94	58.45	52.81
Mauritius	0.259	0.155	0.105	23.71	9.875	4.646	4.589	7.205	7.953	368.5	241.4	149.8	0.534	0.941	1.195	41.51	35.21	30.32
Djibouti	2.641	1.735	0.419	293.2	153.2	33.7	1.698	3.148	5.061	489.9	427.6	318.9	0.074	0.144	0.231	19.97	18.15	14.75
Africa-Eastern	**900.9**	**506.4**	**162.8**	**213.5**	**69.34**	**18.34**	**380.8**	**961.3**	**2090**	**315.2**	**364.9**	**308.2**	**46.59**	**91.76**	**193.7**	**36.83**	**30.98**	**25.33**
Congo, Democratic Republic of	350.7	403	411.6	369.6	208.2	124.9	92.56	205.6	447.8	424.4	498.4	466.7	11.78	23.19	53.98	50.86	48.46	46.12
Angola	72.35	40.35	22.87	275.5	95.52	46.18	23.29	41.98	83.59	378.8	267.8	194.1	3.193	6.861	16.35	49.84	41.15	37.54
Cameroon	48.43	39.2	16.21	208	108.9	39.21	27.49	47.43	93.06	334.7	283	220.2	3.716	7.184	15.08	44.12	40.12	35.13
Chad	66.09	78.82	87.91	377	236.1	155	14.75	28.4	56.13	380	346.9	269.4	2.184	4.48	10.83	53.17	49.72	46.85
Central African Republic	19.45	18.52	10.05	335.9	203.7	85.02	7.446	12.76	26.44	359.1	352.8	347.3	1.006	1.731	3.258	46.82	44.01	38.99
Congo, Republic of	14.7	11.54	6.693	284.4	147	70.33	6.328	10.2	20.4	313.2	245.9	184.8	0.86	1.631	3.777	41.36	37.21	34.33
Gabon	3.051	2.722	1.753	176.4	109.6	65.32	2.237	3.623	6.686	255.3	180.8	136	0.309	0.657	1.364	35.34	32.41	30.12
Equatorial Guinea	2.036	1.911	1.314	272.5	175.7	119	0.842	1.316	1.879	334.5	207.7	151.7	0.121	0.277	0.483	47.32	42.68	30.47
São Tomé and Príncipe	0.529	0.604	0.48	228.3	161	88.96	0.257	0.417	1.116	322.4	263.8	223.3	0.03	0.063	0.164	36.73	34.65	31.71
Africa-Middle	**577.3**	**596.7**	**558.9**	**325.8**	**179.2**	**106.4**	**175.2**	**351.8**	**737.1**	**391.8**	**407.2**	**372.8**	**23.2**	**46.07**	**105.3**	**49.23**	**45.81**	**43.34**
Egypt	47.61	17.91	10.56	55.48	18.58	7.593	197	359.4	547.6	428.4	308.3	183.7	7.966	16.65	32.51	16.56	13.95	11.87
Sudan	75.7	26.57	7.303	147.2	37.77	9.626	73.86	158.8	300.9	409.7	376.3	285.7	5.511	10.64	20.09	27.6	22.98	19.81
Algeria	19.86	9.961	6.915	59.45	26.68	16.17	47.64	101.5	196.2	227.6	167.8	120.3	6.504	15.88	31.6	29.97	25.94	23.42
Morocco	19.03	8.527	3.747	56.53	24.93	9.98	81.05	152.9	237.7	390.5	291.9	200.7	3.206	6.798	11.58	14.69	12.68	10.82
Tunisia	5.906	2.954	2.119	62.81	18.4	7.011	27.34	47.05	72.47	317.5	214.9	130	0.973	1.999	3.749	11.03	9.223	7.901
Libyan Arab Jamahiriya	2.031	0.859	0.639	31.12	10.97	6.206	11.73	24.37	46.14	329.2	205.6	139.2	0.483	1.25	2.622	13.02	10.91	9.913
Africa-Northern	**170.1**	**66.78**	**31.28**	**73.9**	**24.94**	**9.663**	**438.6**	**844.2**	**1401**	**375.5**	**291.3**	**199**	**24.64**	**53.22**	**102.2**	**20.34**	**17.46**	**15.28**

Health

Base Case: Countries in Year 2060 Descending Population Sequence	Deaths and Death Rates from Communicable Diseases						Deaths and Death Rates from Noncommunicable Diseases											
	Other Communicable Diseases						Cardiovascular Diseases						Diabetes					
	Annual Deaths (in thousands)			Age Standardized Death Rates per 100,000			Annual Deaths (in thousands)			Age Standardized Death Rates per 100,000			Annual Deaths (in thousands)			Age Standardized Death Rates per 100,000		
	2010	2035	2060	2010	2035	2060	2010	2035	2060	2010	2035	2060	2010	2035	2060	2010	2035	2060
AFRICA continued																		
South Africa	78.08	28.79	11.08	156.3	55.08	19.13	89.22	122.6	127.6	311.9	205.6	110.5	20.41	34.08	50.2	67.92	58.56	48.99
Namibia	4.244	2.098	0.927	177.2	61.66	20.21	2.222	4.743	8.476	215.4	161.9	100.2	0.291	0.694	1.507	27.31	23.4	19.49
Lesotho	6.877	2.974	0.859	330.2	120.6	34.21	3.547	4.299	7.992	348.6	312.4	237.7	0.47	0.572	1.223	45.26	40.4	34.06
Botswana	2.333	0.921	0.602	124.6	40.08	18.42	2.233	3.473	5.298	232.9	134	78.09	0.305	0.658	1.386	30.72	25.89	23.52
Swaziland	3.847	2.015	0.812	316	119.4	41.69	1.721	2.546	4.188	318.1	232	153.4	0.231	0.418	0.858	42.13	36.61	32.03
Africa-Southern	**95.38**	**36.8**	**14.28**	**165.4**	**59.07**	**20.4**	**98.94**	**137.7**	**153.5**	**306.7**	**205.3**	**114.8**	**21.7**	**36.43**	**55.17**	**63.72**	**54.16**	**45.11**
Nigeria	657.6	330.8	197.7	313.6	101.3	49.11	221.9	443.4	853.5	373.4	343.2	266.7	30.5	59.59	127.8	48.9	42	37.85
Niger	65.76	63.24	33.85	273.5	104.1	33.75	18.61	47.34	123.7	421.9	428.9	449.3	2.748	6.303	14.58	56.74	49.6	42.69
Côte d'Ivoire	52	50.01	24.14	182.6	109.2	42.31	23.74	48.42	107.5	286.9	249.8	207.8	3.307	6.98	15.68	36.12	33.32	28.96
Ghana	66.92	60.71	29	235	135.7	53.94	36.77	71.7	148.1	315.6	271.1	243.6	2.486	5.22	9.475	19.81	18.29	15.95
Mali	74.31	34.99	10.27	313.6	73.44	17.22	21.98	47.64	113.8	481.6	509.9	471.2	3.279	6.27	13.12	66.32	54.16	44.59
Burkina Faso	50.22	52.81	19.16	243.2	127.9	34.17	17.03	40.6	98.86	422.9	407	370.9	2.582	6.228	13.19	59.87	53.34	43.13
Senegal	37.94	32.86	10.86	243.6	112.6	29.21	18.41	35.5	83.88	476.5	423.1	361.8	2.772	5.957	12.98	65.94	59.27	48.85
Guinea	31.09	27.9	15.85	206.7	100.7	42.25	12.91	29.91	62.44	327.1	320.5	274.4	1.791	3.798	8.068	42	37.3	32.58
Benin	20.37	18.61	11	142.8	70.1	31.91	11.11	25.87	60.03	313	288	253.1	1.489	3.38	7.518	38.48	33.7	29.78
Togo	12.22	12.81	12.72	142.3	84.5	57.71	7.505	17.98	40.55	276.5	248.4	204.6	0.993	2.38	5.796	33.67	30.56	28.78
Sierra Leone	25.11	15.91	3.492	382.1	137.1	26.32	11.48	25.57	50.62	699.2	888	795	1.773	3.167	5.792	94.53	85.53	68.63
Liberia	11.63	4.987	1.145	210.6	56.31	12.97	4.639	16.66	34.14	360.4	649.7	606.6	0.55	1.043	1.913	38.43	32.15	26.11
Mauritania	10.04	11.18	7.583	249.3	156.4	74.39	4.965	8.866	18.52	456.6	342.5	286.7	0.754	1.776	3.737	62.2	57.87	52.41
Guinea-Bissau	7.824	6.077	4.922	292	111.1	54.02	3.049	5.707	11.4	390.6	349.2	306.5	0.412	0.737	1.498	49.44	42.19	38.4
Gambia	4.375	3.558	1.453	202	87.51	30.16	2.929	6.297	11.92	493.2	502.2	425.3	0.43	0.826	1.575	64.6	55.7	47.72
Cape Verde	0.468	0.202	0.041	90.21	27.79	3.287	0.668	1.285	2.378	237.7	199.5	124.2	0.139	0.283	0.578	49.1	40.89	32.54
Africa-Western	**1128**	**726.6**	**383.2**	**274**	**104.1**	**42.48**	**417.7**	**872.7**	**1821**	**380.5**	**364.8**	**313.7**	**56**	**113.9**	**243.2**	**48.43**	**42.57**	**37.38**

Health

Base Case: Countries in Year 2060 Descending Population Sequence	Deaths and Death Rates from Communicable Diseases — Other Communicable Diseases — Annual Deaths (in thousands)			Age Standardized Death Rates per 100,000			Deaths and Death Rates from Noncommunicable Diseases — Cardiovascular Diseases — Annual Deaths (in thousands)			Age Standardized Death Rates per 100,000			Diabetes — Annual Deaths (in thousands)			Age Standardized Death Rates per 100,000		
	2010	2035	2060	2010	2035	2060	2010	2035	2060	2010	2035	2060	2010	2035	2060	2010	2035	2060
AMERICAS																		
Haiti	27.19	28.36	17.61	301.7	204	90.41	14.43	24.61	51.5	310.1	272	251.5	2.632	4.994	9.543	55.31	52.76	46.96
Dominican Republic	5.633	2.015	1.126	60.1	15.92	4.878	16.04	28.99	43.89	204.2	140.5	91.3	2.319	4.616	7.967	30.6	25.7	22.7
Cuba	0.909	0.461	0.406	8.469	2.376	0.824	31.88	49.29	57.58	172.6	113.6	75.17	1.88	3.217	3.649	11.11	9.51	8.15
Puerto Rico	1.334	1.062	0.848	22.17	7.983	3.403	9.093	10.67	9.544	118.3	68.04	38.74	2.55	4.051	5.331	36.63	31.66	28.16
Jamaica	1.303	0.573	0.318	44.15	16.62	5.75	6.09	8.554	11.69	201.5	148.8	101.9	0.781	1.337	2.053	28.27	25.48	22.62
Trinidad	0.59	0.213	0.139	49.71	13.25	4.822	3.294	4.322	4.71	267	148.8	91.34	1.231	2.225	3.029	98.59	81.69	74.26
Bahamas	0.195	0.101	0.06	57.29	20.29	7.064	0.597	1.096	1.351	195.4	125.4	73.12	0.126	0.275	0.424	40.98	36.28	32.34
Barbados	0.089	0.06	0.041	30.57	11.68	4.331	0.68	0.999	0.884	163.1	111.5	64.23	0.186	0.364	0.441	45.91	41.21	35.74
Grenada	0.051	0.029	0.024	44.52	18.28	6.663	0.283	0.376	0.643	268.3	195.8	127.3	0.045	0.073	0.155	42.97	37.87	32.61
Saint Vincent and Grenadines	0.065	0.028	0.021	55.39	16.32	5.891	0.265	0.378	0.546	239.1	169.4	108.2	0.109	0.2	0.326	102.5	87.04	75.35
Saint Lucia	0.065	0.028	0.024	37.36	12.37	4.799	0.316	0.416	0.561	186.9	129.6	83.63	0.125	0.221	0.326	83.76	73.74	65.13
America-Caribbean	**37.42**	**32.93**	**20.62**	**96.53**	**67.73**	**35.06**	**82.97**	**129.7**	**182.9**	**213.1**	**167**	**142.1**	**11.98**	**21.57**	**33.25**	**34.24**	**32.59**	**30.82**
Guatemala	13.07	5.168	2.665	78.82	19.78	5.676	10.77	22.62	44.83	128.8	101.9	71.38	2.823	6.127	13.88	35.59	31.25	27.59
Honduras	5.805	2.288	0.895	60.38	19.43	5.972	9.686	20.42	42.51	204.1	164.3	120	1.745	4.031	8.514	38.78	34.6	30.78
El Salvador	4.68	2.332	1.298	64.73	21.83	6.571	10.27	17.07	26.72	148	109.2	74.85	1.71	3.042	5.123	27.16	23.91	20.66
Nicaragua	3.226	2.257	1.312	53.21	29.01	13.45	6.481	14.3	29.54	189.4	157.3	121.8	1.52	3.674	7.212	46.56	43.45	39.82
Costa Rica	0.553	0.23	0.134	12.52	3.505	1.112	5.43	10.83	15.73	126.4	85.28	52.82	0.966	2.305	3.928	23.98	20.58	17.92
Panama	1.003	0.53	0.468	28.55	9.357	3.63	4.746	8.267	11.04	157.3	99.59	57.77	1.034	2.288	4.088	35.12	29.58	25.73
Belize	0.119	0.058	0.051	34	11.81	3.905	0.342	0.694	1.299	177	123.6	77.3	0.06	0.15	0.312	32.44	28.12	23.99
America-Central	**28.46**	**12.86**	**6.823**	**58.41**	**18.96**	**6.3**	**47.72**	**94.2**	**171.7**	**155.9**	**120.1**	**84.69**	**9.857**	**21.62**	**43.06**	**34.89**	**31.28**	**27.89**
USA	63.69	52.69	43.94	15.46	6.826	3.099	884.8	1019	968.2	141	80.02	42.98	74.8	126.6	174.1	14.11	12.67	11.29
Mexico	27.96	13.71	9.286	26.48	9.602	3.603	128.3	231.2	360.8	133.9	90.9	59.72	47.85	101.1	160.7	53.07	46.99	41.75
Canada	4.298	3.724	2.973	10.06	4.25	1.8	83.93	113.9	104.8	114.5	70.81	39.4	9.225	17.52	23.78	13.78	12.53	11.14
America-North	**95.95**	**70.13**	**56.2**	**17.71**	**7.31**	**3.119**	**1097**	**1364**	**1434**	**137.3**	**81.98**	**46.46**	**131.9**	**245.2**	**358.6**	**23.46**	**20.94**	**18.09**
Brazil	86.88	37.57	23.78	46.76	12.78	4.144	377.4	634	811.2	205.7	134.9	82.37	53.2	108.7	174.8	29.66	24.93	21.45
Colombia	19.21	8.558	5.405	39.96	12.65	4.4	71.98	156.3	234.6	194	145.3	99.3	10.17	24.23	40.62	27.56	24.2	21.3
Argentina	18	11.51	10.27	36.44	12.93	5.623	101.3	115.8	124.8	176.3	109.3	63.86	10.45	15.31	22.86	19.79	16.96	15.06
Peru	20.68	11.06	9.318	71.69	22.85	8.891	29.21	57.08	91.06	126.4	88.22	56.59	3.827	8.45	15.47	16.83	14.51	12.88
Venezuela	10.04	4.52	3.352	34.71	10.29	3.885	44.89	90.78	139.8	212.6	145.8	100.9	9.46	21.57	37.11	44.27	38.14	34.55
Ecuador	8.55	5.296	4.104	59.51	24.5	11.72	17.75	35.51	60.75	140.4	106	78.52	3.882	8.598	15.41	33.02	30.09	27.97
Chile	2.521	1.732	1.392	14.16	4.627	1.75	26.17	44.36	50.79	122.5	80.21	47.17	3.755	7.848	11.68	18.58	16.11	14.18
Bolivia	13.5	4.975	2.823	127.9	35.24	12.4	11.75	22.74	39.48	204.8	164.9	118	1.621	3.243	6.324	27.18	23.47	21.12
Paraguay	4.329	1.761	0.961	60.38	19.14	6.43	9.112	18.78	31.74	207	162.1	115.1	2.332	5.136	9.759	54.29	47.71	41.56
Uruguay	0.827	0.348	0.23	19.68	5.288	1.81	11.5	10.87	9.586	170.7	102.6	53.84	0.8	1.005	1.374	12.71	10.65	9.205
Guyana	0.548	0.284	0.116	76.25	35.03	10.96	1.791	2.898	3.108	288.6	227.8	160.5	0.373	0.641	0.732	59.34	54.59	47.68
Suriname	0.224	0.103	0.064	50.22	17.23	5.707	1.195	1.611	1.732	311.9	208.2	128.6	0.161	0.257	0.318	41.76	35.86	31.27
America-South	**185.3**	**87.71**	**61.82**	**47.06**	**14.31**	**5.235**	**704.1**	**1191**	**1599**	**189.8**	**128.8**	**82.3**	**100**	**205**	**336.5**	**28.39**	**24.42**	**21.48**

Health

Base Case: Countries in Year 2060 Descending Population Sequence	Deaths and Death Rates from Communicable Diseases						Deaths and Death Rates from Noncommunicable Diseases												
	Other Communicable Diseases						Cardiovascular Diseases						Diabetes						
	Annual Deaths (in thousands)			Age Standardized Death Rates per 100,000			Annual Deaths (in thousands)			Age Standardized Death Rates per 100,000			Annual Deaths (in thousands)			Age Standardized Death Rates per 100,000		
	2010	2035	2060	2010	2035	2060	2010	2035	2060	2010	2035	2060	2010	2035	2060	2010	2035	2060
ASIA with OCEANIA																		
China	525.1	220.5	116.6	43.57	13.66	5.286	3368	5127	4706	239.8	149.1	72.34	141	235.5	296.4	9.834	7.545	6.046
Japan	25.45	17.51	9.453	8.384	3.291	1.386	400.2	491.2	349.8	92.88	57.42	32.71	15.64	23.14	24.63	4.256	3.797	3.393
Korea, Repub of	7.806	9.409	8.729	15.19	7.136	3.411	82.42	142	141	124.2	76.8	44.39	15.62	33.98	42.84	23.48	20.81	18.41
Taiwan	0.594	0.201	0.088	2.729	0.947	0.316	14.09	23.46	22.1	54.57	33.39	18.53	24.6	52.42	74.71	94.55	83.42	74.48
Korea, Dem. People's Rep.	28.99	19.03	8.51	131.4	69.95	30.57	79.69	110.5	128.8	330.4	269.3	204.5	6.968	10.61	12.8	27.31	25.47	23.46
Hong Kong SAR	0.086	0.056	0.035	2.137	1.021	0.396	4.845	7.406	7.341	34.8	22.92	14.57	9.62	19.33	26.53	72.32	66.88	61.7
Mongolia	1.411	0.532	0.196	64.24	17.89	2.972	6.291	13.24	19.61	406.7	333.7	218.4	0.035	0.064	0.17	1.787	1.761	1.705
Asia-East	**589.5**	**267.2**	**143.6**	**40.34**	**13.31**	**5.259**	**3956**	**5914**	**5374**	**222.2**	**140.3**	**70.29**	**213.5**	**375**	**478.1**	**11.62**	**9.454**	**7.901**
India	1871	570.4	180.2	160.5	39.73	5.538	2608	4910	6186	341.7	280.9	170.7	152.1	283.7	444.5	19.48	16.34	13
Pakistan	412.4	373.2	122.6	185.7	116.8	32.37	274.8	537.1	1052	303.4	246	194.4	15.44	35.15	71.76	16.98	15.98	13.78
Bangladesh	222.9	96.35	42.17	157.8	51.07	16.63	288.1	757.9	1280	372.8	393.4	307.7	16.6	35.89	61.27	20.67	17.84	15.42
Afghanistan	220.5	112	3.763	411	113.3	3.844	99.51	202.6	341.1	726.2	735.9	499.3	3.702	6.854	12.96	29.52	24.36	17.66
Iran (Islamic Republic of)	27.08	8.913	5.502	36.33	12.55	7.125	189.7	310.3	574	422.8	268.1	184.9	7.457	16.04	33.16	16.17	13.49	12.25
Nepal	50.22	46.55	21.31	179.2	107.9	36.87	47.83	99.38	209.6	326	297.4	273.2	3.482	7.479	14.14	22.8	21.5	18.74
Uzbekistan	18.63	7.683	2.381	62.31	26.89	9.256	90.31	181.8	304.7	528.5	443.9	325.7	3.746	7.789	10.94	20.11	18.45	17.05
Sri Lanka	7.212	5.25	3.498	36.64	13.53	5.858	40.27	80.23	88.37	194.4	152.7	107.1	5.145	10.72	14.16	24.76	20.96	17.98
Kazakhstan	6.282	1.731	0.963	41.66	13.99	10.07	86.84	93.44	110.6	608.1	353.3	248.8	1.263	1.619	1.846	8.448	7.216	6.929
Tajikistan	9.309	8.393	5.484	124.1	79.66	44.83	14.9	31.99	64.6	447.3	386.2	319.2	0.554	1.327	2.495	15.15	14.76	15.14
Turkmenistan	3.189	0.993	0.66	54.95	18.29	12.87	18.61	26.24	44.44	606.3	302.9	199.3	0.475	0.938	1.687	14.25	11.24	10.52
Kyrgyzstan	3.108	1.503	0.671	52.12	26.2	12.88	19.3	33.83	51.92	520.2	446.7	340.9	0.357	0.658	0.896	9.165	8.051	7.178
Bhutan	1.169	0.571	0.277	169.1	61.47	18.84	1.305	2.23	3.29	315	226	126.5	0.071	0.14	0.293	16.88	14.09	11.75
Maldives	0.176	0.081	0.047	46.67	19.54	7.284	0.331	0.665	1.289	193.1	143.1	90.74	0.069	0.161	0.358	37.95	32.54	27.2
Asia-South Central	**2853**	**1234**	**389.5**	**158.2**	**52.5**	**11.6**	**3779**	**7268**	**10313**	**357.2**	**303.4**	**206.7**	**210.4**	**408.5**	**670.5**	**19.37**	**16.64**	**13.69**
Indonesia	184.6	111.7	63.21	89.84	36.3	13.62	453.3	879.5	1254	272.1	217.1	155.7	42.87	89.21	137.6	24.65	21.88	19.33
Philippines	73.57	59.5	26.99	93.65	47.81	15.02	130.2	277.1	448.8	272.1	214.2	151.8	12.46	29.34	51.91	24.45	22.33	19.46
Viet Nam	50.98	23.57	11.99	61.91	19.22	5.708	161	343.3	534.7	220	199	142.6	11.87	23.67	37.93	16.55	13.95	11.84
Thailand	55.11	28.92	14.49	82.15	31.81	12.78	112.2	195	209.9	172.9	128.2	87.63	31.57	60.28	69.83	47.59	42.11	36.75
Myanmar	81.89	31.2	17.65	160.8	52.78	26.61	137	288.9	434.4	343.6	330.9	269.7	8.899	17.04	24.03	22.16	19.43	17.66
Malaysia	13.08	11.32	9.286	60.68	24.41	11.33	36.58	76.33	105.3	211.6	139.1	86.57	4.821	11.74	19.42	26.23	22.42	19.45
Cambodia	31.88	19.18	9.117	219.1	90.15	27.48	23.61	55.47	98.49	318.8	307.3	235.6	2.964	6.16	11.37	38.75	32.9	27.43
LAO People's Dem Repub	11.85	4.811	1.193	169	48.96	9.159	10.72	23.49	43.13	357.2	325.8	226.8	0.557	1.17	2.377	17.76	15.4	12.95
Singapore	0.38	0.492	0.479	7.413	3.051	1.326	8.814	19.33	22.49	144.5	92.26	57.47	0.578	1.43	1.899	9.356	8.289	7.259
Timor-Leste	4.431	4.383	3.865	305.8	148	76.24	1.799	4.053	8.184	367.4	312.6	241.5	0.133	0.318	0.761	26.15	24	22.15
Brunei Darussalam	0.062	0.072	0.068	20.57	9.962	4.951	0.386	1.115	2.02	193.7	134.6	100.8	0.106	0.431	0.927	54.05	51.05	48.31
Asia-South East	**507.9**	**295.2**	**158.3**	**94.43**	**38.18**	**14.34**	**1076**	**2163**	**3162**	**258**	**214.9**	**156.7**	**116.8**	**240.8**	**358**	**26.02**	**22.74**	**19.79**

Health

Base Case: Countries in Year 2060 Descending Population Sequence	Deaths and Death Rates from Communicable Diseases						Deaths and Death Rates from Noncommunicable Diseases											
	Other Communicable Diseases						Cardiovascular Diseases						Diabetes					
	Annual Deaths (in thousands)			Age Standardized Death Rates per 100,000			Annual Deaths (in thousands)			Age Standardized Death Rates per 100,000			Annual Deaths (in thousands)			Age Standardized Death Rates per 100,000		
	2010	2035	2060	2010	2035	2060	2010	2035	2060	2010	2035	2060	2010	2035	2060	2010	2035	2060
ASIA with OCEANIA continued																		
Turkey	29.46	13.86	7.744	40.77	19.25	10.76	229.1	379.6	542.9	423.3	281	173.8	10.65	20.73	32.66	18.17	15.3	13.23
Yemen	36.76	19.81	6.869	95.51	33.1	10.45	40.91	94.75	204	482.2	423.5	319.7	1.522	3.824	9.606	18.69	16.46	14.61
Iraq	23.52	9.577	4.622	67.12	20.49	7.849	50.37	90.27	139.9	436.5	298.5	182.7	1.797	3.99	9.604	15.02	12.41	10.68
Saudi Arabia	8.222	7.254	7.858	40.57	20.42	11.97	35.51	87.26	155.2	327.6	218.6	145.7	5.296	19.43	46.04	52.54	47.79	43.77
Syrian Arab Repub	6.072	4.405	3.026	27.53	13.76	6.471	29.66	68.35	143.8	327.2	244.2	170.8	1.686	4.596	10.72	17.7	15.79	13.82
Israel	1.506	1.25	1.297	14.25	5.455	2.44	12.37	15	14.3	105.6	57.2	26.42	3.038	5.651	9.599	28.06	24.12	20.57
Jordan	2.085	0.903	0.481	29	11.22	4.103	10.46	22.48	37.02	357.7	267.5	150.6	0.744	1.871	4.299	25.19	21.74	17.98
Occupied Palestinian Territory	1.507	0.547	0.27	29.99	7.676	2.303	6.146	14.54	31.86	380.3	313.2	215.6	0.518	1.348	3.35	31.9	27.65	23.49
Azerbaijan	3.584	1.095	0.61	42.77	14.81	9.404	32.03	54.28	82.54	426.8	278.7	194.1	1.509	2.662	3.555	18.85	16.33	14.36
United Arab Emirates	0.665	0.653	0.74	30.64	7.009	2.147	3.26	17.4	39.12	225.7	150.7	93.48	0.35	3.03	8.339	27.09	25.23	21.96
Oman	0.398	0.277	0.157	12.33	7.212	3.84	3.466	9.271	14.55	297.5	195.4	112.2	0.531	2.115	4.965	48.18	44.1	37.98
Kuwait	0.294	0.524	0.791	21.47	9.428	4.269	2.58	11.1	25.65	243.2	159.3	129	0.389	2.715	7.1	40.83	37.97	37.01
Lebanon	1.415	0.715	0.464	38.64	16.93	8.02	12.61	18.09	23.9	385.9	251.1	152.3	0.468	0.861	1.42	13.99	12.1	10.53
Armenia	0.906	0.208	0.092	32.3	9.1	4.162	15.18	17.59	20.95	334	217	128.4	1.425	1.73	2.115	35.73	27.33	22.25
Georgia	1.515	0.443	0.193	44.15	19.27	10.56	39.23	40.41	39.15	519.5	394.5	266.8	0.771	0.776	0.668	11.17	9.403	8.294
Bahrain	0.133	0.187	0.25	29.12	13.56	6.049	0.698	2.062	2.482	191.8	122.4	66.55	0.172	0.816	1.525	51.43	47.57	40.84
Qatar	0.13	0.36	0.606	36.08	19.48	10.53	0.759	2.42	3.879	183.8	108.8	86.13	0.163	1.2	3.768	59.12	56.33	56.79
Cyprus	0.078	0.063	0.053	7.836	3.179	1.309	3.436	4.848	5.383	242.5	150.9	93.63	0.045	0.076	0.098	3.549	3.124	2.766
Asia-West	**118.2**	**62.12**	**36.12**	**46.37**	**19.21**	**8.77**	**527.7**	**949.7**	**1557**	**388**	**279.7**	**190.7**	**31.08**	**77.42**	**159.4**	**23.55**	**20.84**	**18.47**
Australia	2.464	1.977	1.672	8.666	3.418	1.404	55.91	78.79	78.68	117.6	72.78	39.43	4.003	7.759	11.74	9.497	8.644	7.712
Papua New Guinea	12.44	7.104	3.91	204.9	71.23	29.24	11.15	26.49	46.31	429	375.4	286.6	0.831	1.982	3.805	30.41	26.69	24.11
New Zealand	0.284	0.162	0.101	6.605	2.53	0.903	12.12	16.37	15.92	141.9	88.83	49.05	0.931	1.646	2.198	12.73	11.5	10.09
Solomon Islands	0.718	0.713	0.569	147.3	83.74	42.16	0.909	2.007	3.838	379.6	330.3	262.2	0.102	0.264	0.579	45.98	43.16	39.66
Fiji	0.707	0.488	0.315	106.8	45.28	18.94	2.325	3.662	4.086	413.7	314.1	211.3	0.253	0.46	0.641	44.65	39.77	33.89
Vanuatu	0.214	0.162	0.123	116.4	48.15	19.1	0.371	0.774	1.355	333.1	254.8	175.6	0.044	0.109	0.237	41.08	35.98	31.06
Micronesia, Federated States of	0.146	0.129	0.094	131.4	67.6	32.01	0.229	0.423	0.696	354	270.8	181.7	0.028	0.062	0.136	44.46	40.57	35.94
Tonga	0.108	0.111	0.091	106.9	60.77	27.68	0.239	0.36	0.599	296.8	221.6	159.2	0.03	0.058	0.12	39.12	36.51	32.49
Samoa	0.16	0.094	0.067	103.8	40.83	18.06	0.358	0.493	0.62	302.6	225.2	141.7	0.044	0.073	0.13	38.8	34.34	29.8
Oceania	**17.24**	**10.94**	**6.943**	**52.81**	**23.17**	**10.67**	**83.62**	**129.4**	**152.1**	**196**	**161.1**	**118.2**	**6.267**	**12.41**	**19.59**	**15.99**	**15.29**	**14.18**

Multination Regional Analysis

Measures of Poverty, Health, Education, Infrastructure, and Governance

Health

Base Case: Countries in Year 2060 Descending Population Sequence	Deaths and Death Rates from Communicable Diseases — Other Communicable Diseases						Deaths and Death Rates from Noncommunicable Diseases — Cardiovascular Diseases						Diabetes					
	Annual Deaths (in thousands)			Age Standardized Death Rates per 100,000			Annual Deaths (in thousands)			Age Standardized Death Rates per 100,000			Annual Deaths (in thousands)			Age Standardized Death Rates per 100,000		
	2010	2035	2060	2010	2035	2060	2010	2035	2060	2010	2035	2060	2010	2035	2060	2010	2035	2060
EUROPE																		
Russian Federation	38.88	10.72	5.236	28.83	10.69	7.511	1271	1144	1124	559	329.8	229.1	10.07	10.17	9.478	4.985	4.652	4.096
Poland	3.565	1.615	0.903	10.21	4.504	2.641	202.2	236	224.6	289.3	179.2	113.1	5.75	8.198	9.623	8.772	7.534	6.751
Ukraine	11.45	3.441	1.217	26.07	10.9	5.728	492	418.3	362.1	573.1	395.2	263.4	2.437	2.054	1.543	3.728	3.36	3.521
Romania	3.562	1.38	0.645	19.68	10.35	6.367	170.5	169.7	175.9	432.5	288.3	181.8	2.172	2.352	2.499	6.22	5.252	4.833
Czech Republic	0.533	0.238	0.141	5.881	2.942	1.827	60	71.03	67.03	284.8	191	124.6	1.471	2.036	2.371	7.419	6.64	6.033
Belarus	1.348	0.428	0.197	14.86	5.461	3.155	90.55	79.24	78.4	555.5	342.6	226.3	0.536	0.544	0.536	3.764	3.179	2.897
Hungary	0.969	0.382	0.191	11.7	5.512	3.175	70.67	64.18	53.99	337.9	213.9	131.7	2.433	2.692	2.846	12.46	10.83	9.588
Bulgaria	0.836	0.327	0.153	12.92	7.146	4.307	78.5	69.58	58.22	477.8	332.8	214.3	1.943	1.933	1.887	12.5	11.11	10.01
Slovak Republic	0.365	0.167	0.108	7.834	3.588	2.35	29.69	37.24	40.97	334.4	217.6	148.9	0.781	1.142	1.365	9.379	8.198	7.512
Moldova, Repub of	1.081	0.569	0.162	27.24	16.5	6.479	31.07	33.71	33.59	568.6	453.5	348.7	0.393	0.423	0.397	7.393	6.933	7.008
Europe-East	**62.59**	**19.27**	**8.952**	**22.64**	**9.059**	**5.793**	**2497**	**2323**	**2219**	**493.3**	**305.8**	**205.9**	**27.98**	**31.55**	**32.55**	**5.983**	**5.406**	**4.919**
United Kingdom	6.221	3.058	2.128	8.451	2.69	0.915	231.5	229.2	193.9	150.4	86.18	45.63	7.438	11.1	15.14	5.223	4.673	4.14
Sweden	1.427	1.092	0.861	7.939	3.144	1.372	41.95	40.21	31.74	153.1	84.63	44.65	1.945	2.839	3.59	8.28	7.436	6.611
Denmark	0.593	0.373	0.242	8.142	3.024	1.162	21.38	23.18	17.42	160.3	97.74	51.34	1.427	2.051	2.387	12.21	10.87	9.441
Ireland	0.296	0.193	0.176	6.167	2.16	0.903	11.11	14.48	17.1	151.5	87.36	53.01	0.492	0.978	1.664	6.92	6.183	5.653
Norway	0.61	0.496	0.396	7.1	3.126	1.436	16.28	19.6	18.05	134.7	87.11	50.71	0.671	1.102	1.511	6.216	5.773	5.222
Finland	0.424	0.261	0.136	5.645	2.029	0.746	22.09	24.48	16.62	166.4	98.13	51.88	0.591	0.868	0.924	5.256	4.761	4.282
Lithuania	0.542	0.205	0.102	15.22	5.95	2.954	25.02	23.43	22.28	370.4	232.4	137.9	0.339	0.362	0.383	5.827	5.025	4.422
Latvia	0.342	0.106	0.05	15.88	5.796	2.888	19.22	16.98	15.32	394.5	243.8	144.7	0.238	0.244	0.273	5.62	4.788	4.252
Estonia	0.173	0.053	0.024	13.22	4.972	2.28	9.728	8.756	7.004	330.8	202.3	115.2	0.284	0.293	0.295	10.96	9.461	8.288
Iceland	0.022	0.017	0.015	5.023	1.914	0.796	0.789	1.071	1.087	127.9	76.9	41.32	0.021	0.043	0.068	3.766	3.483	3.145
Europe-North	**10.65**	**5.854**	**4.131**	**8.522**	**2.887**	**1.082**	**399.1**	**401.4**	**340.5**	**166.9**	**95.87**	**51.29**	**13.44**	**19.88**	**26.24**	**6.13**	**5.469**	**4.851**
Italy	6.211	2.873	1.464	7.379	2.477	0.926	275.1	308.5	304.6	139.7	95.66	62.36	19.89	27	32.52	11.29	10.19	9.198
Spain	6.728	3.882	2.644	9.55	3.546	1.492	141.4	153.2	164	116.6	75.91	48.24	11.52	16.88	24.72	9.546	8.589	7.798
Greece	0.864	0.479	0.307	5.592	2.02	0.801	62.07	69.67	73.56	223.4	142.9	90.68	1.325	1.763	2.227	4.957	4.405	3.999
Portugal	1.944	0.924	0.444	12.74	4.526	1.583	47.92	51.84	52.35	177.6	117.7	75	5.172	6.953	8.552	20.52	18.32	16.33
Serbia	1.101	0.519	0.253	19.52	11.33	6.454	54.19	56.57	54.76	392.2	280.1	184.2	2.158	2.45	2.597	17.05	15.21	13.74
Bosnia and Herzegovina	0.661	0.296	0.155	21.01	9.121	4.526	26.78	34.3	36.93	404.7	275.5	177.4	0.723	0.983	1.138	11.13	9.412	8.313
Croatia	0.469	0.177	0.082	10.12	4.408	2.303	27.59	29.66	26.67	278.8	186.4	120.6	1.025	1.255	1.352	10.71	9.357	8.365
Albania	0.51	0.232	0.136	17.89	7.83	4.261	12.08	19.26	23.26	321.4	229.6	152.1	0.2	0.327	0.444	5.41	4.705	4.18
Maceconia, FYR	0.338	0.165	0.082	21.85	12.66	7.391	11.6	15.93	17.23	394.7	295.7	203.9	0.649	0.951	1.122	21.85	19.54	17.26
Slovenia	0.122	0.057	0.036	5.09	1.393	0.495	8.001	10.01	9.204	173.2	109.5	66.59	0.703	1.166	1.477	15.42	13.69	12.25
Montenegro	0.089	0.038	0.017	16.95	7.823	3.614	3.704	4.567	4.515	373.5	263.8	164	0.157	0.195	0.216	17.08	15.09	12.54
Malta	0.027	0.02	0.014	6.858	3.811	2.264	1.415	2.019	1.814	167.7	110.5	70.3	0.106	0.187	0.225	13.19	12.01	10.89
Europe-South	**19.07**	**9.662**	**5.632**	**9.761**	**3.876**	**1.745**	**671.9**	**755.5**	**768.9**	**174.7**	**118.6**	**77.23**	**43.63**	**60.11**	**76.6**	**11.33**	**10.12**	**9.101**
Germany	11.79	7.775	4.766	9.048	3.586	1.381	413.4	446.8	367	172.3	105.8	56.2	26.9	40.36	51.91	11.74	10.56	9.249
France	12.9	8.531	6.128	10.19	3.82	1.573	178.7	205.6	178.3	98.83	63.72	35.88	12.96	19.53	24.4	8.188	7.398	6.519
Netherlands	2.527	2.026	1.297	10.04	4.212	1.689	48.32	60.78	49.25	131.1	83.83	47.28	4.211	7.207	8.822	11.84	10.7	9.442
Belgium	1.588	0.925	0.603	8.484	3.076	1.191	42.4	44.98	36.83	148.7	95.13	51.68	1.879	2.623	3.232	6.969	6.156	5.34
Austria	0.619	0.288	0.142	7.315	2.594	0.939	35.43	40.65	39.29	153.3	96.22	54.59	4.016	6.044	7.546	20.23	18.28	16.19
Switzerland	0.694	0.526	0.349	6.867	2.772	1.067	24.66	30.03	26.71	110	67.87	37.5	1.793	3.097	4.094	8.701	7.936	7.07
Luxembourg	0.088	0.081	0.068	12.71	6.04	2.908	1.674	2.268	2.885	161.7	108.6	77.22	0.057	0.103	0.149	6.065	5.673	5.326
Europe-West	**30.2**	**20.15**	**13.35**	**9.33**	**3.632**	**1.448**	**744.7**	**831.1**	**700.2**	**139.7**	**86.68**	**47.05**	**51.81**	**78.96**	**100.2**	**10.55**	**9.433**	**8.225**

Multination Regional Analysis

Measures of Poverty, Health, Education, Infrastructure, and Governance

Health

Deaths and Death Rates from Noncommunicable Diseases

Base Case
Source: International Futures
Version 6.32, June 2010

| | Digestive Disorders | | | | | | Malignant Neoplasms | | | | | | Mental Health | | | | | |
	Annual Deaths (in thousands)			Age Standardized Death Rates per 100,000			Annual Deaths (in thousands)			Age Standardized Death Rates per 100,000			Annual Deaths (in thousands)			Age Standardized Death Rates per 100,000		
	2010	2035	2060	2010	2035	2060	2010	2035	2060	2010	2035	2060	2010	2035	2060	2010	2035	2060
World	1909	2460	3247	31.25	21.52	15.84	7389	12424	16923	108.6	101.3	88.99	1311	2620	5003	19.03	20.04	21.12
Africa	256.8	362.3	531.3	47.04	30.47	20.74	538.3	1232	2599	115.9	129.9	125.6	163.8	323.2	633.7	26.56	26.97	27.46
Americas	296	466.1	698.6	30.3	22.76	18.31	1129	1812	2434	102.1	82.93	68.93	294.4	607.3	1142	19.32	19.31	19.63
Asia with Oceania	1001	1247	1584	28.22	18.27	12.73	4046	7516	10090	105.3	95.95	77.3	568.7	1240	2554	17.33	18.05	18.74
Europe	347.2	376.3	425.6	27.39	20.53	17.62	1652	1837	1773	124.9	99.43	81.7	281.6	447	669.9	18.03	18.54	19.03
World	1909	2460	3247	31.25	21.52	15.84	7389	12424	16923	108.6	101.3	88.99	1311	2620	5003	19.03	20.04	21.12
Africa-Eastern	61.94	77.55	97.26	38.28	21.9	12.44	149.3	388.8	856.9	109.7	130.1	116.5	44.83	89.77	181	23.93	23.96	24.09
Africa-Middle	33.47	60.01	104.1	54.22	46.41	38.01	73.3	169.7	391.8	144	167.3	170.1	22.01	42.65	85.71	30.7	30.87	30.99
Africa-Northern	68	104	166.3	52.3	33.46	24.15	95.61	186.9	303	69.73	62.26	52.25	30.61	61.61	119	20.36	20.5	20.61
Africa-Southern	15.98	18.39	22.92	40.22	27.8	18.88	41.75	63.36	102.9	118.5	96.22	84.51	10.14	17.72	31.4	26.49	26.37	26.48
Africa-Western	77.44	102.4	140.7	51.06	31.64	20.06	178.3	423.5	944.8	142.4	152.9	146.2	56.27	111.4	216.6	31.94	32.02	32.05
Africa	256.8	362.3	531.3	47.04	30.47	20.74	538.3	1232	2599	115.9	129.9	125.6	163.8	323.2	633.7	26.56	26.97	27.46
America-Caribbean	11.58	17.83	24.03	32.03	27.33	21.05	39.07	66.86	98.99	93.54	83.56	79.37	8.273	18.1	34.54	19.39	20.1	21.15
America-Central	13.27	20.86	33.73	43.97	30.31	22.84	27.22	55.78	101.5	89.18	77.41	63.7	8.211	17.1	31.61	23.96	24.06	24.66
America-North	145.9	245.2	373.9	25.25	21	17.53	668.7	984.1	1223	98.83	77.56	64.83	219.4	452.8	850.1	23.29	23.32	23.69
America-South	125.2	182.2	266.9	34.37	23.25	18.21	394.3	705.3	1011	108.2	89.52	73.28	58.51	119.2	225.8	14.28	14.18	14.17
Americas	296	466.1	698.6	30.3	22.76	18.31	1129	1812	2434	102.1	82.93	68.93	294.4	607.3	1142	19.32	19.31	19.63
Asia-East	369.5	462.6	589	20.47	12.14	8.344	2365	4027	4702	124.9	110.6	93.33	178.6	393.9	777.3	9.931	9.96	9.945
Asia-South Central	444.6	501.6	586.6	34.84	21.6	13.73	1039	2190	3510	92.32	89.51	70.13	274	593.8	1282	24.34	24.56	24.85
Asia-South East	138.6	202.8	270.5	29.52	20.81	16.32	452.2	943.9	1323	97.08	92.27	76.98	80.59	173.2	328.5	17.38	17.21	17.11
Asia-West	40.38	66.81	117.2	29.76	21.35	16.68	136.9	275.5	451.9	88.23	74.49	61.11	23.72	52.94	116.4	15.31	16.25	16.97
Oceania	8.05	13.12	20.77	20.48	15.68	12.55	52.52	78.96	103.6	110.1	89.81	76.95	11.83	26.31	50.47	19.66	19.62	19.64
Asia with Oceania	1001	1247	1584	28.22	18.27	12.73	4046	7516	10090	105.3	95.95	77.3	568.7	1240	2554	17.33	18.05	18.74
Europe-East	160.9	143.8	134.9	38.86	28.92	26.93	603.2	645.4	570.5	133.3	112.2	93.09	49.17	53.72	53.99	13.24	13.29	13.36
Europe-North	43.91	55.64	75.65	22.21	17.18	14.15	236.3	261.3	287.1	124	89.61	73.77	59.85	105.4	171.1	24.85	24.96	25.04
Europe-South	62.88	72.04	83.18	18.8	14.52	12.05	357.7	400.6	381.3	116.1	92.42	76	68.53	109	172.5	17.14	17.28	17.29
Europe-West	87.79	113.1	139.2	21.03	16.99	13.58	478.9	557.4	560.3	121.7	94.96	78.63	106.1	181.6	275.6	22.45	22.87	23.17
Europe	347.2	376.3	425.6	27.39	20.53	17.62	1652	1837	1773	124.9	99.43	81.7	281.6	447	669.9	18.03	18.54	19.03

Health

Deaths and Death Rates from Noncommunicable Diseases

Base Case: Countries in Year 2060 Descending Population Sequence	Digestive Disorders — Annual Deaths (in thousands)			Digestive Disorders — Age Standardized Death Rates per 100,000			Malignant Neoplasms — Annual Deaths (in thousands)			Malignant Neoplasms — Age Standardized Death Rates per 100,000			Mental Health — Annual Deaths (in thousands)			Mental Health — Age Standardized Death Rates per 100,000		
	2010	2035	2060	2010	2035	2060	2010	2035	2060	2010	2035	2060	2010	2035	2060	2010	2035	2060
AFRICA																		
Ethiopia	17.39	19.61	16.43	41.19	21.81	8.716	42.85	118.9	260.8	123.2	162.3	152.4	11.46	22.63	42.85	24.74	24.77	24.78
Tanzania, United Rep	6.393	6.086	8.397	29.57	12.68	7.166	17.7	47.27	92.73	94.8	110	80.11	5.176	10.87	23.74	20.98	21.06	21.11
Uganda	4.699	6.112	9.884	33.36	18.88	10.91	12.5	32.85	75.84	103.5	120.2	87.01	4.086	8.486	19.8	21.93	22.07	22.07
Kenya	5.121	7.877	12.04	27.24	17.59	10.78	12.7	35.82	92.2	81.69	86.89	80.82	4.396	9.272	20.71	19.17	19.23	19.28
Madagascar	5.178	7.975	10.41	44.46	29.77	18.85	11.3	30.07	69.66	116.2	126.2	131	3.606	7.695	14.99	26.85	26.88	26.94
Mozambique	5.15	4.419	4.047	32.78	18.71	8.312	13.24	32.75	51.09	129.3	163.3	110.9	4.021	7.269	13.2	28.61	28.65	28.86
Malawi	2.176	3.146	4.97	36.52	20.03	14.19	5.677	14.39	40.04	101.1	111.5	127.8	1.563	3.467	7.311	23.02	22.95	23.17
Zambia	2.442	3.494	5.499	36.52	26.82	18.17	5.648	12.55	32.61	103.6	119.2	113.9	1.938	3.605	7.225	24.05	24.01	24.21
Somalia	3.12	4.25	6.073	67.25	41.52	28.33	5.632	12.96	26.21	118.7	124.3	121.1	1.901	3.771	6.971	28.56	28.62	28.72
Rwanda	2.523	3.45	3.425	49.74	31.45	14.66	5.337	15.46	29.24	130.3	171.2	129.3	1.654	3.228	6.223	27.54	27.74	27.85
Zimbabwe	3.964	5.433	8.364	47.13	33.77	28.76	8.029	14.52	34.61	110.5	103.2	108.5	2.663	4.581	8.17	28	28.22	28.69
Burundi	1.818	2.606	3.338	42.44	27.68	17.12	4.31	11.18	29.89	122.1	136	160.6	1.243	2.521	4.919	26.02	26.33	26.43
Eritrea	1.073	1.827	2.934	48.03	32.32	23.21	2.591	6.702	16.64	134.6	133.6	136.6	0.681	1.593	3.622	27.02	27.34	27.56
Comoros	0.13	0.261	0.365	34.8	29.83	20.32	0.337	0.901	2.059	109.4	111.6	114.5	0.095	0.213	0.451	24.22	24.28	24.33
Mauritius	0.465	0.534	0.573	34.24	23.84	17.15	0.952	1.632	2.034	74.35	62.28	52.11	0.178	0.302	0.463	13.59	13.61	13.7
Djibouti	0.301	0.478	0.517	74.94	58.52	33.36	0.483	0.884	1.175	100.6	101.3	79.15	0.169	0.273	0.404	29.34	29.51	29.63
Africa-Eastern	**61.94**	**77.55**	**97.26**	**38.28**	**21.9**	**12.44**	**149.3**	**388.8**	**856.9**	**109.7**	**130.1**	**116.5**	**44.83**	**89.77**	**181**	**23.93**	**23.96**	**24.09**
Congo, Democratic Republic of	17.5	35	64.81	55.99	51.42	43.72	38.18	95.45	236	151.7	193.2	203.6	11.05	21.62	43.56	30.93	31.04	31.08
Angola	4.773	7.247	12.2	55.9	38.82	27.6	9.895	21.01	42.42	143	125.5	97.57	3.447	7.077	14.44	32.56	32.54	32.5
Cameroon	5.135	7.166	9.818	48.48	34.77	23.15	11.7	24.09	49.86	129.4	130.6	116.5	3.627	6.506	12.4	29.59	29.69	29.73
Chad	3.119	5.713	9.907	58.44	49.52	37.63	6.492	15.1	34.51	144.5	158.5	144.7	1.99	4.082	8.77	32.53	32.6	32.71
Central African Republic	1.321	2.038	2.555	51.3	43.82	29.18	3.111	6.318	13.8	136.7	156.2	166.3	0.831	1.38	2.467	29.06	29.11	29.18
Congo, Republic of	1.015	1.625	2.834	42.34	33.77	26.34	2.583	5.078	10.72	118.1	113.8	97.75	0.702	1.273	2.69	25.24	25.33	25.36
Gabon	0.396	0.809	1.367	40.39	38.54	33.03	0.884	1.67	2.885	97.05	81.74	64.92	0.228	0.45	0.934	21.28	21.33	21.35
Equatorial Guinea	0.184	0.358	0.56	56.75	52.86	45.92	0.375	0.767	1.111	134.5	116.9	90.79	0.117	0.226	0.371	31.16	31.12	31.16
São Tomé and Príncipe	0.026	0.047	0.09	28.58	24.03	18.18	0.087	0.179	0.503	102.7	97.58	97.79	0.016	0.032	0.075	14.79	14.74	14.98
Africa-Middle	**33.47**	**60.01**	**104.1**	**54.22**	**46.41**	**38.01**	**73.3**	**169.7**	**391.8**	**144**	**167.3**	**170.1**	**22.01**	**42.65**	**85.71**	**30.7**	**30.87**	**30.99**
Egypt	32.59	48.17	83.53	64.41	40.4	30.44	33.71	60.69	97.03	60.12	50.91	41.55	13.88	27.3	50.15	23.29	23.38	23.49
Sudan	11.92	13.58	16.87	54.3	28.53	16.76	21.2	43.61	71.92	91.98	89.45	72.61	5.42	10.3	18.67	19.79	19.79	19.8
Algeria	6.927	12.27	20.56	28.83	20.59	17.1	18.26	39.91	66.14	78.84	66.03	56.48	4.212	10.23	24.57	17.75	17.91	17.97
Morocco	12.38	22.9	32.66	55.12	43.22	31.68	15.1	27.6	42.82	62.66	53.37	46.33	5.21	9.788	16.84	20.19	20.41	20.58
Tunisia	2.842	4.347	7.335	32.08	20.27	15.12	4.572	8.759	15.01	50.81	41.84	35.59	1.219	2.471	5.381	13.02	13.11	13.17
Libyan Arab Jamahiriya	1.348	2.709	5.339	35.36	23.24	19.89	2.774	6.328	10.04	67.92	56.28	44.52	0.663	1.514	3.373	14.27	14.07	14.04
Africa-Northern	**68**	**104**	**166.3**	**52.3**	**33.46**	**24.15**	**95.61**	**186.9**	**303**	**69.73**	**62.26**	**52.25**	**30.61**	**61.61**	**119**	**20.36**	**20.5**	**20.61**

Health

Deaths and Death Rates from Noncommunicable Diseases

Base Case: Countries in Year 2060 Descending Population Sequence	Digestive Disorders						Malignant Neoplasms						Mental Health					
	Annual Deaths (in thousands)			Age Standardized Death Rates per 100,000			Annual Deaths (in thousands)			Age Standardized Death Rates per 100,000			Annual Deaths (in thousands)			Age Standardized Death Rates per 100,000		
	2010	2035	2060	2010	2035	2060	2010	2035	2060	2010	2035	2060	2010	2035	2060	2010	2035	2060
AFRICA continued																		
South Africa	14.3	16.26	19.62	40.52	28.17	19.16	37.94	56.47	87.74	121.4	97.55	85.51	9.051	15.79	27.34	27.02	27.04	27.2
Namibia	0.354	0.631	1.064	28	20.72	14.07	0.838	2.018	4.667	75	67.7	60.05	0.231	0.53	1.31	17.27	17.37	17.5
Lesotho	0.543	0.524	0.704	46.09	31.34	20.69	1.368	1.898	4.415	126.9	130.3	123.9	0.38	0.506	0.91	28.83	28.72	29.54
Botswana	0.414	0.525	0.933	33.41	20.63	15.51	0.902	1.853	3.747	85.72	73.1	60.63	0.25	0.516	1.143	20.01	20.24	20.33
Swaziland	0.378	0.456	0.598	52.28	35.57	23.18	0.703	1.121	2.367	117.4	95.82	87.25	0.227	0.383	0.697	28.97	28.65	29.16
Africa-Southern	**15.98**	**18.39**	**22.92**	**40.22**	**27.8**	**18.88**	**41.75**	**63.36**	**102.9**	**118.5**	**96.22**	**84.51**	**10.14**	**17.72**	**31.4**	**26.49**	**26.37**	**26.48**
Nigeria	43.08	51.04	73.72	52.75	30.55	21.31	94.33	216.4	469.2	140.9	149	139.3	33.04	63.56	118.7	34.47	34.56	34.63
Niger	3.417	4.942	7.01	53.24	30.79	17.34	8.152	22.17	58.65	158.2	169.2	171.7	2.262	5.488	12.31	31.5	31.54	31.44
Côte d'Ivoire	3.718	6.356	9.279	35.9	27.95	17.26	9.757	22.44	52.05	103.9	106.5	96.48	2.292	4.857	11.19	21.75	21.48	21.38
Ghana	6.354	9.775	11.97	40.79	31.29	20.69	15.7	35.94	79.12	116.8	123.6	133	5.072	8.851	14.1	25.15	25.21	25.26
Mali	3.898	3.586	4.002	59.54	24.68	12.22	9.708	23	52.13	185.1	189.9	178.7	2.847	5.943	12.1	37.24	37.33	37.49
Burkina Faso	3.424	6.385	7.805	58.01	43.44	23.3	7.555	21.08	53.16	158.3	172.7	176.3	2.217	4.94	10.63	32.32	32.66	32.8
Senegal	3.613	5.402	6.55	64.93	43	23.25	8.33	19.35	43.91	183.5	184.4	166.6	2.22	4.503	9.664	36.69	36.61	36.77
Guinea	2.267	3.497	5.023	43.12	29.69	19.39	5.351	13.51	30.22	118	129.4	122.5	1.536	3.285	6.741	26.34	26.48	26.5
Benin	1.669	2.486	3.777	35.53	22.04	14.64	4.361	11.62	28.33	105.9	112.4	112.1	1.184	2.714	6.036	23.53	23.82	23.83
Togo	1.085	1.908	3.514	31.2	22.4	17.87	2.894	7.535	18.17	93.11	94.34	90.42	0.757	1.765	4.161	20.91	20.99	21.07
Sierra Leone	2.267	3.341	3.415	92.23	69	34.87	5.333	12.7	23.84	273.9	364.7	324.1	1.127	2.055	3.881	47.51	47.47	47.49
Liberia	0.634	0.931	0.888	36.45	23.64	11.15	1.747	6.095	12.26	118.1	200.2	185.6	0.385	0.747	1.433	22.41	22.47	22.49
Mauritania	0.927	1.508	2.081	59.84	42.51	28.25	2.222	5.318	11.05	170.4	163.4	152.6	0.558	1.173	2.466	34.67	34.94	34.93
Guinea-Bissau	0.513	0.497	0.681	49.37	24.03	15.85	1.314	2.686	5.538	146.2	142.5	134.9	0.394	0.792	1.585	33.76	33.79	33.88
Gambia	0.503	0.63	0.827	59.9	35.72	23	1.298	2.979	5.928	183.5	197.5	183.3	0.323	0.649	1.231	37.17	37.18	37.28
Cape Verde	0.068	0.093	0.17	22.16	13.27	9.847	0.266	0.628	1.251	89.66	90.42	70.71	0.059	0.121	0.315	17.7	17.7	18.45
Africa-Western	**77.44**	**102.4**	**140.7**	**51.06**	**31.64**	**20.06**	**178.3**	**423.5**	**944.8**	**142.4**	**152.9**	**146.2**	**56.27**	**111.4**	**216.6**	**31.94**	**32.02**	**32.05**

Multinational Regional Analysis

Measures of Poverty, Health, Education, Infrastructure, and Governance

Health

Deaths and Death Rates from Noncommunicable Diseases

Base Case: Countries in Year 2060 Descending Population Sequence	Digestive Disorders — Annual Deaths (in thousands)			Digestive Disorders — Age Standardized Death Rates per 100,000			Malignant Neoplasms — Annual Deaths (in thousands)			Malignant Neoplasms — Age Standardized Death Rates per 100,000			Mental Health — Annual Deaths (in thousands)			Mental Health — Age Standardized Death Rates per 100,000		
	2010	2035	2060	2010	2035	2060	2010	2035	2060	2010	2035	2060	2010	2035	2060	2010	2035	2060
AMERICAS																		
Haiti	3.112	5.115	6.547	54.98	48.65	32.84	4.431	9.445	22.55	91.42	100.3	107.7	1.486	2.898	6.214	31.86	31.9	32.17
Dominican Republic	2.478	3.954	6.136	32.23	21.41	15.59	6.291	12.75	22.52	81.34	67.75	56.54	0.758	1.701	3.62	9.237	9.211	9.241
Cuba	3.008	4.61	5.824	17.77	13.79	11.15	18.36	29.21	33.79	109.5	88.67	73.94	3.714	8.92	17.26	20.02	20.08	20.12
Puerto Rico	1.58	2.096	2.63	25.12	18.77	15.12	4.971	7.238	9.168	73.67	60.05	52.26	1.796	3.655	5.941	24.54	24.66	25.04
Jamaica	0.838	1.186	1.708	29.59	22.98	18.42	2.779	4.099	5.411	103	83.64	67.52	0.208	0.3	0.449	7.281	7.306	7.292
Trinidad	0.318	0.485	0.694	25.04	17.4	14.2	1.13	2.094	2.706	90.4	76.87	63.03	0.174	0.352	0.621	13.75	13.89	14.03
Bahamas	0.088	0.145	0.198	27.5	21.35	16.33	0.303	0.619	0.934	97.62	81.43	69.64	0.047	0.108	0.19	15.05	15.15	15.22
Barbados	0.084	0.133	0.161	21.24	17.25	13.67	0.407	0.745	0.886	104.9	92.44	82.51	0.049	0.094	0.135	12.29	12.28	12.26
Grenada	0.02	0.032	0.04	20.31	16.89	12.69	0.097	0.157	0.29	100.6	84.32	70.54	0.012	0.02	0.039	11.02	11.09	11.07
Saint Vincent and Grenadines	0.023	0.032	0.044	21.04	16.64	11.04	0.123	0.219	0.346	114.7	97.81	82	0.013	0.023	0.038	11.01	11.18	11.07
Saint_Lucia	0.034	0.042	0.045	22.69	16.2	12.9	0.18	0.279	0.38	115.9	95.75	78.61	0.017	0.024	0.032	10.37	10.26	10.41
America-Caribbean	**11.58**	**17.83**	**24.03**	**32.03**	**27.33**	**21.05**	**39.07**	**66.86**	**98.99**	**93.54**	**83.56**	**79.37**	**8.273**	**18.1**	**34.54**	**19.39**	**20.1**	**21.15**
Guatemala	4.898	7.212	12.02	55.73	35.35	25.24	7.445	15.3	31.85	89.14	76.01	62.03	2.615	5.816	11.04	26.71	26.83	27.51
Honduras	2.098	3.108	5.357	41.61	25.94	20.13	4.199	9.052	17.28	85.99	76.46	62.33	1.078	2.217	3.925	18.54	18.47	18.63
El Salvador	2.357	3.453	4.75	37.03	27.96	20.35	5.482	8.576	13.29	86.5	68.28	54.53	2.668	4.961	8.374	41.42	41.83	43.08
Nicaragua	1.891	3.237	4.909	51.61	37.83	29.63	3.144	7.524	13.69	88.99	88.86	76.6	0.77	1.469	2.362	17.4	17.38	17.61
Costa Rica	1.286	2.451	4.072	30.64	22.09	17.23	3.957	8.891	14.43	95.72	81.15	67.05	0.627	1.622	3.774	13.98	14	14.01
Panama	0.701	1.32	2.477	23.22	17.14	14.23	2.871	6.147	10.29	96.29	83.43	71.09	0.436	0.983	2.051	13.88	13.86	13.88
Belize	0.038	0.08	0.152	19.02	15.01	11.09	0.123	0.291	0.658	62.45	53.56	44.49	0.017	0.036	0.09	7.023	7.019	7.018
America-Central	**13.27**	**20.86**	**33.73**	**43.97**	**30.31**	**22.84**	**27.22**	**55.78**	**101.5**	**89.18**	**77.41**	**63.7**	**8.211**	**17.1**	**31.61**	**23.96**	**24.06**	**24.66**
USA	86.53	139.7	212.3	16.78	14.44	12.54	534.2	758.3	915.6	107.1	83.08	68.89	189.9	389.9	736.8	27.99	28.03	28.06
Mexico	49.41	87.68	135	52.44	41.94	35.15	64.16	121.9	190.2	69.17	57.15	48.1	8.771	17.2	32.81	8.707	8.739	8.771
Canada	9.983	17.83	26.59	15.31	13.32	11.63	70.34	103.8	116.7	118.9	93.31	77.05	20.68	45.73	80.49	27.21	27.23	27.23
America-North	**145.9**	**245.2**	**373.9**	**25.25**	**21**	**17.53**	**668.7**	**984.1**	**1223**	**98.83**	**77.56**	**64.83**	**219.4**	**452.8**	**850.1**	**23.29**	**23.32**	**23.69**
Brazil	65.23	85.28	113.4	35.01	21.8	15.9	186.2	326	452.2	102.9	82.35	67.42	31.98	65.57	124.7	16.63	16.68	16.78
Colombia	10.82	20.63	33.45	28.54	20.42	16.21	39.69	82.71	120.3	103.9	87.38	71.46	2.676	5.298	9.056	6.257	6.271	6.277
Argentina	12.41	16.57	25.14	23.91	17.73	14.7	60.71	88.59	119.8	120.7	104.6	86.4	7.713	13.85	25.3	13.95	14.03	14.09
Peru	11.79	19.79	32.95	49.47	35.08	28.46	28.6	59.8	99.63	122.4	104.7	84.75	2.719	5.336	9.687	10.4	10.42	10.46
Venezuela	5.594	9.754	15.98	25.19	17.21	14.07	21.96	44.17	65.93	99.26	80.51	64.59	2.288	4.593	7.951	9.262	9.266	9.266
Ecuador	4.277	8.103	13.99	35.08	29.14	27.36	10.32	19.86	30.64	85.26	69.3	55.24	1.627	3.364	6.189	12.62	12.61	12.63
Chile	7.02	10.66	14.1	35.72	25.78	20.31	21.18	41.15	54.29	106.8	92.54	74.96	5.514	14.26	30.59	25.15	25.25	25.32
Bolivia	5.135	7.344	11.77	78.32	52.55	41.42	12.4	23.01	38.55	195.1	165.1	131.9	1.339	2.504	4.266	17.33	17.41	17.47
Paraguay	1.267	2.121	3.605	27.31	19.45	15.47	4.643	9.046	15.78	103.6	85.8	72.21	0.415	0.823	1.423	8.183	8.116	8.131
Uruguay	1.233	1.355	1.916	20.51	14.03	10.99	7.76	9.554	12.45	138.3	115	98.5	2.13	3.482	6.344	30.11	30.21	30.24
Guyana	0.223	0.26	0.257	33.18	25.38	20.42	0.441	0.829	0.924	69.57	68.99	55.88	0.07	0.095	0.12	9.997	10.02	9.985
Suriname	0.22	0.297	0.348	55.37	41.86	30.55	0.351	0.561	0.663	89.88	76.72	62.1	0.04	0.064	0.082	9.794	9.823	9.83
America-South	**125.2**	**182.2**	**266.9**	**34.37**	**23.25**	**18.21**	**394.3**	**705.3**	**1011**	**108.2**	**89.52**	**73.28**	**58.51**	**119.2**	**225.8**	**14.28**	**14.18**	**14.17**

Health

Deaths and Death Rates from Noncommunicable Diseases

Base Case: Countries in Year 2060 Descending Population Sequence	Digestive Disorders						Malignant Neoplasms						Mental Health					
	Annual Deaths (in thousands)			Age Standardized Death Rates per 100,000			Annual Deaths (in thousands)			Age Standardized Death Rates per 100,000			Annual Deaths (in thousands)			Age Standardized Death Rates per 100,000		
	2010	2035	2060	2010	2035	2060	2010	2035	2060	2010	2035	2060	2010	2035	2060	2010	2035	2060
ASIA with OCEANIA																		
China	293.5	343.6	444.4	21.05	11.84	7.876	1885	3355	4024	129.4	114.9	96.81	141.5	309.9	639	10.11	10.13	10.14
Japan	49.28	76.09	88.92	13.74	11.26	9.559	366.4	458.3	437.2	108.5	89.89	75.25	19.89	36.77	45.95	5.512	5.542	5.563
Korea, Repub of	14.62	27.05	38.15	22.27	19.79	17.21	79.78	155.1	173.5	121.3	106.2	90.73	14.2	42.44	85.02	21.96	21.88	21.89
Taiwan	1.327	2.299	3.183	5.079	3.774	3.033	5.109	9.843	12.72	19.73	15.98	13.2	0	0	0	0	0	0
Korea, Dem. People's Rep.	9.337	11.46	11.56	37.39	29.51	23.1	22.66	34.89	38.08	88.4	86.87	76.21	2.797	4.501	6.846	11.94	12.18	12.21
Hong Kong SAR	0.466	0.978	1.344	3.457	3.319	2.88	2.422	4.181	4.824	18.7	14.95	12.07	0	0	0	0	0	0
Mongolia	1.049	1.051	1.424	56.5	27.31	18.85	4.227	9.401	12.09	260.5	228.1	169.3	0.18	0.283	0.466	8.11	8.114	8.045
Asia-East	369.5	462.6	589	20.47	12.14	8.344	2365	4027	4702	124.9	110.6	93.33	178.6	393.9	777.3	9.931	9.96	9.945
India	310.7	315.9	366.9	33.37	18.73	12.23	736.6	1521	2368	92.55	87.61	65.76	191.1	420.5	911.6	24.56	24.51	24.42
Pakistan	35.08	59.98	70.23	30.24	25.11	14.43	76.19	180.8	361.1	80.27	81.2	69.38	23.5	53.19	124.9	23.4	23.37	23.35
Bangladesh	33.48	42.55	46.41	33.51	20.76	13.01	80.45	209	353.7	94.79	104.9	89.88	18.6	41.21	89.91	22.55	22.48	22.49
Afghanistan	18.45	21.07	19	118.9	65.29	25.63	28.81	61.25	83.38	159.7	162	100.9	12.79	26.32	50.51	53.65	53.05	52.69
Iran (Islamic Republic of)	9.398	14.72	29.97	19.82	12.66	10.39	45.82	91.44	156.9	95.14	76.49	63.56	14.18	29.08	69.14	27.11	27.07	27.14
Nepal	6.471	11.46	13.26	36.11	30.96	18.61	14.45	32.65	67.85	88.57	91.64	91.61	2.554	5.408	11.87	15.96	15.98	16.07
Uzbekistan	9.866	11.73	12.75	47.67	28.04	21.45	12.21	23.11	29.91	59.54	56.07	47.52	3.476	4.797	5.407	13.12	13.13	13.14
Sri Lanka	7.795	9.855	9.748	35.76	26.76	21	14.79	26.25	32.48	69.45	59	51.04	2.792	6.374	9.856	13.39	13.32	13.49
Kazakhstan	7.606	6.512	7.091	49.71	31.12	31.11	19.93	25.93	26.41	134.3	112.6	92.92	2.521	2.857	2.938	16.6	16.84	17.08
Tajikistan	1.545	2.921	4.693	37.82	32.27	27.17	2.574	5.8	10.45	64.28	64.46	61.03	0.997	1.595	1.877	14.76	14.93	15.02
Turkmenistan	1.815	2.117	3.414	47.89	25.39	21.63	2.682	5.122	7.773	73.62	62.15	51.68	0.649	1.006	1.284	13.76	13.85	13.97
Kyrgyzstan	2.118	2.443	2.585	48.61	30.78	23.73	3.315	6.45	9.105	80.87	80.74	72.02	0.728	1.034	1.333	14.53	14.53	14.56
Bhutan	0.165	0.217	0.289	32.47	21.69	11.93	0.356	0.749	1.568	82.24	75.72	61.44	0.115	0.236	0.633	24.58	24.56	24.55
Maldives	0.074	0.155	0.24	38.72	29.86	19.65	0.356	0.817	1.632	187.7	158.5	131.4	0.06	0.159	0.518	34.53	35.71	35.96
Asia-South Central	444.6	501.6	586.6	34.84	21.6	13.73	1039	2190	3510	92.32	89.51	70.13	274	593.8	1282	24.34	24.56	24.85
Indonesia	48.06	70.69	95.64	26.43	18.15	14.43	172	379	546.8	97.22	94.54	78.92	33.44	77.29	152.8	19.69	19.76	19.76
Philippines	19.41	36.05	58.79	34.1	27.69	23.27	40.95	90.21	140.7	72.28	68.76	57.21	4.591	9.476	18.26	7.429	7.438	7.447
Viet Nam	14.77	17.5	23.68	19.56	10.92	7.706	60.04	143.6	212.1	82.28	86.6	69.56	13.3	28.78	62.29	17.38	17.49	17.53
Thailand	29.8	43.11	47.35	43.1	33.88	26.53	99.94	158.5	159.9	145.5	122.7	100.5	14.58	27.71	39.55	21.64	21.65	21.74
Myanmar	15.03	15.67	15.68	33.7	19.4	13.72	38.39	82.58	121.5	91.55	96.95	94.13	8.206	14.79	24.91	18.67	18.68	18.74
Malaysia	5.182	10.04	16.13	26.45	19.68	15.79	20.04	43.3	68.04	104.2	84.88	71.27	2.806	7.669	16.1	14.85	14.81	14.84
Cambodia	4.214	6.072	7.804	44.42	31	20.22	10.41	23.66	39.23	118.2	122	99	2.55	5.007	8.858	24.32	24.65	24.73
LAO People's Dem Repub	1.198	1.486	2.162	31.16	18.37	12.2	3.633	8.433	15.05	110.3	109.5	83.08	0.903	1.996	4.63	25.87	26.02	26.09
Singapore	0.594	1.566	2.295	9.768	8.514	7.261	6.102	12.5	15.05	99.27	76.06	62.12	0.07	0.152	0.195	1.265	1.271	1.271
Timor-Leste	0.295	0.488	0.838	40.57	29.03	22.36	0.574	1.411	3.22	99.02	97.02	90.08	0.128	0.324	0.74	19.44	19.44	19.51
Brunei Darussalam	0.027	0.1	0.18	12.81	11.85	10.61	0.222	0.635	0.883	94.96	75.48	58.42	0.013	0.037	0.106	5.127	5.602	5.202
Asia-South East	138.6	202.8	270.5	29.52	20.81	16.32	452.2	943.9	1323	97.08	92.27	76.98	80.59	173.2	328.5	17.38	17.21	17.11

Health

Deaths and Death Rates from Noncommunicable Diseases

Base Case: Countries in Year 2060 Descending Population Sequence	Digestive Disorders Annual Deaths (in thousands) 2010	2035	2060	Digestive Disorders Age Standardized Death Rates per 100,000 2010	2035	2060	Malignant Neoplasms Annual Deaths (in thousands) 2010	2035	2060	Malignant Neoplasms Age Standardized Death Rates per 100,000 2010	2035	2060	Mental Health Annual Deaths (in thousands) 2010	2035	2060	Mental Health Age Standardized Death Rates per 100,000 2010	2035	2060
ASIA with OCEANIA continued																		
Turkey	13.26	18.6	25.11	21.29	14.21	10.91	61.2	111.3	164.4	101.8	83.62	68.86	7.249	15.37	31.45	12.29	12.29	12.29
Yemen	6.631	10.61	18.84	67.14	42.08	28.64	10.97	26.3	50.24	95.67	91.18	75.22	4.17	9.661	18.74	27.9	27.96	27.97
Iraq	5.439	8.791	17.82	42.22	27.04	19.68	12.4	25.44	51.55	85.96	72.21	60.01	2.711	5.817	13.83	16.43	16.46	16.5
Saudi Arabia	2.957	7.878	15.98	24.97	19.61	16.2	10.61	32.44	55.14	88.33	77.8	60.01	1.288	2.814	6.283	7.383	7.513	7.27
Syriar Arab Repub	1.937	4.789	10.88	20.5	16.68	13.53	4.756	11.2	21.98	44.85	36.76	30.72	3.124	9.224	26.38	32.46	32.56	32.58
Israel	1.338	2.34	4.41	12.35	9.568	8.088	9.675	15.54	24.94	99.58	78.33	66.62	2.104	4.593	9.515	18.71	18.86	18.92
Jordan	0.871	1.679	4.339	29.04	20.08	15.39	3.553	7.764	15.28	106	88.49	73.73	0.527	0.951	1.766	10.66	10.65	10.64
Occupied Palestinian Territory	0.313	0.506	1.078	16.88	10.38	7.429	1.207	2.773	6.185	63.45	52.94	44.69	0.268	0.515	0.983	8.153	8.198	8.191
Azerbaijan	2.976	4.1	6.191	38.24	22.56	18.44	6.924	11.44	14.21	87.17	71.11	61.23	0.79	1.069	1.529	9.44	9.382	9.393
United Arab Emirates	0.245	0.883	1.711	13.12	7.503	4.937	0.982	6.211	13.85	62.61	53.18	39.34	0.084	0.37	0.632	3.442	3.179	2.758
Oman	0.281	0.921	1.951	22.87	19.31	15.52	1.084	3.772	7.018	82.94	77.91	61.39	0.115	0.302	0.706	6.588	6.826	6.509
Kuwait	0.166	0.822	1.986	14.83	12.06	10.6	0.749	3.809	6.164	61.5	54.01	39.57	0.076	0.315	0.952	5.35	5.556	5.312
Lebanon	1.367	2.11	3.263	40.67	30.07	23.83	2.583	4.074	5.858	75.43	60.23	50.18	0.581	1.027	1.92	16.65	16.81	16.94
Armenia	0.856	0.799	1.154	21.72	11.74	9.026	3.736	4.758	5.821	99.79	80.87	69.67	0.207	0.261	0.369	6.217	6.246	6.345
Georgia	1.495	1.259	1.111	22.86	16.47	13.41	5.083	5.031	4.351	81.72	67.25	57.26	0.319	0.287	0.26	6.757	7.07	7.096
Bahrain	0.088	0.383	0.878	26.84	23.53	19.41	0.307	1.292	2.017	82.11	74.49	57.41	0.032	0.077	0.163	5.654	5.795	5.867
Qatar	0.044	0.158	0.211	8.719	7.236	8.515	0.197	1.139	1.467	56.14	50.26	36.64	0.046	0.235	0.823	15.14	12.99	13.57
Cyprus	0.115	0.193	0.274	8.96	7.42	6.516	0.876	1.25	1.477	71.41	55.71	46.61	0.029	0.052	0.071	2.49	2.498	2.509
Asia-West	**40.38**	**66.81**	**117.2**	**29.76**	**21.35**	**16.68**	**136.9**	**275.5**	**451.9**	**88.23**	**74.49**	**61.11**	**23.72**	**52.94**	**116.4**	**15.31**	**16.25**	**16.97**
Australia	5.032	8.636	14.21	12.29	9.973	8.508	39.68	56.9	71.07	108	80.69	66.86	9.084	20.33	38.94	19.64	19.66	19.69
Papua New Guinea	1.772	2.34	3.133	48.27	29.01	20.35	3.808	9.092	16.06	122.4	118.3	102.9	0.68	1.563	3.224	20.96	20.76	20.76
New Zealand	0.775	1.34	2.188	9.701	8.07	6.955	8.051	11.18	13.52	118.6	89.06	75.5	1.889	4.087	7.745	21.52	21.57	21.6
Solomon Islands	0.124	0.223	0.38	45.02	35.24	26.25	0.232	0.572	1.13	84.99	87.4	79.29	0.052	0.099	0.183	13.48	13.17	13.23
Fiji	0.194	0.315	0.4	34.86	27.15	20.43	0.463	0.714	0.927	74.97	63.41	53.18	0.079	0.139	0.207	12.4	12.4	12.5
Vanuatu	0.048	0.091	0.164	39.76	29.58	21.25	0.094	0.192	0.356	72.84	60.65	49.67	0.017	0.035	0.071	10.99	10.63	10.51
Micronesia, Federated States of	0.029	0.056	0.105	42.67	35	27.67	0.056	0.105	0.189	78.28	63.71	52.43	0.01	0.02	0.04	11.46	11.55	11.54
Tonga	0.032	0.058	0.104	38.02	35.14	27.71	0.054	0.088	0.157	65.19	53.98	45	0.008	0.015	0.031	9.214	8.935	9.101
Samoa	0.044	0.058	0.09	35.74	26.18	19.66	0.079	0.119	0.187	64.71	54.88	45.79	0.013	0.021	0.036	9.027	9.166	9.441
Oceania	**8.05**	**13.12**	**20.77**	**20.48**	**15.68**	**12.55**	**52.52**	**78.96**	**103.6**	**110.1**	**89.81**	**76.95**	**11.83**	**26.31**	**50.47**	**19.66**	**19.62**	**19.64**

Health

Base Case: Countries in Year 2060 Descending Population Sequence	Digestive Disorders						Malignant Neoplasms						Mental Health					
	Annual Deaths (in thousands)			Age Standardized Death Rates per 100,000			Annual Deaths (in thousands)			Age Standardized Death Rates per 100,000			Annual Deaths (in thousands)			Age Standardized Death Rates per 100,000		
	2010	2035	2060	2010	2035	2060	2010	2035	2060	2010	2035	2060	2010	2035	2060	2010	2035	2060
EUROPE																		
Russian Federation	78.29	65.84	63.53	40.89	29.02	29.15	268.1	289.6	247.3	129.1	109	90.38	23.54	23.83	22.04	14.07	14.14	14.25
Poland	17.32	21.23	24.22	38.51	21.89	19.03	97.29	120.7	117.8	158.3	131.6	109.3	6.444	8.94	10.14	11.75	11.84	11.92
Ukraine	24.29	18.54	12.84	38.91	32.16	28.54	82.11	71.39	55.1	115.1	96.66	78.1	8.145	7.154	5.864	15.2	15.36	15.46
Romania	14.02	13.17	11.76	44.48	33.95	29.51	41.92	42.98	39.51	125.8	102.8	85.39	2.474	2.934	3.288	8.399	8.457	8.513
Czech Republic	4.498	4.906	4.936	25.65	20.02	17.22	49.83	33.79	31.78	161	129.8	106.7	2.262	3.283	4.023	13.26	13.35	13.38
Belarus	3.528	2.939	2.684	26.57	18.53	16.25	18.49	20.5	19.51	129	110.3	94.1	1.482	1.658	1.826	12.4	12.51	12.67
Hungary	8.645	7.206	6.131	54.92	40.24	32.85	31.85	30.61	27.14	181.9	147.2	121.5	2.752	3.494	4.245	16.66	16.88	17.04
Bulgaria	2.748	2.398	2.056	20.79	17.14	14.57	15.44	13.65	10.84	115.5	96.16	79.03	0.875	0.947	1.057	7.37	7.412	7.458
Slovak Republic	2.633	2.903	2.994	33.96	24.83	21.44	11.96	15.34	14.69	150.5	125.8	103.4	0.707	0.948	1.084	10.45	10.54	10.6
Moldova, Repub of	4.968	4.653	3.777	96.61	78.92	63.17	6.194	6.777	6.825	119.1	114.3	102.3	0.49	0.531	0.427	10.71	10.98	11.05
Europe-East	**160.9**	**143.8**	**134.9**	**38.86**	**28.92**	**26.93**	**603.2**	**645.4**	**570.5**	**133.3**	**112.2**	**93.09**	**49.17**	**53.72**	**53.99**	**13.24**	**13.29**	**13.36**
United Kingdom	29.71	37.43	51.9	23.6	18.21	14.92	152.9	163.8	184.2	125.5	87.34	72.16	37.33	64.7	110.5	24.34	24.4	24.43
Sweden	3.199	4.559	6.391	13.52	11.2	9.733	20.55	22.05	23.74	103.7	73.8	60.68	7.454	12.91	19.95	27.55	27.53	27.52
Denmark	2.836	3.584	4.472	26.04	20.78	16.98	15.27	18	17.86	144.9	117	95.79	3.167	5.252	7.534	26.58	26.62	26.66
Ireland	0.995	1.77	3.072	14.49	11.72	10.49	7.695	12.26	15.64	121.6	97.09	79.18	1.241	2.637	5.042	18.16	18.24	18.26
Norway	1.504	2.327	3.386	13.95	12.26	11.06	10.95	13.66	14.58	122.6	92.62	75.52	2.904	5.181	8.219	25.38	25.37	25.38
Finland	2.362	3.003	3.333	22.55	18.02	14.57	11.15	13.13	12.82	99.51	74.35	62.06	6.361	12.98	17.75	44.89	44.99	45.03
Lithuania	1.674	1.496	1.49	32.42	23.56	19.16	8.359	8.655	8.405	149.9	122.7	102.7	0.492	0.548	0.578	10.65	10.72	10.77
Latvia	0.988	0.867	0.933	25.27	17.29	13.68	5.577	5.665	5.65	136.3	114.2	94.34	0.38	0.412	0.408	12.47	12.69	12.82
Estonia	0.586	0.488	0.46	27.27	19.41	14.76	3.311	3.311	3.198	134.3	111.6	94.61	0.332	0.344	0.358	18.19	18.63	18.71
Iceland	0.061	0.114	0.215	9.902	8.055	7.15	0.536	0.786	0.962	109.1	81.82	66.79	0.184	0.418	0.807	29.66	29.75	29.75
Europe-North	**43.91**	**55.64**	**75.65**	**22.21**	**17.18**	**14.15**	**236.3**	**261.3**	**287.1**	**124**	**89.61**	**73.77**	**59.85**	**105.4**	**171.1**	**24.85**	**24.96**	**25.04**
Italy	26.11	28.41	30.21	17.22	13	10.7	157.5	168.8	151.1	114.6	90.39	74.01	27.9	43.76	63.87	15.31	15.41	15.43
Spain	21	26.32	34.55	20.9	16.68	14.36	100.5	121.6	121.3	114.1	92.26	75.98	30.99	51.19	89.27	24.89	24.98	24.97
Greece	2.844	3.625	4.645	11.53	9.621	8.538	30.19	34.28	35.37	116.4	100.6	82.35	1.662	2.441	3.432	7.06	7.069	7.056
Portugal	4.918	5.382	5.549	23.8	18.64	14.52	23.25	25.56	25.16	111.3	88.74	73.7	3.471	5.002	6.84	15.72	15.81	15.87
Serbia	2.523	2.583	2.577	20.97	17.02	14	14.76	14.41	13.15	129.6	104	85.01	1.362	1.634	1.928	13.11	13.2	13.25
Bosnia and Herzegovina	0.998	1.072	1.013	16	11.26	8.38	6.011	7.241	7.298	97.73	78.13	65.88	0.431	0.659	0.963	7.586	7.599	7.717
Croatia	2.308	2.11	1.94	28.25	19.98	15.84	12.01	11.82	10.65	144.1	112.2	93.59	1.164	1.651	2.111	14.27	14.38	14.44
Albania	0.357	0.472	0.605	9.801	6.78	5.416	3.276	4.732	5.734	90.45	73.88	61.41	0.696	1.339	2.32	19.64	19.56	19.71
Macedonia, FYR	0.356	0.389	0.361	12.66	9.559	7.904	3.195	3.7	3.457	114.7	93.33	75.94	0.192	0.286	0.363	7.306	7.371	7.418
Slovenia	1.154	1.27	1.287	30.67	21.33	16.57	5.18	6.185	5.906	134.8	103.7	86.64	0.427	0.679	0.87	12.02	12.26	12.31
Montenegro	0.188	0.194	0.194	21.09	15.41	11.37	1.18	1.268	1.269	137.5	110.4	91.19	0.109	0.143	0.179	13.83	13.92	14.01
Malta	0.126	0.212	0.251	15.94	13.54	11.6	0.725	0.912	0.895	101.2	80.39	66.45	0.122	0.254	0.35	16.28	16.44	16.46
Europe-South	**62.88**	**72.04**	**83.18**	**18.8**	**14.52**	**12.05**	**357.7**	**400.6**	**381.3**	**116.1**	**92.42**	**76**	**68.53**	**109**	**172.5**	**17.14**	**17.28**	**17.29**
Germany	45.23	57.25	68.89	24.36	20.13	15.92	218.1	247.7	244.1	118.7	93.32	76.92	29.72	46.16	64.12	16.15	16.36	16.4
France	25.61	31.71	39.32	18.71	14.53	11.61	156.2	180.3	186.8	125.3	96.46	80.31	49.06	84.51	131.3	28.89	29.05	29.18
Netherlands	6.198	10.2	13.35	17.58	15.23	12.96	40.38	52.88	51.74	132.2	104.5	85.55	11.43	23.29	36.88	28.65	28.48	28.49
Belgium	4.72	5.689	7.272	19.75	15.59	12.73	27.58	31.15	31.97	125	97.25	80.65	6.79	11.11	17.03	23.97	24.09	24.12
Austria	3.341	3.987	4.574	20.47	16.33	13.22	19.08	22.34	22.74	113.3	85.55	70.01	2.603	4.098	5.778	15.87	16.07	16.13
Switzerland	2.506	3.93	5.297	13.75	11.95	10.15	16.64	21.67	21.37	106.2	83.61	68.73	6.243	12.03	19.67	29.66	29.82	29.85
Luxembourg	0.188	0.316	0.459	21.2	19.64	18.71	0.98	1.374	1.54	114.2	88.2	70.48	0.224	0.435	0.746	23.02	23.03	23.01
Europe-West	**87.79**	**113.1**	**139.2**	**21.03**	**16.99**	**13.58**	**478.9**	**557.4**	**560.3**	**121.7**	**94.96**	**78.63**	**106.1**	**181.6**	**275.6**	**22.45**	**22.87**	**23.17**

Multination Regional Analysis

Measures of Poverty, Health, Education, Infrastructure, and Governance

Health

Base Case
Source: International Futures
Version 6.32, June 2010

	Deaths and Death Rates from Noncommunicable Diseases												Deaths and Death Rates from Injuries					
	Respiratory Conditions						Other Noncommunicable Diseases						Road Traffic Accidents					
	Annual Deaths (in thousands)			Age Standardized Death Rates per 100,000			Annual Deaths (in thousands)			Age Standardized Death Rates per 100,000			Annual Deaths (in thousands)			Age Standardized Death Rates per 100,000		
	2010	2035	2060	2010	2035	2060	2010	2035	2060	2010	2035	2060	2010	2035	2060	2010	2035	2060
World	4102	8146	14213	69.86	59.59	52.16	3.094	4.536	6.306	52.76	42.52	34.39	1317	2467	3151	19.65	26.89	28.45
Africa	337.2	625.3	1330	71.31	62.29	57.9	0.558	0.834	1.478	100.9	79.08	63.77	268.1	509.5	881.1	27.81	30.62	35.74
Americas	404	818	1440	34.98	30.39	27.03	0.588	0.959	1.408	56.73	43.15	32.79	143.4	198.4	209.4	15.3	15.61	13.76
Asia with Oceania	3020	6204	10777	85.85	70.78	59.23	1.569	2.287	2.907	44.8	33.12	23.36	811.7	1678	2001	20.06	30.44	30.79
Europe	336.8	493.3	660.4	21.38	19.52	18.19	0.375	0.453	0.508	26.49	18.86	13.73	92.15	80.24	58.33	11.59	10.41	8.234
World	4102	8146	14213	69.86	59.59	52.16	3.094	4.536	6.306	52.76	42.52	34.39	1317	2467	3151	19.65	26.89	28.45
Africa-Eastern	91.5	163.9	356.9	65.26	54.45	47.22	0.148	0.207	0.357	89.13	66.31	47.95	83.71	175	398.6	26.88	30.96	47.58
Africa-Middle	45.25	85.39	185.1	83.87	78.85	75.4	0.077	0.119	0.223	117	100.3	89.46	46.26	85.52	116.2	36.97	37.29	30.33
Africa-Northern	59.05	126.4	267.6	48.51	41.61	37.53	0.111	0.185	0.335	82.31	62.11	48.71	40.72	86.2	125	20.93	29.12	32.46
Africa-Southern	28.34	44.74	69.88	78.45	66.89	57.78	0.044	0.061	0.083	121.6	90.87	62.94	19.37	26.48	28.85	37.09	40.59	37.55
Africa-Western	113.1	204.8	450.5	87	73.92	68.7	0.178	0.262	0.481	115.7	91.25	74.05	78.08	136.3	212.5	28	26.97	27.09
Africa	337.2	625.3	1330	71.31	62.29	57.9	0.558	0.834	1.478	100.9	79.08	63.77	268.1	509.5	881.1	27.81	30.62	35.74
America-Caribbean	11.03	20.52	35.11	26.15	23.7	22.27	0.023	0.035	0.048	61.05	51.59	43.41	5.563	8.81	9.061	14.38	16.74	14.52
America-Central	9.006	19.69	43.36	26.86	23.6	20.21	0.024	0.042	0.076	76.03	58.38	45.04	6.04	10.22	13.75	14.99	14.91	14.49
America-North	223.6	429	691.8	30.53	27.06	24.43	0.319	0.501	0.656	51.33	39.35	28.62	56.49	65.48	66.93	12.03	10.43	8.537
America-South	160.4	348.8	669.5	41.81	35.62	31.44	0.222	0.382	0.627	60.32	44.46	34.5	75.27	113.9	119.6	19.15	21.29	19.41
Americas	404	818	1440	34.98	30.39	27.03	0.588	0.959	1.408	56.73	43.15	32.79	143.4	198.4	209.4	15.3	15.61	13.76
Asia-East	1741	3685	6384	103	85.16	72.77	0.534	0.729	0.787	29.25	18.13	11.78	376.4	702.9	593.3	22.04	36.59	31.76
Asia-South Central	915.8	1708	2860	82.74	68.33	56.05	0.64	0.843	0.999	50.56	35.72	22.06	309.9	765.9	1128	20.16	31.78	35.84
Asia-South East	279.9	629.3	1155	66.29	60.98	56.09	0.285	0.506	0.725	61.51	49.42	39.28	83.3	124.2	155.5	15	15.49	15.68
Asia-West	68.5	151.2	329.1	48.42	40.71	35.44	0.092	0.177	0.352	65.88	55.11	46.02	39.25	80.54	119.5	20.42	25.89	26.3
Oceania	15.06	30.62	49.65	39	37.27	35.24	0.019	0.032	0.044	44.07	36.21	28.82	2.907	3.972	4.817	9.174	9.197	8.66
Asia with Oceania	3020	6204	10777	85.85	70.78	59.23	1.569	2.287	2.907	44.8	33.12	23.36	811.7	1678	2001	20.06	30.44	30.79
Europe-East	108.2	134.4	163.3	22.33	19.84	18.97	0.085	0.073	0.074	23.16	14.81	11.45	59.6	51.86	36.04	18.27	18.18	15.22
Europe-North	62.67	96.31	133	27.59	24.58	22.17	0.054	0.066	0.073	25.35	16.98	10.89	6.02	5.431	4.557	5.618	4.57	3.599
Europe-South	87.11	133.9	196.3	21.42	20.33	19.12	0.106	0.134	0.159	30.31	23.47	18.31	15.43	13.2	9.988	9.407	7.903	6.475
Europe-West	82.82	134	173.9	16.99	16.02	14.57	0.134	0.185	0.207	29.4	22.06	15.08	12.46	10.81	8.591	6.18	5.027	4.041
Europe	336.8	493.3	660.4	21.38	19.52	18.19	0.375	0.453	0.508	26.49	18.86	13.73	92.15	80.24	58.33	11.59	10.41	8.234

Multination Regional Analysis

Health

Base Case: Countries in Year 2060 Descending Population Sequence	Deaths and Death Rates from Noncommunicable Diseases												Deaths and Death Rates from Injuries					
	Respiratory Conditions						Other Noncommunicable Diseases						Road Traffic Accidents					
	Annual Deaths (in thousands)			Age Standardized Death Rates per 100,000			Annual Deaths (in thousands)			Age Standardized Death Rates per 100,000			Annual Deaths (in thousands)			Age Standardized Death Rates per 100,000		
	2010	2035	2060	2010	2035	2060	2010	2035	2060	2010	2035	2060	2010	2035	2060	2010	2035	2060
AFRICA																		
Ethiopia	25.02	39.37	79.35	68.45	52.84	45.59	0.038	0.05	0.076	92.18	66.3	44.64	18.22	38.64	102.4	24.56	27.76	47.33
Tanzania, United Rep	10.81	18.09	43.99	57.57	42.72	37.9	0.018	0.022	0.04	77.4	51.71	34.97	9.229	25.87	61.85	21.54	33.55	55.64
Uganda	7.688	15.64	36.3	62.15	58.3	41.48	0.013	0.018	0.032	82.67	60.94	37.83	10.57	28.69	73.42	29.3	40.95	71.12
Kenya	8.504	18.17	44.79	52.16	44.45	39.36	0.015	0.024	0.046	71.28	56	40.56	10.12	17.25	36.04	25.81	25.77	38.45
Madagascar	7.401	16.26	32.07	73.3	68.69	60.59	0.011	0.02	0.034	97.65	79.68	63.45	4.683	7.448	13.26	22.93	19.27	21.44
Mozambique	7.953	10.67	22.17	75.42	53.97	47.72	0.013	0.013	0.019	102.2	66.26	42.59	8.815	21.56	51.8	39.31	56.96	100.9
Malawi	3.532	6.8	14.57	62.17	52.58	46.16	0.005	0.009	0.016	81.66	65.38	52.76	2.497	4.339	9.006	20.22	17.23	21.43
Zambia	3.707	6.25	14.44	64.36	57.77	50.26	0.006	0.008	0.015	89.06	70.66	53.87	3.698	6.695	11.39	25.76	27.13	32.1
Somalia	2.579	5.146	10.95	65.91	60.65	58.02	0.006	0.01	0.017	124.1	99.91	86.4	1.985	2.918	3.918	16.96	14.29	12.44
Rwanda	3.298	5.689	11.4	65.73	61.21	50.33	0.005	0.007	0.011	104.5	75.78	47.52	3.753	8.434	18.87	37.56	48.33	76.59
Zimbabwe	5.851	10.67	23.44	75.49	74.56	75.34	0.008	0.012	0.023	98.89	82.21	72.23	6.277	7.814	9.348	48.03	39.25	37.92
Burundi	2.599	5.301	10.62	71.43	65.63	58.27	0.004	0.007	0.012	99.49	81.58	66.72	2.161	2.657	3.064	27.34	18.8	13.44
Eritrea	1.62	3.836	9.095	81.67	78.18	75.28	0.002	0.005	0.01	108.5	93.73	82.59	1.08	1.836	2.935	26.5	21.96	19.52
Comoros	0.227	0.558	1.182	71.26	69.64	65.97	0.001	0.001	0.002	115.4	107.1	89.41	0.094	0.151	0.26	15.86	13.19	13.53
Mauritius	0.527	1.106	1.931	42.65	37.1	33.96	0.001	0.001	0.002	73.84	55	41.38	0.211	0.272	0.254	15.98	16.6	14.42
Djibouti	0.187	0.363	0.612	50.89	47.8	38.72	0.001	0.001	0.001	105.9	89.22	60.89	0.318	0.462	0.754	39.84	43.29	59.89
Africa-Eastern	**91.5**	**163.9**	**356.9**	**65.26**	**54.45**	**47.22**	**0.148**	**0.207**	**0.357**	**89.13**	**66.31**	**47.95**	**83.71**	**175**	**398.6**	**26.88**	**30.96**	**47.58**
Congo, Democratic Republic of	23.09	43.93	94.57	86.89	83.68	79.84	0.041	0.065	0.122	120.7	107.7	97.53	22.66	31.92	39.58	33.72	24.7	17.17
Angola	6.235	12.55	28.4	82.19	71.44	65.08	0.01	0.014	0.028	114.8	78.91	64.28	10.56	30.47	39.85	59.09	94.58	85
Cameroon	7.484	13.16	26.82	79.14	71.1	62.9	0.011	0.017	0.029	107.1	88.26	68.52	5.825	10.23	18.77	31.47	34.76	45.47
Chad	4.166	7.869	18.99	87.42	79.34	80.49	0.007	0.013	0.025	128.4	113.8	102.7	3.146	6.203	9.152	29.1	29.22	23.78
Central African Republic	1.927	3.257	5.993	82.63	79.31	72.59	0.003	0.004	0.007	112.9	99.45	80.18	1.676	2.114	3.063	38.6	31.17	30.58
Congo, Republic of	1.462	2.737	6.441	65.18	61.38	58.79	0.003	0.004	0.008	99.27	82.49	71.13	1.639	3.456	4.476	38.2	49.83	45.76
Gabon	0.576	1.222	2.598	61.98	59.72	57.12	0.001	0.002	0.003	86.64	74.93	64.82	0.489	0.763	0.93	32.72	32.87	29.39
Equatorial Guinea	0.248	0.548	0.946	85.57	80.3	77.88	0	0.001	0.001	112.9	92.13	79.3	0.229	0.332	0.365	40.24	37.25	32.44
São Tomé and Príncipe	0.06	0.124	0.352	71.65	72.26	69.34	0	0	0	72.19	65.88	57.88	0.029	0.038	0.048	17.77	12.75	9.74
Africa-Middle	**45.25**	**85.39**	**185.1**	**83.87**	**78.85**	**75.4**	**0.077**	**0.119**	**0.223**	**117**	**100.3**	**89.46**	**46.26**	**85.52**	**116.2**	**36.97**	**37.29**	**30.33**
Egypt	24.17	50	103.7	50.44	42.74	36.24	0.049	0.076	0.136	89.68	65.29	48.76	8.99	18.87	29.14	12.21	16.85	17.96
Sudan	9.904	18.31	40.38	51.75	41.99	38.81	0.022	0.032	0.058	96.99	71.12	55.78	17.81	40.98	57.74	42.71	63.56	71.4
Algeria	11.75	29.01	63.71	52.78	48.14	46.76	0.016	0.033	0.07	70.16	56.16	48.3	4.547	8.576	12.76	15.17	16.77	15.23
Morocco	9.258	20.1	39.4	43.66	38.51	35.67	0.017	0.03	0.048	74.22	58.28	44.61	6.237	11.5	17.24	22.07	24.88	25.97
Tunisia	2.889	6.062	13.27	33.35	27.79	24.56	0.005	0.008	0.014	51.95	38.23	29.91	2.191	4.417	5.746	21.96	26.66	24.19
Libyan Arab Jamahiriya	1.08	2.934	7.19	29.51	25.19	23.09	0.002	0.005	0.01	54.5	39.48	33.75	0.95	1.851	2.334	18.69	18	14.58
Africa-Northern	**59.05**	**126.4**	**267.6**	**48.51**	**41.61**	**37.53**	**0.111**	**0.185**	**0.335**	**82.31**	**62.11**	**48.71**	**40.72**	**86.2**	**125**	**20.93**	**29.12**	**32.46**

Health

Base Case: Countries in Year 2060 Descending Population Sequence	Deaths and Death Rates from Noncommunicable Diseases						Other Noncommunicable Diseases						Deaths and Death Rates from Injuries					
	Respiratory Conditions												Road Traffic Accidents					
	Annual Deaths (in thousands)			Age Standardized Death Rates per 100,000			Annual Deaths (in thousands)			Age Standardized Death Rates per 100,000			Annual Deaths (in thousands)			Age Standardized Death Rates per 100,000		
	2010	2035	2060	2010	2035	2060	2010	2035	2060	2010	2035	2060	2010	2035	2060	2010	2035	2060
AFRICA continued																		
South Africa	25.72	40.43	60.89	80.49	69.26	60.02	0.04	0.056	0.074	126.7	95.83	66.18	17.05	22.69	23.41	37.38	40.86	36.71
Namibia	0.576	1.298	2.84	49.79	43.41	36.16	0.001	0.002	0.003	68.73	52.42	37.66	0.643	1.336	2.056	32.82	40.06	41.42
Lesotho	0.866	0.984	2.122	78.19	65.89	60.66	0.001	0.001	0.002	109.4	85.62	65.36	0.663	0.866	1.323	37.61	37.44	47.68
Botswana	0.642	1.172	2.474	57.34	46	40.45	0.001	0.001	0.003	73.77	49.02	37.14	0.546	0.814	1.006	30.89	33.55	29.25
Swaziland	0.541	0.853	1.553	82.52	70.54	58.91	0.001	0.001	0.001	108.4	78.16	54.88	0.465	0.774	1.049	42.37	47.71	51.25
Africa-Southern	**28.34**	**44.74**	**69.88**	**78.45**	**66.89**	**57.78**	**0.044**	**0.061**	**0.083**	**121.6**	**90.87**	**62.94**	**19.37**	**26.48**	**28.85**	**37.09**	**40.59**	**37.55**
Nigeria	60.71	97.9	228.5	85.71	67.07	68.08	0.1	0.133	0.25	118.2	88.37	74.94	44.22	80.22	98.13	30.46	31.95	26.47
Niger	5.117	11.31	25.52	95.76	87.75	75.73	0.008	0.014	0.027	124.8	102	81.09	3.448	6.115	11.45	25.07	19.84	18.6
Côte d'Ivoire	6.491	12.89	28.52	68.06	61.08	53.35	0.01	0.017	0.033	88.34	77.31	62.02	3.947	6.121	9.563	21.25	18.21	17.37
Ghana	9.58	20.55	37.63	74.31	73.62	62.89	0.012	0.019	0.028	74.52	62.52	47.76	6.116	8.016	13.41	27.12	21.27	24.6
Mali	6.019	10.56	21.81	110.6	91	76.13	0.01	0.013	0.022	145.8	105.4	78.39	4.24	8.382	21.71	31.43	30.75	47.3
Burkina Faso	4.819	10.96	22.7	97.36	90.27	75.12	0.008	0.014	0.025	132.2	111.7	82.69	3.734	7.234	18.56	26.68	26.32	40.76
Senegal	5.238	10.17	22.01	112.3	98.58	84.29	0.008	0.013	0.023	147.5	123.2	90.95	3.221	4.94	9.429	28.66	23.55	28.26
Guinea	3.476	6.884	14.18	74.43	65.88	57.84	0.005	0.009	0.016	100.5	82.39	66.42	2.461	4.31	8.054	25.03	23.16	26.01
Benin	2.739	6.43	13.85	66.15	63.74	55.47	0.005	0.008	0.016	91.63	75.1	62.23	1.352	2.379	4.64	15.4	13.98	15.94
Togo	1.877	4.419	11.18	60.15	56.15	56.07	0.003	0.006	0.013	81.11	70.68	64.99	0.804	1.059	1.152	13.09	9.194	5.806
Sierra Leone	3.016	4.835	8.524	154.2	130.9	107.2	0.004	0.006	0.009	200.9	166.4	116	2.178	3.804	9.774	45.78	44.31	70.96
Liberia	0.97	1.591	3.035	64.75	50.96	44.5	0.002	0.002	0.003	88.63	65.99	47.1	0.439	0.824	1.914	14.05	14.23	20.83
Mauritania	1.324	3.263	6.741	101.2	105.2	95.5	0.002	0.004	0.008	140.7	127.4	110	0.852	1.084	1.515	28.33	20.57	17.88
Guinea-Bissau	0.794	1.389	2.838	88.03	76.92	71.9	0.001	0.002	0.003	117	90.26	78.67	0.565	0.755	0.977	31.96	22.96	16.59
Gambia	0.77	1.376	2.643	108.6	92.41	81.64	0.001	0.002	0.003	144.1	113.4	89.43	0.434	0.831	1.809	29.13	30.49	42.01
Cape Verde	0.15	0.324	0.728	51.48	47.21	40.35	0	0	0.001	87.6	67.53	48.37	0.076	0.2	0.425	16.45	26.38	35.03
Africa-Western	**113.1**	**204.8**	**450.5**	**87**	**73.92**	**68.7**	**0.178**	**0.262**	**0.481**	**115.7**	**91.25**	**74.05**	**78.08**	**136.3**	**212.5**	**28**	**26.97**	**27.09**

Health

Base Case: Countries in Year 2060 Descending Population Sequence	Deaths and Death Rates from Noncommunicable Diseases												Deaths and Death Rates from Injuries					
	Respiratory Conditions						Other Noncommunicable Diseases						Road Traffic Accidents					
	Annual Deaths (in thousands)			Age Standardized Death Rates per 100,000			Annual Deaths (in thousands)			Age Standardized Death Rates per 100,000			Annual Deaths (in thousands)			Age Standardized Death Rates per 100,000		
	2010	2035	2060	2010	2035	2060	2010	2035	2060	2010	2035	2060	2010	2035	2060	2010	2035	2060
AMERICAS																		
Haiti	1.52	2.744	5.549	29.35	28.72	27.12	0.005	0.009	0.015	94.73	86.9	71.17	0.389	0.585	1	5.726	4.87	5.194
Dominican Republic	2.156	4.581	9.459	27.05	22	19.03	0.004	0.006	0.01	50.41	34.52	25.41	2.969	5.266	5.04	32.46	41.41	34.29
Cuba	3.415	6.199	8.897	19.47	16.27	15.11	0.004	0.005	0.004	27.16	17.88	10.98	1.134	1.687	1.702	8.912	11.66	12.22
Puerto Rico	2.135	3.82	5.653	27.32	23.1	21.28	0.005	0.007	0.009	70.66	52.14	39.48	0.434	0.462	0.428	9.543	8.343	7.002
Jamaica	1.404	2.424	4.294	45.77	41.94	36.69	0.002	0.003	0.004	58.4	48.13	38.32	0.382	0.495	0.598	14.43	13.07	12.93
Trinidad	0.223	0.429	0.725	18.13	15.1	14.04	0.002	0.003	0.004	143.7	102.4	84.54	0.156	0.189	0.163	11.28	11.5	10.16
Bahamas	0.048	0.107	0.202	15.24	13.45	12.24	0	0	0.001	79.4	61.15	45.69	0.052	0.067	0.076	15.41	14.77	12.9
Barbados	0.052	0.093	0.125	13.5	12.58	11.7	0	0.001	0.001	84.36	71.8	57.62	0.015	0.018	0.016	4.737	4.288	3.605
Grenada	0.014	0.023	0.041	13.4	12.67	10.89	0	0	0	76.7	67.46	55.34	0.002	0.002	0.004	1.739	1.598	1.516
Saint Vincent and Grenadines	0.016	0.028	0.043	14.79	13.03	11.18	0	0	0	130.6	104.3	84.41	0.006	0.009	0.009	5.081	5.506	4.926
Saint Lucia	0.044	0.071	0.119	26.37	23.66	21.33	0	0	0	115.8	93.8	76.74	0.025	0.029	0.026	14.56	15.48	14.8
America-Caribbean	**11.03**	**20.52**	**35.11**	**26.15**	**23.7**	**22.27**	**0.023**	**0.035**	**0.048**	**61.05**	**51.59**	**43.41**	**5.563**	**8.81**	**9.061**	**14.38**	**16.74**	**14.52**
Guatemala	2.276	4.423	10.21	23.19	19.92	16.99	0.007	0.011	0.022	71.02	51.74	38.76	0.634	1.403	2.373	5.344	6.123	6.577
Honduras	1.299	2.865	7.096	25.72	23.23	20.6	0.004	0.008	0.015	79.79	64.42	52.15	0.855	1.364	1.89	11.02	11.37	11.71
El Salvador	2.034	3.915	7.263	29.39	26.56	22.7	0.006	0.009	0.013	92.67	69.86	50.56	2.5	4.201	5.707	37.47	41.72	45.47
Nicaragua	1.028	2.486	5.721	28.27	27.88	24.43	0.003	0.007	0.012	89.38	77.55	66.19	0.738	1.096	1.446	14.41	13.11	13.25
Costa Rica	1.347	3.615	7.911	30.98	27	23.94	0.002	0.004	0.007	50.4	36.84	27.46	0.689	1.097	1.227	14.92	15.54	13.33
Panama	0.976	2.267	4.862	31.9	26.86	23.39	0.002	0.004	0.007	67.12	48.74	37.09	0.571	0.948	0.95	17.13	19.49	16.79
Belize	0.046	0.115	0.3	22.88	20.81	18.58	0	0	0.001	59.41	46.4	34.78	0.053	0.106	0.161	19.7	21.63	20.19
America-Central	**9.006**	**19.69**	**43.36**	**26.86**	**23.6**	**20.21**	**0.024**	**0.042**	**0.076**	**76.03**	**58.38**	**45.04**	**6.04**	**10.22**	**13.75**	**14.99**	**14.91**	**14.49**
USA	175.8	318.9	471.1	30.57	26.74	24.12	0.212	0.308	0.357	39.8	29.24	20.18	35.41	36.31	34.27	10.59	8.457	6.721
Mexico	31.99	77.7	173.7	32.93	29.91	27.24	0.084	0.155	0.256	89.24	71.87	58.49	18.54	26.64	30.38	17.68	17.47	15.55
Canada	15.77	32.42	46.99	22.26	20.48	18.76	0.022	0.037	0.043	34.87	26.7	18.5	2.536	2.525	2.278	6.939	5.617	4.511
America-North	**223.6**	**429**	**691.8**	**30.53**	**27.06**	**24.43**	**0.319**	**0.501**	**0.656**	**51.33**	**39.35**	**28.62**	**56.49**	**65.48**	**66.93**	**12.03**	**10.43**	**8.537**
Brazil	86.97	195.9	377	47.15	39.59	34.61	0.105	0.181	0.291	57.13	39.88	29.29	44.52	62.25	59.17	22.4	24.45	21.42
Colombia	16.15	42.42	84.14	43.77	38.89	34.44	0.023	0.046	0.079	58.44	46.49	37.37	8.166	13.91	17.97	17.72	19.92	20.81
Argentina	30.51	49.85	84.84	52.55	45.86	41	0.03	0.04	0.059	56.95	41.21	31.68	3.739	4.858	4.563	9.034	9.281	7.842
Peru	6.841	15.53	33.81	28.73	24.87	22.25	0.015	0.028	0.056	60.14	45.16	35.79	4.193	8.509	10.7	15.08	19.19	18.26
Venezuela	5.098	13.71	29.88	24.19	21.4	20.01	0.017	0.031	0.053	74.36	55.33	44.79	7.524	13.03	14.34	27.57	31.67	28.66
Ecuador	3.043	7.275	15.76	23.56	21.72	20.45	0.008	0.016	0.03	66.68	56.36	49.67	1.599	2.451	2.843	11.74	11.78	10.84
Chile	5.387	12.79	22.64	25.13	22.3	19.67	0.01	0.016	0.022	48.82	33.87	23.99	2.236	3.068	2.899	12.49	13.05	11.46
Bolivia	2.94	5.55	11.43	46.87	39.96	36.08	0.007	0.01	0.019	99.19	73.88	59.84	1.859	3.854	4.92	20.07	26.09	25.89
Paraguay	0.987	2.287	4.722	21.57	19.74	17.4	0.004	0.008	0.014	85.77	69.5	55.6	0.831	1.232	1.53	13.49	13	13.49
Uruguay	2.222	3.045	4.667	33.29	28.66	25.56	0.003	0.002	0.002	45.12	26.7	15.65	0.322	0.409	0.369	8.332	9.024	7.502
Guyana	0.124	0.218	0.271	19.37	18.07	15.61	0.001	0.001	0.001	106.9	91.26	72.54	0.154	0.18	0.209	21.09	22.46	26.94
Suriname	0.095	0.164	0.271	24.57	20.74	17.73	0	0.001	0.001	105	81.23	63.07	0.125	0.153	0.118	28.29	29.66	24.2
America-South	**160.4**	**348.8**	**669.5**	**41.81**	**35.62**	**31.44**	**0.222**	**0.382**	**0.627**	**60.32**	**44.46**	**34.5**	**75.27**	**113.9**	**119.6**	**19.15**	**21.29**	**19.41**

Health

Base Case: Countries in Year 2060 Descending Population Sequence	Deaths and Death Rates from Noncommunicable Diseases												Deaths and Death Rates from Injuries					
	Respiratory Conditions						Other Noncommunicable Diseases						Road Traffic Accidents					
	Annual Deaths (in thousands)			Age Standardized Death Rates per 100,000			Annual Deaths (in thousands)			Age Standardized Death Rates per 100,000			Annual Deaths (in thousands)			Age Standardized Death Rates per 100,000		
	2010	2035	2060	2010	2035	2060	2010	2035	2060	2010	2035	2060	2010	2035	2060	2010	2035	2060
ASIA with OCEANIA																		
China	1572	3334	5895	113.3	91.69	77.13	0.37	0.437	0.436	27.07	15.3	9.041	354.2	677.2	569.8	24.54	41.2	35.35
Japan	70.65	133.8	160.6	15.56	14.52	13.57	0.08	0.13	0.141	21.89	17.16	13.37	9.542	8.752	6.879	5.09	4.126	3.309
Korea, Repub of	17.42	50.3	86.06	26.2	25.2	23.64	0.025	0.05	0.057	39.9	30.7	22.83	7.454	10.1	9.021	12.59	11.01	9.301
Taiwan	45.24	99.86	146.2	173.6	150.2	131.2	0.029	0.063	0.09	112.3	92.82	77.32	1.283	1.174	0.945	5.551	4.626	3.667
Korea, Dem. People's Rep.	17.71	29.51	41.54	74.57	71.76	65.89	0.017	0.024	0.03	70.64	62.86	54.08	2.69	3.698	4.462	11.18	11.63	12.2
Hong Kong SAR	17.79	36.98	52.05	129.1	118.4	109.1	0.011	0.023	0.032	82.64	73.53	64.91	0.047	0.041	0.036	0.827	0.643	0.501
Mongolia	0.447	0.971	2.015	28.9	24.84	21.17	0.001	0.001	0.001	32.87	21.21	13.25	1.189	1.992	2.172	44.29	57.21	61.58
Asia-East	**1741**	**3685**	**6384**	**103**	**85.16**	**72.77**	**0.534**	**0.729**	**0.787**	**29.25**	**18.13**	**11.78**	**376.4**	**702.9**	**593.3**	**22.04**	**36.59**	**31.76**
India	725.8	1319	2114	92.72	75.84	61.02	0.44	0.553	0.596	49.95	32.8	17.77	221	587.1	823.3	20.84	37.33	41.68
Pakistan	59.9	132.9	260.8	63.38	59.8	51.1	0.06	0.092	0.115	41.69	35.85	23.56	14.22	26.65	58.16	10.74	10.47	13.24
Bangladesh	58.76	117.1	211.3	72.17	58.34	53.21	0.043	0.067	0.095	45.63	33.81	24.92	18.19	32.81	56.96	14.35	15.96	20.61
Afghanistan	12.79	19	34.55	80.95	63.95	47.51	0.034	0.037	0.042	160	108.4	59.81	11.84	33.46	83.88	31.49	46.9	75.9
Iran (Islamic Republic of)	18.95	40.07	101.4	41.94	34.88	33.07	0.023	0.032	0.064	45.07	28.99	23.36	31.44	64.81	79.52	49.93	60.53	54.06
Nepal	10.63	22.78	44.37	71.47	67.38	58.44	0.01	0.018	0.029	55	49.56	39.55	2.54	3.955	6.756	10.86	9.732	10.7
Uzbekistan	3.762	7.623	13.99	21.19	18.4	16.81	0.009	0.012	0.016	42.26	29.94	23.27	4.46	8.481	10.66	16.88	22.88	27.02
Sri Lanka	12.89	28.46	40.46	62.05	54.96	49.49	0.012	0.022	0.029	55.71	44.12	34.82	1.062	1.835	2.174	4.922	5.774	6.037
Kazakhstan	6.371	9.44	14.16	44.12	36.85	36.8	0.004	0.003	0.004	29.92	15.04	13.14	3.12	3.631	2.625	20.23	23.68	19.94
Tajikistan	1.366	3.063	6.681	38.41	36.46	33.57	0.002	0.003	0.005	44.14	37.4	30.85	0.422	0.872	1.585	7.071	8.49	11.81
Turkmenistan	1.094	2.173	5.236	33.33	25.39	25.58	0.001	0.001	0.002	32.47	15.66	12.7	0.521	0.735	0.694	10.41	10.51	8.259
Kyrgyzstan	3.122	5.801	10.66	83.45	75.81	71.67	0.002	0.002	0.002	35.17	25.39	20.43	0.874	1.134	1.155	16.81	15.53	14.49
Bhutan	0.275	0.523	1.036	63.39	52.56	41.55	0	0	0	36.06	21.95	11.26	0.116	0.316	0.467	18.9	32.08	31.86
Maldives	0.085	0.19	0.575	53.29	44.08	37.56	0	0	0	68.21	50.01	32.86	0.055	0.124	0.19	20.25	22.92	22.14
Asia-South Central	**915.8**	**1708**	**2860**	**82.74**	**68.33**	**56.05**	**0.64**	**0.843**	**0.999**	**50.56**	**35.72**	**22.06**	**309.9**	**765.9**	**1128**	**20.16**	**31.78**	**35.84**
Indonesia	106.8	243.3	441.1	64.29	60.3	56.43	0.097	0.18	0.267	55.11	45.38	36.96	32.3	46.76	51.18	14.98	14.18	12.2
Philippines	30.08	77.82	168.9	64.64	60.36	55.12	0.036	0.074	0.128	65.22	57.05	46.62	5.997	11.45	19.05	8.259	8.906	9.854
Viet Nam	51.07	108.2	220.9	69.25	62.99	57.79	0.027	0.043	0.06	36.47	26.39	18.93	10.55	21	35.29	12.16	16.86	22.72
Thailand	43.44	94.02	132.2	67.59	63.23	57.82	0.072	0.124	0.142	108.7	88.62	69.47	20.56	23	21.47	30.12	31.59	31.57
Myanmar	27.56	49.74	73.4	68.21	56.99	50.12	0.027	0.036	0.048	60.65	44.39	36.79	7.031	9.975	12.72	14.06	14.37	15.32
Malaysia	10.68	32.64	68.49	65.07	57.74	52.52	0.012	0.025	0.041	61.74	48.03	37.46	3.033	4.596	4.948	11.95	11.45	9.664
Cambodia	5.695	12.34	25.98	78.4	70.44	61	0.009	0.014	0.023	97.64	75.02	55.15	2.481	4.556	6.256	17.29	20.36	20.86
LAO People's Dem Repub	2.951	5.853	13.7	99.3	81.33	72.47	0.002	0.006	0.009	34.06	29.27	24.91	0.917	2.141	3.379	17.43	22.36	23.88
Singapore	1.093	3.696	6.366	18.05	16.78	15.7	0.002	0.006	0.009	34.06	29.27	24.91	0.212	0.274	0.264	3.972	3.102	2.418
Timor-Leste	0.432	1.092	2.675	82.78	82.62	78.65	0.001	0.001	0.002	66.28	55.55	47.58	0.176	0.422	0.848	17.98	18.39	18.63
Brunei Darussalam	0.118	0.522	1.223	63.49	63.58	57.36	0.001	0.001	0.001	96.93	87.2	79.29	0.048	0.069	0.071	13.13	10.95	8.926
Asia-South East	**279.9**	**629.3**	**1155**	**66.29**	**60.98**	**56.09**	**0.285**	**0.506**	**0.725**	**61.51**	**49.42**	**39.28**	**83.3**	**124.2**	**155.5**	**15**	**15.49**	**15.68**

Health

	Deaths and Death Rates from Noncommunicable Diseases												Deaths and Death Rates from Injuries					
	Respiratory Conditions						Other Noncommunicable Diseases						Road Traffic Accidents					
Base Case: Countries in Year 2060 Descending Population Sequence	Annual Deaths (in thousands)			Age Standardized Death Rates per 100,000			Annual Deaths (in thousands)			Age Standardized Death Rates per 100,000			Annual Deaths (in thousands)			Age Standardized Death Rates per 100,000		
	2010	2035	2060	2010	2035	2060	2010	2035	2060	2010	2035	2060	2010	2035	2060	2010	2035	2060
ASIA with OCEANIA continued																		
Turkey	43.43	92.12	189.5	79.34	68.32	61	0.02	0.03	0.043	33.28	23.57	17.32	6.961	11.35	12.65	9.594	11.08	10.05
Yemen	5.048	10.83	26.59	53.27	46.36	41.15	0.013	0.02	0.039	97.24	75.36	59.88	9.235	20.4	34.15	44.53	49.04	50.04
Iraq	5.355	11.35	29.26	44.02	36.72	31.88	0.011	0.016	0.033	68.3	48.7	37.31	10.26	26.62	43.17	46.86	63.37	58.99
Saudi Arabia	2.316	8.269	19.36	22.55	20.93	18.47	0.012	0.034	0.075	98.3	84.35	73.14	4.609	7.248	7.714	19.19	17.98	15.15
Syrian Arab Repub	3.076	8.508	22.54	33.57	30.47	26.84	0.013	0.03	0.067	123.1	103.2	82.76	1.759	3.579	6.672	10.69	10.88	12.38
Israel	2.174	4.255	7.895	18.71	16.1	14.03	0.007	0.012	0.02	63.5	48.28	36.37	0.317	0.393	0.389	4.207	3.654	3.001
Jordan	0.751	1.784	4.262	24.51	21.11	17.21	0.002	0.004	0.008	61.74	45.82	31.73	1.123	2.324	3.387	22.9	25.52	24.66
Occupied Palestinian Territory	0.372	0.932	2.483	22.7	19.84	16.8	0.002	0.003	0.006	69.98	54.39	41.82	0.367	0.712	1.255	15.58	12.43	9.635
Azerbaijan	1.504	2.722	5.429	19.7	14.82	14.57	0.003	0.004	0.005	36.41	22.58	18.68	0.549	0.97	0.805	6.161	8.35	6.851
United Arab Emirates	0.203	1.601	4.247	16.65	13.05	12.07	0.001	0.006	0.02	64.34	57.09	47.43	1.095	2.345	4.216	27.13	24.36	19.21
Oman	0.226	0.957	2.294	20.82	20.16	17.7	0.001	0.004	0.008	88.52	77.76	62.99	0.2	0.36	0.643	8.892	8.341	7.142
Kuwait	0.125	0.864	2.387	13.68	12.83	11.88	0.001	0.004	0.01	66.99	57.23	53.75	0.392	0.711	0.822	16.85	13.59	10.57
Lebanon	1.349	2.494	4.741	40.89	34.95	30.97	0.002	0.003	0.005	65.25	48.69	37.77	1.257	1.89	2.214	35.02	32.55	26.46
Armenia	1.341	1.891	3.305	30.07	23.86	22.65	0.002	0.002	0.003	54.32	32.59	24.16	0.277	0.685	0.727	8.533	17.91	16.7
Georgia	0.588	0.595	0.69	9.799	8.308	7.873	0.001	0.001	0.001	22.87	17.86	13.64	0.429	0.493	0.385	8.926	11.73	10.63
Bahrain	0.12	0.615	1.57	40.34	38.56	33.74	0	0.002	0.004	130.7	114.3	94.53	0.063	0.096	0.07	9.464	6.756	4.657
Qatar	0.056	0.475	0.929	22.55	20.64	20.23	0	0.002	0.005	94.47	85.81	88.18	0.22	0.235	0.117	23.74	18.56	13.85
Cyprus	0.465	0.941	1.535	33.4	30.42	28.56	0	0	0	17.46	13.77	11.16	0.14	0.128	0.103	16.05	12.91	10.2
Asia-West	**68.5**	**151.2**	**329.1**	**48.42**	**40.71**	**35.44**	**0.092**	**0.177**	**0.352**	**65.88**	**55.11**	**46.02**	**39.25**	**80.54**	**119.5**	**20.42**	**25.89**	**26.3**
Australia	9.557	19.18	29.35	22.16	20.01	17.97	0.012	0.021	0.028	30	22.76	16.03	1.378	1.419	1.351	6.131	4.901	3.888
Papua New Guinea	2.494	5.702	11.6	91.99	79.15	72.16	0.003	0.004	0.007	74.18	57.32	47.27	1.021	2.008	2.891	20.2	21.47	20.18
New Zealand	2.167	4.129	5.86	27.7	24.84	22.24	0.002	0.003	0.004	32.33	24.41	16.17	0.411	0.383	0.317	9.374	7.55	5.961
Solomon Islands	0.188	0.384	0.848	68.1	62.06	57.94	0	0.001	0.001	123.7	109	94.04	0.04	0.071	0.119	8.361	8.388	9.296
Fiji	0.41	0.747	1.066	72.42	64.09	54.76	0.001	0.001	0.002	123.3	103.9	81.77	0.021	0.027	0.034	2.624	2.682	3.176
Vanuatu	0.079	0.16	0.343	62.77	52.17	44.51	0	0	0.001	106.6	85.83	67.54	0.013	0.027	0.045	6.301	7.282	8.601
Micronesia, Federated States of	0.046	0.103	0.211	65.14	65.07	55.2	0	0	0	114.4	97.78	78.48	0.007	0.012	0.02	6.39	6.244	6.9
Tonga	0.052	0.099	0.183	59.57	59.81	48.98	0	0	0	99.05	88.16	71.93	0.005	0.009	0.019	4.924	5.029	6.715
Samoa	0.069	0.112	0.19	55.41	50.29	43.43	0.001	0.001	0.001	95.74	77.9	61.63	0.009	0.016	0.021	5.877	7.308	7.624
Oceania	**15.06**	**30.62**	**49.65**	**39**	**37.27**	**35.24**	**0.019**	**0.032**	**0.044**	**44.07**	**36.21**	**28.82**	**2.907**	**3.972**	**4.817**	**9.174**	**9.197**	**8.66**

Health

Base Case: Countries in Year 2060 Descending Population Sequence	Deaths and Death Rates from Noncommunicable Diseases												Deaths and Death Rates from Injuries					
	Respiratory Conditions						Other Noncommunicable Diseases						Road Traffic Accidents					
	Annual Deaths (in thousands)			Age Standardized Death Rates per 100,000			Annual Deaths (in thousands)			Age Standardized Death Rates per 100,000			Annual Deaths (in thousands)			Age Standardized Death Rates per 100,000		
	2010	2035	2060	2010	2035	2060	2010	2035	2060	2010	2035	2060	2010	2035	2060	2010	2035	2060
EUROPE																		
Russian Federation	49.44	61.86	74.88	22.68	19.94	19.52	0.034	0.023	0.022	21.61	12.27	9.661	36.5	31.22	21.26	23.46	23.25	19.22
Poland	10.74	16.83	21.26	16.08	14.64	13.81	0.016	0.02	0.024	26.95	19.34	15.45	5.839	5.382	3.957	13.2	12.01	9.76
Ukraine	22.74	23.48	25.45	27.87	25.16	23.59	0.012	0.007	0.004	24.75	16.14	11.36	8.271	7.049	4.716	16.5	18.4	16.31
Romania	8.463	11	15.51	22.45	20.38	18.89	0.006	0.005	0.006	20.77	14.96	11.84	2.421	2.39	1.864	9.838	10.04	8.792
Czech Republic	2.479	3.571	4.245	12.77	11.92	11.08	0.003	0.004	0.005	18.33	13.92	10.95	0.854	0.704	0.512	7.37	6.344	5.254
Belarus	4.566	5.67	7.861	29.13	25.59	25.18	0.002	0.002	0.002	21.69	12.14	8.608	2.174	2.213	1.578	19.88	22.27	18.76
Hungary	4.428	5.189	5.893	23.02	20.67	19	0.005	0.005	0.005	27.82	19.39	14.28	1.352	1.1	0.772	11.75	10.61	8.834
Bulgaria	1.81	1.976	2.179	11.9	10.84	9.838	0.003	0.003	0.003	26.53	20.85	16.41	0.808	0.593	0.406	9.757	8.968	7.424
Slovak Republic	1.244	1.963	2.684	15.14	13.66	13.07	0.002	0.002	0.003	25.2	18.42	15.2	0.732	0.691	0.536	11.94	10.86	9.13
Moldova, Repub of	2.235	2.841	3.359	41.17	39.78	37.41	0.001	0.001	0.001	30.98	25.85	19.32	0.647	0.52	0.437	14.31	12.36	12.6
Europe-East	**108.2**	**134.4**	**163.3**	**22.33**	**19.84**	**18.97**	**0.085**	**0.073**	**0.074**	**23.16**	**14.81**	**11.45**	**59.6**	**51.86**	**36.04**	**18.27**	**18.18**	**15.22**
United Kingdom	46.97	71.31	99.77	31.88	27.77	24.72	0.035	0.044	0.049	25.52	17.05	10.7	3.019	2.735	2.384	4.623	3.776	3.039
Sweden	3.53	5.289	6.819	14.87	13.28	12.02	0.006	0.007	0.006	23.72	15.61	9.783	0.441	0.405	0.35	4.259	3.511	2.851
Denmark	4.203	6.136	6.829	36	32.65	28.87	0.004	0.005	0.004	34.07	23.97	15.05	0.397	0.38	0.336	6.694	5.596	4.593
Ireland	2.275	4.785	8.609	30.92	28.5	26.64	0.002	0.003	0.005	29.09	20.88	16.29	0.222	0.245	0.239	4.708	3.925	3.219
Norway	2.132	3.655	4.751	20.65	19.43	17.66	0.003	0.004	0.005	23.89	18.27	12.73	0.218	0.225	0.206	4.002	3.267	2.64
Finland	1.497	2.52	2.845	12.2	11.42	10.37	0.002	0.001	0	16.98	7.639	2.612	0.333	0.32	0.263	5.142	4.236	3.433
Lithuania	1.232	1.552	2.029	19.32	17.59	16.35	0.001	0.001	0.001	24.18	16.21	11.55	0.785	0.635	0.44	20.55	18.37	14.8
Latvia	0.398	0.467	0.583	8.788	8.047	7.475	0.001	0.001	0.001	23.43	14.91	11.06	0.433	0.355	0.247	16.76	15.54	12.59
Estonia	0.331	0.39	0.446	12.31	11.32	10.6	0.001	0.001	0.001	27.1	17.54	12.72	0.155	0.112	0.076	10.72	9.394	7.566
Iceland	0.102	0.208	0.336	17.51	15.81	14.11	0	0	0	16.68	10.24	5.232	0.018	0.019	0.017	5.055	4.002	3.159
Europe-North	**62.67**	**96.31**	**133**	**27.59**	**24.58**	**22.17**	**0.054**	**0.066**	**0.073**	**25.35**	**16.98**	**10.89**	**6.02**	**5.431**	**4.557**	**5.618**	**4.57**	**3.599**
Italy	30.58	46.51	63.33	15.95	15.39	14.62	0.045	0.057	0.063	28.67	22.69	18.04	6.088	4.876	3.491	9.601	7.746	6.161
Spain	36.4	56.72	89.43	29.66	28.17	26.7	0.034	0.044	0.057	31.11	23.37	17.67	4.193	3.581	2.663	8.58	7.062	5.704
Greece	5.405	8.833	13.75	19.48	17.98	16.81	0.004	0.006	0.007	18.83	14.57	11.67	1.716	1.444	1.13	13.26	10.94	8.897
Portugal	6.793	10.14	14.47	25.32	23.61	21.97	0.01	0.013	0.016	43.11	34.56	27.73	1.602	1.401	1.078	13.29	11.35	9.295
Serbia	2.822	3.551	4.333	21.32	19.56	17.54	0.004	0.004	0.005	37.15	29.65	22.94	0.541	0.496	0.401	6.603	6.266	5.672
Bosnia and Herzegovina	1.17	1.776	2.448	18.18	15.24	13.39	0.002	0.002	0.002	28.43	20.54	15.95	0.13	0.216	0.201	2.627	3.866	3.858
Croatia	1.491	2.049	2.388	15.08	14	12.92	0.002	0.002	0.002	25.51	18.79	14.46	0.547	0.471	0.354	12.01	11.09	9.223
Albania	0.662	1.261	2.026	17.8	15.42	13.87	0.001	0.001	0.001	30.14	20.33	14.44	0.238	0.361	0.374	7.022	8.455	8.038
Macedonia, FYR	0.704	1.149	1.569	24	22.08	19.84	0.001	0.002	0.002	44.37	36.81	30.15	0.097	0.103	0.092	4.092	3.872	3.721
Slovenia	0.739	1.354	1.77	16.09	15.62	14.63	0.001	0.002	0.002	28.21	20.97	16.57	0.219	0.193	0.148	9.471	7.924	6.409
Montenegro	0.2	0.283	0.364	20.78	18.49	16.1	0.001	0	0	36.44	27.04	19.08	0.05	0.054	0.049	7.46	7.892	7.372
Malta	0.149	0.311	0.403	17.99	17.98	16.99	0	0.001	0.001	40.77	34.06	28.07	0.009	0.007	0.005	1.977	1.485	1.114
Europe-South	**87.11**	**133.9**	**196.3**	**21.42**	**20.33**	**19.12**	**0.106**	**0.134**	**0.159**	**30.31**	**23.47**	**18.31**	**15.43**	**13.2**	**9.988**	**9.407**	**7.903**	**6.475**
Germany	38.24	59.47	75.28	17.51	16.52	14.88	0.058	0.081	0.097	28.28	21.46	15.24	5.017	4.096	3.122	5.596	4.524	3.617
France	22.21	35.97	48.85	13.11	12.22	11.24	0.047	0.062	0.065	29.8	21.81	14.18	4.42	3.943	3.202	6.861	5.578	4.471
Netherlands	8.097	15.43	19.45	22.41	21.64	19.84	0.012	0.018	0.019	34.93	27	18.55	0.784	0.798	0.679	4.23	3.446	2.781
Belgium	8.035	12.36	16.01	29.63	28.08	25.48	0.006	0.008	0.008	24.67	17.82	11.33	1.14	0.992	0.788	9.991	8.098	6.5
Austria	3.344	5.454	7.373	16.5	15.55	14.28	0.007	0.01	0.012	38.45	30.62	23.47	0.664	0.578	0.46	7.187	5.892	4.767
Switzerland	2.667	4.841	6.281	13.57	12.97	11.85	0.004	0.006	0.005	23.46	16.41	10.23	0.407	0.375	0.308	4.887	3.988	3.214
Luxembourg	0.227	0.441	0.68	23.38	22.88	21.79	0	0	0	18.72	14.75	11.79	0.028	0.031	0.031	4.971	3.868	3.008
Europe-West	**82.82**	**134**	**173.9**	**16.99**	**16.02**	**14.57**	**0.134**	**0.185**	**0.207**	**29.4**	**22.06**	**15.08**	**12.46**	**10.81**	**8.591**	**6.18**	**5.027**	**4.041**

Multination Regional Analysis

Measures of Poverty, Health, Education, Infrastructure, and Governance

Base Case
Source: International Futures
Version 6.32, June 2010

Health

Deaths and Death Rates from Injuries

| | Other Unintentionl Injuries | | | | | | Intentional Injuries | | | | | |
| | Annual Deaths (in thousands) | | | Age Standardized Death Rates per 100,000 | | | Annual Deaths (in thousands) | | | Age Standardized Death Rates per 100,000 | | |
	2010	2035	2060	2010	2035	2060	2010	2035	2060	2010	2035	2060
World	2428	2955	4122	35.93	28.13	23.77	1508	2139	2909	22.72	23.63	27.51
Africa	362.5	519.4	738.2	37.03	33.64	30.84	321.9	543.2	872.7	37.91	36.58	37.63
Americas	186.1	265.8	413.7	17.72	14.25	11.57	232.6	332.2	420.1	24.34	29.14	37.25
Asia with Oceania	1532	1837	2580	40.05	30.06	23.66	772.4	1071	1418	15.03	17.98	20.27
Europe	343.3	327.3	383.5	34.23	23.2	20.6	178.3	189.1	195.7	20.66	23.44	29.45
World	2428	2955	4122	35.93	28.13	23.77	1508	2139	2909	22.72	23.63	27.51
Africa-Eastern	124.1	177.1	223.6	39.64	34.09	27.18	97.84	161.9	251.1	37.6	32.8	30.11
Africa-Middle	65.02	110.1	192.7	52.45	52.97	55.4	62.76	143.6	283	65.36	74.43	83.54
Africa-Northern	38.65	46.32	64.75	19.66	15.41	12.54	46.23	62.22	88.34	24.37	22.73	25.18
Africa-Southern	14.69	14.84	16.37	28.93	22.95	15.7	38.1	53.58	65.42	70.66	79.96	93.59
Africa-Western	120	171	240.8	41.34	35.6	31.43	76.95	121.9	184.8	30.88	26.45	23.86
Africa	362.5	519.4	738.2	37.03	33.64	30.84	321.9	543.2	872.7	37.91	36.58	37.63
America-Caribbean	11.56	18.56	29.66	27.03	26.24	24.95	8.738	12.93	15.62	22.3	26.11	29.52
America-Central	8.254	12.93	21.5	21.73	18.97	15.85	15.42	27.22	38.72	37.71	42.07	50.59
America-North	89.41	132.7	204.6	14.97	12.03	9.527	61.63	93.25	126.6	12.93	16.68	22.5
America-South	76.87	101.6	157.9	19.5	14.89	11.87	146.8	198.8	239.2	36.05	41.44	52.43
Americas	186.1	265.8	413.7	17.72	14.25	11.57	232.6	332.2	420.1	24.34	29.14	37.25
Asia-East	458.5	472.2	662.1	27.45	15.71	10.28	307.2	438.9	514.3	17.58	17.69	19.62
Asia-South Central	808.2	1000	1413	54.55	41.47	31.72	338.8	439.1	624.9	21.64	18.64	20.96
Asia-South East	212.6	290	389.5	39.66	33.65	28.54	89.45	124.9	162.5	15.89	15.44	17.24
Asia-West	44.65	61.9	95.2	22.33	18.55	15.98	32.24	61.41	106.5	18.21	20.78	24.43
Oceania	7.54	12.48	20.27	19.4	17.91	16.03	4.662	6.897	9.659	14.32	16.03	19.01
Asia with Oceania	1532	1837	2580	40.05	30.06	23.66	772.4	1071	1418	19.03	17.98	20.27
Europe-East	240.4	173	157.2	67.28	45.32	43.91	125	123.7	121.8	35.59	43.16	57.99
Europe-North	25.65	34.96	49.52	15.04	11.65	9.035	12.26	14.6	16.92	10.85	12.67	15.79
Europe-South	33.25	46.97	67.25	10.95	9.555	8.404	14.75	17.33	18.2	7.508	8.719	10.61
Europe-West	48.72	78.01	115.6	11.71	10.57	8.957	28.8	36.34	41.44	11.55	13.8	16.89
Europe	343.3	327.3	383.5	34.23	23.2	20.6	178.3	189.1	195.7	20.66	23.44	29.45

Education

Literacy

| | Percent of Population 15 and Older | | | |
	2010	2035	2060	% Chg
World	83.33	92.4	97.61	17.1%
Africa	66.61	85.87	95.77	43.8%
Americas	95.28	98.97	99.83	4.8%
Asia with Oceania	81.85	92.1	97.68	19.3%
Europe	99.37	99.92	100	0.6%
World	83.33	92.4	97.61	17.1%
Africa-Eastern	66.98	88.33	96.98	44.8%
Africa-Middle	66	84.23	94.4	43.0%
Africa-Northern	71.33	90.33	99.33	39.3%
Africa-Southern	88.84	98.17	99.97	12.5%
Africa-Western	59.03	80.11	93.42	58.3%
Africa	66.61	85.87	95.77	43.8%
America-Caribbean	86.9	92.79	97	11.6%
America-Central	83.09	93.37	99.36	19.6%
America-North	98.35	99.59	100	1.7%
America-South	93.95	99.64	100	6.4%
Americas	95.28	98.97	99.83	4.8%
Asia-East	94.31	99.01	99.92	5.9%
Asia-South Central	65.89	84.52	95.44	44.8%
Asia-South East	93.34	98.77	99.83	7.0%
Asia-West	84.58	93.7	99.19	17.3%
Oceania	91.64	94.88	97.8	6.7%
Asia with Oceania	81.85	92.1	97.68	19.3%
Europe-East	99.63	100	100	0.4%
Europe-North	100	100	100	0.0%
Europe-South	98.27	99.67	99.99	1.8%
Europe-West	100	100	100	0.0%
Europe	99.37	99.92	100	0.6%

Health

Deaths and Death Rates from Injuries

Education

Base Case: Countries in Year 2060 Descending Population Sequence	Other Unintentional Injuries — Annual Deaths (in thousands)			Other Unintentional Injuries — Age Standardized Death Rates per 100,000			Intentional Injuries — Annual Deaths (in thousands)			Intentional Injuries — Age Standardized Death Rates per 100,000			Literacy — Percent of Population 15 and Older			
	2010	2035	2060	2010	2035	2060	2010	2035	2060	2010	2035	2060	2010	2035	2060	% Chg
AFRICA																
Ethiopia	25.57	39.45	51.2	34.45	31.6	24.68	20.39	34.45	43.14	31.97	28.19	20.19	40.76	69.93	90.75	122.6%
Tanzania, United Rep	13.23	16.42	19.98	31.16	24.08	17.49	9.082	12.85	22.58	25.69	19.29	19.38	84.34	100	100	18.6%
Uganda	14.76	19.81	19.94	41.31	32.4	20.61	16.02	28.27	54.83	59.29	49.44	52	77.71	97.85	100	28.7%
Kenya	13.95	19.02	22.45	35.41	30.1	22.45	9.168	15.27	23.64	28.13	25.08	23.92	80.02	95.39	100	25.0%
Madagascar	7.103	11.9	16.74	33.82	31.59	27.82	3.724	6.694	10.1	20.94	19.13	16.94	73.87	96.01	100	35.4%
Mozambique	10.39	11.72	12.76	45.97	35.08	25.83	7.92	10.61	13.83	42.13	32.08	26.38	49.76	79.39	95.29	91.5%
Malawi	4.613	9.047	14.12	36.39	36.64	34.43	2.842	6.122	10.91	28.3	26.98	26.29	79.68	100	100	25.5%
Zambia	6.2	8.106	9.718	44.66	36.19	28.52	4.105	7.084	11.53	35.7	32.49	32.14	82.69	90.88	98.5	19.1%
Somalia	8.261	12.48	17.95	79.51	68.41	61.75	5.579	9.947	16.89	75.84	69.8	66.3	63.45	84.96	100	57.6%
Rwanda	5.015	6.56	7.237	50.85	42.89	29.86	4.802	8.007	9.908	55.07	51.25	39.72	70.26	100	100	42.3%
Zimbabwe	9.096	12.38	14.47	67.42	63.27	56.96	8.149	11.96	15.64	64.26	60.82	62.27	94.51	100	100	5.8%
Burundi	3.195	5.397	8.951	38.96	39.5	41.12	4.183	7.153	12.05	58.98	57.25	56.97	67.63	95.84	100	47.9%
Eritrea	2.033	3.899	7.011	46.52	46.44	47.14	1.525	2.988	5.442	40.44	38.37	38.02	52.04	72.48	87.65	68.4%
Comoros	0.162	0.293	0.442	25.18	25.01	23.08	0.087	0.17	0.265	15.07	15.37	14.18	75.27	85.97	98.22	30.5%
Mauritius	0.194	0.211	0.26	15.17	10.9	7.908	0.166	0.201	0.231	12.36	14.21	17.32	89.06	97.49	100	12.3%
Djibouti	0.346	0.379	0.342	42.86	36.29	25.82	0.1	0.118	0.127	11.77	10.94	10.29	54.22	70.85	89.07	64.3%
Africa-Eastern	**124.1**	**177.1**	**223.6**	**39.64**	**34.09**	**27.18**	**97.84**	**161.9**	**251.1**	**37.6**	**32.8**	**30.11**	**66.98**	**88.33**	**96.98**	**44.8%**
Congo, Democratic Republic of	38.51	75.24	142.7	58.4	65.52	69.83	42.79	105.5	219	85.08	101.3	110.1	68.99	84.61	96.73	40.2%
Angola	8.514	9.047	13.1	49.43	32.26	28.56	7.199	15.97	29.23	45.67	51.07	61.68	70.42	100	100	42.0%
Cameroon	7.763	10.13	12.03	42.08	35.9	28.86	4.798	7.144	10.45	28.52	25.65	25.27	69.82	80.89	90.76	30.0%
Chad	4.862	8.337	14.86	42.28	39.9	39.14	2.61	5.48	9.887	29.18	29.71	28.19	29.59	62.98	79.69	169.3%
Central African Republic	2.3	3.362	4.456	53.1	51.79	46.34	3.003	5.135	7.161	77.95	81.88	74.39	49.85	65.87	79.71	59.9%
Congo, Republic of	2.043	2.535	3.526	46.66	38.13	35.16	1.641	2.822	4.558	42.39	42.09	46.39	85.71	98.09	100	16.7%
Gabon	0.691	0.961	1.378	46.46	41.93	40.21	0.501	1.067	1.767	33.98	45.8	59.81	85.08	93.33	100	17.5%
Equatorial Guinea	0.29	0.356	0.474	53.32	41.96	41.08	0.202	0.514	0.896	40.53	58.38	79.71	87.48	99.76	100	14.3%
São Tomé and Príncipe	0.054	0.093	0.147	32.67	32.1	29.78	0.013	0.027	0.046	9.542	9.784	9.486	89.26	100	100	12.0%
Africa-Middle	**65.02**	**110.1**	**192.7**	**52.45**	**52.97**	**55.4**	**62.76**	**143.6**	**283**	**63.36**	**74.43**	**83.54**	**66**	**84.23**	**94.4**	**43.0%**
Egypt	10.16	11.07	13.91	13.42	9.872	6.848	2.165	3.393	4.401	2.885	2.92	3.261	74.97	94	100	33.4%
Sudan	14.92	15	16.18	33.86	23.89	18.98	37.43	47.91	66.77	101	79.18	78.24	66.76	85.82	100	49.8%
Algeria	5.627	9.015	17.64	19.43	17.1	16.1	4.729	7.98	13.12	14.58	15.98	18.94	76.53	90.9	99.11	29.5%
Morocco	5.533	7.67	10.72	19.42	16.49	13.35	1.183	1.786	2.396	3.847	4.149	4.603	56.39	85.75	96.24	70.7%
Tunisia	1.41	1.938	3.15	14.45	10.98	8.608	0.386	0.571	0.828	3.678	3.821	4.367	79.35	90.78	99.25	25.1%
Libyan Arab Jamahiriya	0.997	1.632	3.146	20.48	15.24	14.61	0.33	0.581	0.826	5.688	5.992	7.289	87.18	95.23	100	14.7%
Africa-Northern	**38.65**	**46.32**	**64.75**	**19.66**	**15.41**	**12.54**	**46.23**	**62.22**	**88.34**	**24.37**	**22.73**	**25.18**	**71.33**	**90.33**	**99.33**	**39.3%**

Health

Deaths and Death Rates from Injuries

Base Case: Countries in Year 2060 Descending Population Sequence	Other Unintentionl Injuries						Intentional Injuries					
	Annual Deaths (in thousands)			Age Standardized Death Rates per 100,000			Annual Deaths (in thousands)			Age Standardized Death Rates per 100,000		
	2010	2035	2060	2010	2035	2060	2010	2035	2060	2010	2035	2060
AFRICA continued												
South Africa	11.18	10.89	11.3	25.26	19.45	12.51	34.96	48.74	58.74	74.12	85.64	101.7
Namibia	0.533	0.767	1.283	28.81	24.08	18	0.635	1.221	1.967	33.42	36.58	40.42
Lesotho	1.246	1.313	1.345	69.05	58.6	46.35	0.991	1.194	1.332	56.41	50.98	46.92
Botswana	0.856	0.817	1.364	49.96	32.39	25.63	0.775	1.172	1.665	41.87	47.29	58.29
Swaziland	0.87	1.05	1.08	81.21	67.39	48.66	0.737	1.255	1.709	67.76	75.57	84.37
Africa-Southern	**14.69**	**14.84**	**16.37**	**28.93**	**22.95**	**15.7**	**38.1**	**53.58**	**65.42**	**70.66**	**79.96**	**93.59**
Nigeria	71.53	91.09	126.2	47.4	38.15	34.44	45.77	66.33	100.2	35.26	28.65	27.33
Niger	5.019	10.19	18.81	34.35	33.76	33.03	2.526	5.162	9.663	22.07	19.61	17.53
Côte d'Ivoire	5.894	9.167	13.55	31.48	28.6	24.88	5.588	10.22	16.57	35.11	33.7	30.45
Ghana	8.904	13.6	16.98	38.41	36.43	30.54	5.179	8.532	11.66	24.5	23.69	21.27
Mali	6.182	9.79	13.22	42.28	37.75	31.57	3.196	4.576	7.146	25.77	20.01	16.95
Burkina Faso	5.351	8.955	11.7	37.56	35.25	28.47	2.863	5.612	8.193	23.71	22.82	18.82
Senegal	4.681	7.44	9.542	40.95	37.56	30.44	3.543	6.08	8.955	34.35	30.86	26.92
Guinea	3.177	5.072	7.218	30.99	28.21	24.38	1.805	3.245	5.1	21.07	19.29	17.16
Benin	2.125	3.676	5.514	22.53	21.35	19.21	0.944	1.738	2.934	12.67	11.44	10.51
Togo	1.308	2.31	4.039	20.29	20.05	20.11	0.631	1.172	2.084	11.34	10.97	10.98
Sierra Leone	2.473	4.128	5.322	53.34	55.06	43.95	2.024	3.751	4.577	42.13	43.2	32.69
Liberia	0.614	1.12	1.633	18.27	20.99	18.12	1.356	3.093	4.027	53.61	60.77	46.42
Mauritania	1.197	2.069	3.145	40.44	39.88	37.62	0.709	1.14	1.672	25.07	23.02	20.71
Guinea-Bissau	0.82	1.388	2.436	45.27	41.85	41.69	0.425	0.605	1.037	23.54	21.91	20.23
Gambia	0.598	0.913	1.238	40.01	36.02	30.95	0.327	0.538	0.828	24.58	21.43	19.46
Cape Verde	0.11	0.142	0.233	23.87	19.85	15.06	0.064	0.092	0.173	13.56	11.97	15.39
Africa-Western	**120**	**171**	**240.8**	**41.34**	**35.6**	**31.43**	**76.95**	**121.9**	**184.8**	**30.88**	**26.45**	**23.86**

Education

Literacy

Base Case: Countries in Year 2060 Descending Population Sequence	Percent of Population 15 and Older			
	2010	2035	2060	% Chg
AFRICA continued				
South Africa	89.4	98.48	100	11.9%
Namibia	88.48	97.93	100	13.0%
Lesotho	85.26	100	100	17.3%
Botswana	83.12	94.18	100	20.3%
Swaziland	81.39	91.55	98.94	21.6%
Africa-Southern	**88.84**	**98.17**	**99.97**	**12.5%**
Nigeria	74.13	89.12	98.81	33.3%
Niger	23.55	59.72	82.03	248.3%
Côte d'Ivoire	50.7	76.03	92.69	82.8%
Ghana	66.01	79.28	92.05	39.4%
Mali	32.97	68.24	89.77	172.3%
Burkina Faso	27.5	66.37	87.13	216.8%
Senegal	44.75	72.83	91.01	103.4%
Guinea	33.9	72.68	86.49	155.1%
Benin	43.58	73.29	88.79	103.7%
Togo	60.04	78.8	92.48	54.0%
Sierra Leone	37.4	57.05	78.52	109.9%
Liberia	54.5	78.26	94.7	73.8%
Mauritania	58.01	92.39	100	72.4%
Guinea-Bissau	72.33	100	100	38.3%
Gambia	31.59	75.19	87.85	178.1%
Cape Verde	88.91	100	100	12.5%
Africa-Western	**59.03**	**80.11**	**93.42**	**58.3%**

Health

Education

Base Case: Countries in Year 2060 Descending Population Sequence	Deaths and Death Rates from Injuries												Literacy			
	Other Unintentional Injuries						Intentional Injuries						Percent of Population 15 and Older			
	Annual Deaths (in thousands)			Age Standardized Death Rates per 100,000			Annual Deaths (in thousands)			Age Standardized Death Rates per 100,000						
	2010	2035	2060	2010	2035	2060	2010	2035	2060	2010	2035	2060	2010	2035	2060	% Chg
AMERICAS																
Haiti	5.152	7.45	9.613	58.89	56.81	50.07	2.006	3.447	4.458	24.84	26.75	24.06	60.82	77.72	91.73	50.8%
Dominican Republic	1.559	1.699	2.63	17.13	11.17	8.315	1.591	2.347	3.115	17.09	18.68	22.78	90.77	100	100	10.2%
Cuba	3.372	7.433	14.52	19.55	17.52	15.54	2.112	2.691	2.81	15.52	17.53	20.68	100	100	100	0.0%
Puerto Rico	0.729	0.981	1.343	13.8	9.823	7.171	0.747	0.989	1.243	18.13	23.28	31.66	94.67	98.09	100	5.6%
Jamaica	0.45	0.588	0.846	15.76	14.05	11.47	1.894	2.952	3.433	71.44	90.73	115.7	87.06	94.17	100	14.9%
Trinidad	0.15	0.204	0.408	11.58	7.555	6.519	0.251	0.304	0.318	17.44	20.4	25.96	99.72	100	100	0.3%
Bahamas	0.073	0.112	0.182	22.04	17.34	13.02	0.06	0.09	0.109	17.3	22.08	29.08	95.32	99.19	100	4.9%
Barbados	0.014	0.02	0.021	4.671	3.855	2.812	0.021	0.028	0.03	6.475	7.885	9.645	100	100	100	0.0%
Grenada	0.019	0.027	0.044	16.7	15.84	12.52	0.003	0.006	0.009	3.081	3.528	4.034	90.19	99.35	100	10.9%
Saint Vincent and Grenadines	0.02	0.02	0.018	16.65	11.69	7.887	0.014	0.022	0.029	11.86	13.07	15.42	88.39	96.67	100	13.1%
Saint Lucia	0.023	0.026	0.033	13.63	11.15	8.768	0.039	0.055	0.064	23.6	27.16	33.13	92.27	98.64	100	8.4%
America-Caribbean	**11.56**	**18.56**	**29.66**	**27.03**	**26.24**	**24.95**	**8.738**	**12.93**	**15.62**	**22.3**	**26.11**	**29.52**	**86.9**	**92.79**	**97**	**11.6%**
Guatemala	3.682	6.075	9.899	32.98	27.64	22.13	5.907	12.64	20.65	47.04	52.13	61.82	75.94	90.99	99.6	31.2%
Honduras	1.171	1.489	2.134	14.9	12.35	9.991	1.771	2.594	3.987	24.53	21.24	25.55	85.12	95.27	100	17.5%
El Salvador	0.962	1.365	1.974	13.56	11.77	9.264	4.753	7.654	8.682	65.08	82.36	100.1	82.14	93.83	100	21.7%
Nicaragua	1.062	1.583	2.281	20.94	18.72	16.35	1.604	2.22	2.783	28.97	26.36	28.13	80.97	89.88	96.16	18.8%
Costa Rica	0.808	1.748	4.115	17.65	14.78	12.62	0.658	0.984	1.165	13.98	15.92	19.44	97.77	100	100	2.3%
Panama	0.515	0.593	0.943	15.29	9.755	6.947	0.681	1.039	1.308	19.84	23.93	32.21	94.11	98.56	100	6.3%
Belize	0.053	0.078	0.155	18.79	15.09	11.13	0.046	0.094	0.144	17.08	19.59	22.7	78.82	91.47	98.99	25.6%
America-Central	**8.254**	**12.93**	**21.5**	**21.73**	**18.97**	**15.85**	**15.42**	**27.22**	**38.72**	**37.71**	**42.07**	**50.59**	**83.09**	**93.37**	**99.36**	**19.6%**
USA	66.25	96.61	144.3	15.16	12.02	9.406	43.8	66.24	93.08	13.26	17.25	23.45	100	100	100	0.0%
Mexico	15.88	22.61	38.36	15.24	12.42	10.11	13.46	21.03	25.7	12.42	15.61	20.4	93.13	98.3	100	7.4%
Canada	7.277	13.49	21.94	12.38	10.77	8.883	4.38	5.974	7.783	11.59	14.83	19.67	100	100	100	0.0%
America-North	**89.41**	**132.7**	**204.6**	**14.97**	**12.03**	**9.527**	**61.63**	**93.25**	**126.6**	**12.93**	**16.68**	**22.5**	**98.35**	**99.59**	**100**	**1.7%**
Brazil	33.84	45.15	74.22	17.35	12.67	9.574	76.07	92.91	107.1	37.19	41.63	52.36	92.71	100	100	7.9%
Colombia	6.969	9.606	13.46	15.16	12.55	9.935	41.02	60.67	72.51	83.63	98.68	124	95.09	100	100	5.2%
Argentina	8.254	9.664	14.47	17.74	12.18	9.435	6.137	8.803	11.62	14.72	17.58	23.17	98.44	100	100	1.6%
Peru	9.209	11.27	16.22	32.68	23.57	18.04	1.239	1.999	2.637	4.3	4.769	5.842	89.5	95.59	100	11.7%
Venezuela	4.443	6.791	13.02	17.02	12.75	10.74	12.21	18.47	24	41.8	49.27	66.33	95.37	100	100	4.9%
Ecuador	3.645	5.73	8.526	27.08	25.12	24.61	3.955	6.931	9.695	28.13	36	50.14	94.94	100	100	5.3%
Chile	2.767	4.411	7.294	14.35	10.9	8.508	2.724	3.714	4.539	15.27	18.09	23.27	97.74	100	100	2.3%
Bolivia	4.706	5.294	6.357	48.29	36.44	29.15	0.666	1.113	1.544	7.007	7.412	8.941	92.52	100	100	8.1%
Paraguay	2	2.491	2.67	31.11	26.29	20.04	1.748	3	4.012	27.71	31.76	39.06	96.29	100	100	3.9%
Uruguay	0.806	0.905	1.357	16.78	11.02	7.978	0.611	0.781	0.981	15.43	16.92	20.36	99.22	100	100	0.8%
Guyana	0.145	0.165	0.205	20.22	18.05	14.95	0.252	0.254	0.265	34.68	33.39	39.76	98.66	100	100	1.4%
Suriname	0.083	0.095	0.124	19.68	14.82	11.6	0.149	0.194	0.212	33.59	39.18	47.25	90.54	97.35	100	10.4%
America-South	**76.87**	**101.6**	**157.9**	**19.5**	**14.89**	**11.87**	**146.8**	**198.8**	**239.2**	**36.05**	**41.44**	**52.43**	**93.95**	**99.64**	**100**	**6.4%**

Multinational Regional Analysis

Measures of Poverty, Health, Education, Infrastructure, and Governance

Health

Deaths and Death Rates from Injuries

Education

Base Case: Countries in Year 2060 Descending Population Sequence	Other Unintentional Injuries – Annual Deaths (in thousands)			Other Unintentional Injuries – Age Standardized Death Rates per 100,000			Intentional Injuries – Annual Deaths (in thousands)			Intentional Injuries – Age Standardized Death Rates per 100,000			Literacy – Percent of Population 15 and Older			
	2010	2035	2060	2010	2035	2060	2010	2035	2060	2010	2035	2060	2010	2035	2060	% Chg
ASIA with OCEANIA																
China	404.8	383.7	550.1	30.05	16.51	10.48	257.6	377.9	453.1	17.76	17.55	19.31	93.76	99.09	100	6.7%
Japan	37.85	62.49	75.37	12.02	10.13	8.6	30.91	33.66	31.86	17.97	21.32	26.41	100	100	100	0.0%
Korea, Repub of	9.533	18.52	27.82	15.48	13.06	10.98	13.12	21.04	22.48	21.44	24.8	29.28	100	100	100	0.0%
Taiwan	0.761	0.549	0.313	3.085	1.893	1.042	0.777	0.921	1.03	3.018	3.658	4.694	97.92	100	100	2.1%
Korea, Dem. People's Rep.	4.846	6.286	7.84	21.22	19.64	17.93	4.089	4.711	4.904	16.58	16.13	16.81	76.9	86.1	94.6	23.0%
Hong Kong SAR	0.098	0.1	0.084	1.443	1.216	0.903	0.178	0.224	0.269	2.375	3.276	4.344	100	100	100	0.0%
Mongolia	0.586	0.618	0.521	22.95	17.13	11.66	0.485	0.519	0.685	17.94	14.3	19.21	100	100	100	0.0%
Asia-East	**458.5**	**472.2**	**662.1**	**27.45**	**15.71**	**10.28**	**307.2**	**438.9**	**514.3**	**17.58**	**17.69**	**19.62**	**94.31**	**99.01**	**99.92**	**5.9%**
India	620.2	734.4	1020	61.07	45.21	33.38	256.1	313.5	455.4	23.68	19.87	24.33	67.2	86.2	96.63	43.8%
Pakistan	52.39	92.52	158.9	39.23	37.31	32.31	19.83	37.16	59.79	14.93	14.72	13.64	52.06	77.13	92.12	76.9%
Bangladesh	54.37	80.9	120.1	45.84	40.57	35.59	26.62	36.69	43.53	19.69	17.62	15.82	56.18	80.47	92.65	64.9%
Afghanistan	15.76	18.01	15.27	38.74	26.71	15.74	5.96	8.682	13.62	19.11	14.68	13.13	28.7	63.06	89.67	212.4%
Iran (Islamic Republic of)	13.61	16.42	33	22.05	15.89	14.65	5.117	7.161	9.323	6.955	7.295	8.697	85.67	94.01	100	16.7%
Nepal	7.259	12.04	18.47	31.25	30.64	27.59	7.771	14.03	17.89	31.33	33.32	29.22	55.96	76.38	91.79	64.0%
Uzbekistan	6.565	6.973	6.691	24.52	19.25	15.4	3.123	3.717	4.168	11.55	9.717	10.59	97.32	100	100	2.8%
Sri Lanka	21.47	25.78	25.84	104.7	87.44	68.35	4.948	6.484	7.285	23.05	24.98	29.11	93.6	98.72	100	6.8%
Kazakhstan	11.13	6.938	6.797	71.87	39.15	38.88	6.688	7.531	8.465	42.78	47.54	64	100	100	100	0.0%
Tajikistan	1.606	2.213	2.642	23.54	21.69	19	0.608	1.084	1.439	10.23	10.56	10.77	99.94	100	100	0.1%
Turkmenistan	1.514	0.877	1.393	29.37	12.16	10.44	1.01	1.526	2.181	19.88	21.36	28.06	100	100	100	0.0%
Kyrgyzstan	1.918	2.65	2.884	38.34	35.45	32.23	0.877	1.145	1.323	17.23	15.09	15.17	99.63	100	100	0.4%
Bhutan	0.315	0.382	0.674	53.7	39.09	28.46	0.14	0.217	0.319	21.42	22.23	23.81	54.34	75.72	91.79	68.9%
Maldives	0.153	0.203	0.33	51.19	41.44	30.87	0.043	0.094	0.153	16.82	17.07	17.58	98.11	100	100	1.9%
Asia-South Central	**808.2**	**1000**	**1413**	**54.55**	**41.47**	**31.72**	**338.8**	**439.1**	**624.9**	**21.64**	**18.64**	**20.96**	**65.89**	**84.52**	**95.44**	**44.8%**
Indonesia	133.4	182	241.4	63.31	55.55	48.68	28.02	39.18	52.31	12.77	11.92	13.18	93.15	100	100	7.4%
Philippines	8.259	12.01	17.74	10.79	9.487	7.985	12.65	20.21	29.57	15.91	15.79	19.27	93.54	96.75	100	6.9%
Viet Nam	19.48	29.56	48.73	23.97	20.54	17.6	9.661	13.59	19.98	11.37	9.941	10.72	95.27	100	100	5.0%
Thailand	26.04	31.4	32.36	38.7	33.3	26.57	16.88	21.49	23.16	24.01	28.14	33.7	95.23	100	100	5.0%
Myanmar	16.69	22.59	30.23	34.57	30.73	28.27	13.56	16.06	16.89	25.73	22.82	21.46	95.69	100	100	4.5%
Malaysia	3.013	4.553	6.959	12.76	10.05	8.078	3.443	6.134	8.57	13.6	15.49	18.8	93.25	98.99	100	7.2%
Cambodia	2.449	2.886	3.792	16.75	13.74	11.24	3.141	4.712	6.009	22.55	20.89	20.07	76.63	88.71	98.77	28.9%
LAO People's Dem Repub	2.444	3.379	5.438	38.38	39.56	32.3	1.208	1.848	3.094	22.96	19.78	21.42	74.71	87.16	95.41	27.7%
Singapore	0.327	0.721	1.112	6.031	5.344	4.582	0.574	1.06	1.587	10.34	12.28	14.89	95.53	99.76	100	4.7%
Timor-Leste	0.473	0.921	1.638	46.82	41.8	38.23	0.299	0.63	1.276	30.09	27.52	27.67	73.88	83.56	92.52	25.2%
Brunei Darussalam	0.037	0.055	0.078	9.778	8.582	8.528	0.009	0.015	0.021	2.076	3.003	4.438	94.66	97.82	100	5.6%
Asia-South East	**212.6**	**290**	**389.5**	**39.66**	**33.65**	**28.54**	**89.45**	**124.9**	**162.5**	**15.89**	**15.44**	**17.24**	**93.34**	**98.77**	**99.83**	**7.0%**

Multination Regional Analysis

Measures of Poverty, Health, Education, Infrastructure, and Governance

Health

Deaths and Death Rates from Injuries

Education

Base Case: Countries in Year 2060 Descending Population Sequence	Other Unintentionl Injuries						Intentional Injuries						Literacy			
	Annual Deaths (in thousands)			Age Standardized Death Rates per 100,000			Annual Deaths (in thousands)			Age Standardized Death Rates per 100,000			Percent of Population 15 and Older			
	2010	2035	2060	2010	2035	2060	2010	2035	2060	2010	2035	2060	2010	2035	2060	% Chg
ASIA with OCEANIA continued																
Turkey	11.59	16.64	28.49	17.75	14.11	11.73	3.848	5.185	6.741	5.054	5.621	6.968	89.46	95.56	100	11.8%
Yemen	8.837	12.58	16.94	37.91	30.54	25.28	2.586	4.382	7.399	12.68	10.63	10.75	59.51	84.51	96.9	62.8%
Iraq	7.572	9.419	15.56	32.94	24.14	19.03	19.88	41.71	76.8	95.92	97.55	107	78.66	94.13	100	27.1%
Saudi Arabia	6.679	8.292	9.553	27.77	20.47	17.74	1.837	3.034	4.627	6.873	7.899	10.38	84.05	91.81	98.99	17.8%
Syriar Arab Repub	3.032	5.792	10.73	19.63	18.52	16.21	0.436	0.938	1.501	2.341	2.776	3.299	84.13	92.83	98.91	17.6%
Israel	1.022	1.758	3.317	10.24	7.79	6.209	0.902	1.591	2.331	12.02	14.65	19.2	96.48	100	100	3.6%
Jordan	0.97	1.306	2.155	18.68	14.99	9.616	0.389	0.672	0.897	6.62	7.222	8.478	93.66	100	100	6.8%
Occupied Palestinian Territory	0.886	1.416	1.935	25.9	21.65	15.72	0.72	1.799	3.623	27.33	28.08	29.96	95.72	100	100	4.5%
Azerbaijan	1.241	1.011	1.12	13.87	8.229	7.272	0.358	0.472	0.59	3.951	4.083	5.059	100	100	100	0.0%
United Arab Emirates	0.222	0.46	0.297	5.722	4.035	3.271	0.09	0.117	0.08	1.547	1.418	1.5	94.06	100	100	6.3%
Oman	0.28	0.392	0.66	11.89	8.947	6.85	0.088	0.147	0.232	2.953	3.613	4.897	84.32	96.35	100	18.6%
Kuwait	0.235	0.378	0.697	9.286	6.962	8.655	0.081	0.112	0.162	2.431	2.979	3.965	95.5	100	100	4.7%
Lebanon	0.902	1.232	1.899	25.26	20.38	16.72	0.393	0.598	0.825	10.49	11.96	14.46	81.55	91.69	99.2	21.6%
Armenia	0.547	0.501	0.775	15.2	8.625	6.331	0.155	0.177	0.21	4.655	4.647	5.486	99.67	100	100	0.3%
Georgia	0.463	0.412	0.412	8.738	6.805	5.556	0.371	0.353	0.337	7.524	8.331	9.858	79.28	97.84	100	26.1%
Bahrain	0.091	0.118	0.146	12.18	9.657	6.763	0.03	0.04	0.05	3.267	3.831	4.902	88.81	95.38	100	12.6%
Qatar	0.036	0.146	0.45	7.883	7.608	8.464	0.07	0.084	0.078	5.924	7.814	9.343	89.7	93.1	98.2	9.5%
Cyprus	0.041	0.053	0.062	4.171	3.377	2.781	0.005	0.007	0.008	0.568	0.692	0.884	97.71	99.25	100	2.3%
Asia-West	44.65	61.9	95.2	22.33	18.55	15.98	32.24	61.41	106.5	18.21	20.78	24.43	84.58	93.7	99.19	17.3%
Australia	3.979	7.029	11.92	11.87	9.814	7.551	2.31	3.356	4.668	10.06	12.63	16.74	100	100	100	0.0%
Papua New Guinea	2.361	3.626	5.599	48.06	41.3	37.51	1.742	2.669	3.856	32.74	27.95	27.04	60.23	80.82	92.97	54.4%
New Zealand	0.767	1.287	2.191	12.08	10.1	7.492	0.533	0.733	0.908	11.89	14.95	19.62	100	100	100	0.0%
Solomon Islands	0.156	0.213	0.254	27.3	23.63	19.83	0.025	0.048	0.081	6.21	6.109	6.035	70.46	78.95	88.38	25.4%
Fiji	0.172	0.185	0.157	20.72	18.3	13.07	0.028	0.045	0.061	4.057	4.28	4.511	97.34	100	100	2.7%
Vanuatu	0.04	0.053	0.058	17.5	14.41	10.38	0.008	0.017	0.032	4.892	5.055	5.339	79.85	91.45	99.11	24.1%
Micronesia, Federated States of	0.025	0.035	0.038	20.1	17.89	13.17	0.005	0.01	0.019	5.285	5.633	6.139	84.49	90.08	96.72	14.5%
Tonga	0.016	0.026	0.032	14.46	14.32	11.03	0.004	0.008	0.016	4.442	4.898	5.24	100	100	100	0.0%
Samoa	0.025	0.025	0.023	14.7	11.25	7.45	0.006	0.01	0.017	4.501	4.704	4.982	100	100	100	0.0%
Oceania	7.54	12.48	20.27	19.4	17.91	16.03	4.662	6.897	9.659	14.32	16.03	19.01	91.64	94.88	97.8	6.7%

Health

Education

Base Case: Countries in Year 2060 Descending Population Sequence	Other Unintentional Injuries — Annual Deaths (in thousands)			Other Unintentional Injuries — Age Standardized Death Rates per 100,000			Intentional Injuries — Annual Deaths (in thousands)			Intentional Injuries — Age Standardized Death Rates per 100,000			Literacy — Percent of Population 15 and Older			
	2010	2035	2060	2010	2035	2060	2010	2035	2060	2010	2035	2060	2010	2035	2060	% Chg
EUROPE																
Russian Federation	161.2	101.6	89.1	95.63	59.82	62.16	85.81	84.23	85.46	53.06	63.32	87.54	99.66	100	100	0.3%
Poland	11.36	14.42	18.74	21.06	16.33	14.18	6.913	7.528	6.977	15.29	17.99	23	99.74	100	100	0.3%
Ukraine	38.33	27.68	18.08	70.52	57.77	49.03	17.15	15.68	13.71	31.51	37.05	46.54	100	100	100	0.0%
Romania	6.641	5.948	5.354	25.89	20.51	16.64	3.255	3.519	3.281	12.39	14.25	17.37	98.2	100	100	1.8%
Czech Republic	4.256	6.264	8.401	25.19	22.42	20.37	1.723	2.009	2.056	13.32	15.7	19.57	100	100	100	0.0%
Belarus	8.557	5.715	4.597	73.47	45.49	37.7	4.165	4.293	4.22	36.04	41.2	53.07	100	100	100	0.0%
Hungary	4.778	6.051	7.823	26.56	23.17	20.83	2.894	3.093	3.055	22.54	25.53	30.7	99.73	100	100	0.3%
Bulgaria	1.447	1.169	0.981	15.44	12.73	9.941	1.2	1.187	1.157	11.58	13.42	16.17	98.76	100	100	1.3%
Slovak Republic	1.305	1.518	1.846	18.6	14.57	15.07	0.841	0.981	0.922	12.91	14.8	18.43	100	100	100	0.0%
Moldova, Repub of	2.536	2.679	2.237	54.43	53.58	47.01	1.08	1.137	0.963	23.37	23.52	24.44	99.76	100	100	0.2%
Europe-East	**240.4**	**173**	**157.2**	**67.28**	**45.32**	**43.91**	**125**	**123.7**	**121.8**	**35.59**	**43.16**	**57.99**	**99.63**	**100**	**100**	**0.4%**
United Kingdom	11.44	17.14	27	9.49	7.909	6.44	5.221	6.449	7.905	7.641	9.324	12.04	100	100	100	0.0%
Sweden	2.665	4.188	6.156	12.44	10.5	8.854	1.263	1.523	1.752	11.14	13.17	16.36	100	100	100	0.0%
Denmark	1.761	2.764	3.926	16.81	14.31	11.53	0.803	1.023	1.24	11.65	13.89	17.26	100	100	100	0.0%
Ireland	0.5	0.845	1.472	8.23	6.585	5.865	0.406	0.578	0.743	8.811	11.18	15.28	100	100	100	0.0%
Norway	1.643	2.541	3.712	19.7	17.87	14.83	0.487	0.655	0.82	8.899	11.01	14.3	100	100	100	0.0%
Finland	2.684	3.604	4.077	29.7	23.67	17.82	1.052	1.25	1.453	17.24	21.27	27.75	100	100	100	0.0%
Lithuania	2.49	2.028	1.611	59.21	43.42	32.43	1.86	1.936	1.837	46.94	54.61	68.36	100	100	100	0.0%
Latvia	1.514	1.157	0.973	52.06	35.03	25.39	0.736	0.758	0.735	26.32	29.76	36.34	100	100	100	0.0%
Estonia	0.905	0.617	0.484	56.57	38.54	25.26	0.399	0.388	0.394	25.58	30.12	36.64	100	100	100	0.0%
Iceland	0.044	0.072	0.109	9.785	8.127	6.522	0.028	0.037	0.042	7.975	9.388	11.7	100	100	100	0.0%
Europe-North	**25.65**	**34.96**	**49.52**	**15.04**	**11.65**	**9.035**	**12.26**	**14.6**	**16.92**	**10.85**	**12.67**	**15.79**	**100**	**100**	**100**	**0.0%**
Italy	16.74	25.85	38.91	10.38	9.612	8.837	4.593	5.24	5.308	5.776	6.782	8.346	99.87	100	100	0.1%
Spain	8.021	10.67	15.42	10.19	8.619	7.492	4.123	4.94	5.363	7.156	8.522	10.73	98.31	100	100	1.7%
Greece	1.737	1.817	1.976	10.7	8.821	7.587	0.444	0.523	0.569	3.051	3.695	4.713	97.59	100	100	2.5%
Portugal	2.082	2.688	3.52	11.54	10.03	8.591	1.265	1.552	1.677	8.382	9.671	11.32	95.06	98.29	99.91	5.1%
Serbia	0.957	1.077	1.25	9.693	8.642	7.161	1.485	1.772	1.958	15.06	16.96	19.51	90.2	96.31	100	10.9%
Bosnia and Herzegovina	0.709	0.71	0.781	14.87	10.82	8.395	0.482	0.55	0.55	10.05	10.9	12.67	97.77	100	100	2.3%
Croatia	1.404	1.903	2.459	17.79	15.43	13.67	0.94	1.065	1.086	15.35	17.04	19.81	99.61	100	100	0.4%
Albania	0.537	0.558	0.579	16.05	12.23	9.584	0.255	0.306	0.326	7.712	8.537	10.37	100	100	100	0.0%
Macedonia, FYR	0.252	0.361	0.471	9.863	9.283	8.182	0.52	0.634	0.648	22.31	25.49	29.93	99.09	100	100	0.9%
Slovenia	0.643	1.065	1.528	16.61	14.24	12.51	0.501	0.563	0.499	18.49	20.52	24.11	100	100	100	0.0%
Montenegro	0.078	0.091	0.108	10.37	8.55	5.302	0.125	0.159	0.187	16.56	18.15	20.43	88.23	95.06	100	13.3%
Malta	0.092	0.184	0.256	12.61	11.44	10.38	0.019	0.024	0.024	3.706	4.332	5.229	92.39	96.85	100	8.2%
Europe-South	**33.25**	**46.97**	**67.25**	**10.95**	**9.555**	**8.404**	**14.75**	**17.33**	**18.2**	**7.508**	**8.719**	**10.61**	**98.27**	**99.67**	**99.99**	**1.8%**
Germany	16.34	25.33	37.25	9.086	7.919	5.494	11.66	14.38	15.94	9.99	11.91	14.48	100	100	100	0.0%
France	23.28	37.75	56.41	16.06	14.6	12.42	10.57	13.64	16.04	13.42	15.81	19.2	100	100	100	0.0%
Netherlands	2.789	5.198	7.826	8.471	7.76	5.598	1.658	2.085	2.452	8.376	10.31	12.87	100	100	100	0.0%
Belgium	2.423	3.467	4.864	11.69	10.3	8.264	2.037	2.467	2.831	15.48	18.49	22.91	100	100	100	0.0%
Austria	1.953	2.858	4.003	12.36	10.93	9.031	1.454	1.885	2.096	13.02	15.61	19.33	100	100	100	0.0%
Switzerland	1.812	3.167	4.882	10.82	9.577	8.064	1.359	1.792	1.952	13.24	15.98	19.77	100	100	100	0.0%
Luxembourg	0.134	0.235	0.389	16.09	15.3	15.38	0.055	0.09	0.121	8.593	10.06	12.13	100	100	100	0.0%
Europe-West	**48.72**	**78.01**	**115.6**	**11.71**	**10.57**	**8.957**	**28.8**	**36.34**	**41.44**	**11.55**	**13.8**	**16.89**	**100**	**100**	**100**	**0.0%**

Multination Regional Analysis

Measures of Poverty, Health, Education, Infrastructure, and Governance

Education

Base Case
Source: International Futures
Version 6.32, June 2010

	Years of Education, Female Adults (25+)				Years of Education, Male Adults (25+)				Primary Education Enrollment Rate, Net				Lower Secondary Enrollment Rate, Gross			
	Number of Years Completed				Number of Years Completed				Percent of Primary Age Children Enrolled				Total Enrolled as % of Nominal Age Population			
	2010	2035	2060	% Chg	2010	2035	2060	% Chg	2010	2035	2060	% Chg	2010	2035	2060	% Chg
World	5.727	7.584	9.729	69.9%	7.174	8.688	10.37	44.5%	89.19	96	98.64	10.6%	85.05	93.8	94.26	10.8%
Africa	3.17	4.949	7.273	129.4%	4.495	5.943	7.818	73.9%	73.3	86.53	95.49	30.3%	52.51	68.39	82.26	56.7%
Americas	8.727	10.97	13	49.0%	8.802	10.61	12.38	40.6%	95.95	99.45	99.79	4.0%	103.2	105.4	103.6	0.4%
Asia with Oceania	4.945	7.055	9.549	93.1%	6.928	8.622	10.57	52.6%	89.94	97.9	99.7	10.9%	85.6	98.71	96.88	13.2%
Europe	9.86	12.36	14.64	48.5%	10.17	12.81	14.91	46.6%	98.13	99.99	99.99	1.9%	103.6	102	101.3	-2.2%
World	5.727	7.584	9.729	69.9%	7.174	8.688	10.37	44.5%	89.19	96	98.64	10.6%	85.05	93.8	94.26	10.8%
Africa-Eastern	2.289	4.341	7.073	209.0%	3.293	4.883	7.11	115.9%	76.54	88.26	97.98	28.0%	40	62.01	87.58	119.0%
Africa-Middle	2.877	3.738	5.268	83.1%	4.763	5.553	7.062	48.3%	57.15	75.03	85.03	48.8%	32.52	52.15	62.45	92.0%
Africa-Northern	4.531	7.376	10.23	125.8%	6.302	8.553	10.75	70.6%	86.73	96.1	99.92	15.2%	89.07	100.8	103.4	16.1%
Africa-Southern	7.571	10.08	12.68	67.5%	8.092	10.93	13.7	69.3%	89.2	99.8	99.99	12.1%	95.77	98.87	99.92	4.3%
Africa-Western	2.468	4.259	6.826	176.6%	3.745	5.309	7.278	94.3%	64.3	83.06	95.73	48.9%	40.82	61.81	76.39	87.1%
Africa	3.17	4.949	7.273	129.4%	4.495	5.943	7.818	73.9%	73.3	86.53	95.49	30.3%	52.51	68.39	82.26	56.7%
America-Caribbean	6.589	7.933	9.504	44.2%	6.226	7.423	8.841	42.0%	84.36	92.88	95.46	13.2%	83.05	92.38	93.73	12.9%
America-Central	5.029	7.353	9.658	92.0%	5.166	7.037	8.974	73.7%	92.25	97.42	99.86	8.2%	74.52	86.85	96.99	30.2%
America-North	11.26	13.01	14.63	29.9%	11.36	12.62	13.95	22.8%	97.03	99.94	100	3.1%	103.6	100.5	100.6	-2.9%
America-South	6.456	9.511	12.04	86.5%	6.548	9.177	11.5	75.6%	96.28	99.84	99.98	3.8%	107.8	114.6	109	1.1%
Americas	8.727	10.97	13	49.0%	8.802	10.61	12.38	40.6%	95.95	99.45	99.79	4.0%	103.2	105.4	103.6	0.4%
Asia-East	5.835	8.121	10.77	84.6%	7.786	9.496	11.55	48.3%	91.56	99.93	99.98	9.2%	100.1	108.9	99.5	-0.6%
Asia-South Central	3.74	5.671	8.285	121.5%	6.304	7.916	9.93	57.5%	86.77	95.98	99.44	14.6%	73.15	93.53	94.79	29.6%
Asia-South East	5.566	8.097	10.31	85.2%	6.309	8.409	10.22	62.0%	95.52	98.84	99.88	4.6%	83.37	92.25	97.24	16.6%
Asia-West	5.594	8.212	10.92	95.2%	6.854	9.065	11.24	64.0%	88.15	99.19	99.98	13.4%	83.68	98.08	99.96	19.5%
Oceania	9.292	11.49	13.33	43.5%	9.829	11.68	13.08	33.1%	90.16	94.35	99.13	9.9%	92.88	87.23	91.94	-1.0%
Asia with Oceania	4.945	7.055	9.549	93.1%	6.928	8.622	10.57	52.6%	89.94	97.9	99.7	10.9%	85.6	98.71	96.88	13.2%
Europe-East	10.99	13.18	15.17	38.0%	10.86	13.54	15.54	43.1%	96.44	100	99.98	3.7%	97.46	103.2	102.2	4.9%
Europe-North	10.42	13.27	15.39	47.7%	10.65	13.22	15	40.8%	99.09	99.99	100	0.9%	103	99.15	99.99	-2.9%
Europe-South	7.693	10.7	13.39	74.1%	8.387	11.22	13.6	62.2%	99	99.98	100	1.0%	106.1	100.5	99.97	-5.8%
Europe-West	9.547	12.08	14.57	52.6%	10.31	12.88	15.11	46.6%	99.58	100	99.99	0.4%	111.3	103.2	101.9	-8.4%
Europe	9.86	12.36	14.64	48.5%	10.17	12.81	14.91	46.6%	98.13	99.99	99.99	1.9%	103.6	102	101.3	-2.2%

Education

Base Case: Countries in Year 2060 Descending Population Sequence	Years of Education, Female Adults (25+) Number of Years Completed				Years of Education, Male Adults (25+) Number of Years Completed				Primary Education Enrollment Rate, Net Percent of Primary Age Children Enrolled				Lower Secondary Enrollment Rate, Gross Total Enrolled as % of Nominal Age Population			
	2010	2035	2060	% Chg	2010	2035	2060	% Chg	2010	2035	2060	% Chg	2010	2035	2060	% Chg
AFRICA																
Ethiopia	0.65	2.114	5.359	724.5%	1.844	2.698	5.256	185.0%	61.54	78.61	97.98	59.2%	40.32	65.69	94.22	133.7%
Tanzania, United Rep	2.03	5.298	8.685	327.8%	3.3	6.236	9.253	180.4%	91.32	94.66	99.96	9.5%	12.98	41.5	78.79	507.0%
Uganda	3.661	6.238	9.316	154.5%	3.608	5.593	8.056	123.3%	88.73	97.39	100	12.7%	25.05	58.78	97.64	289.8%
Kenya	4.28	6.911	9.757	128.0%	5.495	7.489	9.778	77.9%	78.4	95.02	99.9	27.4%	92.47	101.5	111	20.0%
Madagascar	1.493	2.929	4.802	221.6%	2.646	3.629	5.211	96.9%	92.95	96.67	98.32	5.8%	31.43	47.84	59.6	89.6%
Mozambique	1.348	3.084	6.31	368.1%	1.902	3.916	6.754	255.1%	77.91	89.77	100	28.4%	23.17	52.6	96.17	315.1%
Malawi	2.507	4.603	6.36	153.7%	3.598	5.998	7.527	109.2%	90.36	95	97.32	7.7%	41.14	60.24	76.95	87.0%
Zambia	5.276	7.352	9.521	80.5%	5.865	6.343	7.572	29.1%	89.25	91.01	98.98	10.9%	50.16	59.37	82.25	64.0%
Somalia	1.363	2.963	5.032	269.2%	2.722	4.417	6.537	140.2%	13.62	57.92	76.19	459.4%	35.74	62.87	62.44	74.7%
Rwanda	1.961	3.011	5.62	186.6%	2.652	3.666	6.096	129.9%	81.76	92.27	98.85	20.9%	22.23	53.8	82.87	272.8%
Zimbabwe	5.301	8.391	9.664	82.3%	6.877	8.899	9.396	35.6%	88.77	91.26	96.86	9.1%	61.05	64.85	79.42	30.1%
Burundi	0.788	1.759	3.898	394.7%	1.986	3.059	4.94	143.7%	57.1	71.22	98.08	71.8%	21.07	36.7	58.99	180.0%
Eritrea	1.07	2.164	3.797	254.9%	2.389	3.564	4.876	104.1%	52.75	74.19	92.98	76.3%	49.1	69.21	85.3	73.7%
Comoros	2.051	2.831	4.671	127.7%	3.16	3.461	4.51	42.7%	57.22	74.84	88.06	53.9%	45.03	59.73	71.92	59.7%
Mauritius	5.676	7.949	10.75	89.4%	6.592	8.77	11.48	74.2%	97.12	99.98	99.98	2.9%	98.47	100.3	99.99	1.5%
Djibouti	3.003	3.821	6.755	124.9%	4.102	4.656	6.923	68.8%	39.46	77.36	99.97	153.3%	32.17	62.51	103.1	220.5%
Africa-Eastern	**2.289**	**4.341**	**7.073**	**209.0%**	**3.293**	**4.883**	**7.11**	**115.9%**	**76.54**	**88.26**	**97.98**	**28.0%**	**40**	**62.01**	**87.58**	**119.0%**
Congo, Democratic Republic of	2.172	2.962	4.189	92.9%	4.82	5.72	6.895	43.0%	56.41	67.55	80.07	41.9%	33.11	46.35	55.21	66.7%
Angola	4.67	6.073	9.454	102.4%	5.49	6.107	9.312	69.6%	38.36	95.81	100	160.7%	27.85	78.58	91.99	230.3%
Cameroon	3.143	4.511	6.523	107.5%	4.418	5.498	7.244	64.0%	73.86	84.59	97.5	32.0%	35.54	52.74	77.97	119.4%
Chad	2.51	3.021	4.545	81.1%	3.653	4.087	5.417	48.3%	62.32	72.17	81.18	30.3%	21.33	38.01	46.49	118.0%
Central African Republic	1.493	2.071	3.638	143.7%	3.072	3.467	4.585	49.3%	47.24	67.44	77.22	63.5%	18.24	38.2	54.01	196.1%
Congo, Republic of	4.99	5.826	8.051	61.3%	5.207	5.674	7.506	44.2%	56.25	81.55	96.15	70.9%	57.56	75.21	87.72	52.4%
Gabon	7.356	7.918	10.34	40.6%	8.055	8.278	10.42	29.4%	88.42	98.34	100	13.1%	66.14	86.79	93.49	41.4%
Equatorial Guinea	8.838	9.148	11.7	32.4%	9.249	8.476	10.37	12.1%	89.78	98.42	100	11.4%	47.72	90.66	96.42	102.1%
São Tomé and Príncipe	2.617	3.655	5.046	92.8%	3.503	3.75	4.725	34.9%	94.67	96.87	98.02	3.5%	72.04	80.26	89.2	23.8%
Africa-Middle	**2.877**	**3.738**	**5.268**	**83.1%**	**4.763**	**5.553**	**7.062**	**48.3%**	**57.15**	**75.03**	**85.03**	**48.8%**	**32.52**	**52.15**	**62.45**	**92.0%**
Egypt	5.382	9.258	12.22	127.1%	7.921	11.44	13.71	73.1%	97.18	99.99	100	2.9%	100.8	97.45	99.58	-1.2%
Sudan	1.887	3.909	7.413	292.8%	2.943	4.513	7.274	147.2%	45.45	83.58	100	120.0%	50.48	97.43	104.4	106.8%
Algeria	5.162	8.17	10.64	106.1%	6.936	8.992	10.99	57.3%	99.09	100	99.55	0.5%	111.5	118.3	114.1	2.3%
Morocco	4.628	5.989	8.411	81.7%	5.555	6.478	8.383	50.9%	91.87	98.96	99.93	8.8%	71.79	94.34	101.6	41.5%
Tunisia	4.703	8.371	11.64	147.5%	6.256	8.848	11.36	81.6%	99.98	100	99.97	0.0%	108.2	107.3	103.7	-4.2%
Libyan Arab Jamahiriya	6.127	10.11	12.66	106.6%	7.035	8.915	10.73	52.5%	98.33	99.98	100	1.7%	114.6	97.57	97.64	-14.8%
Africa-Northern	**4.531**	**7.376**	**10.23**	**125.8%**	**6.302**	**8.553**	**10.75**	**70.6%**	**86.73**	**96.1**	**99.92**	**15.2%**	**89.07**	**100.8**	**103.4**	**16.1%**

Education

Base Case: Countries in Year 2060 Descending Population Sequence	Years of Education, Female Adults (25+) Number of Years Completed				Years of Education, Male Adults (25+) Number of Years Completed				Primary Education Enrollment Rate, Net Percent of Primary Age Children Enrolled				Lower Secondary Enrollment Rate, Gross Total Enrolled as % of Nominal Age Population			
	2010	2035	2060	% Chg	2010	2035	2060	% Chg	2010	2035	2060	% Chg	2010	2035	2060	% Chg
AFRICA continued																
South Africa	7.828	10.49	13.13	67.7%	8.442	11.56	14.43	70.9%	89.97	99.99	99.99	11.1%	99.42	100.2	100.1	0.7%
Namibia	5.322	7.201	9.802	84.2%	6.12	7.313	9.783	59.9%	87.55	99.7	100	14.2%	77.82	95.49	102.9	32.2%
Lesotho	5.58	7.578	10.32	84.9%	4.427	6.599	9.103	105.6%	78.49	96.36	99.94	27.3%	49.71	75.06	91.76	84.6%
Botswana	6.222	8.899	11.32	81.9%	6.53	8.793	11.05	69.2%	87.77	100	100	13.9%	92.52	105.3	101.8	10.0%
Swaziland	6.588	8.253	11.14	69.1%	5.824	7.776	10.79	85.3%	80.27	98.92	100	24.6%	59.3	87.17	96.43	62.6%
Africa-Southern	**7.571**	**10.08**	**12.68**	**67.5%**	**8.092**	**10.93**	**13.7**	**69.3%**	**89.2**	**99.8**	**99.99**	**12.1%**	**95.77**	**98.87**	**99.92**	**4.3%**
Nigeria	2.96	5.353	8.353	182.2%	4.154	6.288	8.44	103.2%	67.68	87.34	97.21	43.6%	42.14	66.69	73.62	74.7%
Niger	0.737	1.802	3.971	438.8%	1.421	2.396	4.001	181.6%	44.2	65.78	81.6	84.6%	16.64	37.7	57.47	245.4%
Côte d'Ivoire	2.729	3.36	5.68	108.1%	3.971	4.97	7.535	89.8%	57.5	83.67	100	73.9%	32.8	52.66	84.31	157.0%
Ghana	3.596	5.563	8.076	124.6%	5.411	6.421	8.234	52.2%	67.11	86.1	98.01	46.0%	65.75	77.45	98.96	50.5%
Mali	0.636	2.472	5	686.2%	1.383	2.939	5.271	281.1%	61.4	78.23	99.27	61.7%	43.25	62.69	88.17	103.9%
Burkina Faso	1.881	2.858	5.492	192.0%	3.044	3.76	5.752	89.0%	46.13	69.98	96.04	108.2%	22.58	47.84	75.04	232.3%
Senegal	2.009	3.725	6.706	233.8%	3.03	3.995	6.53	115.5%	71.21	86.8	98.67	38.6%	33.53	57.07	84.08	150.8%
Guinea	1.942	2.899	4.748	144.5%	3.394	4.887	6.469	90.6%	69.54	76.48	88.9	27.8%	43.18	54.3	71.87	66.4%
Benin	1.521	3.16	5.271	246.5%	3.628	5.596	7.411	104.3%	78.02	88.44	96.13	23.2%	44.5	57.49	72.39	62.7%
Togo	2.079	3.806	5.79	178.5%	4.671	6.161	7.355	57.5%	78.53	91.89	98.85	25.9%	57.26	70.81	78.22	36.6%
Sierra Leone	1.664	2.605	5.026	202.0%	3.222	4.13	6.004	86.3%	46.99	67.68	95.2	102.6%	29.31	55.17	82.91	182.9%
Liberia	1.553	3.156	6.544	321.4%	3.272	4.898	7.98	143.9%	45.41	81.58	98.54	117.0%	38.5	81.37	96.95	151.8%
Mauritania	1.462	2.628	4.664	219.0%	2.584	3.708	5.486	112.3%	77.47	86.8	91.35	17.9%	30.65	45.93	54.81	78.8%
Guinea-Bissau	0.226	1.123	2.546	1026.5%	1.571	3.102	4.569	190.8%	47.22	65.6	90.37	91.4%	25.46	47.02	63.47	149.3%
Gambia	1.746	3.747	5.941	240.3%	3.572	5.237	6.736	88.6%	61.32	72.63	91.2	48.7%	59.15	68.11	96.17	62.6%
Cape Verde	4.299	7.217	9.681	125.2%	5.246	7.61	9.817	87.1%	93.55	99.99	99.69	6.6%	93.74	110.9	108.7	16.0%
Africa-Western	**2.468**	**4.259**	**6.826**	**176.6%**	**3.745**	**5.309**	**7.278**	**94.3%**	**64.3**	**83.06**	**95.73**	**48.9%**	**40.82**	**61.81**	**76.39**	**87.1%**

Education

Base Case: Countries in Year 2060 Descending Population Sequence	Years of Education, Female Adults (25+) Number of Years Completed				Years of Education, Male Adults (25+) Number of Years Completed				Primary Education Enrollment Rate, Net Percent of Primary Age Children Enrolled				Lower Secondary Enrollment Rate, Gross Total Enrolled as % of Nominal Age Population			
	2010	2035	2060	% Chg	2010	2035	2060	% Chg	2010	2035	2060	% Chg	2010	2035	2060	% Chg
AMERICAS																
Haiti	2.783	3.152	4.621	66.0%	2.642	3.014	4.301	62.8%	55.79	77.12	87.56	56.9%	44.81	67.42	78.78	75.8%
Dominican Republic	6.126	8.334	11.1	81.2%	5.435	7.081	9.568	75.0%	83.44	98.77	100	19.8%	80.72	104	103	27.6%
Cuba	8.612	10.92	13.13	52.5%	8.49	10.81	12.93	52.3%	99.45	100	99.88	0.4%	102.6	99.63	99.32	-3.2%
Puerto Rico	9.964	12.65	15.05	51.0%	9.242	11.77	13.88	50.2%	99.31	100	99.99	0.7%	105.6	98.24	99.68	-5.6%
Jamaica	6.359	8.295	9.961	56.6%	5.359	7.398	9.295	73.1%	91.6	99.58	100	9.2%	96.17	115.2	111.7	16.1%
Trinidad	8.422	10.49	13.02	54.6%	8.359	10.8	13.71	64.0%	92.85	100	99.92	7.6%	91.73	110.2	103	12.3%
Bahamas	8.679	10.88	13.06	50.5%	9.196	10.67	12.62	37.2%	93.73	99.99	100	6.7%	96.75	98.63	99.36	2.7%
Barbados	8.125	10.5	12.73	56.7%	8.858	11.01	13.03	46.9%	98.28	100	100	1.8%	105.7	97.53	98.85	-6.5%
Grenada	6.962	9.115	11.55	65.9%	7.646	9.1	11.3	47.8%	87.51	100	99.99	14.3%	106.8	117.9	113.1	5.9%
Saint Vincent and Grenadines	6.573	9.67	12.47	89.7%	7.442	10.13	12.53	68.4%	93.24	100	100	7.3%	89.32	99.89	100.7	12.7%
Saint Lucia	7.358	10.42	12.66	72.1%	8.06	10.56	12.55	55.7%	99.25	100	99.99	0.7%	90.61	89.14	100.5	10.9%
America-Caribbean	**6.589**	**7.933**	**9.504**	**44.2%**	**6.226**	**7.423**	**8.841**	**42.0%**	**84.36**	**92.88**	**95.46**	**13.2%**	**83.05**	**92.38**	**93.73**	**12.9%**
Guatemala	3.369	5.843	8.474	151.5%	4.337	6.642	8.697	97.8%	91.51	96.73	99.98	9.3%	58.38	74.89	92.84	59.0%
Honduras	4.895	8.397	10.85	121.7%	4.654	6.606	8.347	79.0%	92.13	97.16	99.88	8.4%	71.16	85.14	97.43	36.9%
El Salvador	5.199	6.984	9.503	82.8%	5.144	6.811	9.181	78.5%	93.43	98.54	100	7.0%	84.64	97.58	102.8	21.5%
Nicaragua	5.583	7.661	9.646	72.8%	4.623	6.306	8.125	75.8%	86	95.27	99.12	15.3%	77.45	94.13	98.6	27.3%
Costa Rica	6.645	9.254	11.54	73.7%	6.649	8.8	11.04	66.0%	95.61	100	100	4.6%	97.82	104.6	104.7	7.0%
Panama	8.64	10.62	12.24	41.7%	8.257	9.89	11.37	37.7%	98.4	99.99	100	1.6%	89.28	97.68	98.83	10.7%
Belize	6.402	8.267	10.47	63.5%	7.056	8.1	10.05	42.2%	95.73	99.99	100	4.5%	98.75	101.1	101.5	2.8%
America-Central	**5.029**	**7.353**	**9.658**	**92.0%**	**5.166**	**7.037**	**8.974**	**73.7%**	**92.25**	**97.42**	**99.86**	**8.2%**	**74.52**	**86.85**	**96.99**	**30.2%**
USA	12.62	14.16	15.52	23.0%	12.55	13.67	14.75	17.5%	96.04	99.92	100	4.1%	101.7	99.76	100.1	-1.6%
Mexico	7.168	9.454	11.51	60.6%	7.744	9.386	11.19	44.5%	99.34	100	100	0.7%	110	102.8	102.5	-6.8%
Canada	12.01	13.99	15.66	30.4%	12.31	13.49	14.7	22.4%	98.71	99.97	99.99	1.3%	100.9	99.31	100	-0.9%
America-North	**11.26**	**13.01**	**14.63**	**29.9%**	**11.36**	**12.62**	**13.95**	**22.8%**	**97.03**	**99.94**	**100**	**3.1%**	**103.6**	**100.5**	**100.6**	**-2.9%**
Brazil	5.485	8.989	12.06	119.9%	5.639	8.406	11.07	97.4%	97.13	99.95	100	3.0%	118	131.3	120.2	1.9%
Colombia	6.026	8.507	10.5	74.2%	5.611	8.182	10.29	83.4%	93.35	99.71	100	7.1%	94.76	94.64	95.54	0.8%
Argentina	9.467	11.88	13.74	45.1%	9.158	11.33	13.19	43.9%	99.09	99.99	100	0.9%	107.4	107.3	103	-4.1%
Peru	7.794	10.7	12.81	64.4%	8.822	11.14	12.98	47.1%	96.31	99.97	100	3.8%	106.4	103.5	102.3	-3.9%
Venezuela	6.38	9.208	11.3	77.1%	6.495	9.015	11.17	74.4%	94.94	100	100	5.3%	91.65	101.2	100.7	9.9%
Ecuador	7.113	9.059	10.52	47.9%	7.386	9.442	10.75	45.5%	96.36	98.23	99.54	3.3%	77.38	78.2	86.51	11.8%
Chile	8.815	11.74	14.07	59.6%	8.835	11.79	14.13	59.9%	91.08	100	100	9.8%	100.2	101.8	100.1	-0.1%
Bolivia	6.013	9.129	11.92	98.2%	6.95	9.624	12.13	74.5%	95.51	99.98	99.95	4.6%	95.81	102.4	101.4	5.8%
Paraguay	6.383	9.629	11.76	84.2%	6.507	9.136	11.06	70.0%	94.82	98.79	100	5.5%	84.39	91.65	97.78	15.9%
Uruguay	8.372	11.17	13.45	60.7%	7.881	10.93	13.47	70.9%	97.66	99.7	100	2.4%	105.6	99.98	101.7	-3.7%
Guyana	6.597	7.888	9.477	43.7%	6.517	8.407	10.23	57.0%	95.09	97.96	99.17	4.3%	114.9	80.74	91.68	-20.2%
Suriname	6.371	8.281	10.91	71.2%	6.893	7.45	9.715	40.9%	93.57	99.94	99.99	6.9%	97.31	111.2	106.3	9.2%
America-South	**6.456**	**9.511**	**12.04**	**86.5%**	**6.548**	**9.177**	**11.5**	**75.6%**	**96.28**	**99.84**	**99.98**	**3.8%**	**107.8**	**114.6**	**109**	**1.1%**

Education

Base Case: Countries in Year 2060 Descending Population Sequence	Years of Education, Female Adults (25+) Number of Years Completed				Years of Education, Male Adults (25+) Number of Years Completed				Primary Education Enrollment Rate, Net Percent of Primary Age Children Enrolled				Lower Secondary Enrollment Rate, Gross Total Enrolled as % of Nominal Age Population			
	2010	2035	2060	% Chg	2010	2035	2060	% Chg	2010	2035	2060	% Chg	2010	2035	2060	% Chg
ASIA with OCEANIA																
China	5.238	7.645	10.45	99.5%	7.338	9.102	11.28	53.7%	90.6	100	99.98	10.4%	100.4	110.6	99.45	-0.9%
Japan	10.03	12.24	14.24	42.0%	10.84	12.9	14.4	32.8%	99.67	99.99	100	0.3%	101.5	98.84	100	-1.5%
Korea, Repub of	10.05	11.27	12.59	25.3%	12.01	13.04	14.21	18.3%	98.55	99.96	99.95	1.4%	99.61	100	99.92	0.3%
Taiwan	8.991	11.98	14.46	60.8%	9.961	12.18	13.98	40.3%	98.23	100	100	1.8%	105.7	100.2	100.8	-4.6%
Korea, Dem. People's Rep.	4.265	5.74	7.701	80.6%	5.288	6.573	8.158	54.3%	79.46	95.45	99.55	25.3%	67.24	90.77	97.37	44.8%
Hong Kong SAR	8.983	9.586	11.66	29.8%	10.07	10.37	12.2	21.2%	95.83	100	99.99	4.3%	103.5	100.9	100	-3.4%
Mongolia	4.64	9.417	12.74	174.6%	5.615	9.478	12.23	117.8%	92.47	100	100	8.1%	102	101.1	100.1	-1.9%
Asia-East	**5.835**	**8.121**	**10.77**	**84.6%**	**7.786**	**9.496**	**11.55**	**48.3%**	**91.56**	**99.93**	**99.98**	**9.2%**	**100.1**	**108.9**	**99.5**	**-0.6%**
India	4.223	6.569	9.686	129.4%	7.195	9.405	12	66.8%	89.79	99.04	100	11.4%	76.71	102.1	99.89	30.2%
Pakistan	1.386	2.207	4.259	207.3%	3.37	3.289	4.669	38.5%	68.86	85.81	98.13	42.5%	42.88	58.87	75.67	76.5%
Bangladesh	1.989	3.872	6.095	206.4%	3.569	4.58	6.336	77.5%	89.83	93.97	98.55	9.7%	65.17	85.02	93.5	43.5%
Afghanistan	0.596	1.441	4.509	656.5%	1.704	2.44	4.724	177.2%	32.61	70.11	97.2	198.1%	29.08	61.38	83.16	186.0%
Iran (Islamic Republic of)	5.148	8.275	11.17	117.0%	7.371	10.72	13.1	77.7%	97.63	99.98	99.98	2.4%	95.03	102.5	101	6.3%
Nepal	1.274	2.049	4.262	234.5%	3.222	3.183	4.602	42.8%	80.73	93.5	98.76	22.3%	74.01	81.57	89.61	21.1%
Uzbekistan	3.672	5.949	8.191	123.1%	4.846	7.32	9.47	95.4%	83.32	100	99.97	20.0%	99.14	107.3	103	3.9%
Sri Lanka	6.805	9.223	11.82	73.7%	7.42	10.06	12.57	69.4%	99.55	100	99.99	0.4%	109.5	106.3	103.3	-5.7%
Kazakhstan	9.284	12.28	14.53	56.5%	10.06	13.09	15	49.1%	95.64	100	100	4.6%	100.5	102	100.2	-0.3%
Tajikistan	9.08	10.05	11.09	22.1%	10.78	12.44	13.38	24.1%	98.84	99.67	100	1.2%	95.63	97.5	99.58	4.1%
Turkmenistan	6.829	9.361	11.49	68.3%	7.707	10.19	12.29	59.5%	97.87	100	100	2.2%	99.05	102.3	101.5	2.5%
Kyrgyzstan	3.524	6.223	8.287	135.2%	4.6	7.088	8.83	92.0%	88.35	99.83	100	13.2%	92.5	100	98.84	6.9%
Bhutan	4.456	5.461	8.968	101.3%	5.407	6.11	9.39	73.7%	76.17	98.97	99.98	31.3%	61	89.57	98.35	61.2%
Maldives	4.693	5.895	8.714	85.7%	5.666	6.774	9.731	71.7%	98	100	99.94	2.0%	131.4	139.5	127.7	-2.8%
Asia-South Central	**3.74**	**5.671**	**8.285**	**121.5%**	**6.304**	**7.916**	**9.93**	**57.5%**	**86.77**	**95.98**	**99.44**	**14.6%**	**73.15**	**93.53**	**94.79**	**29.6%**
Indonesia	5.301	7.978	10.23	93.0%	6.525	8.859	10.61	62.6%	95.16	99.2	99.99	5.1%	81.19	92.45	98.09	20.8%
Philippines	8.361	9.849	11.17	33.6%	7.958	8.975	10.08	26.7%	92.55	97.08	100	8.0%	91.17	93.53	99.67	9.3%
Viet Nam	3.86	6.935	9.665	150.4%	4.945	8.115	10.67	115.8%	96.84	99.8	99.82	3.1%	87.93	102	101.3	15.2%
Thailand	6.654	9.382	12.07	81.4%	7.01	8.675	10.91	55.6%	96.52	100	99.95	3.6%	99.48	100.9	104.3	4.8%
Myanmar	2.964	5.719	8.186	176.2%	3.277	5.617	7.52	129.5%	98.35	99.52	99.86	1.5%	58.71	69.06	78.65	34.0%
Malaysia	8.262	11.47	14.14	71.1%	9.005	11.02	13.11	45.6%	99.94	100	99.99	0.1%	94.19	98.42	98.98	5.1%
Cambodia	2.575	3.698	5.872	128.0%	3.67	4.539	6.264	70.7%	96.1	96.43	99.26	3.3%	52.96	70.17	85.61	61.7%
LAO People's Dem Repub	3.363	5.434	7.935	136.0%	4.444	6.232	8.238	85.4%	84.73	93.79	99.2	17.1%	56.81	77.35	93.26	64.2%
Singapore	8.091	9.612	11.71	44.7%	9.247	10.75	12.6	36.3%	94.99	99.88	99.66	4.9%	81.21	97.07	99.11	22.0%
Timor-Leste	3.877	5.709	7.669	97.8%	4.869	6.256	7.684	57.8%	68.06	81.77	95.56	40.4%	71.03	77.79	85.59	20.5%
Brunei Darussalam	10.63	12.42	14.21	33.7%	10.9	11.85	13.39	22.8%	96.11	100	100	4.0%	111.4	99.32	98.07	-12.0%
Asia-South East	**5.566**	**8.097**	**10.31**	**85.2%**	**6.309**	**8.409**	**10.22**	**62.0%**	**95.52**	**98.84**	**99.88**	**4.6%**	**83.37**	**92.25**	**97.24**	**16.6%**

Multination Regional Analysis

Measures of Poverty, Health, Education, Infrastructure, and Governance

Education

Base Case: Countries in Year 2060 Descending Population Sequence	Years of Education, Female Adults (25+) Number of Years Completed				Years of Education, Male Adults (25+) Number of Years Completed				Primary Education Enrollment Rate, Net Percent of Primary Age Children Enrolled				Lower Secondary Enrollment Rate, Gross Total Enrolled as % of Nominal Age Population			
	2010	2035	2060	% Chg	2010	2035	2060	% Chg	2010	2035	2060	% Chg	2010	2035	2060	% Chg
ASIA with OCEANIA continued																
Turkey	4.856	7.422	9.673	99.2%	6.012	7.997	9.619	63.0%	94.26	100	100	6.1%	88.16	103.4	102.2	15.9%
Yemen	3.778	6.125	9.622	154.7%	5.011	7.282	9.528	90.1%	77.49	94.98	99.99	29.0%	56.29	83.85	99.15	76.1%
Iraq	4.076	6.654	9.843	141.5%	6.224	8.906	11.61	86.5%	90.79	99.93	100	10.1%	63.61	95.5	101.8	60.0%
Saudi Arabia	8.839	11.66	14.61	65.3%	9.513	11.96	14.93	56.9%	63.7	100	99.99	57.0%	87.56	107.4	99.53	13.7%
Syrian Arab Repub	5.532	7.73	9.756	76.4%	7.732	8.953	10.42	34.8%	97.04	99.99	99.97	3.0%	96.33	90.98	93.91	-2.5%
Israel	9.828	12.63	14.98	52.4%	10.01	12.45	14.34	43.3%	98.79	100	100	1.2%	80.76	96.19	100	23.8%
Jordan	8.246	12.54	15.1	83.1%	10.09	13.01	14.94	48.1%	94.29	99.47	99.57	5.6%	96.35	101.7	98.69	2.4%
Occupied Palestinian Territory	5.277	9.263	12.43	135.6%	6.238	9.49	12.09	93.8%	79.88	97.42	99.99	25.2%	99.62	105.3	103.1	3.5%
Azerbaijan	5.583	8.578	11.48	105.6%	6.69	10.03	12.67	89.4%	89.7	100	100	11.5%	92.03	101.5	100.4	9.1%
United Arab Emirates	3.092	7.532	10.99	255.4%	3.618	5.945	9.481	162.1%	91.43	99.85	100	9.2%	96.42	99.72	97.56	1.2%
Oman	8.648	10.78	13.17	52.3%	9.132	10.29	12.4	35.8%	79.34	99.96	100	26.0%	100	101.1	100.3	0.3%
Kuwait	7.858	10.56	13.15	67.3%	7.822	9.216	12.11	54.8%	93.19	99.99	100	7.3%	95.8	100.2	99.59	4.0%
Lebanon	7.145	9.741	12.21	70.9%	7.921	10.04	12.27	54.9%	85.38	99.99	100	17.1%	90.7	100.4	99.73	10.0%
Armenia	5.419	8.125	10.38	91.5%	6.406	9.465	11.8	84.2%	89.32	100	99.97	11.9%	102.1	102.1	100	-2.1%
Georgia	4.854	6.717	8.531	75.8%	5.873	7.878	9.686	64.9%	95.48	100	99.9	4.6%	101.5	102.6	100.7	-0.8%
Bahrain	9.9	12.22	14.44	45.9%	10.29	11.59	13.52	31.4%	99.49	100	100	0.5%	107.8	98.88	100	-7.2%
Qatar	11.53	14.08	16.51	43.2%	11.55	12.08	13.79	19.4%	98.55	99.94	100	1.5%	103	101.7	100.1	-2.8%
Cyprus	9.122	11.31	13.26	45.4%	9.643	11.36	12.84	33.2%	99.95	100	99.93	0.0%	99.1	100	99.86	0.8%
Asia-West	**5.594**	**8.212**	**10.92**	**95.2%**	**6.854**	**9.065**	**11.24**	**64.0%**	**88.15**	**99.19**	**99.98**	**13.4%**	**83.68**	**98.08**	**99.96**	**19.5%**
Australia	11.24	14.3	16.47	46.5%	11.69	14.28	15.89	35.9%	98.5	99.96	100	1.5%	112.4	99.09	100	-11.0%
Papua New Guinea	2.53	4.203	6.436	154.4%	3.403	5.131	7.053	107.3%	58.12	78.77	97.26	67.3%	25.3	52.26	71.18	181.3%
New Zealand	12.19	15.29	17.49	43.5%	12.45	14.94	16.61	33.4%	100	99.93	100	0.0%	105.1	97.5	99.46	-5.4%
Solomon Islands	3.126	4.272	5.739	83.6%	4.163	4.846	5.024	44.7%	63.77	76.09	94.38	48.0%	49.83	65.79	76.96	54.4%
Fiji	5.346	7.462	9.7	81.4%	6.216	7.756	9.626	54.9%	94.21	98.32	100	6.1%	100.5	113.2	110.6	10.0%
Vanuatu	4.795	6.715	9.43	96.7%	5.707	7.274	9.795	71.6%	95.87	99.79	99.99	4.3%	51.1	77.55	101.2	98.0%
Micronesia, Federated States of	5.909	7.688	9.853	66.7%	6.82	8.163	9.592	40.6%	84.22	95.34	99.92	18.6%	103.4	109.9	115.4	11.6%
Tonga	5.421	6.415	8.126	49.9%	6.298	6.906	8.319	32.1%	95.6	99	100	4.6%	93.06	86.65	96.11	3.3%
Samoa	5.679	8.401	10.63	87.2%	6.48	8.316	10.4	60.5%	90.33	99.13	100	10.7%	99.58	102.5	102.8	3.2%
Oceania	**9.292**	**11.49**	**13.33**	**43.5%**	**9.829**	**11.68**	**13.08**	**33.1%**	**90.16**	**94.35**	**99.13**	**9.9%**	**92.88**	**87.23**	**91.94**	**-1.0%**

Education

Base Case: Countries in Year 2060 Descending Population Sequence	Years of Education, Female Adults (25+) Number of Years Completed				Years of Education, Male Adults (25+) Number of Years Completed				Primary Education Enrollment Rate, Net Percent of Primary Age Children Enrolled				Lower Secondary Enrollment Rate, Gross Total Enrolled as % of Nominal Age Population			
	2010	2035	2060	% Chg	2010	2035	2060	% Chg	2010	2035	2060	% Chg	2010	2035	2060	% Chg
EUROPE																
Russian Federation	11.47	13.19	14.79	28.9%	10.92	13.41	15.15	38.7%	94.84	100	99.97	5.4%	91.31	105.1	103.8	13.7%
Poland	10.57	13.51	16.03	51.7%	10.8	13.62	15.75	45.8%	99.35	100	99.97	0.6%	104.2	97.7	98.68	-5.3%
Ukraine	11.46	13.18	14.96	30.5%	10.97	13.91	16.33	48.9%	97.42	100	100	2.6%	104.3	103.1	101.9	-2.3%
Romania	9.829	12.92	15.46	57.3%	10.72	13.44	15.71	46.5%	97.87	100	99.96	2.1%	101.2	104.1	102.6	1.4%
Czech Republic	9.597	13.26	16.15	68.3%	11.12	14.44	16.87	51.7%	97.59	100	100	2.5%	101.9	99.15	98.9	-2.9%
Belarus	11.47	13.52	15.54	35.5%	10.79	12.93	14.81	37.3%	96.67	100	100	3.4%	110.1	105.5	103.5	-6.0%
Hungary	9.261	13.07	16.2	74.9%	10.4	13.88	16.36	57.3%	95.74	100	100	4.4%	99.27	99.8	99	-0.3%
Bulgaria	10.37	12.49	14.35	38.4%	10.63	13.39	15.41	45.0%	98.46	100	99.99	1.6%	96.81	103.9	103	6.4%
Slovak Republic	9.503	13.44	16.65	75.2%	10.98	14.31	16.71	52.2%	98.41	100	100	1.6%	102.6	102.6	100.1	-2.4%
Moldova, Repub of	9.063	11.35	13.34	47.2%	10.04	11.93	13.6	35.5%	98.04	100	99.93	1.9%	99.87	99.79	100.3	0.4%
Europe-East	**10.99**	**13.18**	**15.17**	**38.0%**	**10.86**	**13.54**	**15.54**	**43.1%**	**96.44**	**100**	**99.98**	**3.7%**	**97.46**	**103.2**	**102.2**	**4.9%**
United Kingdom	10.21	13.17	15.36	50.4%	-0.3	12.99	14.85	44.2%	99.5	99.99	100	0.5%	101.7	98.91	100	-1.7%
Sweden	11.93	14.21	16	34.1%	1.-86	13.98	15.51	30.8%	98.54	99.99	99.99	1.5%	103.6	99.64	100.1	-3.4%
Denmark	10.02	12.88	15.06	50.3%	11.56	13.95	15.6	34.9%	98.13	100	100	1.9%	114.8	99.14	100.1	-12.8%
Ireland	9.743	11.89	13.49	38.5%	9.726	11.85	13.36	37.4%	97.72	99.99	99.97	2.3%	105.5	99.49	99.32	-5.9%
Norway	12.09	14.48	16.22	34.2%	12.52	14.49	15.81	26.3%	98.72	100	100	1.3%	101.3	99.85	100.1	-1.2%
Finland	10.7	13.3	15.45	44.4%	11.19	13.55	15.33	37.0%	99.56	99.99	99.99	0.4%	103.2	99.15	100	-3.1%
Lithuania	9.576	13.12	15.86	65.6%	10.36	13.48	15.58	50.4%	97.28	100	99.98	2.8%	101.4	100.6	99.8	-1.6%
Latvia	10.02	14.03	17.25	72.2%	10.5	14.2	17.06	62.5%	97.61	100	99.97	2.4%	103.6	99.71	99.22	-4.2%
Estonia	9.678	13.01	16.19	67.3%	9.819	13.09	15.82	61.1%	98.85	100	99.98	1.1%	111.4	99.97	99.58	-10.6%
Iceland	9.586	12.64	14.85	54.9%	9.98	12.09	13.64	36.7%	98.71	99.98	99.99	1.3%	102.6	99.65	100.1	-2.4%
Europe-North	**10.42**	**13.27**	**15.39**	**47.7%**	**10.65**	**13.22**	**15**	**40.8%**	**99.09**	**99.99**	**100**	**0.9%**	**103**	**99.15**	**99.99**	**-2.9%**
Italy	7.624	11.15	14.32	87.8%	8.418	11.89	14.78	75.6%	99.93	100	100	0.1%	105.8	100	100	-5.5%
Spain	8.326	10.87	12.99	56.0%	8.512	11.18	13.27	55.9%	99.95	100	100	0.1%	115.1	98.86	98.91	-14.1%
Greece	8.597	11.68	14.17	64.8%	10.37	11.96	13.21	27.4%	99.95	100	100	0.1%	102	98.89	99.56	-2.4%
Portugal	5.587	7.688	10.34	85.1%	5.641	7.437	9.717	72.3%	98.28	99.98	99.99	1.7%	97.82	108.3	100.7	2.9%
Serbia	8.541	11.64	14.32	67.7%	10.21	12.53	14.63	43.3%	94.1	99.98	99.99	6.3%	95.67	101	101.8	6.4%
Bosnia and Herzegovina	6.015	8.363	11.38	89.2%	6.845	8.607	11.1	62.2%	91.03	99.99	99.99	9.8%	89.13	106.2	104.2	16.9%
Croatia	6.786	10.34	13.55	99.7%	7.931	11.33	14.14	78.3%	96.75	100	99.98	3.3%	98.79	100.9	100	1.2%
Albania	5.976	8.457	10.78	80.4%	6.905	9.44	11.57	67.6%	96.48	99.36	100	3.6%	99.86	100.4	101.1	1.2%
Macedonia, FYR	6.802	10.18	13.11	92.7%	7.77	11.31	14.09	81.3%	95.41	100	99.99	4.8%	97.46	99.55	100.1	2.7%
Slovenia	7.928	11.77	15.08	90.2%	8.663	12.55	15.67	80.9%	99.24	100	99.96	0.7%	99.35	100.7	100.7	1.4%
Montenegro	6.662	9.716	12.61	89.3%	7.505	10.04	12.48	66.3%	92.12	99.97	100	8.6%	91.86	101.2	101.8	10.8%
Malta	8.739	10.66	12.8	46.5%	9.528	11.6	13.56	42.3%	96	100	99.99	4.2%	108.9	112.4	106.3	-2.4%
Europe-South	**7.693**	**10.7**	**13.39**	**74.1%**	**8.387**	**11.22**	**13.6**	**62.2%**	**99**	**99.98**	**100**	**1.0%**	**106.1**	**100.5**	**99.97**	**-5.8%**
Germany	9.857	11.84	14.16	43.7%	10.79	13.08	15.32	42.0%	100	100	100	0.0%	107.4	101.7	99.08	-7.7%
France	9.219	12.58	15.34	66.4%	9.608	12.81	15.21	58.3%	99.97	100	100	0.0%	112.6	99.52	99.49	-11.6%
Netherlands	9.425	11.24	13.39	42.1%	10.14	11.84	13.73	35.4%	99.71	100	99.99	0.3%	129.9	128.3	124.8	-3.9%
Belgium	9.229	12.39	14.86	61.0%	9.806	12.78	14.95	52.5%	98.99	100	99.99	1.0%	113.2	98.77	99.98	-11.7%
Austria	8.965	11.99	14.65	63.4%	10.57	13.44	15.59	47.5%	99.97	100	99.99	0.0%	105.2	99.2	99.99	-5.0%
Switzerland	10.11	11.88	14.03	38.8%	11.71	13.46	15.36	31.2%	91.92	100	99.98	8.8%	105.8	102.1	101.3	-4.3%
Luxembourg	11.39	13.18	14.95	31.3%	11.76	12.93	14.52	23.5%	97.47	99.99	99.9	2.5%	105.4	100.2	99.86	-5.3%
Europe-West	**9.547**	**12.08**	**14.57**	**52.6%**	**10.31**	**12.88**	**15.11**	**46.6%**	**99.58**	**100**	**99.99**	**0.4%**	**111.3**	**103.2**	**101.9**	**-8.4%**

Education

Infrastructure
Health-Related

Base Case
Source: International Futures
Version 6.32, June 2010

	Upper Secondary Enrollment Rate, Gross — Total Enrolled as % of Nominal Age Population				Tertiary Enrollment Rate, Gross — Total Enrolled as % of Nominal Age Population				Knowledge Society Index — Index: 0-100				Water Safety — Percent Pop with No Access to Improved Drinking Water Sources		
	2010	2035	2060	% Chg	2010	2035	2060	% Chg	2010	2035	2060	% Chg	2010	2035	2060
World	59.83	73.69	81.65	36.5%	28.14	37.15	45.16	50.5%	53.62	60.31	72.22	34.7%	15.17	9.116	6.335
Africa	31.46	43.8	58.98	87.5%	8.635	17.98	27.8	221.9%	12.49	24.57	41.02	228.4%	35.07	24.14	15.89
Americas	81.24	88.58	94.52	16.3%	49.2	53.9	60.31	22.6%	63.13	69.07	76.02	20.4%	5.229	3.452	2.128
Asia with Oceania	54.71	76.71	86.89	58.8%	22.08	35.89	46.97	112.7%	46.54	55.13	73.28	57.5%	14.84	6.354	3.48
Europe	100.8	101.5	102.4	1.6%	62.99	66.57	69.63	10.5%	52.61	66.74	76.57	45.5%	2.379	1.302	0.78
World	59.83	73.69	81.65	36.5%	28.14	37.15	45.16	50.5%	53.62	60.31	72.22	34.7%	15.17	9.116	6.335
Africa-Eastern	14.5	32.06	60.39	316.5%	3.437	15.11	30.52	788.0%	3.845	15.95	36.87	858.9%	46.46	30.19	15.83
Africa-Middle	17.57	28.27	36.98	110.5%	2.953	8.803	12.38	319.2%	6.047	22.46	32.23	433.0%	44.59	35.7	29.21
Africa-Northern	60.12	79.19	88.02	46.4%	19.05	31.54	41.85	119.7%	14.32	28.6	44.45	210.4%	11.8	6.042	3.577
Africa-Southern	87.63	104	108.1	23.4%	15.99	30.28	49.2	207.7%	20.1	37.42	67.53	236.0%	11.36	6.719	3.162
Africa-Western	25.02	37.66	52.49	109.8%	7.933	16.53	25	213.2%	4.956	13.82	21.69	337.7%	39.45	24.07	15.52
Africa	31.46	43.8	58.98	87.5%	8.635	17.98	27.8	221.9%	12.49	24.57	41.02	228.4%	35.07	24.14	15.89
America-Caribbean	67.58	75.56	76.4	13.1%	34.15	36.45	40.08	17.4%	27.73	45.33	58.79	112.0%	15.1	13.53	10.64
America-Central	59.55	73.18	90.23	51.5%	19.79	29.09	39.24	98.3%	14.15	28.63	44.72	216.0%	10.28	6.485	2.731
America-North	85.32	93.37	98.36	15.3%	67.56	69.41	74.15	9.8%	69.76	76.97	82.25	17.9%	0.715	0.397	0.223
America-South	80.34	86.64	92.71	15.4%	33.01	41.87	50.12	51.8%	22.19	39.55	58.1	161.8%	8.835	5.421	3.314
Americas	81.24	88.58	94.52	16.3%	49.2	53.9	60.31	22.6%	63.13	69.07	76.02	20.4%	5.229	3.452	2.128
Asia-East	63.81	92.14	101.5	59.1%	29.71	46.69	59.79	101.2%	54.62	63.8	86.22	57.9%	16.51	7.556	4.379
Asia-South Central	43.85	68.27	80.52	83.6%	13.2	28.63	41.23	212.3%	15.94	34.5	52.68	230.5%	13.55	4.142	2.054
Asia-South East	54.41	65.13	77.43	42.3%	23.15	30.94	38.68	57.1%	22.87	30.62	41.28	80.5%	16.21	10.14	5.922
Asia-West	66.05	80.6	88.89	34.6%	27.31	38.35	47.17	69.6%	28.77	45.51	61.01	112.1%	9.708	6.41	3.929
Oceania	108.7	84.26	87.6	-19.4%	58.11	60.1	65.59	12.9%	70.85	81.16	87.17	23.0%	13.2	10.93	7.402
Asia with Oceania	54.71	76.71	86.89	58.8%	22.08	35.89	46.97	112.7%	46.54	55.13	73.28	57.5%	14.84	6.354	3.48
Europe-East	96.42	101.1	102.2	6.0%	66.74	70.41	68.19	2.2%	46.31	62.11	68.68	48.3%	4.966	3.04	1.987
Europe-North	109.5	102.5	103.9	-5.1%	68.32	72.62	79.21	15.9%	60.15	74.78	81.95	36.2%	0.187	0.053	0.028
Europe-South	100.9	101.4	102.1	1.2%	63.05	64.01	66.08	4.8%	44.81	55.99	68.08	51.9%	1.3	0.665	0.392
Europe-West	102.9	101.4	101.8	-1.1%	53.19	58.95	67.38	26.7%	53.18	68.28	78.54	47.7%	0.049	0	0.001
Europe	100.8	101.5	102.4	1.6%	62.99	66.57	69.63	10.5%	52.61	66.74	76.57	45.5%	2.379	1.302	0.78

Multination Regional Analysis

Measures of Poverty, Health, Education, Infrastructure, and Governance

Education

Infrastructure
Health-Related

Base Case: Countries in Year 2060 Descending Population Sequence	Upper Secondary Enrollment Rate, Gross (Total Enrolled as % of Nominal Age Population)				Tertiary Enrollment Rate, Gross (Total Enrolled as % of Nominal Age Population)				Knowledge Society Index (Index: 0-100)				Water Safety (Percent Pop with No Access to Improved Drinking Water Sources)		
	2010	2035	2060	% Chg	2010	2035	2060	% Chg	2010	2035	2060	% Chg	2010	2035	2060
AFRICA															
Ethiopia	10.82	37.37	72.45	569.6%	3.216	15.08	32.17	900.3%	3.131	12.36	29.84	853.1%	72.63	48.05	25.82
Tanzania, United Rep	7.239	23.23	53.22	635.2%	2.849	20.25	36.42	1178.3%	1.772	17.28	37.51	2016.8%	34.36	11.8	3.618
Uganda	12.58	36.59	77.78	518.3%	5.474	20.23	42.16	670.2%	7.009	20.38	47.07	571.6%	37.42	23.89	5.414
Kenya	29.18	42	70.02	140.0%	3.994	15.46	33.35	735.0%	3.182	12.82	30.52	859.1%	37.39	25.83	13.07
Madagascar	12.5	22.23	32.04	156.3%	2.909	7.563	18.34	530.5%	2.693	5.586	14.97	455.9%	52.2	45.08	27.64
Mozambique	7.455	28.24	71.38	857.5%	2.447	18.9	39.37	1508.9%	6.471	20.02	43.08	565.7%	52.57	25.11	11.38
Malawi	15.91	29.6	47.28	197.2%	1.155	6.507	19.13	1556.3%	0.705	3.572	15.12	2044.7%	24.65	18.81	8.256
Zambia	19.9	30.14	51.69	159.7%	4.945	17.96	28.61	478.6%	2.624	12.59	24.77	844.0%	39.12	24	10.11
Somalia	6.663	16.73	19.36	190.6%	2.491	5.629	10.5	321.5%	0.92	2.422	6.802	639.3%	67.25	55.19	42.3
Rwanda	11.1	27.86	56.48	408.8%	3.464	18.92	35.45	923.4%	1.53	14.91	35.14	2196.7%	24.84	7.132	0
Zimbabwe	31.86	34.3	37.59	49.4%	4.118	12.24	22.53	447.1%	1.572	7.612	17.22	995.4%	19.15	19.29	13.65
Burundi	8.974	15.74	31.25	248.2%	2.158	2.134	5.441	152.1%	3.697	3.628	5.152	39.4%	19.42	18.1	15.84
Eritrea	21.69	33.58	44.97	107.3%	1.27	2.676	6.842	438.7%	1.087	1.158	3.851	254.3%	39.38	34.91	30.16
Comoros	29.31	38.44	46.56	58.9%	1.756	5.184	14.65	734.3%	1.415	3.565	11.14	687.3%	16.38	17.71	17.35
Mauritius	79.77	101.3	102.1	28.0%	20.2	35.73	49.38	144.5%	11.44	31.93	55.42	384.4%	0	0	0
Djibouti	16.48	30.49	72.98	342.8%	4.71	15.82	33.65	614.4%	4.508	13.8	31.88	607.2%	23.44	12.9	5.744
Africa-Eastern	**14.5**	**32.06**	**60.39**	**316.5%**	**3.437**	**15.11**	**30.52**	**788.0%**	**3.845**	**15.95**	**36.87**	**858.9%**	**46.46**	**30.19**	**15.83**
Congo, Democratic Republic of	18.36	24.07	27.73	51.0%	0.882	1.628	2.864	224.7%	0.824	0.961	1.131	37.3%	51.01	42.93	35.94
Angola	13.74	45.67	74.49	442.1%	4.753	23.91	38.37	707.3%	7.374	27.26	39.35	433.6%	39.1	25.34	16.33
Cameroon	21.2	32.7	52.65	148.3%	7.362	17.3	28.06	281.1%	3.031	11.91	23.77	684.2%	31.93	21.05	11.38
Chad	11.82	19.69	26.19	121.6%	1.857	10.83	13.67	636.1%	1.573	7.665	9.326	492.9%	51.6	37.93	31.55
Central African Republic	9.405	17.38	27.34	190.7%	2.217	6.066	15.38	593.7%	3.19	4.782	12.9	304.4%	25.42	25.44	17.59
Congo, Republic of	23.19	30.93	50.48	117.7%	8.481	24.27	29.62	249.3%	2.76	15.41	22.58	718.1%	35.76	24.3	16.32
Gabon	33.81	58.63	73.36	117.0%	10.54	24.37	36.79	249.1%	2.224	17.03	30.12	1254.3%	11.18	8.244	5.552
Equatorial Guinea	17.39	58	72.75	318.3%	6.984	24.19	39.81	470.0%	25.82	48	61.64	138.7%	53.38	38.8	24.91
São Tomé and Príncipe	28.75	32	38.58	34.2%	9.157	13.6	19.02	107.7%	5.657	8.405	13.82	144.3%	20.18	23.63	15.5
Africa-Middle	**17.57**	**28.27**	**36.98**	**110.5%**	**2.953**	**8.803**	**12.38**	**319.2%**	**6.047**	**22.46**	**32.23**	**433.0%**	**44.59**	**35.7**	**29.21**
Egypt	81.14	99.3	99.16	22.2%	19.14	33.44	46.5	142.9%	10.47	26.49	47.16	350.4%	1.371	0	0
Sudan	27.37	64.24	83.89	206.5%	9.979	24.42	34.61	246.8%	6.207	20.56	32.04	416.2%	25.63	9.731	5.266
Algeria	59.11	67.09	75.25	27.3%	22.91	32.75	38.76	69.2%	13.51	25.75	34.58	156.0%	13.62	9.279	6.33
Morocco	38.02	56.83	74.45	95.8%	14.23	27	39.62	178.4%	13.55	25.93	40.82	201.3%	17.61	11.21	6.294
Tunisia	73.24	85.57	93.82	28.1%	32.3	43.51	53.15	64.6%	18.86	36.37	56.48	199.5%	6.016	2.542	1.184
Libyan Arab Jamahiriya	95.43	94.75	96.55	1.2%	55.85	57.55	53.57	-4.1%	29.46	46.15	51.35	74.3%	26.9	18.91	12.25
Africa-Northern	**60.12**	**79.19**	**88.02**	**46.4%**	**19.05**	**31.54**	**41.85**	**119.7%**	**14.32**	**28.6**	**44.45**	**210.4%**	**11.8**	**6.042**	**3.577**

Multinational Regional Analysis

Measures of Poverty, Health, Education, Infrastructure, and Governance

Education

Base Case: Countries in Year 2060 Descending Population Sequence	Upper Secondary Enrollment Rate, Gross Total Enrolled as % of Nominal Age Population				Tertiary Enrollment Rate, Gross Total Enrolled as % of Nominal Age Population				Knowledge Society Index Index: 0-100				Water Safety Percent Pop with No Access to Improved Drinking Water Sources		
	2010	2035	2060	% Chg	2010	2035	2060	% Chg	2010	2035	2060	% Chg	2010	2035	2060
AFRICA continued															
South Africa	95.03	112.4	113.3	19.2%	17.32	31.46	50.67	192.6%	20.93	37.41	68.77	228.6%	10.59	6.271	3.207
Namibia	29.26	45.55	76.4	161.1%	7.8	23.74	43	451.3%	8.587	24.28	47.92	458.1%	12.6	4.529	0.272
Lesotho	27.14	49.43	75.16	176.9%	5.29	17.64	31.98	504.5%	3.529	13.18	26.72	657.2%	20.9	13.66	3.859
Botswana	59.7	81.24	93.38	56.4%	8.628	32.67	51.87	501.2%	14.52	46.36	70.68	386.8%	3.889	0.85	0.343
Swaziland	36.16	66.2	89.83	148.4%	5.6	20.65	39.75	609.8%	7.006	20.84	41.06	486.1%	37.09	23.84	10.96
Africa-Southern	**87.63**	**104**	**108.1**	**23.4%**	**15.99**	**30.28**	**49.2**	**207.7%**	**20.1**	**37.42**	**67.53**	**236.0%**	**11.36**	**6.719**	**3.162**
Nigeria	32.82	49.49	59.45	81.1%	11.29	21.87	27.54	143.9%	6.362	16.06	21.24	233.9%	44.52	20.79	15.68
Niger	5.874	12.54	25.8	339.2%	1.474	4.13	13.65	826.1%	0.93	1.555	9.44	915.1%	51.62	43.16	29.02
Côte d'Ivoire	15.07	25.63	54.69	262.9%	7.305	16.33	26.6	264.1%	4.22	11.37	21.07	399.3%	16.27	11.25	5.793
Ghana	23.45	37.01	64.25	174.0%	6.53	11.67	25.33	287.9%	4.2	8.642	20.98	399.5%	24.32	23.09	9.859
Mali	16.45	26.38	50.86	209.2%	3.338	12.05	26.33	688.8%	1.268	8.305	22.16	1647.6%	47.37	32.92	14.4
Burkina Faso	8.027	16.95	39.76	395.3%	3.235	13.2	27.02	735.2%	1.926	8.891	23.03	1095.7%	38.24	29.58	12.75
Senegal	14.79	27.21	52.03	251.8%	4.627	13.25	28.7	520.3%	0.789	7.939	23.31	2854.4%	24.02	16.97	6.916
Guinea	21.94	29.66	43.13	96.6%	4.263	13.44	22.71	432.7%	2.853	9.973	18.81	559.3%	47.78	33.08	19.07
Benin	21.54	27.8	41.02	90.4%	4.411	11.86	21.7	352.0%	2.334	7.495	16.53	608.2%	31.91	26.89	14.72
Togo	21.68	27.19	34.09	57.2%	3.881	5.884	8.226	112.0%	7.204	7.313	8.589	19.2%	46.13	37.74	33.77
Sierra Leone	26.53	35.86	62.92	137.2%	2.287	12.75	30.12	1217.0%	1.026	8.607	26.9	2521.8%	39.11	23.11	7.674
Liberia	30.67	57.35	79.91	160.5%	14.42	22.12	36.05	150.0%	8.273	15.07	32.92	297.9%	33.8	9.522	0
Mauritania	22.55	31.75	38.03	68.6%	4.912	6.233	11.89	142.1%	2.161	2.801	7.771	259.6%	43.78	44.75	31.1
Guinea-Bissau	12.14	21.37	32.66	169.0%	0.703	1.055	1.513	115.2%	0.511	0.569	0.675	32.1%	39.69	34.12	31.58
Gambia	32.77	42.52	63.28	93.1%	3.679	13.59	25.12	582.8%	1.978	10.14	21.36	979.9%	15.84	6.353	0.529
Cape Verde	47.1	65.33	84.04	78.4%	11.76	28.03	43.37	268.8%	4.504	20.99	42.65	846.9%	18.04	9.94	4.924
Africa-Western	**25.02**	**37.66**	**52.49**	**109.8%**	**7.983**	**16.53**	**25**	**213.2%**	**4.956**	**13.82**	**21.69**	**337.7%**	**39.45**	**24.07**	**15.52**

Infrastructure
Health-Related

Education

Infrastructure
Health-Related

Base Case: Countries in Year 2060 Descending Population Sequence	Upper Secondary Enrollment Rate, Gross (Total Enrolled as % of Nominal Age Population)				Tertiary Enrollment Rate, Gross (Total Enrolled as % of Nominal Age Population)				Knowledge Society Index (Index: 0-100)				Water Safety (Percent Pop with No Access to Improved Drinking Water Sources)		
	2010	2035	2060	% Chg	2010	2035	2060	% Chg	2010	2035	2060	% Chg	2010	2035	2060
AMERICAS															
Haiti	18.37	28.9	37.65	105.0%	2.157	8.334	17.74	722.4%	1.466	5.934	13.75	837.9%	45.2	39.3	26.97
Dominican Republic	66.88	99.78	103.7	55.1%	35.33	43.23	49.24	39.4%	22.68	38.34	53.26	134.8%	4.17	0.715	0.155
Cuba	90.09	94.52	97.06	7.7%	51.7	58.71	56.53	-8.4%	18.67	31.07	46.73	150.3%	8.323	4.688	2.732
Puerto Rico	103.8	96.09	99.15	-4.5%	43.33	52.58	61.86	42.8%	42.12	63.59	76.54	81.7%	1.504	0.854	0.518
Jamaica	75.6	78.39	80.96	7.1%	19.75	28.24	39.25	98.7%	7.553	17.52	32.86	335.1%	7.152	4.98	2.796
Trinidad	81.4	99.68	99.48	22.2%	17.74	44.38	60.04	238.4%	7.055	46.77	65.43	827.4%	7.736	3.428	1.907
Bahamas	83.96	95.3	98.02	16.7%	28.09	42.24	56.4	100.8%	21.21	44.01	70.38	231.8%	2.925	1.876	1.101
Barbados	109.8	92.54	96.44	-12.2%	40.15	49.31	62.54	55.8%	29.74	43.67	69.32	133.1%	0	0	0
Grenada	98.86	113.6	107.6	8.8%	35.78	38.61	46.21	29.2%	30.24	34.79	47.2	56.1%	5.241	3.789	1.188
Saint Vincent and Grenadines	56.82	90.15	96.27	69.4%	33.9	41.4	49.83	47.0%	24.27	34.72	48.95	101.7%	7.894	3.148	1.122
Saint Lucia	78.14	86.99	99.68	27.6%	16.66	31.57	44.63	167.9%	8.524	24.34	43.73	413.0%	1.812	0	0
America-Caribbean	**67.58**	**75.56**	**76.4**	**13.1%**	**34.15**	**36.45**	**40.08**	**17.4%**	**27.73**	**45.33**	**58.79**	**112.0%**	**15.1**	**13.53**	**10.64**
Guatemala	45.96	62.27	88.89	93.4%	12.64	26.34	38.57	205.1%	4.044	16.8	34.66	757.1%	5.199	2.066	0
Honduras	92.39	90.52	100.1	8.3%	18.15	26.65	36.02	98.5%	5.506	16.37	29.56	436.9%	12.54	7.888	3.993
El Salvador	51.08	72.48	85.12	66.6%	20.3	27.85	38.76	90.9%	9.06	20.12	35.97	297.0%	15.24	10.35	5.16
Nicaragua	55.11	66.92	77.66	40.9%	18.27	22.97	29.91	63.7%	5.654	12.84	22.39	296.0%	21.05	18.32	9.327
Costa Rica	62.97	85.41	98.22	56.0%	27.89	39.09	50.4	80.7%	20.64	36.25	55.17	167.3%	2.488	0.668	0.194
Panama	60.76	84.73	95.78	57.6%	45.01	53.12	59.2	31.5%	29.82	48.74	71.41	139.5%	8.673	5.095	3.066
Belize	57.52	67.85	87.05	51.3%	5.081	22.65	43.37	753.6%	7.229	24.94	49.34	582.5%	8.427	4.541	2.034
America-Central	**59.55**	**73.18**	**90.23**	**51.5%**	**19.79**	**29.09**	**39.24**	**98.3%**	**14.15**	**28.63**	**44.72**	**216.0%**	**10.28**	**6.485**	**2.731**
USA	88.35	97.23	100.1	13.3%	82.17	81.12	82.73	0.7%	73.55	80.58	85.16	15.8%	0.036	0	0
Mexico	63.33	80.91	92.39	45.9%	26.61	36.11	46.6	75.1%	17.53	31.42	47.65	171.8%	2.864	1.644	0.997
Canada	128.8	98.4	100	-22.4%	65.45	69.27	75.54	15.4%	61.63	73.55	79.69	29.3%	0.02	0	0
America-North	**85.32**	**93.37**	**98.36**	**15.3%**	**67.56**	**69.41**	**74.15**	**9.8%**	**69.76**	**76.97**	**82.25**	**17.9%**	**0.715**	**0.397**	**0.223**
Brazil	90.61	90.4	95	4.8%	25.02	36.73	48.1	92.2%	24.08	40.28	58.81	144.2%	9.091	5.399	3.271
Colombia	67.92	76.35	83.59	23.1%	30.55	36.21	43.18	41.3%	10.85	22.68	37.54	246.0%	6.175	3.56	1.867
Argentina	70.32	86.38	96.98	37.9%	67.21	72.93	76.61	14.0%	18.93	42.67	67.9	258.7%	3.554	2.034	1.241
Peru	76.88	98.24	101.9	32.5%	35.07	42.4	48.54	38.4%	23.15	35.91	49.4	113.4%	15.17	9.567	5.829
Venezuela	61.9	77.78	87.81	41.9%	40.95	47.38	51.5	25.8%	22.56	38.62	52.76	133.9%	15.1	10.03	6.388
Ecuador	55.87	56.14	66.28	18.6%	19.13	26.8	32.34	69.1%	7.153	16.13	24.09	236.8%	5.296	4.404	3.632
Chile	87.23	97.61	101.1	15.9%	48.42	55.54	62.48	29.0%	35.9	50.32	69.22	92.8%	4.605	2.841	1.729
Bolivia	78.98	94.52	97.53	23.5%	30.9	36.91	39.88	29.1%	15.06	27.19	36.92	145.2%	13.41	5.813	3.301
Paraguay	56.96	69.06	82.19	44.3%	25.36	29.92	37.85	49.3%	13.29	20.76	32.41	143.9%	12.8	8.24	4.194
Uruguay	94.89	100.9	104.1	9.7%	44.26	58.11	69.88	57.9%	18.23	43.44	69.95	283.7%	0	0	0
Guyana	68.27	83.68	86.16	26.2%	14.82	25.26	35.19	137.4%	7.968	17.44	30.96	288.6%	15.74	11.29	6.332
Suriname	51.93	79.16	94.17	81.3%	17.48	35.17	48.39	176.8%	9.324	30.15	53.03	468.7%	7.191	3.762	2.194
America-South	**80.34**	**86.64**	**92.71**	**15.4%**	**33.01**	**41.87**	**50.12**	**51.8%**	**22.19**	**39.55**	**58.1**	**161.8%**	**8.835**	**5.421**	**3.314**

Education

Infrastructure
Health-Related

Base Case: Countries in Year 2060 Descending Population Sequence	Upper Secondary Enrollment Rate, Gross				Tertiary Enrollment Rate, Gross				Knowledge Society Index				Water Safety		
	Total Enrolled as % of Nominal Age Population				Total Enrolled as % of Nominal Age Population				Index: 0-100				Percent Pop with No Access to Improved Drinking Water Sources		
	2010	2035	2060	% Chg	2010	2035	2060	% Chg	2010	2035	2060	% Chg	2010	2035	2060
ASIA with OCEANIA															
China	58.3	91.69	101.8	74.6%	24.56	44.32	58.88	138.8%	27.86	55.46	85.32	206.2%	19	8.491	4.866
Japan	105.3	102	104	-1.2%	57.78	64.56	72.55	25.6%	68.76	85.27	91.22	32.7%	0.04	0	0
Korea, Repub of	92.8	92.51	100.4	8.2%	89.24	80.78	75.66	-15.2%	89.08	100.2	110.6	24.2%	7.473	5.216	3.291
Taiwan	103.1	95.81	99.15	-3.8%	46.92	53.42	61.39	30.8%	44.07	58.83	77.26	75.3%	2.255	1.192	0.623
Korea, Dem. People's Rep.	45.91	65.74	74.49	62.3%	19.75	26.27	31.92	61.6%	14.47	20.1	26.25	81.4%	0	0	0
Hong Kong SAR	78.41	97.92	104	32.6%	37.93	48.32	59.58	57.1%	22.15	40.36	56.49	155.0%	0.753	0.6	0.438
Mongolia	84.39	91.27	98.2	16.4%	46.15	56.83	66.91	45.0%	29.7	41.23	57.31	93.0%	33.27	20.93	11.92
Asia-East	**63.81**	**92.14**	**101.5**	**59.1%**	**29.71**	**46.69**	**59.79**	**101.2%**	**54.62**	**63.8**	**86.22**	**57.9%**	**16.51**	**7.556**	**4.379**
India	44.13	75.92	89.2	102.1%	13.53	31.78	46.31	239.8%	16.6	34.75	55.34	233.4%	11.86	0.471	0
Pakistan	23.39	34.07	51.45	120.0%	7.019	16.1	28.52	306.3%	8.722	16.22	28.83	230.5%	8.824	7.05	2.526
Bangladesh	33.73	54.81	74.21	120.0%	8.27	20.81	30.71	271.3%	11.12	21.55	31.47	183.0%	23.29	10.7	5.223
Afghanistan	13.03	29.49	55.06	322.6%	3.023	18.49	36.47	1106.4%	2.36	16.69	38.99	1552.1%	58.15	35.81	15.84
Iran (Islamic Republic of)	81.35	98.44	97.71	20.1%	26.53	43.32	49.33	85.2%	20.47	42.35	53.23	160.0%	4.968	2.427	1.698
Nepal	27.6	42.62	60.62	119.6%	6.059	11.2	19.71	224.8%	8.49	12.5	20.07	136.4%	11.05	12.86	8.288
Uzbekistan	109.6	108	100.3	-8.5%	17.33	29.91	37.88	112.5%	11.93	23.36	33.46	180.5%	13.07	6.061	2.896
Sri Lanka	75.63	90.85	96.83	28.0%	10.37	25.55	39.16	288.9%	4.519	19.56	36.73	712.8%	19.46	12.2	6.625
Kazakhstan	88.59	89.93	94.47	6.6%	52.46	57.93	56.5	7.7%	27.73	50.86	56.44	103.5%	12.49	7.612	4.97
Tajikistan	56.35	59.77	70.97	25.9%	18.35	24.21	32.54	77.3%	7.208	13.27	22.41	210.9%	38.65	30.11	18.98
Turkmenistan	84.42	98.51	99.48	17.8%	25.37	49.74	58.03	128.7%	17.21	58.56	72.22	319.6%	24.68	15.72	10
Kyrgyzstan	78.55	81.7	88.46	12.6%	45.06	57.29	64.49	43.1%	25.84	31.98	39.51	52.9%	21.52	14.82	9.33
Bhutan	32.5	60.94	94.97	192.2%	7.259	27.28	51.78	612.3%	6.519	28.58	60.92	834.5%	34.32	18.21	9.98
Maldives	25.28	57	81.79	223.5%	27.7	37.8	49.78	79.7%	20.28	32.68	50.49	149.0%	15.47	7.001	2.834
Asia-South Central	**43.85**	**68.27**	**80.52**	**83.6%**	**13.2**	**28.63**	**41.23**	**212.3%**	**15.94**	**34.5**	**52.68**	**230.5%**	**13.55**	**4.142**	**2.054**
Indonesia	50.37	58.78	72.32	43.6%	18.41	26.96	34.99	90.1%	12.06	20.21	29.31	143.0%	20.5	13.33	8.306
Philippines	80.29	78.91	90.61	12.9%	29.25	36.02	43.27	47.9%	20.76	28.33	38.68	86.3%	13.12	7.534	4.098
Viet Nam	47.91	66.62	77.09	60.9%	17.99	27.97	37.82	110.2%	11.78	22.1	34.5	192.9%	13.62	7.316	3.339
Thailand	62.76	76.09	85.46	36.2%	47.06	50.38	55.21	17.3%	29.32	36.06	46.95	60.1%	1.029	0	0
Myanmar	39.44	55.27	66.54	68.7%	12.51	18.9	23.33	86.5%	2.573	10.15	16.82	553.7%	19.53	11.31	6.18
Malaysia	59.03	77.72	88.91	50.6%	32.7	42.19	51.99	59.0%	24.14	39.53	57.87	139.7%	0.657	0	0
Cambodia	19.45	37.36	54.93	182.4%	5.564	19.05	30.18	442.4%	3.923	16.35	27.56	602.5%	56	35.47	18.31
LAO People's Dem Repub	37.78	54.84	76.42	102.3%	9.975	24.4	36.23	263.2%	5.082	18.98	34.88	586.3%	46.22	27.06	15.14
Singapore	41.18	74.08	91.4	122.0%	46.12	56.35	65.34	41.7%	47.5	61	71.69	50.9%	0.032	0.025	0.059
Timor-Leste	38.83	43.51	50.83	30.9%	10.37	18.66	25.12	142.2%	3.955	11.86	19.35	389.3%	40.65	31	19.62
Brunei Darussalam	79.87	86.27	88.93	11.3%	16.43	33.44	47.63	189.9%	8.612	25.2	38.57	347.3%	0.517	0.386	0.452
Asia-South East	**54.41**	**65.13**	**77.43**	**42.3%**	**23.15**	**30.94**	**38.68**	**67.1%**	**22.87**	**30.62**	**41.28**	**80.5%**	**16.21**	**10.14**	**5.922**

Education

Infrastructure Health-Related

Base Case: Countries in Year 2060 Descending Population Sequence	Upper Secondary Enrollment Rate, Gross — Total Enrolled as % of Nominal Age Population				Tertiary Enrollment Rate, Gross — Total Enrolled as % of Nominal Age Population				Knowledge Society Index — Index: 0-100				Water Safety — Percent Pop with No Access to Improved Drinking Water Sources		
	2010	2035	2060	% Chg	2010	2035	2060	% Chg	2010	2035	2060	% Chg	2010	2035	2060
ASIA with OCEANIA continued															
Turkey	69.82	85.85	92.44	32.4%	32.12	41.42	50.15	56.1%	23.89	38.23	53.21	122.7%	3.747	1.395	0.653
Yemen	42.67	68.67	89.11	108.8%	10.87	23.26	33.26	206.0%	6.765	17.75	28.53	321.7%	30.28	19.61	11.46
Iraq	34.2	63.58	82.88	142.3%	19.21	37.8	49.36	156.9%	16.59	35.3	55.13	232.3%	16.87	9.007	5.16
Saudi Arabia	103.8	109.8	98.11	-5.5%	30.97	44.23	53.84	73.8%	16.47	37.01	50.86	208.8%	7.506	5.357	3.441
Syrian Arab Repub	36.17	49.72	65.62	81.4%	16.66	25.6	35.77	114.7%	8.611	17.77	31.01	260.1%	5.959	4.623	1.219
Israel	104.6	95.46	99.99	-4.4%	59.19	66.68	76.58	29.4%	86.82	107	114.2	31.5%	0.077	0	0
Jordan	79.94	94.2	100.3	25.5%	40.46	44.64	54.64	35.0%	29.23	39.51	63.35	116.7%	2.505	0.589	0
Occupied Palestinian Territory	66.79	76.63	88.07	31.9%	36.35	36.55	41.36	13.8%	17.08	25.22	39.57	131.7%	9.882	2.957	0
Azerbaijan	74.93	95.07	97.04	29.5%	21.16	39.29	46.78	121.1%	10.77	34.23	46.11	328.1%	19.97	11.76	7.489
United Arab Emirates	85.85	90.28	92.89	8.2%	34.08	47.26	57.1	67.5%	34.73	56.82	70.13	101.9%	0	0	0
Oman	80.24	103.9	102.2	27.4%	21.84	38.83	54.94	151.6%	28.84	48.3	71.87	149.2%	16.75	12.06	7.603
Kuwait	101.5	106.2	100.3	-1.2%	25.59	48.1	56.43	120.5%	5.142	27.53	41.73	711.6%	0.656	0.453	0.461
Lebanon	70.69	80.54	92.02	30.2%	48.49	57.4	63.91	31.8%	35.29	46.7	61.92	75.5%	0	0	0
Armenia	88.01	101.3	99.13	12.6%	31.91	50.03	60.9	90.8%	21.04	48.83	72.83	246.2%	7.01	1.294	0.365
Georgia	72.47	91.05	95.42	31.7%	49.14	56.44	60.78	23.7%	29.8	42.41	53.25	78.7%	16.08	8.961	5.155
Bahrain	102	101.6	101	-1.0%	37.78	49.97	61.34	62.4%	42.23	61.09	74.5	76.4%	0.777	0.527	0.332
Qatar	98.86	96.69	99.92	1.1%	24.49	47.67	66.12	170.0%	17.61	36.46	52.13	196.0%	0	0	0.05
Cyprus	99.13	95.92	99.34	0.2%	35.82	45.98	56.42	57.5%	27.61	45.23	62.02	124.6%	0	0	0
Asia-West	**66.05**	**80.6**	**88.89**	**34.6%**	**27.81**	**38.35**	**47.17**	**69.6%**	**28.77**	**45.51**	**61.01**	**112.1%**	**9.708**	**6.41**	**3.929**
Australia	132.2	99.75	100	-24.4%	73.94	76.86	83.23	12.6%	72.86	83.97	89.15	22.4%	0.023	0	0
Papua New Guinea	35.58	46.15	60.12	69.0%	4.383	17.04	26.37	501.6%	3.12	13.73	22.26	613.5%	56.13	38.79	24.06
New Zealand	130.2	96.53	99.01	-24.0%	83.6	86.32	92.27	10.4%	63.24	73.51	87.63	38.6%	2.882	2.005	1.225
Solomon Islands	18.31	26.37	37	102.1%	12.5	18.62	25.36	102.9%	8.17	13.45	20.1	146.0%	26.54	20.25	14.02
Fiji	70.74	87.35	103.9	46.9%	16.72	26.46	39.32	135.2%	9.019	19.01	36.32	302.7%	50.29	34.96	20.33
Vanuatu	33.72	56.02	84.46	150.5%	7.888	22.62	39.03	394.8%	4.915	18.53	36.64	645.5%	37.07	24.43	13.09
Micronesia, Federated States of	72.25	68.01	81.38	12.6%	17.13	26.97	38.13	122.6%	10.01	19.33	35.79	257.5%	5.712	5.119	1.362
Tonga	103.2	100.9	114.7	11.1%	6.984	17.19	32.62	367.1%	4.466	13.03	30.05	572.9%	2.723	6.374	0.87
Samoa	72.27	86.89	110.1	52.3%	9.305	23.79	43.88	371.6%	9.23	23.93	47.22	411.6%	11.09	5.651	1.844
Oceania	**108.7**	**84.26**	**87.6**	**-19.4%**	**58.11**	**60.1**	**65.59**	**12.9%**	**70.85**	**81.16**	**87.17**	**23.0%**	**13.2**	**10.93**	**7.402**

Multination Regional Analysis

Measures of Poverty, Health, Education, Infrastructure, and Governance

Education

Infrastructure
Health-Related

Base Case: Countries in Year 2060 Descending Population Sequence	Upper Secondary Enrollment Rate, Gross — Total Enrolled as % of Nominal Age Population				Tertiary Enrollment Rate, Gross — Total Enrolled as % of Nominal Age Population				Knowledge Society Index — Index: 0-100				Water Safety — Percent Pop with No Access to Improved Drinking Water Sources		
	2010	2035	2060	% Chg	2010	2035	2060	% Chg	2010	2035	2060	% Chg	2010	2035	2060
EUROPE															
Russian Federation	97.98	107	106.9	9.1%	72.19	75.39	68.09	-5.7%	46.25	64.85	66.81	44.5%	2.35	1.077	0.853
Poland	100.6	97.24	98.48	-2.1%	67.87	73.93	77.89	14.8%	51.66	64.96	76.55	48.2%	1.676	0.527	0.281
Ukraine	97.61	95.06	98.13	0.5%	70.36	69.97	68	-3.4%	43.64	52.67	60.39	38.4%	3.233	1.264	0.648
Romania	80.57	98.03	98.97	22.8%	47.76	56.19	61.78	29.4%	31.55	41.68	52.95	67.8%	40.21	28.71	18.18
Czech Republic	97.25	99.4	99.34	2.1%	49.67	52.62	56.3	13.3%	47.77	58.12	69.97	46.5%	0	0	0
Belarus	75.52	82.43	89.84	19.0%	68.42	79.87	83.88	22.6%	56.28	72.34	82.69	46.9%	0	0	0
Hungary	97.13	100.5	99.16	2.1%	65.39	63.92	63.33	-3.2%	49.23	61.48	75.21	52.8%	1.015	0.262	0.123
Bulgaria	116.5	93.48	98.5	-15.5%	47.31	54.53	61.1	29.1%	30.57	39.16	51.83	69.5%	0.709	0.113	0
Slovak Republic	97.01	98.73	99.51	2.6%	44.24	52.98	58.23	31.6%	32.97	48.43	60.35	83.0%	0	0	0
Moldova, Repub of	82.24	78.67	91.83	11.7%	36.45	38.72	45.39	24.5%	25.02	29.5	39.55	58.1%	7.682	5.434	2.609
Europe-East	**96.42**	**101.1**	**102.2**	**6.0%**	**66.74**	**70.41**	**68.19**	**2.2%**	**46.31**	**62.11**	**68.68**	**48.3%**	**4.966**	**3.04**	**1.987**
United Kingdom	108.7	103.7	105.4	-3.0%	61.1	66.63	74.91	22.6%	52.91	69.89	77.69	46.8%	0.063	0	0
Sweden	102.2	99.46	100	-2.2%	83.55	85.51	89.68	7.3%	85.79	98.82	103.3	20.4%	0.033	0	0
Denmark	122.8	99.34	100	-18.6%	81.27	86.28	82.83	14.2%	70.54	84.03	89.75	27.2%	0.059	0	0
Ireland	119.8	107.4	107.3	-10.4%	60.42	67.25	73.19	21.1%	44.66	59.24	66.59	49.1%	0.765	0.302	0.212
Norway	120	99.91	100	-16.7%	79.65	79	80.61	1.2%	66.14	68.97	73.57	11.2%	0.017	0	0
Finland	118.2	99.28	100	-15.4%	94.57	92.82	95.01	0.5%	84.47	97.34	102.1	20.9%	2.583	1.28	0.693
Lithuania	95.07	96.77	101.8	7.1%	81.64	87.33	91.31	11.8%	63.87	74.23	90.28	41.3%	0.733	0	0
Latvia	95.13	99.24	98.89	4.0%	78.97	86.43	90.34	14.4%	60.45	74.32	91.21	50.9%	0	0	0
Estonia	96.12	99.99	99.37	3.4%	71.11	77.3	83.7	17.7%	60.23	74.08	88.77	47.4%	0	0	0
Iceland	114.2	104.5	105	-8.1%	72.83	73.56	76.24	4.7%	73.94	82.54	89.16	20.6%	0	0	0
Europe-North	**109.5**	**102.5**	**103.9**	**-5.1%**	**68.32**	**72.62**	**79.21**	**15.9%**	**60.15**	**74.78**	**81.95**	**36.2%**	**0.187**	**0.053**	**0.028**
Italy	96.75	98.48	99.7	3.0%	65.54	65.77	67.61	3.2%	39.91	50.81	65.03	62.9%	1.063	0.62	0.403
Spain	123	109.8	110.1	-10.5%	69	70.7	72.92	5.7%	56.41	66.13	75.93	34.6%	0.094	0	0
Greece	105.2	98.27	99.4	-5.5%	89.17	76.01	65.08	-27.0%	34.21	48.82	59.93	75.2%	1.014	0.481	0.321
Portugal	79.65	107.5	99.82	25.3%	59.41	62.56	67.59	13.8%	46.8	55.55	68.63	46.6%	2.418	1.352	0.783
Serbia	79.05	91.88	96.03	21.5%	37.22	40.76	46.93	26.1%	27.1	37.01	51.43	89.8%	6.151	3.737	2.053
Bosnia and Herzegovina	69.98	91.55	94.26	34.7%	18.52	35.73	47.43	156.1%	5.441	25.78	45.2	730.7%	2.999	0	0
Croatia	88.91	100.4	100	12.5%	41.12	48.43	55.58	35.2%	31.15	44.76	60.51	94.3%	0	0	0
Albania	57.98	74.54	85.42	47.3%	20.41	31.72	42.33	107.4%	14.53	28.83	43.74	201.0%	3.478	0.736	0.015
Macedonia, FYR	78.31	95.64	99.93	27.6%	30.95	35.65	42.62	37.7%	16.19	24.52	36.95	128.2%	6.889	4.909	3.048
Slovenia	99.03	99.18	99.94	0.9%	82.23	81.29	81.28	-1.2%	61.39	75.02	84.76	38.1%	1.494	0.486	0.204
Montenegro	74.74	83.26	93.01	24.4%	34.3	40.36	49.82	45.2%	28.08	37.26	53.98	92.2%	6.179	3.496	1.763
Malta	92.94	98.72	99.64	7.2%	33.78	43.44	53.42	58.1%	25.31	40.24	58.54	131.3%	0.014	0	0
Europe-South	**100.9**	**101.4**	**102.1**	**1.2%**	**63.05**	**64.01**	**66.08**	**4.8%**	**44.81**	**55.99**	**68.08**	**51.9%**	**1.3**	**0.665**	**0.392**
Germany	97.53	102	102.4	5.0%	47.74	54.36	63.86	33.8%	53.24	70.79	81.58	53.2%	0.06	0	0
France	112	99.44	99.43	-11.2%	57.48	61.84	69.59	21.1%	53.46	66.36	76.98	44.0%	0.049	0	0
Netherlands	106.2	108.8	110.9	4.4%	59.71	63.36	69.42	16.3%	57.87	69.34	74.68	29.0%	0.02	0	0
Belgium	104.7	98.85	99.89	-4.6%	63.41	63.42	68.02	7.3%	48.55	62.6	74.5	53.5%	0.058	0.003	0
Austria	100.2	99.59	99.98	-0.2%	55.7	68.84	78.07	40.2%	49.31	65.58	75.73	53.6%	0.024	0	0
Switzerland	81.57	101.1	100.7	23.5%	48.3	56.61	67.57	39.9%	54.02	68.86	78.96	46.2%	0.001	0	0
Luxembourg	89.37	99.63	99.87	11.7%	15.99	36.15	54.21	239.0%	23.67	41.24	57.83	144.3%	0.033	0.057	0.125
Europe-West	**102.9**	**101.4**	**101.8**	**-1.1%**	**53.19**	**58.95**	**67.38**	**26.7%**	**53.18**	**68.28**	**78.54**	**47.7%**	**0.049**	**0**	**0.001**

Multination Regional Analysis

Measures of Poverty, Health, Education, Infrastructure, and Governance

Base Case
Source: International Futures Version 6.32, June 2010

Infrastructure Health-Related

	Sanitation — Percent Pop with No Access to Improved Sanitation Sources			Household Use of Solid Fuels — Percent of Population			Urban Residential Outdoor Air Pollution — Micrograms per cc of Particulate Matter 2.5mc or Less		
	2010	2035	2060	2010	2035	2060	2010	2035	2060
World	36.94	24.89	16.42	37.98	22.28	13.97	28.24	17.27	9.943
Africa	51.43	34.25	22.41	65.99	47.75	30.3	29.37	18.91	11.32
Americas	13.28	9.352	6.47	12.3	7.891	5.079	15.42	8.614	5.09
Asia with Oceania	44.36	28.19	17.54	42.52	19.41	9.725	33.23	19.95	11.03
Europe	4.863	3.222	2.518	6.47	3.733	2.413	14.83	8.125	4.779
World	36.94	24.89	16.42	37.98	22.28	13.97	28.24	17.27	9.943
Africa-Eastern	59.91	36.54	19.4	86.68	57.51	25.69	19.62	13.28	7.567
Africa-Middle	63.77	51.65	39.84	79.16	68.26	61.02	29.45	22.53	14.93
Africa-Northern	28	17.63	11.57	19.99	10.65	5.809	46.47	27.08	14.76
Africa-Southern	35.88	25.26	15.35	20.34	11.17	4.577	11.36	6.325	3.355
Africa-Western	56.35	33.99	22.1	78.74	51.98	32.26	31.34	20.7	12.85
Africa	51.43	34.25	22.41	65.99	47.75	30.3	29.37	18.91	11.32
America-Caribbean	23.73	22.91	19.27	32.72	31.56	28.37	13.37	8.301	5.686
America-Central	25.42	17.63	10.46	42.95	28.64	14.76	20.94	12.62	7.603
America-North	4.927	3.685	2.722	7.519	4.979	3.177	14.3	7.883	4.542
America-South	20.43	13.15	8.766	12.34	5.998	3.394	16.29	8.915	5.258
Americas	13.28	9.352	6.47	12.3	7.891	5.079	15.42	8.614	5.09
Asia-East	43.73	29.61	18.91	33.09	11.49	4.888	32.04	17.2	8.805
Asia-South Central	54.23	32.58	19.69	53.55	24.5	11.94	35.95	23.2	12.87
Asia-South East	30.58	20.52	13.51	49.1	28.07	15.39	30.73	18.03	10.8
Asia-West	15.08	10.54	7.346	11	5.977	3.388	31.04	17.85	9.292
Oceania	11.72	9.314	6.804	22.7	16.77	10.64	9.599	5.784	3.519
Asia with Oceania	44.36	28.19	17.54	42.52	19.41	9.725	33.23	19.95	11.03
Europe-East	8.634	6.117	4.694	7.181	3.981	2.923	13.4	7.627	4.431
Europe-North	2.955	1.923	1.601	4.946	2.967	1.799	10.73	5.612	3.378
Europe-South	3.547	2.289	1.961	7.594	4.498	2.79	20.91	11.34	6.679
Europe-West	1.398	1.009	1.041	4.784	3.105	1.838	13.7	7.403	4.527
Europe	4.863	3.222	2.518	6.47	3.733	2.413	14.83	8.125	4.779

Infrastructure Resource-Related

	Water Use per Capita — Thousands of Cubic Meters			Crop Yield — Annual Metric Tons per Hectare		
	2010	2035	2060	2010	2035	2060
World	0.613	0.602	0.597	3.253	3.733	4.051
Africa	0.235	0.2	0.179	2.324	2.94	3.296
Americas	0.923	0.91	0.907	3.187	3.575	3.812
Asia with Oceania	0.629	0.655	0.699	3.855	4.326	4.754
Europe	0.646	0.704	0.782	3.721	4.075	4.237
World	0.613	0.602	0.597	3.253	3.733	4.051
Africa-Eastern	0.141	0.131	0.132	2.576	3.408	3.812
Africa-Middle	0.023	0.02	0.017	2.189	2.714	3.002
Africa-Northern	0.698	0.68	0.706	2.681	2.973	3.474
Africa-Southern	0.267	0.265	0.261	1.612	1.769	1.738
Africa-Western	0.099	0.095	0.091	2.238	2.951	3.365
Africa	0.235	0.2	0.179	2.324	2.94	3.296
America-Caribbean	0.441	0.409	0.386	3.524	3.607	3.494
America-Central	0.231	0.201	0.187	3.107	3.349	3.507
America-North	1.442	1.448	1.437	2.251	2.715	2.904
America-South	0.455	0.46	0.476	3.158	3.893	4.507
Americas	0.923	0.91	0.907	3.187	3.575	3.812
Asia-East	0.504	0.531	0.552	5.246	5.544	5.493
Asia-South Central	0.735	0.757	0.813	2.782	3.631	4.397
Asia-South East	0.578	0.556	0.557	3.275	3.819	4.275
Asia-West	0.783	0.77	0.773	5.704	5.927	6.293
Oceania	0.883	0.876	0.999	1.456	1.877	2.24
Asia with Oceania	0.629	0.655	0.699	3.855	4.326	4.754
Europe-East	0.599	0.682	0.819	2.818	3.231	3.352
Europe-North	0.282	0.291	0.305	2.874	3.195	3.324
Europe-South	1.147	1.302	1.501	3.821	4.438	4.813
Europe-West	0.525	0.535	0.549	5.565	5.648	5.584
Europe	0.646	0.704	0.782	3.721	4.075	4.237

Infrastructure
Health-Related

Infrastructure
Resource-Related

Base Case: Countries in Year 2060 Descending Population Sequence	Sanitation — Percent Pop with No Access to Improved Sanitation Sources			Household Use of Solid Fuels — Percent of Population			Urban Residential Outdoor Air Pollution — Micrograms per cc of Particulate Matter 2.5mc or Less			Water Use per Capita — Thousands of Cubic Meters			Crop Yield — Annual Metric Tons per Hectare		
	2010	2035	2060	2010	2035	2060	2010	2035	2060	2010	2035	2060	2010	2035	2060
AFRICA															
Ethiopia	81.01	49.41	25.32	92.27	63.67	23.17	36.28	24.58	12.38	0.078	0.074	0.081	2.536	3.386	4.734
Tanzania, United Rep	46.2	11.63	4.811	91.33	33.68	10.11	11.63	7.035	3.955	0.134	0.125	0.123	3.603	4.487	5.102
Uganda	52.63	31.25	6.898	92.45	61	10.43	5.797	4.194	3	0.01	0.01	0.01	3.502	4.856	6.165
Kenya	53.94	36.32	21.41	66.09	37.64	14.19	17.05	11.06	6.354	0.046	0.042	0.04	2.46	2.996	3.089
Madagascar	65.82	58.19	34.24	94.37	90.17	61.48	16.7	11.68	7.895	0.802	0.753	0.732	2.414	3.122	3.785
Mozambique	62.04	27.38	12.92	92.2	47.06	14.03	13.71	9.405	5.01	0.032	0.031	0.031	2.363	3.222	3.63
Malawi	34.27	22.61	11.95	90.39	69.05	32.93	16.53	10.57	7.587	0.079	0.081	0.084	3.496	5.198	6.127
Zambia	42.29	25.92	11.99	82.64	52.95	19.81	21.91	17.05	11.67	0.148	0.139	0.128	0.892	1.114	1.184
Somalia	68.89	56.85	43.28	93.9	87.88	76.6	14.13	8.915	5.448	0.394	0.35	0.317	2.71	3.127	2.831
Rwanda	55.28	26.69	10.02	92.86	56.14	16.09	14.34	11	5.832	0.017	0.016	0.016	5.126	6.375	7.02
Zimbabwe	44.16	38.14	27.36	69.93	61.93	42	12.58	9.483	6.74	0.325	0.323	0.314	1.314	1.655	1.779
Burundi	60.93	47.76	32.28	94.14	89.06	72.87	15.15	9.681	6.245	0.038	0.037	0.032	3.355	5.481	5.315
Eritrea	75.67	62.22	48.62	62.58	59.6	53.79	25.68	17.11	10.98	0.068	0.063	0.06	2.286	3.012	3.207
Comoros	67.53	57.83	45.7	77.43	72.67	61.83	16.18	11.71	7.801	0.016	0.015	0.014	1.513	2.126	1.764
Mauritius	5.569	2.73	1.906	4.503	2.27	1.186	8.154	4.463	3	0.5	0.511	0.546	1.435	1.841	2.607
Djibouti	18.08	11.67	2.974	12.78	8.353	3.033	23.74	21.57	11.22	0.026	0.025	0.025	2.204	2.528	2.647
Africa-Eastern	**59.91**	**36.54**	**19.4**	**86.68**	**57.51**	**25.69**	**19.62**	**13.28**	**7.567**	**0.141**	**0.131**	**0.132**	**2.576**	**3.408**	**3.812**
Congo, Democratic Republic of	67.33	57.14	45.25	93.79	87.87	79.66	24.93	20.47	14.54	0.01	0.009	0.008	2.996	4.354	4.729
Angola	59.01	41.75	26.93	32.63	15.49	9.173	34.6	21.45	11.29	0.022	0.019	0.018	3.825	5.163	6.12
Cameroon	45.68	32.69	19.73	77.4	52.94	25.96	29.94	19.97	12.42	0.061	0.058	0.058	1.19	1.643	2.279
Chad	78.17	58.11	46.11	81.71	61.01	59.46	52.24	43.36	26.36	0.024	0.021	0.02	1.088	1.468	2.002
Central African Republic	72.09	64.73	44.69	94.53	90.81	72.87	22.54	16.81	11.13	0.01	0.01	0.009	0.82	0.987	1.125
Congo, Republic of	63.31	46.53	31.3	63.41	38.5	26.74	35.25	24.9	14.61	0.01	0.009	0.009	6.174	6.725	6.68
Gabon	60.58	46.44	30.75	27.47	23.08	16.42	3.638	3	3	0.085	0.075	0.069	1.715	1.813	1.729
Equatorial Guinea	44.57	34.13	22.93	4.959	4.098	3.171	4.124	3	3	0.217	0.194	0.182	0.899	0.947	0.922
São Tomé and Príncipe	56.64	55.11	37.9	80.74	81.11	62.38	20.87	14.89	10.01	0.283	0.263	0.243	0.994	1.329	1.438
Africa-Middle	**63.77**	**51.65**	**39.84**	**79.16**	**68.26**	**61.02**	**29.45**	**22.53**	**14.93**	**0.023**	**0.02**	**0.017**	**2.189**	**2.714**	**3.002**
Egypt	27.16	17.63	11.24	4.284	1.893	0.927	54.35	28.31	14.65	0.904	0.812	0.781	10.25	10	10.02
Sudan	58.23	30.72	18.5	82.6	38.49	18.81	85.33	49.27	24.91	1.051	1.019	1.039	0.789	1.048	1.426
Algeria	6.745	4.547	4.252	4.612	2.591	1.768	28.23	18.25	11.35	0.189	0.203	0.223	1.307	1.777	2.396
Morocco	25.78	18.7	12.07	6.326	3.971	2.1	10.28	6.177	3.329	0.428	0.438	0.493	1.714	2.296	3.172
Tunisia	13.15	7.094	4.506	4.322	1.886	0.943	13.72	6.553	3.353	0.273	0.289	0.34	1.186	1.616	2.274
Libyan Arab Jamahiriya	1.599	0	1.124	4.231	1.966	1.434	39.13	21.98	13.32	0.739	0.734	0.783	0.838	1.099	1.552
Africa-Northern	**28**	**17.63**	**11.57**	**19.99**	**10.65**	**5.809**	**46.47**	**27.08**	**14.76**	**0.698**	**0.68**	**0.706**	**2.681**	**2.973**	**3.474**

Infrastructure Health-Related / Infrastructure Resource-Related

Base Case: Countries in Year 2060 Descending Population Sequence	Sanitation — Percent Pop with No Access to Improved Sanitation Sources 2010	2035	2060	Household Use of Solid Fuels — Percent of Population 2010	2035	2060	Urban Residential Outdoor Air Pollution — Micrograms per cc of Particulate Matter 2.5mc or Less 2010	2035	2060	Water Use per Capita — Thousands of Cubic Meters 2010	2035	2060	Crop Yield — Annual Metric Tons per Hectare 2010	2035	2060
AFRICA continued															
South Africa	32.23	22.28	13.62	15.07	7.498	3.051	9.649	5.332	3	0.272	0.273	0.269	1.472	1.632	1.669
Namibia	71.33	48.52	28.43	56.56	29.77	10.59	22.84	12.34	5.623	0.149	0.138	0.132	0.798	0.852	0.831
Lesotho	60.35	41.42	22.51	70.26	47.18	19.58	20.03	11.12	4.784	0.028	0.027	0.026	1.936	2.192	1.997
Botswana	53.92	35.92	22.71	37.21	12.72	6.816	30.45	12.74	5.342	0.108	0.104	0.1	1.443	1.573	1.408
Swaziland	50.8	34.26	17.6	60.9	36.28	12.61	15.84	9.692	4.145	0.919	0.853	0.834	2.41	2.593	2.784
Africa-Southern	**35.88**	**25.26**	**15.35**	**20.34**	**11.17**	**4.577**	**11.36**	**6.325**	**3.355**	**0.267**	**0.265**	**0.261**	**1.612**	**1.769**	**1.738**
Nigeria	45.35	16.09	14.13	72.15	30.63	23.18	25.89	16.57	10.02	0.061	0.056	0.049	3.969	5.647	6.197
Niger	83.61	68.21	41.92	94.47	90.19	69.86	64.86	40.37	24.22	0.156	0.145	0.135	1.266	1.909	2.288
Côte c'Ivoire	61.3	45.85	27.86	77.02	57.96	30.7	22.5	15.76	9.072	0.051	0.045	0.041	1.346	1.647	1.772
Ghana	78.51	64.55	36.9	83.31	76.22	34.58	16.16	11.54	8.006	0.045	0.042	0.04	3.766	5.085	6.005
Mali	50.89	30.3	9.291	93.86	76.53	30.65	70.84	37.83	21.8	0.487	0.451	0.443	1.161	1.533	2.058
Burkina Faso	84.59	63.7	32.66	94.23	78.1	30.27	45.01	32.05	19.14	0.061	0.058	0.058	1.32	1.879	2.421
Senegal	42.64	29.14	14.42	55.14	40.79	16.38	45.53	29.14	16.81	0.192	0.182	0.174	1.393	1.779	1.947
Guinea	77.61	52.71	31.38	92.88	67.8	35.08	33.6	23.69	15.37	0.161	0.137	0.123	2.849	3.102	2.959
Benin	63.49	49.02	27.57	92.31	79.4	43.29	19.02	11.43	7.298	0.016	0.014	0.013	3.486	4.928	5.851
Togo	61.02	46.53	39.61	93.38	82.64	78.05	15.72	10.23	6.597	0.027	0.027	0.024	0.957	1.548	1.589
Sierra Leone	56.58	34.57	14.51	92.61	66.74	22.67	26.06	22.32	13.9	0.068	0.064	0.067	3.636	4.556	5.858
Liberia	66.31	35.87	17.11	94.34	59.06	19.01	20.7	17.07	9.922	0.033	0.032	0.03	1.788	2.276	2.397
Mauritania	61.22	61.73	39.33	58.11	61.96	46.75	46.23	27.82	16.8	0.563	0.528	0.5	1.854	2.401	2.737
Guinea-Bissau	63.01	50.31	42	94.71	91.59	87.17	32.74	17.28	10.13	0.113	0.1	0.09	1.074	1.288	1.245
Gambia	42.36	25.71	14.07	90.14	59.33	26.65	42.24	29.97	19.85	0.02	0.018	0.017	1.825	2.052	1.935
Cape Verde	52.85	36.24	22.77	32.28	14.74	6.37	26.22	16.93	9.304	0.04	0.039	0.039	4.125	5.594	6.587
Africa-Western	**56.35**	**33.99**	**22.1**	**78.74**	**51.98**	**32.26**	**31.34**	**20.7**	**12.85**	**0.099**	**0.095**	**0.091**	**2.238**	**2.951**	**3.365**

Infrastructure Health-Related / Infrastructure Resource-Related

Base Case: Countries in Year 2060 Descending Population Sequence	Sanitation — Percent Pop with No Access to Improved Sanitation Sources			Household Use of Solid Fuels — Percent of Population			Urban Residential Outdoor Air Pollution — Micrograms per cc of Particulate Matter 2.5mc or Less			Water Use per Capita — Thousands of Cubic Meters			Crop Yield — Annual Metric Tons per Hectare		
	2010	2035	2060	2010	2035	2060	2010	2035	2060	2010	2035	2060	2010	2035	2060
AMERICAS															
Haiti	69.32	61.96	44.97	92.65	88.65	71.07	19.36	13.96	9.185	0.116	0.11	0.104	2.386	2.849	2.675
Dominican Republic	20.54	13.2	8.699	6.802	3.085	1.596	9.132	5.32	3	0.387	0.382	0.376	1.77	2.057	2.08
Cuba	1.77	0	0	21.59	11.1	6.124	7.645	3	3	0.747	0.788	0.881	1.137	1.308	1.463
Puerto Rico	4.086	2.323	1.805	4.526	2.511	1.48	12.12	5.188	5.702	0.757	0.725	0.711	10.51	10.23	9.656
Jamaica	19.32	14.33	10.01	29.23	20.31	12.36	17.37	10.04	5.702	0.161	0.157	0.155	3.351	3.387	3.245
Trinidad	0	0	0	4.32	1.959	1.226	43.94	25.38	12.72	0.241	0.241	0.247	1.591	1.664	1.665
Bahamas	0.329	0.22	0.565	4.878	3.041	1.72	22.27	12.63	7.049	0.301	0.286	0.283	9.267	9.082	8.971
Barbados	0.074	0	0.029	4.742	2.934	1.597	14.97	7.789	3.958	0.339	0.338	0.364	2.479	2.414	2.237
Grenada	4.44	4.618	2.553	20.07	15.77	7.592	9.323	5.733	3.189	0.288	0.289	0.278	1.714	1.866	1.778
Saint Vincent and Grenadines	12.64	6.775	4.034	25.87	12.19	6.049	12.41	6.127	3.051	0.088	0.089	0.087	1.333	1.411	1.325
Saint Lucia	10.17	6.667	4.691	4.556	2.592	1.532	13.66	7.485	4.124	0.064	0.065	0.068	3.231	3.409	3.341
America-Caribbean	**23.73**	**22.91**	**19.27**	**32.72**	**31.56**	**28.37**	**13.37**	**8.301**	**5.686**	**0.441**	**0.409**	**0.386**	**3.524**	**3.607**	**3.494**
Guatemala	13.14	7.485	4.062	62.27	36.01	16.8	29.67	16.91	9.675	0.16	0.143	0.135	2.567	2.86	3.033
Honduras	29.02	20	13.14	50	30.19	16.02	20.11	12.12	7.568	0.119	0.109	0.101	2.173	2.168	1.924
El Salvador	36.29	27.15	16.32	21.78	14.84	6.792	16.27	10.14	5.88	0.188	0.178	0.175	1.976	2.041	2.082
Nicaragua	51.18	42.59	26.26	55.81	48.18	27.17	13.92	9.032	5.972	0.257	0.24	0.228	0.922	1.004	0.947
Costa Rica	7.363	4.242	3.016	11.4	5.964	3.316	15.86	7.942	4.329	0.626	0.552	0.554	8.091	7.894	8.37
Panama	24.86	17.24	11.34	15.8	7.481	4.151	16.2	8.799	4.75	0.264	0.255	0.243	2.081	2.261	2.054
Belize	49.87	35.98	22.81	13.05	7.504	3.756	6.871	4.177	3	0.543	0.511	0.517	3.939	5.213	6.143
America-Central	**25.42**	**17.63**	**10.46**	**42.95**	**28.64**	**14.76**	**20.94**	**12.62**	**7.603**	**0.231**	**0.201**	**0.187**	**3.107**	**3.349**	**3.507**
USA	0.204	0.308	0.653	4.904	3.468	2.332	13.47	7.379	4.227	1.673	1.674	1.623	2.928	3.523	3.732
Mexico	19.85	14.29	9.876	15.77	9.73	6.134	17.7	9.76	5.698	0.775	0.781	0.806	2.245	2.711	2.882
Canada	0.134	0.334	0.761	4.907	3.458	2.271	10.9	6.392	4.035	1.473	1.531	1.577	1.579	1.912	2.098
America-North	**4.927**	**3.685**	**2.722**	**7.519**	**4.979**	**3.177**	**14.3**	**7.883**	**4.542**	**1.442**	**1.448**	**1.437**	**2.251**	**2.715**	**2.904**
Brazil	22.68	13.74	8.839	9.643	4.103	2.124	11.19	5.533	3	0.327	0.32	0.311	2.159	2.381	2.314
Colombia	12.37	7.83	5.159	11.7	6.657	3.714	9.485	4.997	3	0.236	0.227	0.23	4.202	4.504	4.867
Argentina	8.185	5.304	3.862	4.235	2.131	1.269	33.98	18.35	10.43	0.802	0.89	0.987	1.657	2.259	2.751
Peru	33.72	23.33	15.48	33.1	15.47	8.97	27.54	16.04	9.543	0.739	0.759	0.808	3.525	4.86	6.175
Venezuela	27.52	18.15	12.08	17.1	7.744	4.604	4.861	3	3	0.321	0.324	0.349	2.892	3.881	5.252
Ecuador	9.398	8.146	7.074	4.458	3.302	2.445	11.09	7.116	4.603	1.337	1.301	1.283	4.726	6.004	6.479
Chile	8.368	5.434	3.892	4.558	2.346	1.345	23.23	12.38	6.918	0.801	0.816	0.86	5.672	6.841	7.631
Bolivia	49.6	32.09	20.88	30.42	12.22	6.866	40.11	26.58	15.65	0.157	0.162	0.167	1.399	1.796	2.16
Paraguay	18.02	12.09	7.728	45.45	26.97	13.85	37.06	21.88	12.98	0.085	0.078	0.076	2.66	3.275	3.649
Uruguay	0	0	0	4.24	1.847	0.895	69.65	37.05	20.2	0.976	1.149	1.408	2.941	4.114	5.505
Guyana	28.25	21.76	14.76	8.575	5.586	3.175	14.27	11.42	7.18	2.378	2.878	3.863	1.352	1.75	2.394
Suriname	6.111	2.826	1.91	24.26	11.97	6.201	12.8	7.545	4.1	1.553	1.618	1.7	4.707	5.046	4.912
America-South	**20.43**	**13.15**	**8.766**	**12.34**	**5.998**	**3.394**	**16.29**	**8.915**	**5.258**	**0.455**	**0.46**	**0.476**	**3.158**	**3.893**	**4.507**

Infrastructure Health-Related | **Infrastructure Resource-Related**

Base Case: Countries in Year 2060 Descending Population Sequence	Sanitation — Percent Pop with No Access to Improved Sanitation Sources			Household Use of Solid Fuels — Percent of Population			Urban Residential Outdoor Air Pollution — Micrograms per cc of Particulate Matter 2.5mc or Less			Water Use per Capita — Thousands of Cubic Meters			Crop Yield — Annual Metric Tons per Hectare		
	2010	2035	2060	2010	2035	2060	2010	2035	2060	2010	2035	2060	2010	2035	2060
ASIA with OCEANIA															
China	50.33	33.55	21.1	36.98	12.15	4.92	34.02	18.1	9.107	0.443	0.47	0.486	6.326	7.315	7.258
Japan	0.213	0.119	0.587	4.779	3.009	1.878	18.95	10.38	6.431	0.701	0.734	0.788	10.35	10.37	9.92
Korea, Repub of	3.962	3.074	2.614	4.709	3.147	2.056	21.85	11.95	6.929	0.388	0.395	0.441	10.41	10.52	10.56
Taiwan	5.231	3.307	2.428	8.71	4.908	2.771	14.44	7.153	3.914	3.159	3.239	3.357	2.255	2.747	2.91
Korea, Dem. People's Rep.	38.12	26.98	17.32	54.57	37.24	22.7	32.58	18.89	9.987	0.416	0.437	0.449	4.457	4.828	4.792
Hong Kong SAR	2.913	3.07	2.776	3.845	3.378	2.341	13.76	8.324	4.946	0.686	0.669	0.67	2.264	2.239	2.182
Mongolia	34.51	21.07	13.08	60.73	23.27	10.25	47.88	27.73	14.36	0.175	0.175	0.175	0.662	0.789	0.827
Asia-East	**43.73**	**29.61**	**18.91**	**33.09**	**11.49**	**4.888**	**32.04**	**17.2**	**8.805**	**0.504**	**0.531**	**0.552**	**5.246**	**5.544**	**5.493**
India	60.4	34.79	21.47	51.08	14.94	5.975	31.43	18.93	9.841	0.6	0.619	0.676	2.698	3.752	5.188
Pakistan	40.19	32.8	19.2	65.22	53.68	27.99	57.93	39.79	21.78	1.094	1.097	1.117	3.001	4.147	5.557
Bangladesh	54.81	29.29	17.95	84.5	45.44	22.49	65.51	45.33	27.82	0.562	0.534	0.53	6.186	6.815	7.155
Afghanistan	63.76	36.4	12.56	84.92	58.7	15.38	21.16	13.79	6.522	0.751	0.718	0.715	1.422	1.938	2.711
Iran (Islamic Republic of)	14.52	9.086	6.688	4.216	1.785	1.198	20.33	11.63	6.898	1.101	1.145	1.289	3.452	4.624	5.934
Nepal	63.95	53.62	32.23	80.12	73.02	46.45	17.94	12.83	7.706	0.385	0.379	0.386	4.012	5.723	6.901
Uzbek'stan	24.79	14.61	9.647	12.49	6.043	3.306	26.42	14.95	8.465	2.272	2.344	2.481	2.613	3.713	4.669
Sri Lanka	7.885	4.401	3.147	64.05	32.51	17.08	42.14	25.66	14.76	0.652	0.668	0.683	3.079	3.246	3.319
Kazakhstan	25.68	17.91	12.36	9.563	3.864	3.01	7.938	4.811	3	2.423	2.391	2.777	0.834	0.79	0.87
Tajikistan	42.51	33.46	22.37	19.71	14.77	8.331	24.1	18.05	12.62	1.895	1.961	2.143	2.577	3.753	5.328
Turkmenistan	12.77	7.043	5.266	3.711	1.214	0.843	23.75	10.61	6.295	5.386	5.633	5.839	2.467	3.443	4.014
Kyrgyzstan	37.32	25.31	17.31	34.19	19.96	11.92	10.55	6.641	4.149	2.046	2.188	2.435	2.551	3.711	4.803
Bhutan	27.59	15.94	8.665	42.87	17.41	6.145	13.13	9.283	4.336	0.704	0.765	0.734	1.804	2.382	2.49
Maldives	38.9	25.77	14.95	8.964	4.597	1.734	15.87	9.245	4.567	0.01	0.01	0.01	2.253	2.791	2.622
Asia-South Central	**54.23**	**32.58**	**19.69**	**53.55**	**24.5**	**11.94**	**35.95**	**23.2**	**12.87**	**0.735**	**0.757**	**0.813**	**2.782**	**3.631**	**4.397**
Indonesia	41.08	28.73	19.27	51.04	28.5	16.97	41.98	24.93	15.24	0.385	0.397	0.416	3.228	4.017	4.551
Philippines	25.81	18.53	12.78	41.91	24.7	14.16	12.12	8.105	5.188	0.346	0.325	0.315	3.728	4.061	4.093
Viet Nam	35.42	22.74	14.62	53.35	25.45	12.35	26.85	16.09	9.506	0.869	0.826	0.83	6.987	7.33	7.634
Thailand	1.155	0.594	0.97	21.77	13.65	7.842	35.33	20.45	11.91	1.321	1.301	1.352	3.295	3.187	3.201
Myanmar	18.26	4.082	0.346	90.44	58.6	30.44	28.03	16.14	9.947	0.673	0.7	0.707	3.199	3.791	3.837
Malaysia	5.6	3.566	2.704	4.633	2.62	1.567	10.69	5.681	3.009	0.359	0.345	0.337	0.652	0.674	0.63
Cambodia	78.45	48.98	25.89	88.1	55.17	21.75	22.08	15.84	9.592	0.294	0.286	0.3	1.683	2.305	3.229
LAO People's Dem Repub	65.12	38.75	24.03	89.15	36.63	15.49	22.74	15.8	9.469	0.516	0.533	0.572	3.777	5.202	6.062
Singapore	0.244	0.634	1.176	4.751	3.541	2.434	23.97	13.93	8.041	0.044	0.043	0.044	2.327	2.234	2.383
Timor-Leste	42.74	33.86	22.8	63.31	49.24	32.21	37.87	29.91	20.83	0.373	0.343	0.32	4.906	6.178	7.097
Brunei Darussalam	2.111	2.289	2.635	5.095	4	3.578	32.39	21.59	13.71	0.241	0.239	0.254	2.245	3.028	4.311
Asia-South East	**30.58**	**20.52**	**13.51**	**49.1**	**28.07**	**15.39**	**30.73**	**18.03**	**10.8**	**0.578**	**0.556**	**0.557**	**3.275**	**3.819**	**4.275**

Infrastructure Health-Related / Infrastructure Resource-Related

Base Case: Countries in Year 2060 Descending Population Sequence	Sanitation — Percent Pop with No Access to Improved Sanitation Sources			Household Use of Solid Fuels — Percent of Population			Urban Residential Outdoor Air Pollution — Micrograms per cc of Particulate Matter 2.5mc or Less			Water Use per Capita — Thousands of Cubic Meters			Crop Yield — Annual Metric Tons per Hectare		
	2010	2035	2060	2010	2035	2060	2010	2035	2060	2010	2035	2060	2010	2035	2060
ASIA with OCEANIA continued															
Turkey	11.25	6.592	4.672	10.21	5.162	2.986	18.09	9.138	4.982	0.572	0.631	0.74	3.052	4.304	5.583
Yemen	51.36	34.82	21.86	32.07	16.98	8.79	25.74	16.18	8.512	0.314	0.284	0.27	3.708	4.161	4.239
Iraq	18.32	8.889	5.252	4.705	1.733	0.828	53.49	26.82	12.05	1.627	1.537	1.478	1.227	1.423	1.453
Saudi Arabia	4.174	3.07	2.355	4.878	2.984	2.122	47.97	28.19	13.2	0.756	0.722	0.747	2.009	2.545	3.462
Syrian Arab Repub	8.217	7.302	3.71	4.463	3.297	1.591	35.67	21.61	12.3	1.029	0.9	0.828	1.948	2.08	1.995
Israel	4.053	2.311	1.653	4.652	2.473	1.262	15.79	7.272	3.833	0.29	0.246	0.224	10.58	10	9.057
Jordan	6.261	3.802	2.308	4.367	2.166	0.913	23.27	14.62	7.942	0.189	0.176	0.171	5.395	6.145	6.577
Occupied Palestinian Territory	28.37	15.06	8.121	52.11	22.6	8.492	25.68	15.61	9.205	0.496	0.458	0.448	10.91	11.57	13.04
Azerbaijan	23.31	14.39	10.14	7.656	2.77	1.794	27.04	14.44	8.261	2.13	2.24	2.326	2.431	3.355	3.713
United Arab Emirates	0.307	0	0	4.011	1.711	0.942	52.6	25.35	13.18	0.509	0.458	0.459	7.985	6.984	7.058
Oman	11.26	8.617	5.97	4.619	3.058	1.867	48.03	29.26	15.72	0.529	0.493	0.487	7.158	7.164	7.81
Kuwait	2.595	2.08	2.133	4.882	3.185	2.892	41.81	24.36	12.18	0.172	0.161	0.158	10.77	9.95	10.09
Lebanon	1.648	0.573	0.637	4.364	2.383	1.307	18.26	10.41	5.844	0.385	0.354	0.364	10.58	10.69	11.37
Armenia	15.29	7.717	5.161	4.188	1.268	0.606	30.66	17.77	9.83	1.004	1.121	1.233	3.277	4.541	5.693
Georgia	4.987	1.696	1.83	36.8	17.57	9.942	34.11	21.14	12.39	0.866	1.134	1.445	2.762	3.675	4.489
Bahrain	2.73	2.315	2.016	4.531	3.121	1.977	29.07	17.12	9.864	0.412	0.385	0.378	2.195	2.153	2.098
Qatar	0	0.138	0.835	3.833	2.661	2.695	21.71	13.2	7.556	0.353	0.322	0.332	10.34	9.685	9.585
Cyprus	0.076	0	0.639	4.581	3.031	2.055	29.65	15.33	8.575	0.287	0.28	0.289	6.351	6.248	5.956
Asia-West	**15.08**	**10.54**	**7.346**	**11**	**5.977**	**3.388**	**31.04**	**17.85**	**9.292**	**0.783**	**0.77**	**0.773**	**5.704**	**5.927**	**6.293**
Australia	0.031	0.022	0.441	4.727	3.033	1.854	9.011	5.026	3	1.283	1.346	1.589	0.954	1.224	1.686
Papua New Guinea	48.63	31	19.39	82.79	51.07	29.52	10.29	6.718	3.895	0.017	0.016	0.016	3.514	4.035	4.139
New Zealand	3.306	2.347	1.822	4.829	3.164	1.865	8.653	4.452	3	0.544	0.614	0.771	1.161	1.622	2.36
Solomon Islands	61.45	46.71	32.81	68.08	51.58	36.1	18.46	14.69	9.419	0.326	0.315	0.304	2.546	3.551	4.32
Fiji	26.73	17.77	10.12	46.57	27.51	11.93	10.58	6.3	3.316	0.086	0.092	0.109	0.957	1.304	1.853
Vanuatu	29.64	19	10.45	75.89	41.81	18.05	9.296	5.552	3	0.288	0.277	0.276	0.541	0.741	0.936
Micronesia, Federated States of	21.37	18.62	11.09	36.56	30.48	14.52	27.38	23.15	12.77	0.293	0.286	0.271	2.245	2.861	3.099
Tonga	7.847	13.63	6.382	47.14	49.93	22.69	23.84	16.44	10.05	0.277	0.258	0.243	0.709	0.887	0.876
Samoa	0	0	0	34.7	18.58	8.109	23.37	14.72	8.48	0.296	0.305	0.338	0.48	0.665	0.889
Oceania	**11.72**	**9.314**	**6.804**	**22.7**	**16.77**	**10.64**	**9.599**	**5.784**	**3.519**	**0.883**	**0.876**	**0.999**	**1.456**	**1.877**	**2.24**

Multination Regional Analysis

Measures of Poverty, Health, Education, Infrastructure, and Governance

Infrastructure Health-Related / Infrastructure Resource-Related

Base Case: Countries in Year 2060 Descending Population Sequence	Sanitation — Percent Pop with No Access to Improved Sanitation Sources			Household Use of Solid Fuels — Percent of Population			Urban Residential Outdoor Air Pollution — Micrograms per cc of Particulate Matter 2.5mc or Less			Water Use per Capita — Thousands of Cubic Meters			Crop Yield — Annual Metric Tons per Hectare		
	2010	2035	2060	2010	2035	2060	2010	2035	2060	2010	2035	2060	2010	2035	2060
EUROPE															
Russian Federation	11.7	8.393	6.31	6.838	3.569	3.005	10.41	6.347	3.655	0.562	0.613	0.733	1.099	1.103	1.182
Polanc	5.52	3.599	2.862	4.413	2.409	1.612	23.56	12.24	7.054	0.323	0.383	0.453	3.617	4.244	4.344
Ukraine	3.509	2.195	1.954	4.9	2.84	1.882	14.1	7.593	4.068	0.859	1.079	1.393	2.138	2.271	2.342
Romaria	7.661	5.396	4.122	20.35	11.74	7.531	9.568	5.632	3.381	0.317	0.37	0.426	3.277	3.593	3.531
Czech Republic	1.826	1.191	1.323	4.53	2.763	1.9	14.38	8.017	4.795	0.201	0.268	0.372	2.443	3.477	4.46
Belarus	14.83	10.18	7.136	4.203	2.055	1.392	4.172	3	3	0.306	0.371	0.432	2.782	3.146	3.14
Hungary	4.813	3.003	2.432	4.667	2.555	1.613	12.12	6.382	3.786	2.231	2.637	3.112	4.521	4.75	4.621
Bulgaria	0.852	0.594	0.935	12.98	8.19	5.235	39.2	22.73	12.72	0.987	1.236	1.494	2.15	2.281	2.224
Slovak Republic	0.678	0.05	0.646	4.249	2.288	1.583	7.131	3.802	3	0.205	0.251	0.299	3.508	4.597	4.916
Moldova, Repub of	30.2	22.5	15.12	13.75	9.47	5.392	17.36	11	7.101	0.583	0.644	0.709	2.65	2.851	2.76
Europe-East	**8.634**	**6.117**	**4.694**	**7.181**	**3.981**	**2.923**	**13.4**	**7.627**	**4.431**	**0.599**	**0.682**	**0.819**	**2.818**	**3.231**	**3.352**
United Kingdom	2.961	1.957	1.63	4.76	2.856	1.696	10.61	5.484	3.232	0.199	0.197	0.195	6.072	6.314	6.072
Sweden	0.149	0.01	0.387	4.76	2.926	1.787	8.086	4.188	3	0.307	0.308	0.302	2.689	2.779	2.605
Denmark	2.832	1.889	1.521	4.886	3.069	1.825	12.92	6.24	3.641	0.133	0.148	0.154	5.448	6.506	6.803
Ireland	2.754	2.022	2.016	4.597	2.903	2.073	11.66	6.648	4.336	0.289	0.27	0.262	3.06	3.135	3.146
Norway	1.735	1.516	1.421	4.705	3.464	2.431	12.18	7.297	4.312	0.529	0.54	0.588	2.451	2.858	3.603
Finland	0.135	0	0.385	4.627	2.89	1.708	11.7	6.146	3.657	0.459	0.476	0.475	2.395	2.561	2.422
Lithuania	5.696	3.594	2.722	4.361	2.34	1.437	12.74	6.648	3.699	1.077	1.511	2.375	1.739	2.467	3.537
Latvia	20.5	14.17	9.339	8.63	4.227	2.465	10.15	5.115	3	0.115	0.136	0.151	1.13	1.303	1.268
Estonia	2.668	1.356	1.163	13.92	7.367	4.137	8.96	4.658	3	1.122	1.369	1.497	1.537	1.752	1.7
Iceland	0	0	0.232	4.386	2.767	1.695	10.75	5.522	3.088	0.582	0.571	0.561	2.223	2.276	2.082
Europe-North	**2.955**	**1.923**	**1.601**	**4.946**	**2.967**	**1.799**	**10.73**	**5.612**	**3.378**	**0.282**	**0.291**	**0.305**	**2.874**	**3.195**	**3.324**
Italy	4.027	2.625	2.157	4.786	2.929	1.928	18.82	9.979	5.836	0.745	0.792	0.87	5.521	5.587	5.401
Spain	0.195	0	0.662	4.691	2.97	2.036	23.09	12.53	7.643	0.897	0.93	0.999	2.867	2.915	2.774
Greece	3.349	2.454	2.25	4.548	3.061	2.212	25.31	13.7	8.248	0.814	0.851	0.901	3.707	3.781	3.629
Portugal	6.595	4.491	3.19	4.831	3.079	1.86	19.2	10.11	5.343	1.093	1.133	1.197	2.552	2.601	2.518
Serbia	11.77	8.216	5.636	15.13	9.244	5.577	24.86	13.89	7.612	6.495	8.53	10.61	5.034	6.46	7.124
Bosnia and Herzegovina	5.028	1.939	0.544	44.91	21.91	9.787	13.04	7.391	4.012	1.146	1.393	1.815	3.31	4.68	6.183
Croatia	0	0	0	11.06	5.801	3.464	14.02	6.946	3.778	1.981	2.672	3.385	3.314	4.686	5.381
Albania	8.232	5.047	3.874	30.69	15.67	9.067	33.57	20.32	11.77	0.562	0.59	0.612	2.216	2.41	2.49
Macedonia, FYR	11.44	8.034	5.7	32.8	19.73	11.88	14.48	8.67	5.119	1.164	1.268	1.495	3.161	3.587	4.068
Slovenia	4.277	2.368	1.818	7.391	3.782	2.233	19.25	9.142	5.172	0.473	0.526	0.612	6.159	7.028	7.555
Montenegro	12.05	7.873	4.781	22.47	12.43	5.758	30.43	17.33	9.577	0.359	0.402	0.449	2.223	3.033	3.638
Malta	4.607	3.491	2.826	4.716	3.208	2.159	20.45	11.54	6.715	0.051	0.052	0.06	5.795	6.494	6.997
Europe-South	**3.547**	**2.289**	**1.961**	**7.594**	**4.498**	**2.79**	**20.91**	**11.34**	**6.679**	**1.147**	**1.302**	**1.501**	**3.821**	**4.438**	**4.813**
Germany	0.232	0.19	0.497	4.815	3.168	1.831	13.24	7.294	4.476	0.478	0.504	0.532	6.13	6.33	6.051
France	3.264	2.164	1.695	4.759	2.929	1.729	9.392	4.782	3	0.57	0.569	0.568	5.251	5.445	5.234
Netherlands	0.26	0.445	0.807	4.86	3.461	2.148	24.3	14.08	8.563	0.562	0.531	0.534	11	10.51	10.19
Belgium	3.201	2.198	1.782	4.743	3.021	1.782	16.22	8.578	5.108	0.766	0.745	0.739	2.361	2.254	2.086
Austria	0.106	0	0.381	4.661	2.987	1.848	22.98	11.97	7.314	0.463	0.481	0.513	5.012	5.098	4.825
Switzerland	0.159	0.219	0.582	4.684	3.305	2.053	17.15	9.136	5.409	0.345	0.35	0.364	6.89	6.902	6.498
Luxembourg	1.543	1.622	1.828	4.742	3.939	3.382	10.43	6.843	4.621	0.135	0.135	0.142	2.309	2.999	4.203
Europe-West	**1.398**	**1.009**	**1.041**	**4.784**	**3.105**	**1.838**	**13.7**	**7.403**	**4.527**	**0.525**	**0.535**	**0.549**	**5.565**	**5.648**	**5.584**

Multination Regional Analysis

Measures of Poverty, Health, Education, Infrastructure, and Governance

Infrastructure
Resource-Related / Transportation

Base Case
Source: International Futures Version 6.32, June 2010

	Energy Demand per Capita (Barrels of Oil Equivalent)			Electricity Use (Annual KWH Per Capita)			Annual Carbon Emissions (Billions of Tons)			Road Density (Kilometers per 1,000 Hectares)			Cars, Buses, and Freight Vehicles (Total Per 1,000 Persons)		
	2010	2035	2060	2010	2035	2060	2010	2035	2060	2010	2035	2060	2010	2035	2060
World	11.98	16.44	17.76	2777	4722	7354	8.333	10.89	8.609	6.484	8.874	12.98	145.2	300.9	459
Africa	3.588	5.45	6.851	607.1	1232	2858	0.36	0.788	0.998	1.544	3.06	5.619	33.16	86.56	220.9
Americas	26.37	30.08	29.41	6538	8102	10565	2.235	2.828	2.25	4.215	9.538	18.65	350.9	515.6	661.7
Asia with Oceania	8.22	15	18.91	1798	4375	8102	4.073	5.549	4.276	7.231	9.85	14.2	72.92	283.4	496.1
Europe	26.62	31.8	28.62	6547	10378	12702	1.647	1.702	1.069	12.03	15.21	21	449.3	608.9	698.6
World	11.98	16.44	17.76	2777	4722	7354	8.333	10.89	8.609	6.484	8.874	12.98	145.2	300.9	459
Africa-Eastern	0.958	2.907	6.784	190.6	735.7	3118	0.021	0.133	0.349	1.466	2.885	6.227	10.82	33.78	282.6
Africa-Middle	3.391	5.298	4.016	185.3	772.8	1304	0.016	0.044	0.02	0.774	1.819	2.895	16.34	63.08	91.74
Africa-Northern	7.073	11.25	13.13	1085	2645	5439	0.149	0.278	0.226	1.031	3.365	7.389	63.26	230.4	492.9
Africa-Southern	14.67	19.3	25.34	4504	6213	11561	0.123	0.168	0.206	3.024	5.803	13.93	157.3	428.5	685.9
Africa-Western	1.994	3.615	4.264	167	644.5	1586	0.051	0.164	0.197	2.026	3.303	4.888	19.98	38.55	72.81
Africa	3.588	5.45	6.851	607.1	1232	2858	0.36	0.788	0.998	1.544	3.06	5.619	33.16	86.56	220.9
America-Caribbean	8.267	12.71	13.16	1239	3342	5859	0.032	0.05	0.044	8.167	9.902	12.32	103.2	280.4	384.2
America-Central	4.548	8.32	11.15	918.9	2358	5313	0.015	0.038	0.049	2.816	4.977	8.737	89.6	230	467.6
America-North	44.94	47.46	43.19	11433	12394	13402	1.907	2.19	1.662	6.014	14.04	27.87	566.8	655.8	741.4
America-South	9.421	15.57	18.44	2107	4614	8672	0.281	0.55	0.494	1.929	5.156	10.51	158.4	422.6	630.2
Americas	26.37	30.08	29.41	6538	8102	10565	2.235	2.828	2.25	4.215	9.538	18.65	350.9	515.6	661.7
Asia-East	12.15	24.9	33.58	2993	7956	13984	2.476	2.702	1.834	6.606	11.31	21.41	106.3	480	638.7
Asia-South Central	3.655	8.628	12.56	686.8	2292	5816	0.776	1.701	1.596	9.079	10.15	11.65	20.96	161.5	460.6
Asia-South East	5.811	8.221	9.469	954.9	1911	3807	0.332	0.429	0.268	4.138	5.498	7.307	86	172.7	316.5
Asia-West	16.56	20.15	18.49	3067	5105	7665	0.38	0.595	0.524	6.382	10.21	14.88	131	329.2	499.3
Oceania	41.38	38.78	33.51	8442	10050	10424	0.11	0.122	0.054	2.251	8.237	19.6	522.3	541.1	577
Asia with Oceania	8.22	15	18.91	1798	4375	8102	4.073	5.549	4.276	7.231	9.85	14.2	72.92	283.4	496.1
Europe-East	23.48	31.06	22.99	5110	8415	9883	0.736	0.735	0.386	4.959	8.568	11.33	285	552.1	673.2
Europe-North	34.82	37.18	34.69	9057	13524	15368	0.227	0.225	0.146	14.27	19.3	30.52	523.5	609.8	677.5
Europe-South	19.57	24.7	24.27	5702	8846	12898	0.279	0.306	0.209	13.28	14.5	17.17	542.1	641.8	732.2
Europe-West	32.32	34.66	34.3	8049	12279	14180	0.422	0.457	0.344	20.63	22.21	29.02	585.5	650.1	707.8
Europe	26.62	31.8	28.62	6547	10378	12702	1.647	1.702	1.069	12.03	15.21	21	449.3	608.9	698.6

Infrastructure
Resource-Related

Infrastructure
Transportation

Base Case: Countries in Year 2060 Descending Population Sequence	Energy Demand per Capita (Barrels of Oil Equivalent)			Electricity Use (Annual KWH Per Capita)			Annual Carbon Emissions (Billions of Tons)			Road Density (Kilometers per 1,000 Hectares)			Cars, Buses, and Freight Vehicles (Total Per 1,000 Persons)		
	2010	2035	2060	2010	2035	2060	2010	2035	2060	2010	2035	2060	2010	2035	2060
AFRICA															
Ethiopia	0.602	2.357	5.655	64.6	514.8	2613	0.003	0.029	0.078	0.526	2.041	5.543	6.394	19.28	201
Tanzania, United Rep	0.915	4.034	10.38	105.4	968.4	4953	0.003	0.028	0.075	0.979	2.632	7.359	7.592	59.34	570.7
Uganda	1.173	4.079	12.48	51.1	833.2	5734	0.002	0.022	0.074	3.177	5.371	10.85	8.739	49.56	551.9
Kenya	1.281	3.097	6.465	186.9	713.6	2999	0.004	0.018	0.042	1.257	2.54	5.606	18.26	38.2	268
Madagascar	0.785	1.545	2.905	38.11	266.7	975.3	0.001	0.005	0.012	0.94	1.63	2.857	7.274	9.093	26.18
Mozambique	0.975	3.835	9.586	503.3	1628	4472	0.001	0.008	0.026	0.497	1.804	6.254	7.273	45.11	521.8
Malawi	0.692	1.465	2.561	110.6	320.2	1157	0.001	0.003	0.007	1.526	2.985	5.316	6.261	8.114	32.07
Zambia	1.165	3.36	5.842	742.5	1410	2675	0.001	0.006	0.011	1.291	2.182	4.06	26.53	65.51	226.3
Somalia	0.703	1.393	1.784	71.97	257.3	550.3	0	0.002	0.003	0.424	0.958	1.689	5.986	7.51	10.56
Rwanda	0.776	3.478	8.939	94.65	804.6	4265	0	0.005	0.013	5.67	8.228	12.38	8.243	35.43	293.7
Zimbabwe	2.308	2.933	3.245	1002	1008	1399	0.003	0.004	0.004	2.489	2.489	2.825	27.26	29.91	55.7
Burundi	0.371	0.656	0.816	225.6	243.1	364.4	0	0.001	0.001	4.629	6.002	7.437	8.448	5.497	4.174
Eritrea	0.676	1.001	0.925	79.67	193.3	409	0	0.001	0.001	0.474	1.334	2.571	4.269	4.848	7.02
Comoros	1.1	1.501	1.767	40.3	254.6	793.5	0	0	0	4.243	6.021	8.219	3.594	4.311	9.774
Mauritius	6.008	13.82	20.19	396.9	3842	10740	0.001	0.002	0.002	10.26	13.46	17.93	155.4	364.4	495.8
Djibouti	1.709	4.035	7.266	83.04	817	3354	0	0.001	0.001	1.482	2.41	4.864	23.43	61.69	344.2
Africa-Eastern	**0.958**	**2.907**	**6.784**	**190.6**	**735.7**	**3118**	**0.021**	**0.133**	**0.349**	**1.466**	**2.885**	**6.227**	**10.82**	**33.78**	**282.6**
Congo, Democratic Republic of	0.388	0.819	0.992	107.3	189.7	267.3	0.001	0.007	0.013	0.737	1.271	1.995	8.339	6.817	4.819
Angola	13.95	23.72	16.47	338	2766	5200	0.009	0.021	-0.01	0.72	3.802	6.712	36.75	319.4	486.6
Cameroon	2.2	4.075	6.307	259.8	851.4	2340	0.002	0.007	0.013	1.206	2.237	4.145	11.92	33.62	158.9
Chad	1.896	3.045	2.654	52.03	451.8	772.6	0	0	-0.001	0.39	1.085	1.73	7.223	15.17	17.09
Central African Republic	0.67	1.334	1.819	101.7	286.1	804.2	0	0.001	0.001	0.445	0.806	1.529	8.704	9.577	19.01
Congo, Republic of	4.504	8.19	7.613	316.7	1539	2712	0.001	0.004	0.003	0.715	2.348	3.827	26.13	121.7	199.5
Gabon	12.72	16.2	14.47	1359	3878	6213	0.001	0.003	0.002	0.922	4.244	7.409	148.2	314.4	477
Equatorial Guinea	73.26	65.21	37.61	1142	8315	14174	0.002	0.001	-0.002	2.304	10.31	16.71	244.4	409.8	569.7
São Tomé and Príncipe	1.922	2.411	2.242	59.02	387.1	982	0	0	0	3.575	4.729	6.052	30.92	23.48	21.59
Africa-Middle	**3.391**	**5.298**	**4.016**	**185.3**	**772.8**	**1304**	**0.016**	**0.044**	**0.02**	**0.774**	**1.819**	**2.895**	**16.34**	**63.08**	**91.74**
Egypt	5.479	10.67	15.93	1412	3223	7158	0.054	0.11	0.11	1.28	4.099	9.843	40.78	228.7	581.3
Sudan	2.578	6.512	8.574	170.9	1236	3178	0.015	0.04	0.035	0.208	1.772	4.405	14.91	104.2	314.8
Algeria	13.31	15.82	12.56	1063	2568	4164	0.04	0.053	0.021	0.754	2.899	5.305	100.9	281.8	443.9
Morocco	3.771	7.388	9.694	783.3	1977	4454	0.016	0.03	0.033	1.565	3.418	6.579	71.45	217.4	512
Tunisia	6.555	13.39	18.39	1455	4025	8891	0.007	0.016	0.017	1.579	5.011	11.29	123	470.1	726.9
Libyan Arab Jamahiriya	38.41	44.54	26.76	3712	7255	8655	0.017	0.03	0.01	0.994	5.648	9.991	303.2	624	713.5
Africa-Northern	**7.073**	**11.25**	**13.13**	**1085**	**2645**	**5439**	**0.149**	**0.278**	**0.226**	**1.031**	**3.365**	**7.389**	**63.26**	**230.4**	**492.9**

Infrastructure
Resource-Related

Infrastructure
Transportation

Base Case: Countries in Year 2060 Descending Population Sequence	Energy Demand per Capita (Barrels of Oil Equivalent)			Electricity Use (Annual KWH Per Capita)			Annual Carbon Emissions (Billions of Tons)			Road Density (Kilometers per 1,000 Hectares)			Cars, Buses, and Freight Vehicles (Total Per 1,000 Persons)		
	2010	2035	2060	2010	2035	2060	2010	2035	2060	2010	2035	2060	2010	2035	2060
AFRICA continued															
South Africa	16.2	21	27.35	5021	6752	12401	0.12	0.159	0.193	3.266	6.121	14.78	167.8	458.7	710.5
Namibia	4.796	9.312	15.06	1539	3037	7215	0.001	0.002	0.004	0.704	2.694	8.391	87.29	332.8	769.4
Lesotho	1.266	3.151	6.267	55.31	604.2	2423	0	0.001	0.001	2.031	2.71	4.246	20.71	43.43	181.6
Botswana	7.772	20.68	28.1	1903	7610	14174	0.002	0.005	0.006	1.044	7.515	18.69	155.2	413.9	578
Swaziland	3.127	6.877	11.28	167.3	1581	5374	0	0.001	0.001	2.202	4.015	7.774	79.47	239.3	618.1
Africa-Southern	**14.67**	**19.3**	**25.34**	**4504**	**6213**	**11561**	**0.123**	**0.168**	**0.206**	**3.024**	**5.803**	**13.93**	**157.3**	**428.5**	**685.9**
Nigeria	2.922	5.246	5.342	184	840.6	1672	0.038	0.116	0.106	2.335	4.225	6.104	24.05	57.84	69.29
Niger	0.609	1.174	1.516	116.5	266.9	676.7	0.001	0.003	0.007	0.233	0.836	1.948	7.86	8.225	14.23
Côte d'Ivoire	1.502	2.998	3.778	210.4	661.2	1673	0.003	0.008	0.01	2.539	3.271	4.252	30.07	41.97	78.07
Ghana	1.308	2.092	3.382	308.1	533.3	1523	0.003	0.007	0.013	2.557	3.229	4.541	18.62	18.95	61.98
Mali	0.929	2.114	4.143	38.84	389.4	1883	0.001	0.005	0.012	0.251	1.013	3.087	7.441	14.32	107.7
Burkina Faso	0.971	2.178	4.213	40.78	399.2	1940	0.001	0.005	0.012	3.382	3.767	4.621	7.233	13.94	107.8
Senegal	1.496	2.707	4.813	202.8	597.2	2187	0.002	0.006	0.012	0.874	2.169	4.893	33.24	39	139.9
Guinea	1.012	2.36	3.477	43.52	441.7	1552	0.001	0.004	0.007	1.842	2.56	3.726	13.62	22.54	67.61
Benin	0.971	2.023	2.761	117.5	425	1239	0.001	0.003	0.006	1.848	2.939	4.595	8.343	12.51	39.02
Togo	0.857	1.226	0.894	120.5	252.8	381.7	0	0.001	0.001	1.519	2.771	4.221	15.87	11.33	5.9
Sierra Leone	0.643	2.124	5.584	132.3	534.9	2595	0	0.002	0.005	1.718	2.854	5.652	12.21	23.05	196.7
Liberia	0.41	1.987	5.06	252.1	853.8	2291	0	0.001	0.003	1.043	1.919	4.1	11.65	24.65	161.4
Mauritania	1.433	1.771	1.544	66	310	672.6	0.001	0.001	0.001	0.199	0.647	1.24	12.89	10.21	14.18
Guinea-Bissau	0.488	0.692	0.498	163.1	185.6	218.7	0	0	0	1.051	1.672	2.583	6.629	5.15	4.049
Gambia	1.078	2.611	4.363	44.54	491.6	1958	0	0.001	0.001	3.485	4.742	6.465	7.433	17.87	97.72
Cape Verde	2.269	6.421	12.79	108.8	1412	5801	0	0	0.001	3.573	5.498	9.262	13.77	108.3	511.1
Africa-Western	**1.994**	**3.615**	**4.264**	**167**	**644.5**	**1586**	**0.051**	**0.164**	**0.197**	**2.026**	**3.303**	**4.888**	**19.98**	**38.55**	**72.81**

Multination Regional Analysis

Measures of Poverty, Health, Education, Infrastructure, and Governance

Infrastructure Resource-Related / Infrastructure Transportation

Base Case: Countries in Year 2060 Descending Population Sequence	Energy Demand per Capita (Barrels of Oil Equivalent)			Electricity Use (Annua. KWH Per Capita)			Annual Carbon Emissions (Billions of Tons)			Road Density (Kilometers per 1,000 Hectares)			Cars, Buses, and Freight Vehicles (Total Per 1,000 Persons)		
	2010	2035	2060	2010	2035	2060	2010	2035	2060	2010	2035	2060	2010	2035	2060
AMERICAS															
Haiti	1.079	1.921	2.458	79.74	366.7	1075	0.001	0.002	0.003	1.902	4.301	7.227	7.199	9.247	23.3
Dominican Republic	7.59	15.36	17.81	1505	4302	8331	0.007	0.016	0.015	3.001	6.958	12.34	139.2	613.5	728.2
Cuba	7.507	12.11	14.26	1332	3177	6653	0.008	0.011	0.009	5.561	6.8	8.948	42.73	200	485.9
Puerto Rico	10.36	22.86	31.98	868.5	7753	14174	0.001	0.006	0.007	28.65	29.41	29.41	315.5	426.4	516.5
Jamaica	9.523	10.33	10.6	2506	2936	4739	0.003	0.003	0.003	19.1	19.1	19.1	159.4	249.7	499.1
Trinidad	61.63	77.44	50.09	5703	12963	14245	0.009	0.007	0.003	16.99	23.43	23.43	170.1	366.4	520.4
Bahamas	8.674	17.23	24.37	720.4	5950	14174	0.001	0.001	0.001	2.565	8.214	19.68	230.7	422.5	585.1
Barbados	8.098	15.24	23.26	565.6	4330	13094	0	0.001	0.001	37.21	37.21	37.21	381.9	529.8	640.5
Grenada	5.528	9.265	13.32	338.2	2270	6394	0	0	0	33.15	33.15	33.15	216.8	326.5	578.9
Saint Vincent and Grenadines	4.745	10.28	15.18	271	2555	7341	0.003	0.003	0.003	21.31	21.31	21.31	152.3	415.1	646.8
Saint Lucia	5.781	11	15.08	357.4	2817	7300	0	0	0	19.52	19.52	19.52	117.6	292.7	526.5
America-Caribbean	**8.267**	**12.71**	**13.16**	**1239**	**3342**	**5859**	**0.032**	**0.05**	**0.044**	**8.167**	**9.902**	**12.32**	**103.2**	**280.4**	**384.2**
Guatemala	3.566	7.34	10.77	651	2030	5071	0.004	0.015	0.023	1.647	4.465	9.128	68.81	214.2	532.6
Honduras	3.205	5.974	7.684	707.1	1605	3485	0.003	0.007	0.008	1.432	3.133	5.85	66.75	154.5	354.1
El Salvador	4.576	8.097	11.07	873.6	2197	5158	0.002	0.004	0.005	5.056	7.208	10.46	65.26	177.5	453.9
Nicaragua	2.919	4.445	4.93	466.7	1028	2165	0.001	0.003	0.003	1.541	2.445	3.805	43.28	67.55	143.8
Costa Rica	7.997	14.64	19.34	2001	4669	9463	0.002	0.002	0.002	7.423	9.483	12.37	234.1	559.9	746.8
Panama	9.665	19.62	26.31	1954	6075	13846	0.002	0.006	0.007	2.114	7.11	16.56	153.9	482.2	644
Belize	4.587	10.02	16.04	279.3	2540	7902	0	0.001	0.001	1.497	4.046	9.494	165.1	460.2	783.4
America-Central	**4.548**	**8.32**	**11.15**	**918.9**	**2358**	**5313**	**0.015**	**0.038**	**0.049**	**2.816**	**4.977**	**8.737**	**89.6**	**230**	**467.6**
USA	54.02	56.76	50.51	14045	14606	14606	1.62	1.876	1.503	7.694	17.32	33.53	685.1	731.4	775.2
Mexico	11.79	16.43	18.06	2178	4498	8213	0.128	0.179	0.141	2.243	5.528	10.39	220.9	436.4	636.3
Canada	68.64	62.75	49.56	17342	17765	17765	0.159	0.135	0.018	2.721	11.25	26.65	597.1	669.7	736.3
America-North	**44.94**	**47.46**	**43.19**	**11433**	**12394**	**13402**	**1.907**	**2.19**	**1.662**	**6.014**	**14.04**	**27.87**	**566.8**	**655.8**	**741.4**
Brazil	8.494	15.08	18.94	2241	4814	9137	0.112	0.237	0.24	2.367	5.556	10.93	194.8	524.7	734.5
Colombia	7.318	10.59	12.64	1111	2497	5153	0.023	0.054	0.037	1.726	3.659	6.9	70.63	208.2	496.7
Argentina	13.31	23	27.01	3011	7300	14012	0.05	0.079	0.073	1.417	6.727	16.15	237.4	532.9	667.5
Peru	5.522	12.21	16.61	1153	3695	8005	0.014	0.032	0.03	1.03	4.28	9.749	74.19	320.9	577.2
Venezuela	19.09	25.07	22.38	3313	6040	9194	0.048	0.081	0.056	1.528	5.591	11.22	112.3	361.3	566
Ecuador	8.826	10.12	8.678	872	1992	3102	0.01	0.012	0.003	1.779	3.389	4.854	63.92	136.4	223.9
Chile	12.77	20.89	25.32	3371	6902	12961	0.018	0.034	0.034	1.613	6.343	15.12	182.2	429	605
Bolivia	5.853	10.14	11.17	573.2	2018	4231	0.003	0.01	0.008	0.748	2.586	5.309	52.97	240.7	491.8
Paraguay	4.026	6.515	9.21	955.2	1766	3690	0.001	0.004	0.005	0.918	2.247	4.886	89.79	171.2	404.1
Uruguay	8.295	19.31	29.97	2472	7272	14174	0.002	0.006	0.007	5.019	10.31	20.24	240.1	614.2	723.1
Guyana	2.663	5.39	7.743	141.5	1151	3540	0	0.001	0.001	0.564	1.729	4.275	39.29	104.3	378.3
Suriname	5.032	12.22	17.93	308.9	3212	9133	0.001	0.001	0.001	0.642	3.984	10.44	292.9	722.8	823.1
America-South	**9.421**	**15.57**	**18.44**	**2107**	**4614**	**8672**	**0.281**	**0.55**	**0.494**	**1.929**	**5.156**	**10.51**	**158.4**	**422.6**	**630.2**

Infrastructure Resource-Related / **Infrastructure Transportation**

Base Case: Countries in Year 2060 Descending Population Sequence	Energy Demand per Capita (Barrels of Oil Equivalent)			Electricity Use (Annual KWH Per Capita)			Annual Carbon Emissions (Billions of Tons)			Road Density (Kilometers per 1,000 Hectares)			Cars, Buses, and Freight Vehicles (Total Per 1,000 Persons)		
	2010	2035	2060	2010	2035	2060	2010	2035	2060	2010	2035	2060	2010	2035	2060
ASIA with OCEANIA															
China	9.541	23.92	34.05	2310	7541	14174	1.881	2.081	1.395	4.01	9.453	20.68	47.55	475.4	648.3
Japan	30.36	35.27	34.49	8771	13426	14174	0.349	0.342	0.229	31.84	31.84	31.84	592.9	657.1	713.1
Korea, Repub of	34.62	38.86	36.72	8277	11743	14363	0.131	0.138	0.082	10.95	15.97	23.77	340.9	460.8	577.8
Taiwan	19.26	26.8	31.22	634.4	5670	14174	0.076	0.096	0.091	9.038	14.93	24.73	447.4	555	587.3
Korea, Dem. People's Rep.	5.61	7.025	6.944	908.2	1437	2239	0.024	0.028	0.022	2.376	3.643	5.004	25.78	59.77	146.6
Hong Kong SAR	23.6	23.63	21.14	7092	11310	14174	0.013	0.013	0.008	22.11	38.84	54.15	1	1	1
Mongolia	4.124	8.476	13.45	1467	2844	5564	0.003	0.005	0.006	0.252	1.895	6.488	56.21	252.6	657.6
Asia-East	**12.15**	**24.9**	**33.58**	**2993**	**7956**	**13984**	**2.476**	**2.702**	**1.834**	**6.606**	**11.31**	**21.41**	**106.3**	**480**	**638.7**
India	3.189	9.275	15.34	600.6	2508	7229	0.48	1.139	1.034	10.13	11.27	12.71	16.07	199.6	600.1
Pakistan	2.813	4.115	5.262	528.7	997.3	2348	0.043	0.102	0.114	3.543	5.096	7.387	15.99	32.02	139.2
Bangladesh	1.195	3.421	5.006	192.1	797.5	2218	0.015	0.057	0.066	16.62	16.68	16.68	3.989	11.73	53.32
Afghanistan	1.201	4.416	11.55	52.79	922.3	5536	0.002	0.023	0.069	0.76	2.612	8.481	9.388	67.27	617.5
Iran (Islamic Republic of)	12	21.15	19.58	2399	6165	8683	0.129	0.202	0.178	1.532	6.277	10.8	92.06	361	542.4
Nepal	0.832	1.677	2.209	114.1	354.5	963.4	0.001	0.005	0.007	1.465	3.141	5.126	5.396	8.054	22.35
Uzbekistan	7.53	11.46	11.12	1951	2925	3307	0.034	0.053	0.052	2.063	3.39	5.156	18.65	96.57	331.5
Sri Lanka	2.87	6.901	10.28	528.1	1868	4797	0.005	0.012	0.014	14.83	14.83	14.83	63.42	218.5	500.1
Kazakhstan	32.82	49.07	29.24	4538	10092	10563	0.051	0.074	0.037	0.807	6.455	11.16	163.1	525.3	644.1
Tajikistan	2.183	3.287	3.926	2386	2386	2386	0.002	0.002	0.001	2.025	2.579	3.459	2.874	10.39	56.95
Turkmenistan	25.91	51.33	36.98	2814	11190	14174	0.014	0.028	0.021	1.109	9.642	18.12	400.4	847.5	851.3
Kyrgyzstan	3.038	4.232	4.409	1929	2034	2038	0.002	0.003	0.002	1.041	1.829	3.031	39.86	64.92	109.3
Bhutan	3.172	10.44	19.89	167.7	2589	10250	0	0.001	0.001	2.007	5.164	12.09	27.53	302.5	637
Maldives	3.418	8.231	13.98	168.6	1865	6705	0	0	0.001	4.072	10.98	20.07	14.52	46.44	88.47
Asia-South Central	**3.655**	**8.628**	**12.56**	**686.8**	**2292**	**5816**	**0.776**	**1.701**	**1.596**	**9.079**	**10.15**	**11.65**	**20.96**	**161.5**	**460.6**
Indonesia	4.699	7.267	8.571	640.5	1536	3126	0.113	0.114	0.037	2.319	3.744	5.607	125.1	219.2	291.2
Philippines	3.557	6.331	7.875	700.1	1607	3551	0.026	0.068	0.077	6.88	7.754	8.598	40.06	106.6	307.6
Viet Nam	3.472	6.617	9.716	677.2	1609	3632	0.035	0.042	0.004	6.778	7.173	7.793	10.43	55.77	284.8
Thailand	9.674	11.99	12.52	2059	3191	5690	0.079	0.093	0.078	3.739	5.353	8.281	111.9	268.8	563
Myanmar	2.07	2.859	2.596	127.1	475.7	1103	0.004	0.009	0.001	0.592	1.649	2.828	5.889	13.16	33.55
Malaysia	19.17	23.9	23.63	3453	6014	10270	0.053	0.077	0.054	3.094	7.059	13.25	292.5	550	698.3
Cambodia	1.415	4.283	6.458	113.9	916.2	2901	0.002	0.008	0.009	2.246	3.601	5.436	33.3	111.3	252.5
LAO People's Dem Repub	1.628	5.164	10.22	75.16	1099	4387	0.001	0.004	0.006	1.532	3.009	6.006	46.31	201.1	512.6
Singapore	73.68	60.82	45.98	9641	12302	14174	0.017	0.012	0.001	54.29	57.93	61.1	1	1	1
Timor-Leste	1.772	3.629	3.816	85.03	705.2	1703	0	0.001	0.001	2.417	3.914	5.706	15.03	33.92	74.43
Brunei Darussalam	88.4	71.9	39.6	8785	11989	14174	0.002	0.002	0	7.184	14.91	19.55	414.3	522.6	631.6
Asia-South East	**5.811**	**8.221**	**9.469**	**954.9**	**1911**	**3807**	**0.332**	**0.429**	**0.268**	**4.138**	**5.498**	**7.307**	**86**	**172.7**	**316.5**

Infrastructure
Resource-Related

Base Case: Countries in Year 2060 Descending Population Sequence	Energy Demand per Capita (Barrels of Oil Equivalent)			Electricity Use (Annual KWH Per Capita)			Annual Carbon Emissions (Billions of Tons)		
	2010	2035	2060	2010	2035	2060	2010	2035	2060
ASIA with OCEANIA continued									
Turkey	8.983	14.93	16.93	2082	4384	7934	0.073	0.125	0.116
Yemen	2.921	5.675	7.41	249.7	1084	2700	0.007	0.021	0.031
Iraq	4.283	11.65	18.03	1470	4226	9040	0.028	0.072	0.114
Saudi Arabia	49.55	47.86	30.8	6973	9738	11508	0.106	0.154	0.097
Syrian Arab Repub	6.159	7.854	9.288	1459	1994	3377	0.02	0.03	0.03
Israel	23.92	35.49	44.89	7310	13401	14174	0.019	0.033	0.039
Jordan	7.15	10.98	18.36	1912	3376	8741	0.007	0.011	0.016
Occupied Palestinian Territory	2.68	6.103	11	140	1355	4896	0.001	0.004	0.007
Azerbaijan	10.98	22.12	18.94	3324	7156	7628	0.012	0.019	0.008
United Arab Emirates	73.33	72.28	48.84	15404	17001	17001	0.041	0.045	0.031
Oman	34.56	37.91	34.15	4295	8567	14174	0.009	0.014	0.007
Kuwait	104.3	89.41	40.31	15747	15747	15747	0.026	0.031	0.013
Lebanon	13.28	19.35	20.85	2574	5277	9939	0.005	0.008	0.007
Armenia	4.987	17.35	26.09	1770	7073	13697	0.002	0.005	0.006
Georgia	4.374	9.643	11.77	1912	3668	5370	0.002	0.003	0.003
Bahrain	88.37	80.27	53.03	12366	14961	14961	0.004	0.004	-0.001
Qatar	263.3	221.2	88.54	15108	15108	15108	0.015	0.013	0.001
Cyprus	23.09	28.99	27	5608	9952	14174	0.002	0.002	0.001
Asia-West	**16.56**	**20.15**	**18.49**	**3067**	**5105**	**7665**	**0.38**	**0.595**	**0.524**
Australia	60.08	57.61	49.82	11566	14490	14490	0.102	0.106	0.038
Papua New Guinea	3.249	5.688	6.087	73.75	792.2	2001	0.002	0.004	0.003
New Zealand	25.34	29.84	31.34	9758	11714	14605	0.005	0.01	0.011
Solomon Islands	1.62	3.213	3.739	73.11	611.3	1645	0	0	0
Fiji	3.015	5.829	10.17	158.8	1276	4437	0	0.001	0.001
Vanuatu	3.055	6.318	9.302	143.7	1335	4322	0	0	0
Micronesia, Federated States of	4.269	7.158	10.03	222.5	1561	4716	0	0	0
Tonga	4.154	5.765	7.694	183.4	1142	3546	0	0	0
Samoa	3.815	8.656	14.21	204.1	2044	6803	0	0	0
Oceania	**41.38**	**38.78**	**33.51**	**8442**	**10050**	**10424**	**0.11**	**0.122**	**0.054**

Infrastructure
Transportation

Base Case: Countries in Year 2060 Descending Population Sequence	Road Density (Kilometers per 1,000 Hectares)			Cars, Buses, and Freight Vehicles (Total Per 1,000 Persons)		
	2010	2035	2060	2010	2035	2060
ASIA with OCEANIA continued						
Turkey	5.696	7.9	10.67	126.7	410.4	645
Yemen	1.502	2.971	4.996	34.68	98.11	221.9
Iraq	1.457	5.311	12.09	71.67	369.8	616
Saudi Arabia	1.854	7.584	13.44	218.3	400.6	565.7
Syrian Arab Repub	2.304	4.018	6.635	46.83	102.8	317
Israel	9.185	17.83	36.92	308.8	417	488.2
Jordan	1.181	3.755	11.58	133.1	409.9	786.7
Occupied Palestinian Territory	133.6	138.5	138.5	1	1	1
Azerbaijan	7.911	11.67	11.67	136.8	658.8	749.7
United Arab Emirates	2.132	13.36	26.22	245.9	404	562.1
Oman	2.069	8.087	18.45	223.8	403.7	570.5
Kuwait	4.91	16.03	21.08	441.6	521.8	601.7
Lebanon	7.238	10.65	15.45	365.5	628.1	685.3
Armenia	2.852	8.528	16.89	20.3	348.1	553
Georgia	3.118	4.809	6.972	94.79	415.6	637.9
Bahrain	50.25	50.86	50.86	357.7	252.8	221.2
Qatar	14.13	37.73	42.74	526.9	606.3	691.5
Cyprus	13.65	15.9	19.73	750.5	804.4	823.9
Asia-West	**6.382**	**10.21**	**14.88**	**131**	**329.2**	**499.3**
Australia	2.391	11.23	28.66	681.2	732.9	776.5
Papua New Guinea	0.557	1.629	3.055	27.14	70.29	123
New Zealand	4.086	9.519	21.99	720.5	789	819
Solomon Islands	0.624	1.51	2.867	12.21	27.55	79.89
Fiji	1.966	3.093	6.005	70.46	153.7	520.8
Vanuatu	1.075	2.596	5.757	41.29	145.4	505.4
Micronesia, Federated States of	0.718	2.526	6.284	104.1	200.8	559.9
Tonga	9.067	9.067	9.067	19.8	45.59	221.3
Samoa	8.229	8.522	9.015	73.45	296.9	690.1
Oceania	**2.251**	**8.237**	**19.6**	**522.3**	**541.1**	**577**

Infrastructure Resource-Related

Infrastructure Transportation

Base Case: Countries in Year 2060 Descending Population Sequence	Energy Demand per Capita (Barrels of Oil Equivalent)			Electricity Use (Annual KWH Per Capita)			Annual Carbon Emissions (Billions of Tons)			Road Density (Kilometers per 1,000 Hectares)			Cars, Buses, and Freight Vehicles (Total Per 1,000 Persons)		
	2010	2035	2060	2010	2035	2060	2010	2035	2060	2010	2035	2060	2010	2035	2060
EUROPE															
Russian Federation	32.8	42.07	25.93	6438	10569	10618	0.436	0.417	0.174	1.101	6.693	10.86	281.2	566.2	666
Poland	17.79	25.53	24.69	3914	7683	11767	0.089	0.096	0.045	14.09	15.33	15.34	440.3	678.6	758.6
Ukraine	12.68	16.53	14.93	3539	4710	5366	0.09	0.084	0.065	3.026	4.814	6.97	155.4	438.7	637.3
Romania	11.46	16.67	17.29	2747	4914	8066	0.027	0.035	0.027	8.884	9.39	10.23	219.9	484.4	679.3
Czech Republic	25.56	29.1	25.99	6961	9236	12392	0.032	0.029	0.017	10.67	12.39	14.96	424.6	563.8	676.4
Belarus	9.85	20.2	22.05	3838	8030	10698	0.019	0.025	0.021	5.219	9.71	12.73	195.8	562.5	690.9
Hungary	19.25	25.48	25.69	3991	7533	12604	0.016	0.018	0.012	17.16	17.16	17.16	384	577.9	692.1
Bulgaria	11	15.38	16.85	4602	5711	7881	0.013	0.014	0.012	4.063	6.09	9.708	413.1	664.7	794.4
Slovak Republic	21.27	28.15	25.16	5734	9097	11947	0.011	0.015	0.01	9.889	12.84	14.76	340.2	523	646.4
Moldova, Repub of	1.995	3.63	5.166	1588	1611	2303	0.002	0.003	0.003	3.8	3.8	4.158	57.19	73.83	162.9
Europe-East	**23.48**	**31.06**	**22.99**	**5110**	**8415**	**9883**	**0.736**	**0.735**	**0.386**	**4.959**	**8.568**	**11.33**	**285**	**552.1**	**673.2**
United Kingdom	23.16	27.54	28.8	6853	12192	14174	0.152	0.168	0.141	16.47	20.68	31.41	528.7	598.8	660.4
Sweden	47.82	53.87	50.32	16034	18261	18261	0.013	0.018	0.01	10.15	17.62	32.29	533.2	625.1	707.5
Denmark	30.36	34.22	35.05	7210	12182	14174	0.012	0.008	0.004	17.23	20.41	31.12	457.8	558.5	653.5
Ireland	28.84	33.69	29.63	7138	11607	14174	0.013	0.016	0.012	14.88	21.26	28.79	469.4	569.4	666.6
Norway	174.4	128.4	74.9	25083	25083	25083	0.011	-0.014	-0.042	4.721	14.91	31.08	564.5	641.3	717.7
Finland	48.82	51.37	48.31	17069	18435	18435	0.014	0.016	0.011	3.459	12.12	29.8	550.4	639.7	717.1
Lithuania	19.94	26.65	27.38	3637	7345	13288	0.004	0.006	0.004	13.13	14.22	15.64	516	750.7	813.8
Latvia	13.54	23.19	27.55	3288	7813	14174	0.002	0.003	0.003	11.86	14.75	17.29	436.5	700.5	771.2
Estonia	26.36	34.06	34.82	6304	10574	14217	0.005	0.005	0.004	13.67	16.35	20.38	531.3	705.8	766.8
Iceland	98.11	75.92	61.45	29390	29390	29390	0	0	0	2.812	12.88	32.04	734	769	799.2
Europe-North	**34.82**	**37.18**	**34.69**	**9057**	**13524**	**15368**	**0.227**	**0.225**	**0.146**	**14.27**	**19.3**	**30.52**	**523.5**	**609.8**	**677.5**
Italy	23.65	27.8	26.75	5977	9120	14039	0.128	0.127	0.084	16.22	16.22	17.7	663.2	722.3	767.6
Spain	18.92	25.47	24.89	6601	10291	14174	0.078	0.094	0.065	13.54	15.32	18.77	559.3	652.9	727.2
Greece	19.04	26.25	25.61	5932	10636	14174	0.023	0.027	0.019	9.651	14.13	19.66	517.1	612.5	699.1
Portugal	18.31	22.84	23.56	4832	7382	11728	0.019	0.021	0.015	9.112	10.94	14.6	497.9	635.6	729.2
Serbia	11.82	14.28	14.58	4276	4824	6664	0.007	0.008	0.006	5.272	6.15	8.574	264.5	469.9	736.4
Bosnia and Herzegovina	9.541	15.7	16.72	2586	4898	7579	0.008	0.009	0.004	4.488	6.867	9.701	41.51	261.9	533.7
Croatia	13.72	19.74	21.5	3807	6449	10383	0.007	0.008	0.006	5.412	8.388	12.71	377.7	610.2	737
Albania	5.965	11.25	13.48	1422	3317	6250	0.001	0.003	0.002	6.454	7.609	8.742	109.7	399.8	691.6
Macedonia, FYR	9.315	11.28	11.3	3644	3848	5097	0.003	0.003	0.003	5.352	5.596	6.989	183.4	319.7	595.7
Slovenia	22.24	30.87	32.9	7667	11816	14174	0.004	0.004	0.004	19.84	20.57	21.68	546.4	655.5	729.2
Montenegro	5.115	10.1	16.15	295.8	2536	8042	0	0.001	0.001	64.92	64.92	64.92	188	460.7	786.8
Malta	19.79	24.69	24.95	5248	8118	12556	0.001	0.001	0.001	69.59	69.59	69.59	593.1	513.1	456.3
Europe-South	**19.57**	**24.7**	**24.27**	**5702**	**8846**	**12898**	**0.279**	**0.306**	**0.209**	**13.28**	**14.5**	**17.17**	**542.1**	**641.8**	**732.2**
Germany	29.6	32.91	33.76	7676	12395	14174	0.211	0.2	0.147	18.39	20.3	29.18	594	659.5	715.1
France	31.03	32.96	32.38	8231	11983	14174	0.101	0.142	0.12	17.28	18.41	25.21	607.4	674.1	732
Netherlands	44.38	44.79	41.66	7639	12259	14174	0.047	0.05	0.033	30.44	30.44	30.44	496.4	552.4	613.4
Belgium	45.28	44.3	41.79	8940	12333	14174	0.028	0.026	0.017	49.61	49.61	49.61	543.1	601.5	657.6
Austria	30.74	32.63	31.18	8568	12753	14174	0.02	0.019	0.013	13.3	17.2	26.52	567.8	644.6	718.4
Switzerland	26.69	29.53	29.32	9246	12832	14174	0.012	0.016	0.012	18.27	21.25	30.32	577.6	642.5	709.5
Luxembourg	73.59	65.72	45.86	15681	15681	15681	0.003	0.003	0.002	22.28	27.58	32.45	729.8	730.8	730.9
Europe-West	**32.32**	**34.66**	**34.3**	**8049**	**12279**	**14180**	**0.422**	**0.457**	**0.344**	**20.63**	**22.21**	**29.02**	**585.5**	**650.1**	**707.8**

Multination Regional Analysis

Measures of Poverty, Health, Education, Infrastructure, and Governance

Base Case
Source: International Futures
Version 6.32, June 2010

Infrastructure

	Communication									Other			Governance			
	Mobile Phone Usage			Internet Usage			Broadband Usage			R&D Expenditures			Freedom House Index (Inverted)			
	Percent of Population			Percent of Population			Percent of Population			Percent of GDP			Index Range: 2-14			
	2010	2035	2060	2010	2035	2060	2010	2035	2060	2010	2035	2060	2010	2035	2060	% Chg
World	66.43	119.8	120	17.26	38.43	48.79	10.05	68.46	99.55	2.055	2.413	2.973	8.39	9.554	10.22	21.8%
Africa	41.01	119.5	120	6.547	25.29	31.29	5.64	57.97	99.07	0.464	0.74	1.35	7.26	8.847	10.04	38.3%
Americas	85.26	119.9	120	31.84	52.33	60.7	15.08	78.72	99.84	2.218	2.484	2.68	11.92	12.61	13.19	10.7%
Asia with Oceania	60.71	119.9	120	13.58	36.56	51.96	8.671	67.41	99.65	2.136	2.426	3.308	7.306	8.753	9.368	28.2%
Europe	110.1	120	120	34.47	61.89	68.57	17.67	85.36	99.95	1.86	2.629	2.927	11.57	12.05	12.33	6.6%
World	66.43	119.8	120	17.26	38.43	48.79	10.05	68.46	99.55	2.055	2.413	2.973	8.39	9.554	10.22	21.8%
Africa-Eastern	29.89	119.4	120	3.416	23.24	32.32	5.416	56.9	99.18	0.208	0.398	1.085	7.697	10.05	11.9	54.6%
Africa-Middle	32.47	119.4	120	7.714	23.93	25.15	5.489	57.05	98.69	0.355	0.798	0.955	4.614	5.527	6.133	32.9%
Africa-Northern	59.37	119.9	120	12.16	31.65	41.49	6.15	61.82	99.57	0.407	0.797	1.419	4.75	5.369	5.883	23.9%
Africa-Southern	94.31	120	120	16.1	39.2	65.68	6.648	66.59	99.86	0.964	1.507	3.001	12.82	13.67	13.75	7.3%
Africa-Western	33.78	119.4	120	3.738	23.14	26.27	5.399	56.49	98.88	0.105	0.223	0.397	8.585	10.22	11.24	30.9%
Africa	41.01	119.5	120	6.547	25.29	31.29	5.64	57.97	99.07	0.464	0.74	1.35	7.26	8.847	10.04	38.3%
America-Caribbean	56.66	119.5	120	15.01	36.08	43.14	7.054	65	99.41	0.948	1.695	2.192	6.163	6.914	7.194	16.7%
America-Central	60.67	119.9	120	12.27	31.26	40.99	6.285	61.61	99.52	0.241	0.718	1.418	10.3	11.08	12.02	16.7%
America-North	94.53	120	120	47.92	67.43	70.74	22.39	90.62	99.96	2.458	2.781	2.836	13.53	13.77	14	3.5%
America-South	80.23	119.9	120	17.34	40.12	54.26	8.521	69.27	99.81	0.743	1.38	2.272	10.85	12.11	13.06	20.4%
Americas	85.26	119.9	120	31.84	52.33	60.7	15.08	78.72	99.84	2.218	2.484	2.68	11.92	12.61	13.19	10.7%
Asia-East	81.45	120	120	17.56	47.78	75.23	12.59	78.27	99.96	2.655	3.017	4.192	4.424	5.1	5.512	24.6%
Asia-South Central	40.75	119.8	120	9.262	29.83	42.95	5.866	61.33	99.55	0.743	1.236	2.032	9.714	11.54	11.73	20.8%
Asia-South East	57.29	119.9	120	12.32	28.52	35.04	6.151	60.24	99.38	0.567	0.727	1.104	7.954	8.97	9.958	25.2%
Asia-West	71.47	119.9	120	17.96	40.34	49.98	8.153	67.56	99.66	1.151	1.703	2.323	6.591	7.118	7.601	15.3%
Oceania	91.22	119.8	120	38.42	58.88	60.31	15.49	82.94	99.69	2.049	2.793	2.891	13.06	13.4	13.79	5.6%
Asia with Oceania	60.71	119.9	120	13.58	36.56	51.96	8.671	67.41	99.65	2.136	2.426	3.308	7.306	8.753	9.368	28.2%
Europe-East	105.4	120	120	24.73	49.47	56.77	9.097	74.15	99.88	1.021	1.901	2.307	8.326	8.976	9.256	11.2%
Europe-North	115.7	120	120	45.41	74.68	75.91	27.52	97.17	100	2.102	2.99	3.036	13.92	13.99	14	0.6%
Europe-South	114.5	120	120	33.97	59.28	70.96	17.64	83.45	99.95	1.056	1.721	2.423	13.41	13.65	13.8	2.9%
Europe-West	110.7	120	120	43.73	72.88	76	25.56	94.92	100	2.269	3.088	3.237	14	14	14	0.0%
Europe	110.1	120	120	34.47	61.89	68.57	17.67	85.36	99.95	1.86	2.629	2.927	11.57	12.05	12.33	6.6%

Multination Regional Analysis

Measures of Poverty, Health, Education, Infrastructure, and Governance

Infrastructure — Communication · Infrastructure — Other · Governance

Base Case: Countries in Year 2060 Descending Population Sequence	Mobile Phone Usage (Percent of Population)			Internet Usage (Percent of Population)			Broadband Usage (Percent of Population)			R&D Expenditures (Percent of GDP)			Freedom House Index (Inverted) (Index Range: 2-14)			
	2010	2035	2060	2010	2035	2060	2010	2035	2060	2010	2035	2060	2010	2035	2060	% Chg
AFRICA																
Ethiopia	30.91	119.7	120	0.778	22.55	30.32	5.395	56.52	99.17	0.181	0.29	0.7	6.417	8.831	11.58	80.5%
Tanzania, United Rep	34.29	119.8	120	3.509	24.92	39.57	5.436	58.14	99.53	0.094	0.326	1.126	9.394	13.2	14	49.0%
Uganda	29.61	119.7	120	3.479	24.79	42.66	5.482	58.21	99.57	0.418	0.604	1.565	7.248	9.508	12.31	69.8%
Kenya	35.35	119.6	120	7.682	23.45	31.85	5.425	56.45	99.18	0.123	0.234	0.689	10.24	12.31	14	36.7%
Madagascar	16.39	118.1	120	2.981	21.36	23.85	5.314	55.46	98.71	0.14	0.172	0.291	10.07	11.66	14	39.0%
Mozambique	37.38	119.8	120	1.919	24.09	37.67	5.423	57.8	99.49	0.588	0.751	1.46	9.516	13.96	14	47.1%
Malawi	26.48	119.3	120	3.643	21.32	24.57	5.381	55.7	98.79	0.072	0.112	0.277	8.395	10.04	12.61	50.2%
Zambia	31.52	119.7	120	6.164	23.74	30.57	5.437	57.18	99.19	0.022	0.169	0.538	8.252	10.17	12.19	47.7%
Somalia	21.14	119.1	120	0.251	21.14	22.17	5.281	55.13	98.5	0.071	0.101	0.142	3.033	3.524	4.004	32.0%
Rwanda	30.23	119.8	120	2.671	23.96	35.85	5.419	57.52	99.4	0.049	0.241	0.948	5.246	7.471	9.657	84.1%
Zimbabwe	18.74	118.6	120	8.685	22.81	25.53	5.538	57.02	99.01	0.137	0.188	0.331	3.017	3.338	3.772	25.0%
Burundi	23.43	118.8	120	1.61	20.42	21.44	5.296	54.92	98.47	0.308	0.304	0.33	6.281	7.443	9.522	51.6%
Eritrea	9.248	113.9	120	2.883	20.74	21.62	5.262	54.9	98.45	0.067	0.078	0.111	2.99	3.261	3.741	25.1%
Comoros	10.68	112.9	120	5.787	21.32	23.14	5.263	55.01	98.56	0.094	0.111	0.197	7.9	8.413	9.968	26.2%
Mauritius	88.38	120	120	20.4	44.13	62.43	6.853	69.09	99.9	0.399	1.067	2.106	14	14	14	0.0%
Djibouti	34.37	119.6	120	6.908	24.99	33.25	5.583	57.63	99.3	0.174	0.313	0.768	6.223	7.187	8.698	39.8%
Africa-Eastern	**29.89**	**119.4**	**120**	**3.416**	**23.24**	**32.32**	**5.416**	**56.9**	**99.18**	**0.208**	**0.398**	**1.085**	**7.697**	**10.05**	**11.9**	**54.6%**
Congo, Democratic Republic of	28.51	119.5	120	10.21	20.4	21.06	5.288	54.92	98.41	0.042	0.06	0.079	4.276	5.326	6.033	41.1%
Angola	51.36	119.9	120	4.403	35.79	40.54	6.238	65.29	99.63	0.361	0.95	1.181	5.244	6.289	6.74	28.5%
Cameroon	35.85	119.7	120	2.28	24.24	29.25	5.43	56.94	99.08	0.166	0.276	0.541	4.051	4.625	5.362	32.4%
Chad	13.16	118	120	1.803	22.49	23.05	5.285	55.83	98.58	0.117	0.18	0.19	4.924	5.606	5.797	17.7%
Central African Republic	21.36	118.9	120	11.15	21.24	23.18	5.32	55.28	98.62	0.251	0.273	0.357	5.125	5.952	7.207	40.6%
Congo, Republic of	39.53	119.8	120	15.24	28.5	30.72	5.648	59.66	99.19	0.044	0.301	0.421	7.169	8.155	8.63	20.4%
Gabon	83.39	120	120	14.84	41.35	44.55	5.949	63.32	99.6	0.015	0.345	0.564	6.982	7.321	7.628	9.3%
Equatorial Guinea	61.26	119.9	120	6.693	72.2	75.84	9.404	78.8	99.96	2.153	3	3.163	3.015	3.178	3.265	8.3%
São Tomé and Príncipe	29.84	119.1	120	12.63	22.18	23.88	6.817	58.59	98.96	0.129	0.159	0.239	12.32	13.18	14	13.6%
Africa-Middle	**32.47**	**119.4**	**120**	**7.714**	**23.93**	**25.15**	**5.489**	**57.05**	**98.69**	**0.355**	**0.798**	**0.955**	**4.614**	**5.527**	**6.133**	**32.9%**
Egypt	52.95	119.9	120	17.64	33.03	48.28	6.071	62.25	99.72	0.271	0.679	1.525	5.143	6.017	6.82	32.6%
Sudan	35.96	119.8	120	3.784	26.77	32.56	5.609	59.33	99.35	0.357	0.605	0.899	2.085	2.631	2.995	43.6%
Algeria	72.61	119.9	120	10.6	32.48	36.45	6.137	61.51	99.46	0.466	0.737	0.948	5.062	5.615	5.957	17.7%
Morocco	77.1	120	120	10.74	29.11	37.6	6.805	61.92	99.58	0.564	0.888	1.333	7.165	8.138	9.174	28.0%
Tunisia	91.99	120	120	14.92	38.33	55.13	6.48	66.21	99.84	0.68	1.231	2.148	5.128	5.939	6.632	29.3%
Libyan Arab Jamahiriya	71.72	119.9	120	6.729	48.38	54.19	6.786	69.69	99.79	0.3	1.138	1.468	2.039	2.3	2.393	17.4%
Africa-Northern	**59.37**	**119.9**	**120**	**12.16**	**31.66**	**41.49**	**6.15**	**61.82**	**99.57**	**0.407**	**0.797**	**1.419**	**4.75**	**5.369**	**5.883**	**23.9%**

Multination Regional Analysis

Measures of Poverty, Health, Education, Infrastructure, and Governance

Infrastructure
Communication / **Other**

Governance

Base Case: Countries in Year 2060 Descending Population Sequence	Mobile Phone Usage (Percent of Population)			Internet Usage (Percent of Population)			Broadband Usage (Percent of Population)			R&D Expenditures (Percent of GDP)			Freedom House Index (Inverted) Index Range: 2-14			
	2010	2035	2060	2010	2035	2060	2010	2035	2060	2010	2035	2060	2010	2035	2060	% Chg
AFRICA continued																
South Africa	100.7	120	120	16.24	39.84	68.99	6.749	66.93	99.9	0.992	1.485	3.087	13.2	14	14	6.1%
Namibia	49.13	119.9	120	12.19	31.48	48.51	5.659	61.29	99.71	0.352	0.696	1.633	11.08	12.75	14	26.4%
Lesotho	39.12	119.7	120	6.305	23.67	29.57	5.46	57.01	99.15	0.022	0.144	0.474	11.34	13.7	14	23.5%
Botswana	70.56	120	120	29.91	58.52	76	7.136	80.98	99.98	0.969	2.254	3.192	12.26	14	14	14.2%
Swaziland	42.6	119.8	120	11.74	29.73	41.23	5.502	59.66	99.55	0.331	0.589	1.222	4.007	4.56	5.232	30.6%
Africa-Southern	**94.31**	**120**	**120**	**16.1**	**39.2**	**65.68**	**6.648**	**66.59**	**99.86**	**0.964**	**1.507**	**3.001**	**12.82**	**13.67**	**13.75**	**7.3%**
Nigeria	38.76	119.8	120	2.909	24.24	26.61	5.405	57	98.9	0.1	0.246	0.36	8.202	10.01	11.01	34.2%
Niger	18.4	118.6	120	1.642	20.89	22.67	5.313	55.3	98.59	0.064	0.092	0.17	10.19	11.96	14	37.4%
Côte d'Ivoire	30.22	119.5	120	6.897	23.19	26.61	5.354	56.38	98.94	0.135	0.218	0.393	4.024	4.595	5.348	32.9%
Ghana	39.33	119.1	120	2.845	22.09	26.02	5.469	55.94	98.88	0.111	0.153	0.36	12.39	13.84	14	13.0%
Mali	23.08	119.2	120	3.725	22.1	27.44	5.359	56.17	99.02	0.091	0.159	0.439	12.14	14	14	15.3%
Burkina Faso	20.4	119.1	120	3.092	22.17	27.66	5.339	56	98.97	0.112	0.178	0.467	7.038	8.316	10.58	50.3%
Senegal	34.69	119.5	120	8.376	22.82	28.64	5.612	56.94	99.12	0.025	0.099	0.415	11.09	12.62	14	26.2%
Guinea	18.87	119	120	4.049	22.45	26.13	5.35	56.07	98.89	0.1	0.178	0.365	5.066	6.032	7.161	41.4%
Benin	26.84	119.1	120	4.486	22.08	24.89	5.386	55.93	98.8	0.109	0.156	0.296	12.21	13.88	14	14.7%
Togo	24.67	117.8	120	10.79	21	21.51	5.319	55.13	98.46	0.475	0.468	0.456	5.061	5.627	6.029	19.1%
Sierra Leone	40.1	119.8	120	2.026	22.18	30.25	5.35	56.13	99.11	0.066	0.162	0.599	9.39	12.59	14	49.1%
Liberia	37.31	119.9	120	0.602	21.98	29.05	5.322	56.08	99.11	0.047	0.151	0.531	7.623	12.05	14	83.7%
Mauritania	46.53	119.2	120	5.409	21.73	22.66	5.397	55.28	98.56	0.142	0.131	0.17	5.053	5.082	5.576	10.4%
Guinea-Bissau	23.86	118	120	4.78	20.39	20.86	5.298	54.96	98.4	0.053	0.059	0.068	8.178	8.873	9.769	19.5%
Gambia	41.01	119.7	120	11.57	22.77	27.74	5.427	56.51	99.05	0.102	0.196	0.457	8.232	10.01	12.14	47.5%
Cape Verde	49.86	119.9	120	11.84	28.64	42.92	6.15	61.29	99.68	0.222	0.528	1.316	14	14	14	0.0%
Africa-Western	**33.78**	**119.4**	**120**	**3.738**	**23.14**	**26.27**	**5.399**	**56.49**	**98.88**	**0.105**	**0.223**	**0.397**	**8.585**	**10.22**	**11.24**	**30.9%**

Infrastructure / Governance

Base Case: Countries in Year 2060 Descending Population Sequence	Mobile Phone Usage (Percent of Population)			Internet Usage (Percent of Population)			Broadband Usage (Percent of Population)			R&D Expenditures (Percent of GDP)			Freedom House Index (Inverted) (Index Range: 2-14)			
	2010	2035	2060	2010	2035	2060	2010	2035	2060	2010	2035	2060	2010	2035	2060	% Chg
AMERICAS																
Haiti	22.16	118.6	120	6.883	21.99	24.25	5.333	55.53	98.72	0.105	0.143	0.259	3.025	3.343	3.907	29.2%
Dominican Republic	79.09	120	120	19.03	38.08	52.92	7.048	67.4	99.86	0.427	1.068	1.879	12.27	14	14	14.1%
Cuba	28.7	119.7	120	11.16	34.99	46.28	5.97	62.23	99.65	0.462	0.832	1.469	2.026	2.258	2.487	22.8%
Puerto Rico	111.2	120	120	29.14	68.69	76	11.64	86.68	99.99	1.637	2.821	3.195	4.287	4.706	5.088	18.7%
Jamaica	95.83	120	120	15.38	31.04	38.72	7.552	63	99.63	0.047	0.233	0.688	10.94	11.71	12.87	17.6%
Trinidad	100.9	120	120	23.41	70.06	76	9.39	90.36	99.99	0.243	1.945	2.325	10.19	11.66	12.45	22.2%
Bahamas	97.82	120	120	40.68	57.26	76	8.791	76.42	99.97	1.361	2.164	3.187	13.99	14	14	0.1%
Barbados	102.8	120	120	19.57	47.35	71.73	19.98	83.62	99.98	1.073	1.582	2.949	14	14	14	0.0%
Grenada	74.53	119.9	120	16.22	34.14	45.26	9.216	66.15	99.77	0.649	0.838	1.449	12.99	13.84	14	7.8%
Saint Vincent and Grenadines	91.35	120	120	15.43	35.94	49	9.634	69.18	99.85	0.186	0.624	1.366	13.2	14	14	6.1%
Saint Lucia	102.2	120	120	26.05	37.79	48.84	11.67	71.54	99.88	0.391	0.76	1.395	13.11	14	14	6.8%
America-Caribbean	**56.66**	**119.5**	**120**	**15.01**	**36.08**	**43.14**	**7.054**	**65**	**99.41**	**0.948**	**1.695**	**2.192**	**6.163**	**6.914**	**7.194**	**16.7%**
Guatemala	65.38	119.9	120	10.95	30.23	40.03	5.915	60.47	99.57	0.057	0.334	0.881	8.059	9.111	10.26	27.3%
Honduras	44.45	119.8	120	10.79	27.17	33.77	5.605	58.53	99.33	0.061	0.256	0.625	10.14	11.57	12.99	28.1%
El Salvador	65.51	119.9	120	12.59	30.84	40.38	6.441	61.45	99.61	0.095	0.35	0.895	11.08	12.27	13.75	24.1%
Nicaragua	41.7	119.6	120	10.5	24.81	28.55	5.667	57.47	99.1	0.049	0.156	0.366	10.06	11.19	12.5	24.3%
Costa Rica	61.63	119.9	120	18.26	41.05	57.39	7.694	69.16	99.89	0.444	1.01	1.925	14	14	14	0.0%
Panama	96.65	120	120	14.91	48.06	74.7	8.017	74.25	99.95	0.459	1.395	2.881	13.39	14	14	4.6%
Belize	75.35	119.9	120	16.72	35.69	51.22	7.92	66.3	99.82	0.539	0.935	1.787	13.05	14	14	7.3%
America-Central	**60.67**	**119.9**	**120**	**12.27**	**31.26**	**40.99**	**6.285**	**61.61**	**99.52**	**0.241**	**0.718**	**1.418**	**10.3**	**11.08**	**12.02**	**16.7%**
USA	102	120	120	58.15	75.79	76	26.42	97.83	100	2.617	2.924	2.944	13.99	14	14	0.1%
Mexico	75.86	120	120	17.32	41.15	52.45	8.013	67.92	99.83	0.41	0.844	1.494	12.05	13.05	14	16.2%
Canada	86.54	120	120	52.71	75.85	76	31.89	97.91	100	2.01	2.774	2.802	14	14	14	0.0%
America-North	**94.53**	**120**	**120**	**47.92**	**67.43**	**70.74**	**22.39**	**90.62**	**99.96**	**2.458**	**2.781**	**2.836**	**13.53**	**13.77**	**14**	**3.5%**
Brazil	80.08	120	120	16.28	40.57	56.1	8.89	70.41	99.88	1.053	1.583	2.414	11.17	12.68	13.99	25.2%
Colombia	80.61	120	120	14	31.97	40.36	6.777	62.91	99.65	0.213	0.477	0.958	8.128	8.975	9.866	21.4%
Argentina	97.52	120	120	21.13	51.77	75.36	10.17	76.12	99.96	0.623	1.602	2.918	12.29	13.89	14	13.9%
Peru	58.7	119.9	120	15.43	38.39	51.63	8.067	68.71	99.85	0.193	0.745	1.492	11.36	12.91	14	23.2%
Venezuela	83.16	120	120	26.32	44.04	56.32	8.006	69.35	99.84	0.336	1.003	1.705	9.13	10.27	11.02	20.7%
Ecuador	75.72	119.9	120	13.55	30.33	32.26	5.773	59.04	99.16	0.152	0.3	0.419	10.03	10.63	11.04	10.1%
Chile	99.05	120	120	26.82	49.06	71.21	11.92	79.59	99.97	0.665	1.437	2.68	14	14	14	0.0%
Bolivia	54.37	119.9	120	12.05	30.01	36.72	5.794	61.01	99.5	0.294	0.605	0.965	10.16	11.94	13.15	29.4%
Paraguay	60.43	119.9	120	10.78	27.58	34.58	5.764	58.81	99.36	0.115	0.287	0.679	10.18	11.33	12.71	24.9%
Uruguay	83.53	120	120	20.03	51.83	76	9.563	77.93	99.97	0.475	1.577	2.921	14	14	14	0.0%
Guyana	72.21	119.9	120	15.56	27.33	33.99	6.085	59.41	99.39	0.264	0.415	0.793	12.34	13.63	14	13.5%
Suriname	89.64	120	120	13.38	40.25	56.09	6.717	66.76	99.84	0.595	1.177	2.061	13.26	14	14	5.6%
America-South	**80.23**	**120**	**120**	**17.34**	**40.12**	**54.26**	**8.521**	**69.27**	**99.81**	**0.743**	**1.38**	**2.272**	**10.85**	**12.11**	**13.06**	**20.4%**

Multination Regional Analysis

Measures of Poverty, Health, Education, Infrastructure, and Governance

Infrastructure
Communication

Infrastructure
Other

Governance

Base Case: Countries in Year 2060 Descending Population Sequence	Mobile Phone Usage Percent of Population			Internet Usage Percent of Population			Broadband Usage Percent of Population			R&D Expenditures Percent of GDP			Freedom House Index (Inverted) Index Range: 2-14			
	2010	2035	2060	2010	2035	2060	2010	2035	2060	2010	2035	2060	2010	2035	2060	% Chg
ASIA with OCEANIA																
China	78.55	120	120	13.3	45.13	76	9.895	76.1	99.97	1.567	2.578	4.202	3.168	3.967	4.563	44.0%
Japan	104.4	120	120	46.01	76	76	28.53	97.39	100	3.398	4.385	4.304	13.02	14	14	7.5%
Korea, Repub of	108.3	120	120	44.87	63.48	76	36.79	97.33	100	3.508	4.3	4.878	13.09	14	14	7.0%
Taiwan	113.5	120	120	37.05	55.61	76	28.6	93.78	100	1.201	2.065	3.19	13.05	14	14	7.3%
Korea, Dem. People's Rep.	23.85	119.4	120	15.38	25.86	28.85	5.565	57.46	99.05	0.241	0.353	0.521	2.042	2.246	2.456	20.3%
Hong Kong SAR	120.3	120	120	65.76	74.29	76	39.2	97.63	100	0.982	1.522	1.71	3.308	3.394	3.576	8.1%
Mongolia	57.77	119.9	120	11.2	29.04	41.98	5.948	61.18	99.64	0.266	0.569	1.287	12.6	14	14	11.1%
Asia-East	**81.45**	**120**	**120**	**17.56**	**47.78**	**75.23**	**12.59**	**78.27**	**99.96**	**2.655**	**3.017**	**4.192**	**4.424**	**5.1**	**5.512**	**24.6%**
India	42.77	119.9	120	9.583	30.88	48.56	5.931	62.49	99.74	0.822	1.235	2.174	11.45	14	14	22.3%
Pakistan	33.17	119.5	120	6.744	24.22	29.28	5.591	57.22	99.12	0.678	0.735	0.973	5.093	5.598	6.503	27.7%
Bangladesh	34.18	119.8	120	2.7	23.9	28.76	5.399	56.73	99.05	0.628	0.734	0.963	8.397	10.52	12.38	47.4%
Afghanistan	27.67	119.7	120	11.62	25.3	41.87	5.422	57.93	99.55	0.117	0.351	1.255	5.128	6.736	8.629	68.3%
Iran (Islamic Republic of)	47.14	119.9	120	25.71	46.79	54.31	6.459	68.93	99.85	0.727	1.554	1.955	4.08	4.697	4.952	21.4%
Nepal	19.17	118.2	120	4.101	21.76	23.81	5.364	55.6	98.71	0.66	0.662	0.73	6.115	6.865	8.134	33.0%
Uzbekistan	37.08	119.8	120	9.241	26.97	33.07	5.765	59.37	99.35	0.199	0.423	0.759	3.169	3.798	4.279	35.0%
Sri Lanka	49.97	119.9	120	9.614	29.65	38.95	6.292	61.64	99.6	0.21	0.495	1.018	10.3	11.9	13.44	30.5%
Kazakhstan	79.17	120	120	10.39	53.33	58.3	7.048	75.06	99.94	0.317	1.534	1.825	5.144	6.047	6.255	21.6%
Tajikistan	29.35	119.5	120	0.458	23.24	26.75	5.491	56.61	98.96	0.078	0.16	0.35	5.133	5.756	6.524	27.1%
Turkmenistan	49.58	119.9	120	1.572	68.19	76	7.929	83.2	99.98	0.84	2.802	3.19	2.098	2.539	2.657	26.6%
Kyrgyzstan	35.16	119.6	120	13.05	24.07	27.49	5.569	57.26	99.04	0.261	0.359	0.538	5.139	5.972	6.75	31.3%
Bhutan	40.76	119.9	120	8.758	35.84	60.5	6.098	64.99	99.86	0.332	0.951	2.309	5.181	6.307	7.388	42.6%
Maldives	97.93	120	120	13.01	31.5	46.49	7.185	64.23	99.77	0.333	0.692	1.518	5.107	5.929	6.851	34.1%
Asia-South Central	**40.75**	**119.8**	**120**	**9.262**	**29.83**	**42.95**	**5.866**	**61.33**	**99.55**	**0.743**	**1.236**	**2.032**	**9.714**	**11.54**	**11.73**	**20.8%**
Indonesia	52.09	119.9	120	11.32	27.37	32.35	5.748	58.92	99.3	0.084	0.265	0.553	9.256	10.42	11.51	24.4%
Philippines	74.21	119.9	120	12.2	27.16	34.03	5.88	59.5	99.41	0.139	0.331	0.713	11.26	12.65	14	24.3%
Viet Nam	43.54	119.8	120	13.83	26.54	34.35	6.182	61.07	99.55	0.217	0.421	0.85	3.119	3.747	4.339	39.1%
Thailand	79.83	120	120	16.17	33.23	42.48	6.044	61.44	99.6	0.262	0.529	1.062	11.07	12.09	13.33	20.4%
Myanmar	27.3	119.6	120	0.249	22.48	24.36	5.405	56.04	98.74	0.087	0.159	0.262	2.126	2.59	2.958	39.1%
Malaysia	102.9	120	120	28.14	44.57	60.57	8.68	71.46	99.91	0.667	1.252	2.144	8.076	8.913	9.688	20.0%
Cambodia	34.43	119.8	120	2.103	25.14	31.46	5.51	58.16	99.3	0.131	0.326	0.666	5.128	6.42	7.459	45.5%
LAO People's Dem Repub	37.45	119.8	120	12.95	26.62	37.33	5.515	58.85	99.47	0.159	0.415	0.998	3.075	3.857	4.558	48.2%
Singapore	113	120	120	53.46	75.97	76	29.38	97.66	100	2.599	2.885	2.905	7.014	7.314	7.701	9.8%
Timor-Leste	20.95	119.4	120	12.48	24.06	26.73	5.393	56.9	98.92	0.177	0.273	0.399	10.07	11.31	12.42	23.3%
Brunei Darussalam	91.88	120	120	73.98	75.65	76	7.844	80.42	99.95	-0.041	0.271	0.468	4.961	5.13	5.19	4.6%
Asia-South East	**57.29**	**119.9**	**120**	**12.32**	**28.52**	**35.04**	**6.151**	**60.24**	**99.38**	**0.567**	**0.727**	**1.104**	**7.954**	**8.97**	**9.958**	**25.2%**

Multination Regional Analysis

Measures of Poverty, Health, Education, Infrastructure, and Governance

Infrastructure — Communication / Infrastructure — Other / Governance

Base Case: Countries in Year 2060 Descending Population Sequence	Mobile Phone Usage (Percent of Population)			Internet Usage (Percent of Population)			Broadband Usage (Percent of Population)			R&D Expenditures (Percent of GDP)			Freedom House Index (Inverted) (Index Range: 2-14)			
	2010	2035	2060	2010	2035	2060	2010	2035	2060	2010	2035	2060	2010	2035	2060	% Chg
ASIA with OCEANIA continued																
Turkey	89.15	120	120	15.84	38.51	51.35	8.473	68.84	99.85	0.722	1.221	1.918	10.08	11.39	12.43	23.3%
Yemen	32.69	119.7	120	13.15	25.57	30.67	5.455	57.88	99.16	0.182	0.357	0.623	6.101	7.269	8.268	35.5%
Iraq	37.11	119.8	120	19.32	38.39	55.72	6.085	65.12	99.82	0.486	1.103	2.042	4.108	4.839	5.412	31.7%
Saudi Arabia	88.61	120	120	21.63	57.67	65.47	6.441	71.35	99.88	0.065	0.827	1.336	2.004	2.165	2.262	12.9%
Syrian Arab Repub	40.77	119.7	120	16.29	27.26	33.34	5.614	58.27	99.28	0.315	0.448	0.775	2.025	2.205	2.454	21.2%
Israel	118	120	120	34.37	72.76	76	28.07	97.44	100	4.686	5.971	5.892	12.04	13.39	14	16.3%
Jordan	89.25	120	120	13.31	31.57	54.53	6.521	63.07	99.79	0.293	0.64	1.917	7.182	8.328	9.789	36.3%
Occupied Palestinian Territory	55.66	119.9	120	15.42	28.16	39.34	5.755	59.52	99.52	0.28	0.507	1.112	7.629	8.845	10.24	34.2%
Azerbaijan	78.09	120	120	5.873	42.2	49.2	7.012	70.73	99.88	0.327	1.144	1.533	5.363	6.446	6.84	27.5%
United Arab Emirates	115.2	120	120	45.46	75.76	76	15.18	96.01	100	2.587	3.185	3.185	4.065	4.426	4.688	15.3%
Oman	91.16	120	120	23.58	60.1	76	8.551	76.64	99.95	1.583	2.316	3.189	5.065	5.429	5.836	15.2%
Kuwait	108.3	120	120	36.32	75.5	76	8.597	86.22	99.98	0.1	0.428	0.615	7.003	7.415	7.381	5.4%
Lebanon	65.85	119.9	120	20.01	42.75	59.27	10.89	72.95	99.92	0.758	1.324	2.24	5.095	5.673	6.206	21.8%
Armenia	50.72	119.9	120	11.08	45.69	74.12	6.46	72.7	99.96	0.269	1.432	2.993	7.265	9.366	10.45	43.8%
Georgia	66.6	119.9	120	10.03	32.06	41.22	6.133	62.7	99.68	0.334	0.725	1.238	9.328	10.99	12.14	30.1%
Bahrain	116	120	120	33.57	75.67	76	13.96	89.89	99.99	2.58	3.188	3.188	6.078	6.408	6.857	12.8%
Qatar	113.4	120	120	37.9	75.89	76	52.07	99.95	100	0.087	0.284	0.481	5.248	5.469	5.425	3.4%
Cyprus	113.8	120	120	35.75	65.05	76	12.86	83.65	99.98	0.519	1.388	2.075	14	14	14	0.0%
Asia-West	**71.47**	**119.9**	**120**	**17.96**	**40.34**	**49.98**	**8.153**	**67.56**	**99.66**	**1.151**	**1.703**	**2.323**	**6.591**	**7.118**	**7.601**	**15.3%**
Australia	112.9	120	120	48.73	75.75	76	19.39	95.24	100	2.181	2.966	2.982	14	14	14	0.0%
Papua New Guinea	23.66	119.5	120	9.387	24.8	27.91	5.485	57.56	99.03	0.157	0.304	0.466	10.28	12.2	13.56	31.9%
New Zealand	110.5	120	120	45.29	61.68	76	15.92	86.39	99.99	1.237	1.959	2.771	14	14	14	0.0%
Solomon Islands	26.2	119.4	120	3.974	23.59	26.5	5.617	56.94	98.95	0.155	0.239	0.386	10.28	11.51	12.89	25.4%
Fiji	46.85	119.8	120	12.5	28.02	37.53	6.386	59.95	99.5	0.315	0.479	1.012	9.011	9.939	11.44	27.0%
Vanuatu	31.8	119.7	120	12.27	28.13	37.07	5.72	59.45	99.46	0.287	0.5	0.986	12.24	13.89	14	14.4%
Micronesia, Federated States of	89.86	120	120	18.92	29.6	38.63	8.243	63.72	99.63	0.433	0.581	1.072	14	14	14	0.0%
Tonga	51.42	119.8	120	11.21	26.9	34.01	6.058	58.22	99.3	0.361	0.431	0.811	7.923	8.282	9.366	18.2%
Samoa	44.79	119.9	120	10.88	32.7	46.88	6.035	62.38	99.73	0.399	0.755	1.539	12.26	13.98	14	14.2%
Oceania	**91.22**	**119.8**	**120**	**38.42**	**58.88**	**60.31**	**15.49**	**82.94**	**99.69**	**2.049**	**2.793**	**2.891**	**13.06**	**13.4**	**13.79**	**5.6%**

Multination Regional Analysis

Measures of Poverty, Health, Education, Infrastructure, and Governance

Base Case: Countries in Year 2060 Descending Population Sequence	Infrastructure Communication — Mobile Phone Usage (Percent of Population)			Internet Usage (Percent of Population)			Broadband Usage (Percent of Population)			Infrastructure Other — R&D Expenditures (Percent of GDP)			Governance — Freedom House Index (Inverted) (Index Range: 2-14)			
	2010	2035	2060	2010	2035	2060	2010	2035	2060	2010	2035	2060	2010	2035	2060	% Chg
EUROPE																
Russian Federation	110.1	120	120	31.54	54.47	57.28	8.603	76.06	99.93	1.227	2.227	2.37	5.103	5.759	5.9	15.6%
Poland	107	120	120	21.94	52.57	66.49	10.35	77.72	99.96	0.677	1.508	2.311	14	14	14	0.0%
Ukraine	96.71	120	120	12.14	34.07	41.2	6.459	63.56	99.64	0.904	1.239	1.615	9.202	10.38	11.23	22.0%
Romania	96.54	120	120	17.97	41.02	51.87	8.68	69.09	99.85	0.604	1.083	1.702	11.21	12.38	13.34	19.0%
Czech Republic	118.1	120	120	28.87	56.53	68.96	15.77	82.4	99.97	1.657	2.22	2.912	14	14	14	0.0%
Belarus	86.99	120	120	16.32	49.29	62.27	7.258	71.76	99.92	1.081	2.018	2.716	3.094	3.567	3.801	22.9%
Hungary	112.5	120	120	24.66	53.44	69.8	13.91	81.24	99.97	0.954	1.689	2.624	14	14	14	0.0%
Bulgaria	107.7	120	120	19.37	39.55	51.14	15.31	76.54	99.93	0.549	0.949	1.617	13.24	14	14	5.7%
Slovak Republic	109.5	120	120	26.41	56.03	67.2	12.53	81.9	99.98	0.617	1.441	2.109	14	14	14	0.0%
Moldova, Repub of	54.33	119.8	120	8.905	24.44	29.1	5.827	57.52	99.14	0.552	0.616	0.855	9.165	10.16	11.63	26.9%
Europe-East	**105.4**	**120**	**120**	**24.73**	**49.47**	**56.77**	**9.097**	**74.15**	**99.88**	**1.021**	**1.901**	**2.307**	**8.326**	**8.976**	**9.256**	**11.2%**
United Kingdom	116	120	120	44.36	75.9	76	26.53	97.65	100	1.805	2.839	2.863	14	14	14	0.0%
Sweden	114.9	120	120	54.37	76	76	32.77	98.97	100	3.69	4.486	4.398	14	14	14	0.0%
Denmark	113.4	120	120	51.32	76	76	35.1	98.78	100	2.51	3.359	3.348	14	14	14	0.0%
Ireland	116	120	120	43.02	75.82	76	19.11	96.32	100	1.311	1.952	2.036	14	14	14	0.0%
Norway	115.9	120	120	59.89	75.94	76	35.99	99.18	100	1.695	1.791	1.887	14	14	14	0.0%
Finland	114.3	120	120	49.91	76	76	35.27	98.84	100	3.481	4.388	4.308	14	14	14	0.0%
Lithuania	121.4	120	120	22.95	52.62	72.5	15.86	83.78	99.98	0.915	1.707	2.836	12.21	13.52	14	14.7%
Latvia	108.6	120	120	22.67	55.32	76	11.58	81.66	99.98	0.736	1.74	2.915	13.28	14	14	5.4%
Estonia	117.1	120	120	37.02	60.38	76	24.99	94.87	100	1.248	2.263	3.138	14	14	14	0.0%
Iceland	116.1	120	120	63.1	75.94	76	43.33	99.42	100	2.977	3.466	3.449	14	14	14	0.0%
Europe-North	**115.7**	**120**	**120**	**45.41**	**74.68**	**75.91**	**27.52**	**97.17**	**100**	**2.102**	**2.99**	**3.036**	**13.92**	**13.99**	**14**	**0.6%**
Italy	120.6	120	120	39.39	61.56	75.47	19.69	85.45	99.98	1.041	1.607	2.446	13.96	14	14	0.3%
Spain	114.4	120	120	33.77	65.5	76	20.85	89.27	99.99	1.217	1.993	2.628	13.99	14	14	0.1%
Greece	113.4	120	120	33.5	70.17	76	10.64	80.81	99.97	0.557	1.407	1.832	13.07	13.87	14	7.1%
Portugal	117	120	120	35.88	52.23	66.34	18.75	83.16	99.97	1.115	1.638	2.446	13.92	14	14	0.6%
Serbia	108.8	120	120	25.78	36.26	46.33	10.19	68.49	99.81	1.209	1.446	1.981	11.18	12.1	13.21	18.2%
Bosnia and Herzegovina	78.7	120	120	12.83	37.36	49.94	6.633	65.92	99.82	0.068	0.631	1.36	9.154	10.59	11.7	27.8%
Croatia	107.5	120	120	22.37	47.11	61.02	9.604	72.32	99.92	0.97	1.539	2.324	12.15	13.4	14	15.2%
Albania	85.38	120	120	4.001	34.54	44.69	6.16	63.45	99.72	0.445	0.851	1.415	10.23	11.67	12.82	25.3%
Macedonia, FYR	92.85	120	120	23.23	32.87	40.14	6.766	62.02	99.59	0.243	0.444	0.875	10.16	11	12.04	18.5%
Slovenia	111.3	120	120	33.77	66.97	76	19.98	91.54	99.99	1.597	2.578	3.09	14	14	14	0.0%
Montenegro	107.6	120	120	23.38	35.95	51.77	7.733	65.42	99.8	0.57	0.933	1.817	6.247	6.956	7.816	25.1%
Malta	108.2	120	120	30.44	55.1	69.61	21.83	86.74	99.99	0.629	1.222	2.089	14	14	14	0.0%
Europe-South	**114.5**	**120**	**120**	**33.97**	**59.28**	**70.96**	**17.64**	**83.45**	**99.95**	**1.056**	**1.721**	**2.423**	**13.41**	**13.65**	**13.8**	**2.9%**
Germany	112.7	120	120	45.93	74	76	22.44	94.7	100	2.514	3.456	3.529	14	14	14	0.0%
France	106.4	120	120	36.96	70.29	76	24.93	93.63	100	2.09	2.828	3.134	14	14	14	0.0%
Netherlands	113	120	120	54.34	75.71	76	36.61	98.27	100	1.741	2.552	2.595	14	14	14	0.0%
Belgium	111.3	120	120	43.32	71.24	76	29.24	95.58	100	1.864	2.628	2.899	14	14	14	0.0%
Austria	116.4	120	120	49.46	76	76	24.97	95.56	100	2.338	3.111	3.116	14	14	14	0.0%
Switzerland	112.9	120	120	45.74	76	76	35.07	98.64	100	2.651	3.258	3.253	14	14	14	0.0%
Luxembourg	117.4	120	120	49.91	75.64	76	37.76	98.51	100	1.709	1.803	1.897	14	14	14	0.0%
Europe-West	**110.7**	**120**	**120**	**43.73**	**72.88**	**76**	**25.56**	**94.92**	**100**	**2.269**	**3.088**	**3.237**	**14**	**14**	**14**	**0.0%**

Multination Regional Analysis

Measures of Poverty, Health, Education, Infrastructure, and Governance

Governance

Base Case
Source: International Futures
Version 6.32, June 2010

	Polity Democracy Index (Index Range: 1-20)				Economic Freedom Index (Index Range: 1-10)				Government Corruption Perception Index (Index Range: 1-10)				Economic Integration Index (Index Range: 0-100)				Globalization Index (Index Range: 0-100)			
	2010	2035	2060	% Chg	2010	2035	2060	% Chg	2010	2035	2060	% Chg	2010	2035	2060	% Chg	2010	2035	2060	% Chg
World	12.95	13.9	15.09	16.5%	7.412	7.521	7.86	6.0%	3.654	4.886	6.262	71.4%	11.24	12.52	13.25	17.9%	37.34	46.51	52.29	40.0%
Africa	10.95	11.97	13.4	22.4%	6.303	6.698	7.468	18.5%	2.665	3.044	3.874	45.4%	9.376	10.57	9.158	-2.3%	43.86	49.64	49.63	13.2%
Americas	18.42	18.93	19.4	5.3%	7.747	7.875	8.105	4.6%	5.064	6.717	7.873	55.5%	7.704	11.89	14.12	83.3%	41.58	52.62	60.76	46.1%
Asia with Oceania	11.19	12.69	14.38	28.5%	7.089	7.322	7.785	9.8%	3.254	4.743	6.754	107.6%	7.182	9.201	11.75	63.6%	31.72	40.74	48.85	54.0%
Europe	18.74	19.21	19.47	3.9%	7.44	7.624	7.935	6.7%	5.508	7.501	8.464	53.7%	21.66	22.69	20.48	-5.4%	55.05	71.12	76.26	38.5%
World	12.95	13.9	15.09	16.5%	7.412	7.521	7.86	6.0%	3.654	4.886	6.262	71.4%	11.24	12.52	13.25	17.9%	37.34	46.51	52.29	40.0%
Africa-Eastern	11.8	12.58	14.16	20.0%	6.189	7.039	8.03	29.7%	2.525	2.879	4.193	66.1%	6.184	8.229	7.324	18.4%	39.64	46.9	52.58	32.6%
Africa-Middle	6.721	7.78	9.111	35.6%	4.851	4.742	5.067	4.5%	2.133	2.466	2.617	22.7%	23.4	21.17	19.18	-18.0%	42.5	50.8	49.17	15.7%
Africa-Northern	5.836	7.891	10.48	79.6%	6.269	6.725	7.173	14.4%	3.148	4.03	5.447	73.0%	8.223	8.493	8.4	2.2%	50.01	48.47	45.34	-9.3%
Africa-Southern	18.51	19.28	19.48	5.2%	7.158	7.56	8.107	13.3%	4.567	5.926	9.511	108.3%	5.908	7.501	10.79	82.6%	40.03	43.76	65.87	64.6%
Africa-Western	13.91	14.38	15.27	9.8%	5.899	6.375	6.795	15.2%	2.346	2.619	3.049	30.0%	13.79	15.57	10.14	-26.5%	45.42	53.44	47.09	3.7%
Africa	10.95	11.97	13.4	22.4%	6.303	6.698	7.468	18.5%	2.665	3.044	3.874	45.4%	9.376	10.57	9.158	-2.3%	43.86	49.64	49.63	13.2%
America-Caribbean	11.45	12.7	14.04	22.6%	6.903	7.219	7.531	9.1%	3.489	4.51	5.425	55.5%	7.988	10.7	12.8	60.2%	32.38	45.2	54.92	69.6%
America-Central	17.93	18.38	18.96	5.7%	7.373	7.778	8.155	10.6%	3.136	3.826	5.186	65.4%	11.96	12.97	12.09	1.1%	53.27	54.58	54.66	2.6%
America-North	19.53	19.69	19.9	1.9%	8.004	8.232	8.511	6.3%	6.566	8.698	9.167	39.6%	7.681	12.72	15.81	105.8%	52.96	68.38	75.43	42.4%
America-South	17.89	18.77	19.43	8.6%	6.026	6.395	6.727	11.6%	3.722	5.14	7.085	90.4%	7.6	8.326	8.465	11.4%	28.24	35.73	45.91	62.6%
Americas	18.42	18.93	19.4	5.3%	7.747	7.875	8.105	4.6%	5.064	6.717	7.873	55.5%	7.704	11.89	14.12	83.3%	41.58	52.62	60.76	46.1%
Asia-East	5.595	7.823	10.51	87.8%	7.171	7.355	7.811	8.9%	3.87	6.644	9.895	155.7%	5.752	9.146	13.82	140.3%	29.62	50.58	68.73	132.0%
Asia-South Central	15.48	15.83	16.51	6.7%	6.453	7.231	7.84	21.5%	2.756	3.742	5.664	105.5%	3.049	4.88	5.761	88.9%	30.5	32.77	39.18	28.5%
Asia-South East	13.89	14.73	15.83	14.0%	6.964	7.146	7.438	6.8%	2.723	3.252	4.222	55.0%	21.72	18.42	14.68	-32.4%	38.18	39.4	39.54	3.6%
Asia-West	9.441	10.51	12.33	30.6%	6.934	7.15	7.362	6.2%	3.499	4.814	6.159	76.0%	10.14	12.67	14.86	46.5%	34.66	43.73	47.51	37.1%
Oceania	19.7	19.63	19.69	-0.1%	7.902	8.115	8.447	6.9%	7.322	7.852	7.806	6.6%	10.65	14.16	15.84	48.7%	59.29	74.11	74.99	26.5%
Asia with Oceania	11.19	12.69	14.38	28.5%	7.089	7.322	7.785	9.8%	3.254	4.743	6.754	107.6%	7.182	9.201	11.75	63.6%	31.72	40.74	48.85	54.0%
Europe-East	17.34	18.16	18.8	8.4%	6.609	6.934	7.082	7.2%	3.069	5.21	6.296	105.1%	13.41	15.16	16.45	22.7%	45.36	52.38	54.06	19.2%
Europe-North	19.91	19.96	19.96	0.3%	7.929	8.201	8.544	7.8%	8.422	9.854	10	18.7%	28.01	29.09	24.73	-11.7%	69.91	90.63	91.68	31.1%
Europe-South	19.45	19.61	19.77	1.6%	7.132	7.311	7.486	5.0%	5.195	6.773	8.54	64.4%	10.76	13.42	12.56	16.7%	47	65.33	77.02	63.9%
Europe-West	19.73	19.93	19.77	0.2%	7.482	7.666	7.968	6.5%	7.962	9.757	10	25.6%	24.86	25.76	21.89	-11.9%	68.33	88.72	91.51	33.9%
Europe	18.74	19.21	19.47	3.9%	7.44	7.624	7.935	6.7%	5.508	7.501	8.464	53.7%	21.66	22.69	20.48	-5.4%	55.05	71.12	76.26	38.5%

Governance

Base Case: Countries in Year 2060 Descending Population Sequence	Polity Democracy Index (Index Range: 1-20)				Economic Freedom Index (Index Range: 1-10)				Government Corruption Perception Index (Index Range: 1-10)				Economic Integration Index (Index Range: 0-100)				Globalization Index (Index Range: 0-100)			
	2010	2035	2060	% Chg	2010	2035	2060	% Chg	2010	2035	2060	% Chg	2010	2035	2060	% Chg	2010	2035	2060	% Chg
AFRICA																				
Ethiopia	10.95	11.69	13.63	24.5%	5.584	6.366	7.18	28.6%	2.227	2.537	3.654	64.1%	4.848	7.596	5.753	18.7%	43.14	46.3	52.37	21.4%
Tanzania, United Rep	12.14	13.32	15.26	25.7%	6.222	7.199	8.115	30.4%	2.925	3.547	5.687	94.4%	5.863	6.934	7.475	27.5%	35.44	46.38	61.55	73.7%
Uganda	6.261	8.067	11.02	76.0%	6.889	7.771	8.86	28.6%	2.529	3.078	5.705	125.6%	4.134	7.135	6.394	54.7%	49.25	56.88	65.78	33.6%
Kenya	17.97	18.26	19.09	6.2%	6.969	7.515	8.377	20.2%	2.12	2.417	3.636	71.5%	3.542	6.045	5.575	57.4%	36.5	44.97	37.77	3.5%
Madagascar	16.8	16.59	16.71	-0.5%	5.998	6.315	6.828	13.8%	2.802	2.896	3.227	15.2%	4.165	9.599	8.959	115.1%	36.31	45.04	47.05	29.6%
Mozambique	15.87	16.37	17.77	12.0%	5.909	6.543	7.9	33.7%	2.825	3.357	5.348	89.3%	10.97	12.63	12.25	11.7%	42.27	48.29	61.44	45.4%
Malawi	16	16.23	16.55	3.4%	5.643	6.018	6.587	16.7%	2.819	2.927	3.37	19.5%	3.85	7.508	5.019	30.4%	35.18	43.91	46.34	31.7%
Zambia	14.96	15.26	16.3	9.0%	7.028	7.74	8.469	20.5%	2.627	3.008	3.98	51.5%	15.83	16.57	12.45	-21.4%	39.94	48.72	54.53	36.5%
Somalia	3.265	4.701	6.628	103.0%	5.16	5.454	5.714	10.7%	2.103	2.183	2.292	9.0%	3.462	10.58	12.16	251.2%	14.98	26.13	27.75	85.2%
Rwanda	7.112	8.513	11.08	55.8%	5.821	6.803	7.705	32.4%	3.124	3.632	5.521	76.7%	1.072	3.031	4.306	301.7%	33.45	44.28	57.89	73.1%
Zimbabwe	3.413	5.316	7.619	123.2%	3.485	3.608	3.809	9.3%	2.594	2.732	3.114	20.0%	9.779	10.95	9.863	0.9%	45.18	49.83	49.72	10.0%
Burundi	8.984	9.372	10.5	16.9%	5.043	5.301	5.722	13.5%	2.307	2.342	2.458	6.5%	1.496	8.407	13.09	775.0%	33.25	43.34	45.97	38.3%
Eritrea	3.243	4.478	6.191	90.9%	5.105	5.214	5.454	6.8%	2.597	2.628	2.715	4.5%	11.91	15.57	16.46	38.2%	41.45	47.82	47.95	15.7%
Comoros	15.78	15.25	15.51	-1.7%	5.378	5.495	5.844	8.7%	2.368	2.413	2.642	11.6%	1.843	6.705	8.71	372.6%	49.95	58.03	48.44	-3.0%
Mauritius	19.98	20	20	0.1%	7.404	7.808	8.178	10.5%	4.303	6.031	8.75	103.3%	9.442	12.6	14.98	58.7%	62.2	56.43	61.4	-1.3%
Djibouti	11.98	12.65	14.49	21.0%	5.808	6.188	6.77	16.6%	2.581	2.955	4.174	61.7%	7.888	9.88	10.27	30.2%	37.98	47.54	56.39	48.5%
Africa-Eastern	11.8	12.58	14.16	20.0%	6.189	7.039	8.03	29.7%	2.525	2.879	4.193	66.1%	6.184	8.229	7.324	18.4%	39.64	46.9	52.58	32.6%
Congo, Democratic Republic of	6.088	6.896	7.985	31.2%	4.746	5.141	5.767	21.5%	2.11	2.16	2.21	4.7%	21.32	29.3	30.9	44.9%	43	50.15	51.46	19.7%
Angola	8.234	10.02	12.45	51.2%	3.58	3.884	3.979	11.1%	2.212	3.792	4.41	99.4%	32.66	23.62	22.59	-30.8%	45.51	58.71	43.77	-3.8%
Cameroon	6.252	7.721	9.884	58.1%	5.838	6.179	6.606	13.2%	2.218	2.515	3.225	45.4%	4.619	6.235	4.97	7.6%	34.69	45.54	44.68	28.8%
Chad	8.095	9.015	10.1	24.8%	5.362	5.627	5.627	4.9%	1.683	1.859	1.886	12.1%	34.29	24.36	16.94	-50.6%	44.73	50.27	44.56	-0.4%
Central African Republic	9.004	9.486	10.67	18.5%	4.615	4.891	5.244	13.6%	2.411	2.501	2.758	14.4%	2.138	6.758	5.898	175.9%	37.15	43.35	45.25	21.8%
Congo. Republic of	6.289	7.984	10.11	60.8%	4.781	5.084	5.195	8.7%	2.382	3.031	3.312	39.0%	34.2	27.13	23	-32.7%	49.67	55.61	58.15	17.1%
Gabon	6.422	8.554	11.12	73.2%	5.684	5.782	5.845	2.8%	2.873	3.593	4.018	39.9%	21.35	16.81	18.69	-12.5%	53.71	51.25	53.69	0.0%
Equatorial Guinea	5.535	8.148	10.62	91.9%	7.377	7.577	7.639	3.6%	2.227	4.557	4.989	124.0%	21.57	16.65	27.53	27.6%	49.25	64.59	74.25	50.8%
São Tomé and Príncipe	10.18	10.7	11.64	14.3%	5.606	5.74	5.977	6.6%	2.461	2.541	2.755	11.9%	10.95	13.15	9.82	-10.3%	42.23	46.95	47.22	11.8%
Africa-Middle	6.721	7.78	9.111	35.6%	4.851	4.742	5.067	4.5%	2.133	2.466	2.617	22.7%	23.4	21.17	19.18	-18.0%	42.5	50.8	49.17	15.7%
Egypt	4.481	7.016	10.13	126.1%	6.53	6.991	7.459	14.2%	3.505	4.578	6.822	94.6%	7.066	8.305	9.142	29.4%	61.36	54.34	48.91	-20.3%
Sudan	4.304	6.27	8.944	107.8%	5.761	6.371	6.723	16.7%	2.161	2.86	3.68	70.3%	7.288	5.848	6.073	-16.7%	36.56	47.79	44.94	22.9%
Algeria	12.24	13.59	15.02	22.7%	5.47	5.704	5.816	6.3%	2.848	3.582	4.151	45.8%	10.1	6.209	5.572	-44.8%	38.41	32.17	32.96	-14.2%
Morocco	4.387	6.463	9.207	109.9%	6.225	6.598	6.988	12.3%	3.284	3.945	5.196	58.2%	5.945	7.2	7.658	28.8%	54.44	50.91	46.7	-14.2%
Tunisia	6.435	8.754	11.63	80.7%	6.597	7.047	7.427	12.6%	5.042	6.539	9.019	78.9%	11.97	12.64	12.84	7.3%	61.25	58.53	57.07	-6.8%
Libyan Arab Jamahiriya	3.581	6.469	9.538	166.4%	6.817	7.254	7.337	7.6%	2.69	4.839	5.631	109.3%	9.685	13.46	6.502	-32.9%	14.62	38.64	42.98	194.0%
Africa-Northern	5.836	7.891	10.48	79.6%	6.269	6.725	7.173	14.4%	3.148	4.03	5.447	73.0%	8.223	8.493	8.4	2.2%	50.01	48.47	45.34	-9.3%

Multination Regional Analysis

Measures of Poverty, Health, Education, Infrastructure, and Governance

Governance

Base Case: Countries in Year 2060 Descending Population Sequence	Polity Democracy Index (Index Range: 1-20)				Economic Freedom Index (Index Range: 1-10)				Government Corruption Perception Index (Index Range: 1-10)				Economic Integration Index (Index Range: 0-100)				Globalization Index (Index Range: 0-100)			
	2010	2035	2060	% Chg	2010	2035	2060	% Chg	2010	2035	2060	% Chg	2010	2035	2060	% Chg	2010	2035	2060	% Chg
AFRICA continued																				
South Africa	19.05	19.93	20	5.0%	7.18	7.576	8.142	13.4%	4.606	5.983	10	117.1%	5.144	6.479	10.39	102.0%	37.76	41.22	67.76	79.4%
Namibia	15.98	16.71	18.07	13.1%	6.841	7.292	7.836	14.5%	4.325	5.246	7.751	79.2%	8.461	6.957	7.639	-9.7%	43.78	49.21	47.18	7.8%
Lesotho	17.89	18.22	18.92	5.8%	6.699	7.193	7.805	16.5%	3.429	3.736	4.603	34.2%	41.91	38.13	25.28	-39.7%	63.69	70.58	59.54	-6.5%
Botswana	19.04	19.97	19.91	4.6%	7.102	7.628	7.951	12.0%	6.184	9.62	10	61.7%	10.99	13.79	15.85	44.2%	56.84	54.7	70.52	24.1%
Swaziland	1.53	4.202	7.718	404.4%	6.226	6.575	6.998	12.4%	2.695	3.386	5.076	88.3%	26.52	26.15	20.33	-23.3%	61.17	59.27	53.38	-12.7%
Africa-Southern	**18.51**	**19.28**	**19.48**	**5.2%**	**7.158**	**7.56**	**8.107**	**13.3%**	**4.567**	**5.926**	**9.511**	**108.3%**	**5.908**	**7.501**	**10.79**	**82.6%**	**40.03**	**43.76**	**65.87**	**64.6%**
Nigeria	14.04	14.84	15.78	12.4%	5.912	6.448	6.678	13.0%	1.925	2.312	2.614	35.8%	17.78	17.83	12.13	-31.8%	45.95	59.87	48.83	6.3%
Niger	13.83	13.7	14.2	2.7%	5.123	5.415	5.846	14.1%	2.406	2.482	2.692	11.9%	2.862	9.631	7.177	150.8%	47.87	48.21	46.13	-3.6%
Côte d'Ivoire	13.89	14.17	15.35	10.5%	5.885	6.223	6.647	12.9%	1.908	2.129	2.597	36.1%	10.35	12.13	9.992	-3.5%	38.64	28.2	21.12	-45.3%
Ghana	17.84	17.69	18.2	2.0%	6.437	6.799	7.544	17.2%	3.528	3.64	4.193	18.8%	8.267	11.23	8.824	6.7%	42.85	48.55	49.65	15.9%
Mali	15.89	16.03	16.89	6.3%	5.946	6.397	7.128	19.9%	2.905	3.087	3.838	32.1%	7.162	12.64	8.8	22.9%	50.44	55.88	53.03	5.1%
Burkina Faso	10.01	10.64	12.39	23.8%	5.641	6.04	6.642	17.7%	3.404	3.586	4.361	28.1%	-0.1	4.856	2.978	3078.0%	40.37	45.62	49.03	21.5%
Senegal	17.78	17.61	18.38	3.4%	5.871	6.201	6.795	15.7%	3.208	3.391	4.219	31.5%	5.577	6.781	5.628	0.9%	37.93	44.99	50.42	32.9%
Guinea	9.084	9.947	11.43	25.8%	5.422	5.823	6.289	16.0%	1.909	2.118	2.621	37.3%	4.795	9.057	8.24	71.8%	49.69	50.84	40.79	-17.9%
Benin	15.94	16.09	16.51	3.6%	5.911	6.182	6.645	12.4%	2.912	3.038	3.413	17.2%	5.448	11.17	7.969	46.3%	50.32	56.73	51.22	1.8%
Togo	8.15	8.993	9.993	22.6%	6.131	6.386	6.56	7.0%	2.403	2.453	2.489	3.6%	14.43	14.28	15.51	7.5%	55.8	60.23	44.12	-20.9%
Sierra Leone	14.82	14.8	16.1	8.6%	5.864	6.633	7.598	29.6%	2.416	2.671	3.843	59.1%	3.051	5.218	6.083	99.4%	35.28	43.91	52.15	47.8%
Liberia	9.989	11.03	13.14	31.5%	4.78	5.805	6.862	43.6%	2.215	2.494	3.512	58.6%	41.94	34.78	26.27	-37.4%	60.43	57.04	58.2	-3.7%
Mauritania	4.282	5.661	7.429	73.5%	6.304	6.203	6.36	0.9%	3.112	3.082	3.186	2.4%	26.02	23.18	16.19	-37.8%	48.17	52.93	49.89	3.6%
Guinea-Bissau	9.014	9.386	9.978	10.7%	4.972	5.09	5.207	4.7%	2.258	2.274	2.298	1.8%	6.375	10.15	14.44	126.5%	50.57	58.33	60.26	19.2%
Gambia	5.261	6.755	9.034	71.7%	5.437	5.891	6.469	19.0%	2.719	2.972	3.669	34.9%	19.87	19.34	15.36	-22.7%	44.13	49.38	52.76	19.6%
Cape Verde	11.81	13.11	14.91	26.2%	5.969	6.543	7.203	20.7%	2.709	3.53	5.638	108.1%	8.435	8.584	8.924	5.8%	59.68	69.1	79.67	33.5%
Africa-Western	**13.91**	**14.38**	**15.27**	**9.8%**	**5.899**	**6.375**	**6.795**	**15.2%**	**2.346**	**2.619**	**3.049**	**30.0%**	**13.79**	**15.57**	**10.14**	**-26.5%**	**45.42**	**53.44**	**47.09**	**3.7%**

Multination Regional Analysis

Measures of Poverty, Health, Education, Infrastructure, and Governance

Governance

Base Case: Countries in Year 2060 Descending Population Sequence	Polity Democracy Index (Index Range: 1-20)				Economic Freedom Index (Index Range: 1-10)				Government Corruption Perception Index (Index Range: 1-10)				Economic Integration Index (Index Range: 0-100)				Globalization Index (Index Range: 0-100)			
	2010	2035	2060	% Chg	2010	2035	2060	% Chg	2010	2035	2060	% Chg	2010	2035	2060	% Chg	2010	2035	2060	% Chg
AMERICAS																				
Haiti	8.075	8.799	10.18	26.1%	6.567	6.834	7.307	11.3%	1.808	1.912	2.221	22.8%	3.296	5.597	5.726	73.7%	50.78	58.2	60.64	19.4%
Dominican Republic	17.97	18.64	19.67	9.5%	6.419	6.982	7.34	14.3%	3.113	4.829	7.004	125.0%	9.011	9.256	9.723	7.9%	40.25	45.85	57.67	43.3%
Cuba	3.532	6.144	9.326	164.0%	6.504	6.83	7.168	10.2%	3.868	4.847	6.541	69.1%	2.966	4.943	7.372	148.6%	7.449	21.8	34.96	369.3%
Puerto Rico	17.23	18.08	18.15	5.3%	7.216	7.537	7.848	8.8%	6.497	9.648	10	53.9%	4.021	9.302	14.47	259.9%	22.87	53.53	65.92	188.2%
Jamaica	19	19.22	19.57	3.0%	7.372	7.562	7.914	7.4%	3.519	3.942	5.083	44.4%	17.72	16.39	12.33	-30.4%	49.18	43.39	45.54	-7.4%
Trinidad	19	20	20	0.0%	7.067	7.527	7.855	11.2%	4.15	8.541	10	141.0%	30.91	26.92	33.45	8.2%	34.97	64.94	74.29	112.4%
Bahamas	16.94	17.98	18.03	6.4%	7.186	7.464	7.825	8.9%	5.759	7.908	10	73.6%	11.24	14.01	17.16	52.7%	46.12	55.69	71.58	55.2%
Barbados	16.27	17.32	17.98	10.5%	6.629	6.842	7.211	8.8%	6.948	8.306	10	43.9%	10.14	12.84	16.14	59.2%	65.54	63.52	78.78	20.2%
Grenada	15.04	16.04	17.42	15.8%	6.647	6.788	7.111	7.0%	3.456	3.96	5.595	61.9%	33.59	28.61	21.18	-36.9%	59.21	64.86	64.47	8.9%
Saint Vincent and Grenadines	14.35	15.7	17.25	20.2%	6.515	6.889	7.306	12.1%	3.518	4.632	6.559	86.4%	37.63	33.44	25.3	-32.8%	57.87	68.03	60.81	5.1%
Saint Lucia	15.17	16.31	17.6	16.0%	6.679	6.948	7.299	9.3%	3.949	4.886	6.534	65.5%	35.89	32.2	24.66	-31.3%	75.75	60.38	60.76	-19.8%
America-Caribbean	**11.45**	**12.7**	**14.04**	**22.6%**	**6.903**	**7.219**	**7.531**	**9.1%**	**3.489**	**4.51**	**5.425**	**55.5%**	**7.988**	**10.7**	**12.8**	**60.2%**	**32.38**	**45.2**	**54.92**	**69.6%**
Guatemala	18.02	18.52	19.23	6.7%	7.078	7.444	7.871	11.2%	2.509	3.198	4.609	83.7%	6.056	7.404	7.122	17.6%	56.43	50.54	46.15	-18.2%
Honduras	17.11	17.73	18.38	7.4%	7.008	7.387	7.801	11.3%	2.622	3.11	4.064	55.0%	14.8	14.51	12.38	-16.4%	58.11	66.34	64.38	10.8%
El Salvador	16.98	17.59	18.58	9.4%	7.558	7.888	8.329	10.2%	4.228	4.856	6.263	48.1%	7.168	7.83	7.491	4.5%	58.98	48.84	47.71	-19.1%
Nicaragua	17.94	18.17	18.44	2.8%	6.947	7.229	7.605	9.5%	2.603	2.863	3.399	30.6%	14.18	13.32	10.41	-26.6%	56.6	63.29	66.33	17.2%
Costa Rica	19.99	20	20	0.1%	7.445	7.834	8.186	10.0%	4.342	5.815	8.223	89.4%	13.11	13.19	12.99	-0.9%	43.57	52.22	59.91	37.5%
Panama	19.02	19.65	19.64	3.3%	7.795	8.357	8.835	13.3%	3.806	6.267	10	162.7%	20.11	21.8	23.66	17.7%	23.75	43.47	69.77	193.8%
Belize	14.43	15.39	16.85	16.8%	7.084	7.444	7.883	11.3%	3.711	4.77	7.046	89.9%	16.11	16.63	16.32	1.3%	62.97	57.65	54.55	-13.4%
America-Central	**17.93**	**18.38**	**18.96**	**5.7%**	**7.373**	**7.778**	**8.155**	**10.6%**	**3.136**	**3.826**	**5.186**	**65.4%**	**11.96**	**12.97**	**12.09**	**1.1%**	**53.27**	**54.58**	**54.66**	**2.6%**
USA	20	20	20	0.0%	8.067	8.311	8.595	6.5%	7.445	10	10	34.3%	6.752	12.32	16.08	138.2%	58.89	74.53	79.89	35.7%
Mexico	18.06	18.72	19.55	8.3%	6.894	7.142	7.397	7.3%	3.516	4.605	6.272	78.4%	9.166	9.9	9.202	0.4%	31.09	44.71	55.99	80.1%
Canada	20	20	20	0.0%	8.062	8.267	8.568	6.3%	8.336	10	10	20.0%	18.71	20.75	19.08	2.0%	69.2	89.11	92.17	33.2%
America-North	**19.53**	**19.69**	**19.9**	**1.9%**	**8.004**	**8.232**	**8.511**	**6.3%**	**6.566**	**8.698**	**9.167**	**39.6%**	**7.681**	**12.72**	**15.81**	**105.8%**	**52.96**	**68.38**	**75.43**	**42.4%**
Brazil	18.11	19.09	20	10.4%	5.951	6.288	6.586	10.7%	3.797	5.28	7.572	99.4%	5.223	6.118	6.561	25.6%	16.25	30.6	44.22	172.1%
Colombia	17.08	17.78	18.54	8.5%	5.692	5.926	6.183	8.6%	4.071	4.736	5.98	46.9%	9.081	8.517	5.841	-35.7%	49.82	36.85	34.27	-31.2%
Argentina	18.11	19.06	18.88	4.3%	5.818	6.197	6.474	11.3%	3.098	5.672	9.149	195.3%	7.04	9.347	10.75	52.7%	26.78	46.11	67.09	150.5%
Peru	19.06	19.79	20	4.9%	7.321	7.782	8.137	11.1%	3.722	5.136	7.075	90.1%	6.143	6.08	6.332	3.1%	47.31	36.88	44.19	-6.6%
Venezuela	16.15	17.31	18.44	14.2%	4.867	5.122	5.269	8.3%	2.42	4.136	5.943	145.6%	11.53	10.93	11.93	3.5%	33.1	39.96	50.73	53.3%
Ecuador	16.1	16.7	17.19	6.8%	5.833	5.942	6.093	4.5%	2.485	2.826	3.089	24.3%	13.08	10.01	8.412	-35.7%	37.17	27.61	23.96	-35.5%
Chile	19.12	19.94	19.94	4.3%	8.052	8.473	8.86	10.0%	7.448	9.469	10	34.3%	20.08	19.44	16.45	-18.1%	28.92	62.45	62.32	115.5%
Bolivia	18.06	18.85	19.62	8.6%	6.41	6.864	7.198	12.3%	2.536	3.37	4.333	70.9%	17.26	12.9	9.604	-44.4%	59.49	60.33	55.44	-6.8%
Paraguay	18.1	18.69	19.25	6.4%	6.475	6.743	7.125	10.0%	2.142	2.57	3.589	67.6%	9.461	10.42	9.675	2.3%	50.01	36.43	30.97	-38.1%
Uruguay	20	20	20	0.0%	7.08	7.63	8.123	14.7%	6.193	9.091	10	61.5%	5.87	8.059	11.89	102.6%	30.44	48.56	67.54	121.9%
Guyana	16.01	16.48	17.29	8.0%	6.141	6.374	6.736	9.7%	2.589	2.994	4.001	54.5%	35.23	33.84	26.02	-26.1%	69.75	74.55	76.71	10.0%
Suriname	14.39	15.42	17.05	18.5%	6.593	7.012	7.355	11.6%	3.371	4.93	7.295	116.4%	2.357	5.038	8.076	242.6%	46.91	63.24	58.81	25.4%
America-South	**17.89**	**18.77**	**19.43**	**8.6%**	**6.026**	**6.395**	**6.727**	**11.6%**	**3.722**	**5.14**	**7.085**	**90.4%**	**7.6**	**8.326**	**8.465**	**11.4%**	**28.24**	**35.73**	**45.91**	**62.6%**

Governance

Base Case: Countries in Year 2060 Descending Population Sequence	Polity Democracy Index (Index Range: 1-20)				Economic Freedom Index (Index Range: 1-10)				Government Corruption Perception Index (Index Range: 1-10)				Economic Integration Index (Index Range: 0-100)				Globalization Index (Index Range: 0-100)			
	2010	2035	2060	% Chg	2010	2035	2060	% Chg	2010	2035	2060	% Chg	2010	2035	2060	% Chg	2010	2035	2060	% Chg
ASIA with OCEANIA																				
China	3.487	6.252	9.432	170.5%	6.365	7.17	7.76	21.9%	3.462	5.364	10	188.9%	7.635	9.209	14.02	83.6%	27.74	49.27	69.22	149.5%
Japan	20	20	20	0.0%	7.538	7.8	8.107	7.5%	7.225	10	10	38.4%	1.934	6.739	11.37	487.9%	44.45	69.71	74.1	66.7%
Korea, Repub of	18.1	18.41	18.75	3.6%	7.309	7.582	7.876	7.8%	5.172	7.605	10	93.3%	6.844	9.869	12.96	89.4%	39.08	54.79	66.34	69.8%
Taiwan	20	20	20	0.0%	7.682	8.034	8.421	9.6%	5.886	8.194	10	59.9%	3.862	7.276	11.57	199.6%	39.19	51.39	65.04	66.0%
Korea, Dem. People's Rep.	1.477	3.76	6.53	342.1%	6.025	6.27	6.514	8.1%	2.76	3.059	3.507	27.1%	2.091	3.487	5.095	143.7%	7.48	13.54	17.42	132.9%
Hong Kong SAR	18.38	18.79	18.96	3.2%	8.96	8.841	8.717	-2.7%	8.693	9.848	10	15.0%	59.42	53.19	39.71	-33.2%	80.27	88.58	88.68	10.5%
Mongolia	20	20	20	0.0%	7.281	7.947	8.682	19.2%	3.099	3.916	5.838	38.4%	16.31	18.49	24.97	53.1%	58.61	69.47	74.49	27.1%
Asia-East	**5.595**	**7.823**	**10.51**	**87.8%**	**7.171**	**7.355**	**7.811**	**8.9%**	**3.87**	**6.644**	**9.895**	**155.7%**	**5.752**	**9.146**	**13.82**	**140.3%**	**29.62**	**50.58**	**68.73**	**132.0%**
India	18.92	19.46	20	5.7%	6.578	7.393	8.029	22.1%	2.981	4.189	6.807	128.3%	1.777	3.182	5.333	200.1%	25.96	26.57	40.11	54.5%
Pakistan	5.269	6.741	9.014	71.1%	6.045	6.307	6.755	11.7%	2.139	2.374	3.094	44.6%	1.291	2.842	2.755	113.4%	36.37	32.77	23.2	-36.2%
Bangladesh	15.88	16.02	16.7	5.2%	6.212	6.849	7.383	18.9%	1.74	2.116	2.826	62.4%	0.581	2.53	2.998	416.0%	47.93	54.31	39.55	-17.5%
Afghanistan	3.282	5.153	8.354	154.5%	5.539	6.288	7.096	28.1%	2.526	3.153	5.575	120.7%	3.335	7.168	8.155	144.5%	37.82	46.72	63.99	69.2%
Iran (Islamic Republic of)	4.528	7.203	10.17	124.6%	6.174	6.603	6.759	9.5%	3.046	5.27	6.343	108.2%	5.606	13.28	8.882	58.4%	25.11	41.8	43.79	74.4%
Nepal	4.225	5.53	7.59	79.6%	5.598	5.852	6.275	12.1%	2.514	2.614	2.896	15.2%	0.339	3.091	3.554	948.4%	48.72	57.21	49.16	0.9%
Uzbekistan	1.457	3.882	6.911	374.3%	5.896	6.373	6.747	14.4%	2.302	2.904	3.801	65.1%	4.989	4.186	7.69	54.1%	40.04	32.5	27.25	-31.9%
Sri Lanka	15.12	16.12	17.52	15.9%	6.224	6.643	7.05	13.3%	3.293	4.04	5.427	64.8%	5.376	6.279	6.34	17.9%	54.39	65.57	54.11	-0.5%
Kazakhstan	4.561	7.469	10.12	121.9%	7.176	7.784	7.919	10.4%	2.862	6.056	6.763	136.3%	23.86	24.34	31.51	32.1%	38.25	54.23	57.91	51.4%
Tajikistan	7.298	8.839	10.84	48.5%	5.638	5.947	6.313	12.0%	2.133	2.343	2.843	33.3%	8.875	8.734	6.163	-30.6%	51.07	60.81	63.19	23.7%
Turkmenistan	1.621	4.928	8.12	400.9%	6.805	7.54	7.745	13.8%	2.351	7.599	9.636	309.9%	7.978	15.62	16.66	108.8%	32.09	63.47	71.25	122.0%
Kyrgyzstan	7.285	8.808	10.65	46.2%	6.763	7.184	7.555	11.7%	2.331	2.612	3.109	33.4%	13.09	12.09	10.41	-20.5%	58.95	63.54	65.31	10.8%
Bhutan	2.463	5.044	8.708	253.6%	6.228	6.874	7.404	18.9%	6.15	7.812	10	62.6%	5.457	8.233	11.38	108.5%	39.1	56.69	82.99	112.3%
Maldives	12.85	13.95	15.85	23.3%	6.232	6.678	7.155	14.8%	3.008	3.967	6.178	105.4%	4.704	6.865	9.05	92.4%	43.51	54.63	58.37	34.2%
Asia-South Central	**15.48**	**15.83**	**16.51**	**6.7%**	**6.453**	**7.231**	**7.84**	**21.5%**	**2.756**	**3.742**	**5.664**	**105.5%**	**3.049**	**4.88**	**5.761**	**88.9%**	**30.5**	**32.77**	**39.18**	**28.5%**
Indonesia	18.02	18.47	18.9	4.9%	6.403	6.716	7.021	9.7%	2.276	2.729	3.466	52.3%	3.798	3.992	4.307	13.4%	39.13	35.09	36.51	-6.7%
Philippines	17.94	18.12	18.6	3.7%	7.095	7.503	7.957	12.1%	2.568	3.065	4.068	58.4%	8.413	9.16	8.137	-3.3%	43.71	37.29	39.7	-9.2%
Viet Nam	3.416	5.653	8.57	150.9%	6.354	6.854	7.328	15.3%	2.663	3.218	4.37	64.1%	17.79	17.42	14.4	-19.1%	64.83	70.88	49.16	-24.2%
Thailand	19	19.51	20	5.3%	6.983	7.234	7.556	8.2%	3.822	4.492	5.876	53.7%	17.3	17.09	14.88	-14.0%	15.36	24.88	33.78	119.9%
Myanmar	2.348	4.255	6.678	184.4%	4.103	4.424	4.635	13.0%	1.835	2.028	2.302	25.4%	1.275	1.615	3.219	152.5%	-0.193	9.686	12.49	6571.5%
Malaysia	13.26	14.78	16.35	23.3%	6.929	7.231	7.517	8.5%	5.171	6.697	9.048	75.0%	25.73	26.78	24.47	-4.9%	39.27	43.23	56.23	43.2%
Cambodia	11.99	12.73	14.09	17.5%	5.618	6.233	6.699	19.2%	2.33	2.852	3.765	61.6%	13.68	15.74	14.62	6.9%	51.86	53.19	57.36	10.6%
LAO People's Dem Repub	3.369	5.521	8.474	151.5%	5.749	6.381	6.955	21.0%	3.334	4.019	5.583	67.5%	7.402	11.47	10.93	47.7%	40.4	49.51	60.55	49.9%
Singapore	8.481	10.68	12.49	47.3%	8.709	8.822	8.922	2.4%	9.368	10	10	6.7%	79.3	74.49	58.43	-26.3%	79.23	93.91	94.72	19.6%
Timor-Leste	15.97	16.21	16.66	4.3%	5.823	6.097	6.303	8.2%	2.606	2.862	3.2	22.8%	2.716	7.195	7.447	174.2%	37.99	45.67	49.18	29.5%
Brunei Darussalam	19.08	19.24	19.4	1.7%	7.589	7.673	7.643	0.7%	9.336	10	10	7.1%	17.77	17.47	21.51	21.0%	59.64	71.42	79.81	33.8%
Asia-South East	**13.89**	**14.73**	**15.83**	**14.0%**	**6.964**	**7.145**	**7.438**	**6.8%**	**2.723**	**3.252**	**4.222**	**55.0%**	**21.72**	**18.42**	**14.68**	**-32.4%**	**38.18**	**39.4**	**39.54**	**3.6%**

Governance

Base Case: Countries in Year 2060 Descending Population Sequence	Polity Democracy Index (Index Range: 1-20)				Economic Freedom Index (Index Range: 1-10)				Government Corruption Perception Index (Index Range: 1-10)				Economic Integration Index (Index Range: 0-100)				Globalization Index (Index Range: 0-100)			
	2010	2035	2060	% Chg	2010	2035	2060	% Chg	2010	2035	2060	% Chg	2010	2035	2060	% Chg	2010	2035	2060	% Chg
ASIA with OCEANIA continued																				
Turkey	17.07	17.81	18.66	9.3%	6.266	6.626	6.919	10.4%	3.534	4.892	6.782	91.9%	2.659	4.797	6.26	135.4%	21.87	31.58	40.44	84.9%
Yemen	8.235	9.805	11.89	44.4%	5.837	6.253	6.596	13.0%	2.723	3.193	3.904	43.4%	7.75	6.776	6.297	-18.7%	55.72	47.22	29.31	-47.4%
Iraq	1.535	4.348	7.872	412.8%	6.468	6.969	7.361	13.8%	2.349	3.999	6.508	177.1%	2.733	6.491	9.14	234.4%	9.446	24.58	44.63	372.5%
Saudi Arabia	0.729	4.133	7.467	924.3%	7.159	7.383	7.53	5.2%	3.383	5.178	6.294	86.0%	14.8	13.59	22.77	53.9%	33.59	57.4	72.54	116.0%
Syrian Arab Repub	3.458	5.661	8.414	143.3%	5.433	5.637	5.93	9.1%	3.437	3.793	4.667	35.8%	4.915	5.861	7.417	50.9%	38.31	29.9	27.21	-29.0%
Israel	20	20	20	0.0%	6.93	7.303	7.729	11.5%	6.273	10	10	59.4%	11.88	14.89	19.96	68.0%	64.67	82.84	80.95	25.2%
Jordan	8.401	10.51	13.01	54.9%	7.385	7.844	8.49	15.0%	5.786	6.705	10	72.8%	16.67	14.27	13.93	-16.4%	47.01	56.77	62.2	32.3%
Occupied Palestinian Territory	12.79	14.25	15.98	24.9%	6.123	6.493	6.988	14.1%	2.623	3.233	4.854	85.1%	10.61	10.88	8.254	-22.2%	59.42	66.7	64.69	8.9%
Azerbaijan	3.509	6.268	9.353	166.5%	6.378	6.965	7.158	12.2%	2.588	4.748	5.762	122.6%	41	37.62	24.94	-39.2%	68.61	69.41	55.15	-19.6%
United Arab Emirates	2.623	5.659	8.839	237.0%	7.461	7.726	7.875	5.5%	6.766	10	10	47.8%	11.5	18.94	25.79	124.3%	48.17	74.73	84.09	74.6%
Oman	2.654	5.743	8.727	228.8%	7.423	7.653	7.903	6.5%	6.651	8.62	10	50.4%	12.65	11.22	14.28	12.9%	36.93	57.2	74.39	101.4%
Kuwait	3.64	6.606	9.468	160.1%	7.113	7.303	7.293	2.5%	4.611	7.494	5.217	13.1%	14.31	20.48	38.21	167.0%	42.27	72.67	88.18	108.6%
Lebanon	15.17	16.41	17.74	16.9%	6.747	7.083	7.406	9.8%	3.283	4.797	7.251	120.9%	17.07	16.35	15.52	-9.1%	67.11	80.5	73.72	9.8%
Armenia	15.14	16.47	17.75	17.2%	7.318	8.331	8.869	21.2%	3.05	6.148	10	227.9%	33.65	25.59	24.08	-28.4%	55.55	80.65	85.08	53.2%
Georgia	17.01	17.52	18.23	7.2%	6.693	7.238	7.607	13.7%	2.423	3.475	4.851	100.2%	12.05	11.26	11.15	-7.5%	59.44	71.67	64.55	8.6%
Bahrain	3.681	6.513	9.347	153.9%	6.885	7.015	7.224	4.9%	6.36	8.847	10	57.2%	29.87	28.83	27.92	-6.5%	73.17	85.13	86.95	18.8%
Qatar	0.8	4.133	7.467	833.4%	8.144	8.317	8.238	1.2%	10	10	10	0.0%	6.528	26.8	36.52	459.4%	42.86	74.52	83.54	94.9%
Cyprus	20	20	20	0.0%	7.407	7.622	7.847	5.9%	5.836	7.944	10	71.4%	22.75	23.71	21.89	-3.8%	65.57	69.03	73.42	12.0%
Asia-West	**9.441**	**10.51**	**12.33**	**30.6%**	**6.934**	**7.15**	**7.362**	**6.2%**	**3.499**	**4.814**	**6.159**	**76.0%**	**10.14**	**12.67**	**14.86**	**46.5%**	**34.66**	**43.73**	**47.51**	**37.1%**
Australia	20	20	20	0.0%	7.86	8.081	8.41	7.0%	8.807	10	10	13.5%	9.938	13.75	15.86	59.6%	65.91	86.65	90.32	37.0%
Papua New Guinea	19.82	19.58	19.63	-1.0%	6.341	6.805	7.122	12.3%	2.338	2.735	3.167	35.5%	19.97	19.69	13.1	-34.4%	43.42	50.7	44.22	1.8%
New Zealand	20	20	20	0.0%	8.438	8.675	9.091	7.7%	9.532	10	10	4.9%	15.23	16.47	16.36	7.4%	51.98	66.99	82.28	58.3%
Solomon Islands	17.82	17.4	17.47	-2.0%	5.733	6.026	6.344	10.7%	2.532	2.757	3.151	24.4%	13.61	13.4	11.49	-15.6%	50.54	52.06	52.15	3.2%
Fiji	16.04	16.55	17.63	9.9%	6.288	6.541	7.007	11.4%	3.986	4.426	5.849	46.7%	19.31	18.29	15.53	-19.6%	62.53	64.61	52	-16.8%
Vanuatu	12.57	13.62	15.31	21.8%	6.136	6.49	6.93	12.9%	2.884	3.455	4.753	64.8%	31.92	29.19	20.9	-34.5%	59.02	61.26	65.97	11.8%
Micronesia, Federated States of	13.76	14.54	15.89	15.5%	6.4	6.586	6.964	8.8%	3.276	3.674	4.988	52.3%	3.731	4.75	6.952	86.3%	45.19	51.25	60.48	33.8%
Tonga	13.52	14.05	15.29	13.1%	6.282	6.399	6.756	7.5%	3.081	3.269	4.288	39.2%	6.895	8.635	8.623	25.1%	43.62	50.42	56.58	29.7%
Samoa	13.49	14.63	16.26	20.5%	6.345	6.752	7.216	13.7%	3.184	4.139	6.237	95.9%	5.738	6.46	7.666	33.6%	56.81	69.26	83.06	46.2%
Oceania	**19.7**	**19.63**	**19.69**	**-0.1%**	**7.902**	**8.115**	**8.447**	**6.9%**	**7.322**	**7.852**	**7.806**	**6.6%**	**10.65**	**14.16**	**15.84**	**48.7%**	**59.29**	**74.11**	**74.99**	**26.5%**

Multination Regional Analysis

Measures of Poverty, Health, Education, Infrastructure, and Governance

Governance

Base Case: Countries in Year 2060 Descending Population Sequence	Polity Democracy Index (Index Range: 1-20)				Economic Freedom Index (Index Range: 1-10)				Government Corruption Perception Index (Index Range: 1-10)				Economic Integration Index (Index Range: 0-100)				Globalization Index (Index Range: 0-100)			
	2010	2035	2060	% Chg	2010	2035	2060	% Chg	2010	2035	2060	% Chg	2010	2035	2060	% Chg	2010	2035	2060	% Chg
EUROPE																				
Russian Federation	17.13	18.08	18.88	10.2%	6.393	6.813	6.873	7.5%	2.665	5.397	5.814	118.2%	13.42	16.7	20.09	49.7%	37.28	50.39	51.43	38.0%
Poland	20	20	20	0.0%	6.775	7.107	7.313	7.9%	3.658	5.813	7.894	115.8%	9.471	11.09	11.7	23.5%	65.14	63.11	66.36	1.9%
Ukraine	16.1	16.94	17.92	11.3%	5.715	6.029	6.255	9.4%	2.715	3.68	4.76	75.3%	10.41	10.59	13.39	28.6%	37	33.99	33.88	-8.4%
Romania	19.12	20	20	4.6%	6.463	6.751	6.991	8.2%	3.17	4.431	6.064	91.3%	8.853	9.454	9.221	4.2%	64.83	62.31	58.3	-10.1%
Czech Republic	20	20	20	0.0%	7.019	7.195	7.344	4.6%	4.495	6.022	7.899	75.7%	20.91	20.69	18.61	-11.0%	45.27	57.99	71.72	58.4%
Belarus	3.546	6.337	9.5	167.9%	6.724	7.215	7.415	10.3%	2.904	5.467	7.394	154.6%	8.717	9.348	11	26.2%	35.08	51.27	64.73	84.5%
Hungary	20	20	20	0.0%	7.404	7.688	7.92	7.0%	4.954	6.875	9.34	88.5%	23.5	22.5	20.58	-12.4%	57.26	60.22	68.76	20.1%
Bulgaria	19.09	19.82	20	4.8%	6.553	6.791	7.053	7.6%	4.168	5.206	6.961	67.0%	20.56	18.92	16.97	-17.5%	73.77	82.76	67.27	-8.8%
Slovak Republic	19.21	20	19.65	2.3%	7.5	7.788	7.933	5.8%	4.693	6.786	8.461	80.3%	17.96	18.44	17.85	-0.6%	62.96	56.92	60.95	-3.2%
Moldova, Repub of	18.01	18.36	18.98	5.4%	6.548	6.824	7.285	11.3%	2.929	3.161	3.866	32.0%	14.89	14.94	11.04	-25.9%	48.69	54.87	43.93	-9.8%
Europe-East	**17.34**	**18.16**	**18.8**	**8.4%**	**6.609**	**6.934**	**7.082**	**7.2%**	**3.069**	**5.21**	**6.296**	**105.1%**	**13.41**	**15.16**	**16.45**	**22.7%**	**45.36**	**52.38**	**54.06**	**19.2%**
United Kingdom	20	20	20	0.0%	8.088	8.366	8.725	7.9%	8.48	10	10	17.9%	29.45	29.94	24.15	-18.0%	65.41	88.9	88.55	35.4%
Sweden	20	20	20	0.0%	7.391	7.672	7.997	8.2%	9.296	10	10	7.6%	32.9	33.57	28.59	-13.1%	92.06	108.6	107.1	16.3%
Denmark	20	20	20	0.0%	7.715	7.946	8.293	7.5%	9.355	10	10	6.9%	24.74	26.7	25	1.1%	86.22	105.2	106.1	23.1%
Ireland	20	20	20	0.0%	8.087	8.364	8.57	6.0%	7.262	10	10	37.7%	31.4	34.78	32.87	4.7%	64.87	87.19	91.74	41.4%
Norway	20	20	20	0.0%	7.649	7.782	8.012	4.7%	9.188	10	10	8.8%	17.18	19.39	21.79	26.8%	81.72	97.21	104.5	27.9%
Finland	20	20	20	0.0%	7.767	8.034	8.386	8.0%	9.71	10	10	3.0%	21.84	24	22.76	4.2%	60.39	82.5	88.21	46.1%
Lithuania	20	20	20	0.0%	7.487	7.817	8.091	8.1%	5.021	7.109	10	99.2%	12.84	12.87	13.87	8.0%	67.69	67.39	75.43	11.4%
Latvia	18.24	19.19	18.75	2.8%	7.424	7.84	8.143	9.7%	4.471	7.105	10	123.7%	11.86	13.41	14.81	24.9%	72.49	78.31	83.66	15.4%
Estonia	16.26	17.46	17.49	7.6%	7.994	8.368	8.709	8.9%	6.748	9.453	10	48.2%	26.12	25.67	24.36	-6.7%	72.84	77.72	77.66	6.6%
Iceland	20	20	20	0.0%	7.902	8.138	8.457	7.0%	10	10	10	0.0%	24.66	26.82	27.36	10.9%	63.21	72.41	72.14	14.1%
Europe-North	**19.91**	**19.96**	**19.96**	**0.3%**	**7.929**	**8.201**	**8.544**	**7.8%**	**8.422**	**9.854**	**10**	**18.7%**	**28.01**	**29.09**	**24.73**	**-11.7%**	**69.91**	**90.63**	**91.68**	**31.1%**
Italy	20	20	20	0.0%	7	7.134	7.302	4.3%	4.699	5.075	8.18	74.1%	6.87	9.649	10.08	46.7%	40.24	57.37	73.92	83.7%
Spain	20	20	20	0.0%	7.465	7.67	7.863	5.3%	6.81	8.779	10	46.8%	17.62	19.01	15.43	-12.4%	46.96	72.68	86.82	84.9%
Greece	20	20	20	0.0%	7	7.172	7.323	4.6%	4.393	6.403	8.695	97.9%	4.444	9.193	11.68	162.8%	49.39	75.2	83.86	69.8%
Portugal	20	20	20	0.0%	7.158	7.348	7.569	5.7%	6.281	7.641	9.763	55.4%	16.02	16.13	13.02	-18.7%	75.3	80.07	86.97	15.5%
Serbia	16.16	17.25	18.52	14.6%	5.676	5.859	6.099	7.5%	2.922	3.644	5.161	76.6%	7.161	8.861	11.13	55.4%	37.85	42.87	50.66	33.8%
Bosnia and Herzegovina	13.93	15.15	16.82	20.7%	6.219	6.663	6.966	12.0%	2.996	4.433	6.316	110.8%	10.07	10.14	11.5	14.2%	64.27	78.61	68.76	7.0%
Croatia	17.17	18.48	19.23	12.0%	6.286	6.531	6.756	7.5%	3.512	5.027	7.123	102.8%	12.28	12.95	13.3	8.3%	42.56	45.81	52.65	23.7%
Albania	17.08	17.84	18.8	10.1%	6.755	7.176	7.507	11.1%	2.513	3.602	5.112	103.4%	8.275	8.918	10.19	23.1%	55.19	71.58	62.77	13.7%
Macedonia, FYR	19.11	19.96	20	4.7%	6.112	6.25	6.491	6.2%	2.779	3.263	4.359	56.9%	11.66	11.23	9.986	-14.4%	69.49	73.18	54.67	-21.3%
Slovenia	20	20	20	0.0%	6.78	7.03	7.262	7.1%	6.395	8.996	10	56.4%	12.52	16	18.02	43.9%	48.26	66.2	74.54	54.5%
Montenegro	14.55	15.86	17.52	20.4%	6.168	6.449	6.832	10.8%	3.642	4.614	6.978	91.6%	4.876	8.102	9.603	96.9%	65.6	71.65	58.04	-11.5%
Malta	17.09	18.07	18.42	7.8%	7.39	7.55	7.756	5.0%	6.639	8.084	10	50.6%	34.01	32.14	26.79	-21.2%	51.07	58.27	66.34	29.9%
Europe-South	**19.45**	**19.61**	**19.77**	**1.6%**	**7.132**	**7.311**	**7.486**	**5.0%**	**5.195**	**6.773**	**8.54**	**64.4%**	**10.76**	**13.42**	**12.56**	**16.7%**	**47**	**65.33**	**77.02**	**63.9%**
Germany	20	20	20	0.0%	7.643	7.871	8.22	7.5%	8.109	10	10	23.3%	14.14	17.15	18.24	29.0%	65.35	86.22	88.97	36.1%
France	19.18	19.8	19.37	1.0%	7.095	7.262	7.554	6.5%	7.463	9.423	10	34.0%	18.79	20.08	17.42	-7.3%	63.24	83.92	88.35	39.7%
Netherlands	20	20	20	0.0%	7.675	7.833	8.107	5.6%	8.538	10	10	17.1%	52.78	49.22	34.4	-34.8%	92.56	110.9	110.7	19.6%
Belgium	20	20	20	0.0%	7.248	7.4	7.683	6.0%	7.261	9.25	10	37.7%	84.27	74.29	47.52	-43.6%	82.13	100	99.45	21.1%
Austria	20	20	20	0.0%	7.564	7.736	8.003	5.8%	8.718	10	10	14.7%	24.2	25.4	22.76	-6.0%	58.86	79.77	82.62	40.4%
Switzerland	20	20	20	0.0%	8.245	8.452	8.766	6.3%	9.328	10	10	7.2%	31.57	32.91	26.35	-16.5%	77.51	94.51	91.78	18.4%
Luxembourg	20	20	20	0.0%	7.638	7.688	7.751	1.5%	8.357	10	10	19.7%	95.41	92.15	65.94	-30.9%	110.7	127.1	123.9	11.9%
Europe-West	**19.73**	**19.93**	**19.77**	**0.2%**	**7.482**	**7.666**	**7.968**	**6.5%**	**7.962**	**9.757**	**10**	**25.6%**	**24.86**	**25.76**	**21.89**	**-11.9%**	**68.33**	**88.72**	**91.51**	**33.9%**

Index

Page numbers followed by the letter n indicate entries in notes,
and page numbers followed by the letter b indicate entries in boxes.

Aben, Katja K. H. 83

Acemoglu, Daron 116

adult mortality 2–3; global goals for
reduction of 6, 59–60, 145; IFs
adjusted base case forecasts 145;
in IFs integrated scenario analysis
151–2, 154; impact of road traffic
accidents 85, 86–7; patterns
affecting life expectancy measure
13, 56; WHO definition 13

Advisory Committee to the United
States Surgeon General 82

Afghanistan 2, 28n, 153

Africa 28n, 61, 110, see also
North Africa; sub-Saharan Africa;
individual countries

age: and accumulation of
noncommunicable diseases
10; as factor in analysing risks
45–6, 109, 110; in global goals
for disease reduction 58–9;
in IFs approach to health and
productivity 122, 134; and
longevity 23, 124–5, 141, 143;
in measurement of morbidity and
mortality 13, 16, 23, 33, 58, 101;
and population in IFs integrated
scenarios 148

agriculture 49, 159; effects
of chemicals 90; increased
productivity in low mortality
scenario 131–2, 133, 135; IPCC on
risks from global warming 105, see
also crop production

Ahluwalia, Montek S. 76

AIDS see HIV/AIDS

air pollution 4, 6, 7, 24

air pollution (indoor) 64, 72,
92, 94, 95, 97–8, 111, 158;
alternative scenarios 99–100; from
solid fuel use 73, 91, 98–9

air pollution (outdoor urban) 73,
91, 92, 95, 100–2, 111, 158

alcohol use/abuse 74, 109, 143,
144, 148

Alma Ata Declaration (1978) 5, 26

Alsan, Marcella 126

alternative health futures 6, 7, 8,
30, 38, 157, 160; adult BMI and
related mortality 80–2; biological
context and human activity
139–40, 148, 154–5; childhood
undernutrition and mortality 77–8;
complexity and uncertainties 136,
159; disease burden patterns
149–52; economic consequences
153–4; education 68–9; GDP per
capita 67–8; integrated scenario
analysis 146–54, 155, 157; time
and technology 69–70; tobacco use
and related mortality 84–5; vehicle
ownership and fatality rates 86–7,
see also global health futures

AngloAmerican Mining 120

"Anglo-Saxon" societies 24–5

Angola 153

antibiotics 23, 24, 90, 91, 142, 143

antiretroviral therapy 65, 120

Arora, Suchit 115

Ashraf, Quamrul H. 117, 123

Asia 78, 83, see also Central Asia;
East Asia; South Asia; individual
countries

Australia 83

avian flu 143

Baldacci, Emmanuele 122

Bangladesh 11–12, 12–13, 76, 122

Barro, Robert J. 121

Becker, Gary 115, 118

behavioral changes: in Becker's
theory of human capital 115; and
decline in transmission of HIV 65;
proximate risk factors of health
outcomes 16, 72, 73

behavioral risks: in "Anglo-Saxon"
societies 25; and decline in life
expectancy in Russian Federation
24

Bill and Melinda Gates Foundation 26

biology: certainty of death 9; in
IFs integrated scenario analysis
146, 147; interaction of human
activity with 139–40, 144, 148,
155; interactions affecting health
17, 27; and uncertainties about
technology 6, 23–4, 138–9, 145

Bloom, David E. 115, 126

body mass index (BMI) 73, 78, 79,
80, 158; alternative scenarios
80–2; and risk of diabetes 35, 47

Bongaarts, John 28n

Botswana 2, 53, 148

Bozzoli, Carlos 122

Brazil 141, see also BRICS

breast cancer 80

Brenkert, Antoinette 106

BRICS (Brazil, Russia, India and
China) 58, 141, 153

Brundtland, Gro Harlem 30

Caldwell, John 19, 25

Campbell-Lendrum, Diarmid 90–1,
104

Canada 24–5, 83

cancers 3, 14; due to pollution 98,
144; health risks predisposing
people to 72, 78, 80

Canning, David 115, 126

capabilities see human capabilities
framework

capital: and GDP per capita
68; in IFs approach to health
and economic growth 118,
123–6, 133–4, 134; in theories
of economic growth 115, 117,
119, 132

carbon dioxide 105, 106–7, 108

cardiopulmonary diseases 100, 101,
102

cardiovascular disease 3, 14, 35;
attributable to environmental
factors 94; and BMI risk factor
78, 81; as disability affecting
productivity 120; due to urban
air pollution 91, 100, 101; health
risks predisposing people to 72;
in IFs base case forecasts 60, 102,
143; in IFs combined risk analysis
110; as potential outcome of
heat and cold stress 104; and
reductions in cause-specific
mortality 48; smoking as risk
factor 82, 85; stagnation of gains
in U.S. mortality rate 23, 144

Caribbean 59, 63, 69, 81, 101;
effect of mortality changes
on GDP 135; in IFs integrated
scenario analysis 152; working-
age demographics 129

Carson, Rachel 90

Carter, Nicholas 76

Central African Republic 153

Central Asia 60, 101; diabetes-
related mortality rates 81; effect
of mortality changes on GDP 128;
in IFs integrated scenario analysis
151, 152; life expectancy rates in
former communist countries 53

Central Europe 96

cerebrovascular disease 80

Doak, Colleen M. 78–9

Doll, Richard 82

Donora, Pennsylvania 90

drugs: emergence of diseases resistant to 23, 27, 140; markets and prices 5, *see also* pharmaceutical treatments

East Asia 59, 63, 80, 84, 87, 101; effect of mortality changes on GDP 128; in IFs integrated scenario analysis 150, 151, 154; working-age demographics 12

Eastern Europe 83, 96

Ebi, Kristie L. 104, 106

economic activity, as driver of urban air quality 100

economic changes: and changing health patterns 30, 38; consequences of alternative health futures 153–4; due to changing age structures of populations 130; in IFs integrated scenario analysis 149; role in decline of life expectancy 24

economic crisis: debt in Latin America 76; as threat to financial support for health incentives 143

economic development: environmental risk factors 111; expected in South Asia 77; leading to sedentary lifestyles 79; and progress in human development 28; in theory of epidemiologic transition 3

economic dislocation, induced by climate change 104, 105

economic growth: alternative scenarios for global life expectancy 68, 155; as distal driver of health outcomes 4; forward linkages from health to 117–26, 128, 129–35, 136, 157, 159; possibility of future slowing of 148; relationship with health in different models 115–17, 159

economic systems: and health modeling 49, 114, 157; model in extended IFs system 31–2, 70; time-related influence on health risks 73

education: alternative health futures 68–9; and better health outcomes for women 19, 20; as driver of health outcomes 7, 17, 19–20, 22, 27, 35, 52–3; expenditures affected by increased spending on elderly 132; and GDP per capita

68–9; in IFs approach to health and productivity 119, 121, 122–3; link with environmental health risk factors 97; model in extended IFs system 30, 32; in Sen's human capabilities framework 9, 115; in theory of epidemiologic transition 3

elderly people: affected by reductions in noncommunicable diseases 126, 150; in IFs integrated scenario analysis 153, 154, 155; increase impacting on economic growth 129, 132, 133, 154, 155; increasing expenditures on 124, 132, 159; potential health impacts of climate change 104; projected increase in 101

endemic diseases 4

endometrial cancer 80

energy systems 49, 73

environment: empirical evidence of impact on human health 92–5; health risks in GISMO forecasting system 63, 63–4; historical relationship with human health 90–1; human-based change and drivers relating to 4, 6, 20, 27, 139, 158; IFs model 32, 39; MDG for sustainability 5; and noncommunicable diseases 10, 143; proximate health risk factors 20, 72–3, 74, 108–11, 112; risk factors now and in future 95–108, 111–12, 144, 159; risk factors and risk transition 91–2, 102, 111, *see also* climate change; social environment

environmental footprints 136

epidemiologic transition 3–4, 4, 7, 13, 157, 159; health risk transition within 73, 92, 111, 144, 158, 159–60; post-World War II era 116, 128, 142; questions left unaddressed by 9, 22–3

Equatorial Guinea 153

ethical issues, and technological interventions 23

Ethiopia 76

Europe: diabetes-related mortality rates 81; effect of mortality changes on GDP 128; heat wave in 2003 104; historical studies of industrial revolution 115; IFs forecasts in relation to global goals 59, 60; in IFs integrated scenario analysis 151, 152; levels of particulate matter concentrations 101; life expectancy rates in former communist countries 53; mortality

registration coverage 28n, *see also* Eastern Europe; Southern Europe; Western Europe; individual countries

European Commission (EC) 32

Ezzati, Majid 17, 27, 41, 91, 100, 102, *see also* Comparative Risk Assessment (CRA) project

families: financing of education and old-age support 125; formation strategies 118

family planning programs 128, 159

famines 76

Fernández-Villaverde, Jesús 125–6

fertility: in IFs approach to health and economic growth 117–19, 128–9, 129, 132, 135, 158–9; in population forecasting 33, 69, 158–9

Fewtrell, Lorna 95–6

Filmer, Deon 25–6

Fishman, Steven 46

Fogel, Robert W. 28, 115, 121

foods: factors causing malnutrition and undernutrition 74–5, 76–7, 105; global impacts of population increases on 131; impacts of climate change on production 105, 106–7; importance of calorie availability 74–5, 76–7; negative effects of globalization 5; risk factors in unhealthy diets 10, 78, 143, 144, *see also* childhood undernutrition; nutritional deficiencies; undernutrition

forecasting: global health outcomes 8, 29–30, 37–8, 49; health model in extended IFs system 31, 31–2; IFs base case 52–60, 70; purposes of 6–7, 29–30, 37–8; structural models 34–9, 49, 66, 70; time limits 156

foreign aid 132–3, 135

foreign direct investment (FDI) 125, 126

Framework Convention on Tobacco Control (2003) 5, 143

France 61

Fraser Institute 137n

Frongillo, Edward A. 75

Gabon 153

Gately, Dermot 43, 86

Gates, Bill and Melinda *see* Bill and Melinda Gates Foundation

GDP per capita: and education in alternative health futures 67–9; in GISMO modeling system 36–7; in IFs approach to health and economic growth 121, 126, 128, 134, 135, 159; in IFs integrated scenario analysis 154; in low mortality scenario 135; relationship with life expectancy 18–19, 147–8; and studies on public health spending 25–6, *see also* income

gender: differences in population BMI 80; as factor in health outcomes 19, 20, 25; factors in smoking rates 84, 84–5, 85; in GISMO forecasts of mortality rates 63; life expectancy of males in IFs forecasts 54

genetic technologies 23, 139

Ghana 153

Global Burden of Disease (GBD) project (WHO): ambitious goals 13; approach used in IFs model 31, 39–40, 53, 69–70, 70, 145, 155, 157; categories of diseases 39, 46; concern over childhood underweight 75; distal drivers in health outcomes model 7, 16, 17, 17–18, 20, 23, 38, 39–40, 69; forecasting aims and analyses 6–7, 11; as landmark structural model 34, 34–5, 49, 66; limitation in comparative risk assessments 35–6; measures showing impact of disability 13, 15–16, 34, 120, 135; mortality forecast for diabetes 79; program on environmental burden of disease 112n; regional forecasts of death and disability 62–3; road traffic accident forecasts 66–7

Global Fund to Fight AIDS, Tuberculosis, and Malaria 26

global health: agenda 5; drivers of health outcomes 4–5; initiatives 26–7, 27, 139, 142; key problems today 2; positive statements on improvements 60; questions on changing patterns 52; "silent crisis" of climate change 103; theory of epidemiologic transition 3–4

global health futures: all-cause mortality models 32–3; IFs models for forecasting 6, 29–30, 70, 146, 152–3, 155, 156; structural models 34–9, 49; uncertainty surrounding 27–8, 154–5, *see also* alternative health futures

global health governance 5, 26, 26–7, 142–3, 155, 159

Global Humanitarian Forum (2009) 104

Global Integrated Sustainability Model (GISMO) (Hilderink and Lucas) 36–7, 63–4, 106

Global Model of Ambient Particulates (GMAPS) 100–1

Global Urban Air quality Model 100–1

global warming 6, 7, 27, 92, 139, 158, 159

Global Water Supply and Sanitation Assessment (WHO and UNICEF, 2000) 96

Gompertz, Benjamin 12b

Gosling, Simon 104

governments 25, 156

Grantham-McGregor, Sally 121b

Graunt, John 1

Great Britain, advances in human health 1; economic effect of great plagues 115; *see also* United Kingdom

groundwater, overuse of 159

Habicht, Jean-Pierre 75

Hajat, Shakoor 104

Hammer, Jeffrey S. 26

health: fundamental questions 9, *see also* global health

health expenditure: as factor in health outcomes 19, 24–6, 114, 134; in IFs approach to child mortality 41, 44; in IFs approach to health and economic growth 122, 123, 124, 126, 134; link with environmental health risk factors 97

health futures *see* alternative health futures; global health futures

health outcomes: CSDH goals 5–6, 54, 59–60, 159, 160; distal drivers influencing 4, 7, 16–17, 17–20, 27, 52–3, 70; forecasting 6, 8, 29–30, 37–8, 49; proximate drivers 4, 7, 16–17, 18, 20–2, 27, 35–6; relationships between proximate and distal factors 72–3, 154; role of alternative scenario analyses 87–8, 108; super-distal drivers influencing 4–5, 17, 22–7,

27, 39, 91; time and human-based changes 20, 23–4, 27, 69–70, 78

health risk factors: combined risk analysis 109–10; comparative risk analysis 108–9; IFs approach to combined risk analysis 110–11, 158; related to noncommunicable diseases 143–4; used in IFs base case forecasts 53, 70, 72–3, 73–4, *see also* Comparative Risk Assessment (CRA) project

health systems 17, 19, 20, 24–5, 26, 27, 159; disruption in Russian Federation 148; evolution in time 73; human-based changes 5, 6, 39; poor quality in "Anglo-Saxon" societies 25

hearing loss 48

Henley, Jane 82

high-income/richer countries: better health outcomes over time 22; decline in smoking rates 143; demographics of labor supply 129, 130, 131; IFs adjusted forecasts for noncommunicable diseases 145; IFs forecasts of vehicle ownership and road fatalities 87; IFs life expectancy forecasts 53, 54, 127; impacts of obesity 78, 81; increase in old-age dependency 159; mortality differences with sub-Saharan Africa 3, 57; potential gains in life expectancy 110; primary causes of deaths 2; rise in portion of retired citizens 52

Hilderink, Henk *see* Global Integrated Sustainability Model (GISMO)

Hirsch, Gary B. 50n

historical patterns: life expectancy 53–4, 55, 140–1; limited success of disease control 142; smoking 82, 84

HIV/AIDS: adults affected by reductions in 126; in countries undergoing epidemiological transition 144; data for measures of occurrence 14; in different theories of economic growth 115; as disability affecting productivity 120; expenditures on treatment 25, 124; global goals for halting and reversing incidence of 5, 58, 60; global health initiatives against 26, 139, 142; growing concerns and uncertainties 4, 10, 23, 27, 28, 64–6, 138, 143; in IFs approach to health and economic

growth 118, 148; in IFs forecasts for deaths by communicable diseases 55, 60, 142, 144, 158; in IFs integrated scenario analysis 151; impact on life expectancy in African countries 2, 13, 53, 141; as key factor in patterns of life expectancy 53, 54–5, 148; special models 33, 36, 41, 42–3; UNAIDS and IFs forecasts compared 64–6

Homer, Jack B. 36, 50n

hormonally active agents 90

human activity/agency 30; directed at proximate risk factors 108–9; and environmental change 27, 139; and failures in fight against disease 143; in IFs forecasts for NCDs and CDs 144; in IFs integrated scenario analysis 146, 155; interaction with biological systems 139–40, 148, 154–5; to mediate effects of climate change 104; super-distal factors linked to 4–5, 17, 23, 23–4, 27, 39, 139; and technology 4, 6, 20, 23, 27, 139; and uncertainties around forecasting 6, 27, 138

human capabilities framework 9, 115

human capital 115, 118, 119

human development: in extended IFs system 30, 39, 114, 126, 158–9; relationship with health 1, 7, 9, 17, 29–30, 38, 135, 138, 157, 160; super-distal drivers influencing 17

Human Development Index (HDI) 116, 135

human genome, potential to advance life expectancy 6, 138–9, 147, 159

human papilloma virus 28n

Huynen, Maud M. T. E. 91, 155n

hybrid health modeling approach 7, 36, 38–9, 49; IFs system 39–49, 146, 157

hygiene 73, 92, 94, 95–7, 158

hypertensive disease 80

Iglesias, Ana 106

income: as driver of health outcomes 7, 16, 17, 18–19, 22, 25, 27, 52–3; in IFs approach to health and productivity 122, 125; levels and convergence of mortality rates 144; link with environmental health risk factors

95, 97; link with food availability and undernutrition 74, 76; relationship with health 18–19, 24, 52, 68, 73, 116; relationship with road traffic deaths 43; relationship with vehicle ownership and accidents 85–6, 87; and worldwide increase in tobacco use 83, *see also* GDP per capita

India 76, 77, 87, 122, 144, 151, *see also* BRICS

indigenous populations 160

infant mortality: in developing countries 2; drop in world rate 2; and GDP per capita 18; global goals and IFs forecasts for reduction of 5, 58, 59; in IFs approach to health and economic growth 118; IFs forecasts 64, 126–7; in IFs integrated scenario analysis 151; poor showing of United States 24, *see also* child mortality

infectious diseases *see* communicable diseases; sexually transmitted infectious diseases

injuries: in changing disease burden 58, 126, 151; cumulative years of life lost due to 69–70; in GBD typology 35; and new challenges for global initiatives 26; risk reduction in IFs combined risk analysis 111; as significant cause of deaths 2; in WHO classification system 11

Inoue, Mie 83, 84, 85

insecticide, use against mosquitoes 134, 139

Intergovernmental Panel on Climate Change (IPCC) 105, 112n

International Futures (IFs) global modeling system 6, 15; adjustment of base case forecasts 141, 144–6; aims and availability of 156–7; approach to combined risk analysis 110–11; base case forecasts 52–60, 67, 70, 79, 138, 140, 155; extensions to include proximate risk factors 44–8, 70, 73–4, 110–11; GBD model foundation 31, 39–40; health model 30, 31, 31–2, 114; larger model for alternative global futures 30–2; special structural models 41–4, 44; and UNPD life expectancy forecasts 61–2, 70; variables for hybrid and integrated system 39, 158

International Health Regulations (IHRs) 5, 28n, 142, 142–3

International Institute of Applied Systems Analysis (IIASA) 33

International Monetary Fund (IMF) 18

International Road Federation 66

internet 136

interventions: in debate over drivers of health improvement 17; demographic and economic impacts 126–9, 134, 135; in IFs model for combined risk analysis 108, 110–11; models to help identify opportunities for 30, 38, 39; relating to proximate risk factors of health outcomes 20, 44; in smoking scenarios 84, 85; and uncertainties in IFs forecasts 52, 70, 159; understanding costs and benefits 7

intestinal nematode infections 94, 95, 96

Investing in Health see World Development Report (World Bank, 1993)

Iraq 28n

ischaemic heart disease 80

Jamison, Dean T. 6, 121

Japan 4, 13, 56, 83, 143, 145

Japanese encephalitis 94, 95, 96

Johnson, Simon 116

Joint United Nations Programme on HIV/AIDS (UNAIDS) 36, 42, 55, 64–6, 122

Kalemi-Ozcan, Sebnem 119b

Kenya 65

Kiemeney, Lambertus A. 83

Kopits, Elizabeth 66, 86

Kovats, R. 104

Krueger, Dirk 125–6

labor: effects of disability on 119–20; in IFs approach to health and economic growth 117–19, 123, 125, 129–30, 134; in models of economic growth 115, 116, 117

Latin America 59, 63, 69, 76, 101; effect of mortality changes on GDP 135; health demographics affecting economic growth 129, 131; in IFs integrated scenario

analysis 152; rise in obesity and overweight 78, 80, 81

Lau, Lawrence J. 121

lead pollution 91, 92

less-developed countries *see* developing countries

Lester, Ashley 117, 123

life expectancy: alternative economic growth scenarios 68, 121; association with GDP per capita 18–19; "best-practice" societies 20–1; at birth (LEB) 5–6, 12; decline in conflict-torn countries 2; decline for post-Soviet Russian men 13, 24, 53; demographic and economic effects of interventions 127–9; gains in Great Britain since 1650 1; and GDP per capita in alternative scenario 147–8; global goals 5–6, 59–60; historical patterns 53–4, 55, 140–1; IFs adjusted base case forecasts 145–6; in IFs approach to health and productivity 122–3, 126, 133, 135; IFs base case forecasts 53–6, 60, 70, 143; in IFs integrated scenario analysis 152–3, 155; IFs and UNPD forecasts 33, 61–2, 70; impact of technology and time-related changes 23–4, 69–70; London in 1650 1; potential of human genome to advance 6, 138–9, 147, 159; potential impact of reversing BMI trends 81–2; in scenario without main health risks 110; slow progress in leading countries 144; and summarizing mortality rates 12–13; in theory of epidemiologic transition 3; use of years of life lost (YLL) measure 13, 14, 58

lifestyles: shaped by changing economic systems 73; unhealthy 6, 21, 79

liver cancer 15

living standards 17, 18, 19

Loncar, Dejan 34, 39, 41, 47, 48, 50n

London 1, 90

longevity: ethical issues around technology for 23; forecasts for 2100 143; in IFs integrated scenario analysis 153; and measures of life expectancy 13, 23, 140–1; and rise in incentive to save 124–5, 133

Lopez, Alan D. 13, 34, 41, 83, 84, 85

Los Angeles 100

low-income/poorer countries: challenges around IHRs 142–3; confidence regarding mortality improvements 159; effect of recession of pandemics 4; health burden from global climate change 105; health spending and child health outcomes 25, 44; impact of environmental risks 94; limited economic and technological potential 145; potential gains in life expectancy 110; potential impact of reversing BMI trends 82; research into disease prevalence 14; slow progress compared with richer countries 22, *see also* developing countries

Lucas, Paul *see* Global Integrated Sustainability Model (GISMO)

lung cancer 34, 41, 82, 91, 102

lymphatic filariasis 95

Maeusezahl-Feuz, Mirjam 98

malaria 39, 40, 46, 95; global initiatives in fight against 5, 26, 58, 142, 143; in IFs forecasts for deaths by communicable diseases 55, 60, 144, 158; prevention measures 4, 142; resurgence of 138, 148

malignant neoplasms 35, 85

malnutrition 7, 75, 78, 91, 95, 105

maternal conditions 35, 46, 55, 56

maternal mortality 5, 10

Mathers, Colin D. 13, 34, 39, 41, 47, 48, 50n, 51n

McKeown, Thomas 18

McMichael, Anthony J. 103

measles 28n, 46, 55

Mehta, Sumi 98

mental health 39, 48, 122

mercury 91

Mexico 141

micronutrients 134

Middle East 53, 59, 78, 87, 101, 154

middle-income countries: confidence regarding mortality improvements 159; demographics of labor supply 130, 158; growing health risk factor 158; growth in vehicle ownership and road deaths 86, 87; impacts of obesity 78; pattern of smoking rates 84, 143; patterns of life expectancy 141, 153; slow pace of reduction in noncommunicable diseases 143

Millennium Development Goals (MDGs) 5, 58–9, 63–4, 95, 96, 98

minorities 160

morbidity: data for measuring 11, 13–15; historical collection of statistics 10; and human biological vulnerablities 17; in IFs approach to health and economic growth 124, 125, 126, 131; influence of distal drivers 44; and mortality combined as single statistic 15–16; relationship with mortality 13–14, 29, 49, 58, 131; shift in predominant causes 3, 58; in structural models 35, 36

mortality: aggregate models 38; all-cause models 32–3; alternative scenarios for adult BMI 80–2; alternative scenarios for tobacco use 84–5; biological clarity of 9; from communicable and noncommunicable diseases 2–3; in comparative risk analysis 108–9; and competing risks 17; convergence of rates across income levels 144; data for measuring 10–12; deaths due to environmental factors 93–4, 95–6, 101, 102, 158; in GBD forecasting models 7, 35, 49, 145; historical collection of statistics 10; in IFs approach to health and economic growth 117–19, 122, 125, 126, 128, 129–30, 131, 134, 135; IFs base case forecasts 55–6, 70, 81; in IFs integrated scenario analysis 148, 151; influence of distal drivers 44; measures for summarizing 12–13; patterns in theory of epidemiologic transition 3–4, 9; projections for tobacco-related deaths 82; related to road traffic accidents 85–6; relationship with morbidity 13–14, 29, 49, 58, 131; threat of high rates due to AIDS 28; trends affected by time 23; from weather-related conditions 104, *see also* adult mortality; infant mortality

Mozambique 65

Mugabe, Robert 143

Multiple Indicator Cluster Survey (MICS) 14

Murray, Christopher J. L. 13, 34

musculoskeletal conditions 48

sexual behaviors 73, 74, 109

sexually transmitted infectious diseases 72

Shibuya, Kenji 83, 84, 85

"sick building syndrome" 98

Sierra Leone 2

Singapore 61

slum areas 92, 160

Smeed, R. J. (Smeed's Law) 43, 86

Smith, Kirk R. 9, 17, 27, 91, 92, 95, 98, 100, 102

smog 90

smoking 7, 38; in base case and alternative scenarios 87, 88; and chronic diseases 41–2, 47, 60; GBD model for impact of 35, 41, 47; as health risk factor 72, 73, 74, 81, 143, 144, 158; in IFs combined risk analysis 110; IFs special model for 41, 41–2; stages of prevalence and associated mortality 83, *see also* tobacco use

Snow, Dr. John 90

Soares, Rodrigo 123

social accounting matrix (SAM) 117, 125

social change, time-related influence on health risks 73

social development 3, 28

social environment 4–5, 16, 20, 24–7, 139, 148

social inequalities 23, 25

social systems, as influence on health outcomes 24–5, 25

socio-political changes 30, 38; with changing age structures of populations 130; model in extended IFs system 32, 39; with reduction in domestic conflict 155

solar ultraviolet radiation 91

solid fuel use 73, 91, 98–9, 109, 110

Solow, Robert Merton 136n

Somalia 122, 153

Sommer, Martin 43, 86

South Africa 66, 141, 148

South Asia 87, 101, 159; alternative scenarios for life expectancy 68, 69, 77–8; child mortality due to diarrheal diseases 97; child mortality related to climate change 108; forecast for obesity rates 80; GISMO forecasts of child mortality 63; IFs base case forecasts for child mortality

145; IFs forecasts in relation to global goals 59, 60, 126; in IFs integrated scenario analysis 150, 151, 152–3, 154; levels of solid fuel use 98, 99; nutritional shortfalls and undernutrition levels 75, 77; patterns of life expectancy 53; population as vulnerable to noncommunicable diseases 144; working-age demographics 129

Southern Europe 83

Sridhar, Devi 26

stem cell research and treatments 23

stomach cancer 82

"stunting" 120–1, 122–3, 131, 132, 134

sub-Saharan Africa 28n, 70, 83, 87; alternative scenarios for life expectancy 68–9, 77, 123; antiretroviral treatment campaigns 120; child mortality due to diarrheal diseases 97; child mortality related to climate change 108; effect of mortality changes on GDP 128, 129, 135; GISMO forecasts of child mortality 63, 64; health demographics affecting economic growth 127, 129, 130, 131, 159; IFs adjusted base case forecasts for mortality 145; in IFs comparisons of changing disease burden 56–7, 58; IFs forecasts in relation to global goals 59, 60, 126, 127; in IFs integrated scenario analysis 150, 151, 152, 152–3, 153, 154; IFs and UNPD forecasts of child mortality 62; impact of AIDS on life expectancy 2, 53; increases in overweight and obesity 78, 80, 81; levels of solid fuel use 98, 99; mortality differences with high-income countries 3; nutritional shortfalls and undernutrition levels 75, 77, 88; worst figures for life expectancy 4

Summers, Lawrence H. 18

Sweden 12, 140–1

systems dynamics approaches 36

Tajikistan 153

Tamerius, James D. 104

technological advance: and biological limits 23–4, 145, 147; debates over economics and ethics of 23; dimensions in

integrated scenario analysis 146, 147, 155; and elders' consumption of health care resources 124; as function of human activity 4, 6, 20, 23, 139; and increase in food production 76; and reduction in communicable diseases 24, 142; and time as proxy for 7, 16, 20, 22–3, 27, 69–70, 73; varying influences on obesity rates 81

technology transfer 24, 26, 142

technophysio evolution 28, 115, 121

Thun, Michael 82

timber, overuse of resources 136

time: as factor in GBD formulations 7, 16, 23, 145; as factor in savings and capital growth 133; historical increase in longevity 140–1; lag between BMI and cause-specific mortality 80–1; limits in health forecasting 156; period between stages in adult smoking prevalence 8; in Preston's study of cross-country income/health relationship 19, 23–4; as variable in drivers of health outcomes 7, 16, 20, 22–3, 27, 35, 69–70; as variable in IFs combined risk analysis 110–11, 158

tobacco use 10, 23, 24; alternative scenarios 84–5; drivers and forecasts 82–4; as proximate health risk factor 72, 109, 110, *see also* smoking

trachoma 94, 95, 96

tropical forests 136

tuberculosis 5, 26, 34, 55, 142

tuna, overuse of resources 136

Turkey 141

UNAIDS *see* Joint United Nations Programme on HIV/AIDS (UNAIDS)

uncertainties: around global health futures 27–8, 154–5; around human-based factors 6, 23, 27

undernutrition: danger of overuse of fossil groundwater 159; due to climate change affecting crop production 106, 107, 158; due to economic and environmental decline 104, 106; in IFs risk analysis 46–7, 73, 74, 110, 158, *see also* childhood undernutrition

UN Food and Agricultural Organization (FAO) 63, 77

UNICEF (United Nations Children's Fund) 96, 137n

United Kingdom 24–5, 61, 82, 83

United Nations 31

United Nations Declaration of Universal Human Rights 5

United Nations Development Programme (UNDP) 137n

United Nations Environment Programme (UNEP), *Global Environmental Outlook-4* 32

United Nations International Children's Fund 14

United Nations Population Division (UNPD) 33, 40, 53, 64; and IFs life expectancy forecasts 61–2, 70, 143; World Population Prospects database 10

United States Census Bureau 33

United States Centers for Disease Control (CDC) 36, 38

United States of America 21, 24, 25, 82, 83; rise in levels of obesity and overweight 78, 79, 144; trend in cardiovascular disease mortality rates 23, 144

urban areas 96, 104, *see also* air pollution (outdoor urban)

urbanization 64, 92

U.S. Agency for International Development 14

U.S. Army 121

U.S. National Institute of Aging 13vaccination 4, 16, 23, 24, 26, 28n, 142

vaccines 5

vehicle ownership and fatality rates 66–7, 85–7, 88

violence 69, 70

vulnerable populations 10

Wang, Jia 121

water systems 4; cholera outbreak linked with 90; environmental risk factor 27, 63–4, 72, 73, 91, 94, 95–7, 111; improvement of 7, 16; MDG for environmental sustainability 5, 95; unsafe water in IFs combined risk analysis 110, 158, *see also* sanitation systems

Weil, David N. 117, 121, 123

welfare 25, 118

Western Europe 83

WHO *see* World Health Organization

Wilkinson, Richard G. 22

women: affected by diseases related to indoor air pollution 98; education and better health outcomes 19, 20; forecasts for obesity rates 80; gaps between countries in health and life expectancy 4; historical patterns in smoking rates 82, 84; life expectancy of Japanese 4, 56, 143, 145; as often excluded from health improvements 160, *see also* fertility; maternal conditions; maternal mortality

Woodruff, Rosalie 104

World Bank 18, 19, 63; approach to combined risk analysis 109–10; Disease Control Priorities project 34, 109; estimates of PM concentrations 101; global health initiatives 26; road traffic fatalities forecasts 66–7, 85, 86; study of private savings rates 125

World Commission on Environment and Development, 1987 (Brundtland) 30

World Development Report (World Bank, 1993) 19, 34

World Health Organization (WHO): aims and organization 5; approach to combined risk analysis 109–10; as central in fight against communicable diseases 142, 143; development of structural models 34; estimates of disease from air pollution 98, 100, 102; forecasts for obesity rates 79, 80; importance in post-World War II era 24; International Classification of Diseases (ICD) system 10–11; push for global health governance 26–7; recent figures for underweight children 75; reports on smoking and tobacco use 82, 83; study on cause-of-death data 11; World Health Survey (WHS) 14, *see also* Commission on Social Determinants of Health (CSDH, 2008); Comparative Risk Assessment (CRA) project; Global Burden of Disease (GBD) project; Global Water Supply and Sanitation Assessment

World War I 83

years lived with disability (YLD) measure 15, 34, 48, 58, 62–3, 122

years of life lost (YLL) 13, 15, 34, 48, 62–3; and changing disease burden 58, 126–7, 149, 151; comparative risk analysis of global scenarios 108–9, 110

Yemen 12, 13

Young, Alwyn 119b

young people 83, 130

Zimbabwe 2, 143

Author Notes

Barry B. Hughes is Johns Evans Professor at the Josef Korbel School of International Studies and Director of the Frederick S. Pardee Center for International Futures, University of Denver. He initiated and leads the development of the International Futures forecasting system and is the Series Editor for the Patterns of Potential Human Progress series.

Randall Kuhn is Assistant Professor and Director of the Global Health Affairs Program at the Josef Korbel School of International Studies, University of Denver. His research in Bangladesh, South Africa, and Sri Lanka explores the effects of economic, political, and demographic forces on health and well-being along with the pathways from health to societal change.

Cecilia M. Peterson is a doctoral candidate at the Josef Korbel School of International Studies, University of Denver. Building on her background in biostatistics and public health, her research interests are focused on modeling long-term health outcomes.

Dale S. Rothman is Associate Professor at the Josef Korbel School of International Studies and Associate Director of the Frederick S. Pardee Center for International Futures, University of Denver. His work focuses on global long-term interactions between environment and human development.

José R. Solórzano is a Senior Consultant for the Frederick S. Pardee Center for International Futures. Currently his main focus is the technical design and implementation of the International Futures modeling system across all volumes in the Pardee Center's Patterns of Potential Human Progress series.

Patterns of Potential Human Progress

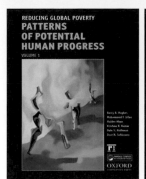 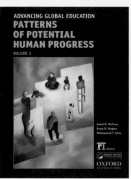 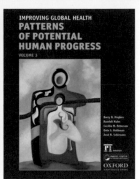

The **Patterns of Potential Human Progress Series** explores prospects for human development—how it appears to be unfolding globally and locally, how we would like it to evolve, and how better to ensure that we move it in desired directions.

Each year the series releases an issue-specific volume with extensive analysis and 50-year country, regional, and global forecasts.

Titles in the Series
Reducing Global Poverty (Vol 1, 2009)
Advancing Global Education (Vol 2, 2010)
Improving Global Health (Vol 3, 2011)

Forthcoming
Transforming Global Infrastructure (Vol 4, *scheduled for 2012*)
Enhancing Global Governance (Vol 5, *scheduled for 2013*)

Barry B. Hughes, Series Editor

**Paradigm Publishers and
Oxford University Press India**

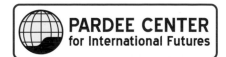

Frederick S. Pardee Center for International Futures
Josef Korbel School of International Studies
University of Denver

For more information about IFs and the PPHP series, go to **www.ifs.du.edu** or email **pardee.center@du.edu**